NURSE'S READY REFERENCE

MEDICATIONS

Springhouse Corporation
Springhouse, Pennsylvania

Staff

The clinical procedures described and recommended in this publication are based on research and consultation with medical and nursing authorities. To the best of our knowledge, these procedures reflect currently accepted clinical practice; nevertheless, they can't be considered absolute and universal recommendations. For individual application, treatment recommendations must be considered in light of the patient's clinical condition and, before administration of new or infrequently used drugs, in light of the latest package-insert information. The authors and the publisher disclaim responsibility for any adverse effects resulting directly or indirectly from the suggested procedures, from any undetected errors, or from the reader's misunderstanding of the text.

Printed in the United States of America.

RRMED-031196

A member of the Reed Elsevier plc group

Library of Congress Cataloging-in-Publication Data

Medications.
p. cm. – (Nurse's ready reference)
Includes index.
1. Drugs – Handbooks, manuals, etc.
2. Nursing – Handbooks, manuals, etc. 3. Chemotherapy – Handbooks, manuals, etc.
I. Springhouse Corporation. II. Series.
[DNLM: 1. Drugs – administration & dosage – nurses' instruction.
2. Drugs – administration & dosage – handbooks.
QV 39 M4895 1994]
RM301.12.M43 1994
615'.1 – dc20
DNLM/DLC 93-39712
ISBN 0-87434-599-5 CIP

Contents

If you're like most nurses today, your time is precious. You can't afford to go searching through dense pharmacology manuals in order to keep up with the latest information in drug therapy. Yet, to perform your duties with skill and confidence and to prevent potentially dangerous adverse reactions, you need the current drug information at your fingertips. Fortunately, *Medications*, the latest book in the Nurse's Ready Reference series, provides just that.

A useful tool for both the practicing and student nurse, *Medications* contains concise information on over 640 of the most commonly used over-the-counter and prescription drugs. Compact and flexible, *Medications* is designed for use in any clinical or academic setting. Its spiral binding lets you lay the book flat, and its fold-out easel back lets you prop it up and use the book flip-chart style. Arranged alphabetically, the entries are printed on both sides of the pages, with a convenient letter guide at the bottom. All entries have been updated to reflect the latest available information, and newly approved drugs have been included.

Each entry follows a standard, easy-to-use format, beginning with the drug's generic name and major brand names. Where drugs are available in different salt forms, brand names have been grouped accordingly and separated by a semicolon (;). A single dagger (†) identifies drugs available only in Canada; an open diamond (◇), drugs available without a prescription. A single asterisk (*) identifies drugs whose liquid formulation may contain alcohol; a double asterisk (**) identifies drugs that contain tartrazine dye (FD&C Yellow No. 5), a coloring agent that can provoke a severe allergic reaction in susceptible people.

Under the *General* section, you'll find each drug's classification, pregnancy risk category and, if applicable, its controlled substance schedule. Classification identifies the drug's therapeutic use along with its pharmacologic grouping, which appears in parentheses. Pregnancy risk category refers to the five categories (A, B, C, D, or X) established by the Food and Drug Administration to indicate a drug's potential for causing birth defects. The categories are defined as follows:

- A: Adequate studies in pregnant women have failed to show a risk to the fetus in the first trimester of pregnancy, and there is no evidence of risk in later trimesters.
- B: Animal studies have not shown an adverse effect on the fetus, but no adequate studies in pregnant women exist.
- C: Animal studies have shown an adverse effect on the fetus, but there are no adequate studies in humans. Or there are no adequate studies in animals or humans. Pregnancy risk is unknown.
- D: There is evidence of risk to the human fetus, but the potential benefits in pregnant women may be acceptable.
- X: Studies in animals or humans show fetal abnormalities, or adverse reaction reports indicate evidence of fetal risk. The risks involved clearly outweigh potential benefits.

(continued)

Any drug with a potential for abuse is indicated by its accompanying controlled substance schedule. The schedules defined by the Drug Enforcement Agency rank from II to V. Category II indicates a drug with a very high risk of severe physical or psychological dependence, and no renewals permitted; III, low to moderate risk of physical dependence or high psychological dependence, with up to five renewals permitted; IV, low potential for physical or psychological dependence; and V, very low risk.

Mechanism of action summarizes the drug's pharmacodynamics and pharmacokinetics. The next section, *Indications and dosage,* gives the drug's major indications and general dosage recommendations for adults and children; it also details dosage and administration tips for any special preparations, such as solutions or extended-release capsules. Dosages for elderly patients or patients with renal impairment are also included for some drugs.

Adverse reactions lists undesirable drug effects grouped according to affected body systems, as follows: blood; central nervous system (CNS); cardiovascular (CV); eyes, ears, nose, and throat (EENT); gastrointestinal (GI); genitourinary (GU); hepatic; metabolic; respiratory; skin; or other (adverse reactions not specific to a single body system.) Common adverse reactions appear in *italics*, and life-threatening adverse reactions appear in ***boldface italics.*** The next section, *Interactions*, lists each drug's confirmed, *clinically significant* interactions with other drugs.

Nursing diagnoses lists the NANDA-approved nursing diagnoses most relevant to the drug's therapy. *Nursing interventions* contains the most relevant and vital recommendations for preparing and administering drugs, monitoring patients, preventing and treating adverse reactions and interactions, and patient teaching. Instructions for I.V. use have been highlighted.

In a time when nurses are expected to know more and work harder and more efficiently than ever before, *Medications* is an essential addition to your professional library. It will save you time, hone your skills, and help ensure that you're providing the best possible care for your patient.

U

V

Guide to Abbreviations

The following abbreviations are used repeatedly in this book:

ABG . . . . arterial blood gas
ACE . . . . angiotensin-converting enzyme
AIDS . . . . . . acquired immunodeficiency syndrome
ALT . . . . alanine aminotransferase
AST . . . . aspartate aminotransferase
ATP . . . . adenosine triphosphate
AV . . . . atrioventricular
b.i.d. . . . . . . twice daily
BUN . . . . blood urea nitrogen
cAMP . . . . . cyclic adenosine monophosphate
CBC . . . . complete blood count
CDC . . . . Centers for Disease Control and Prevention
CHF . . . . congestive heart failure
CK . . . . creatine kinase
CMV . . . . . . cytomegalovirus
CNS . . . . central nervous system
COPD . . . . . chronic obstructive pulmonary disease
CPR . . . . cardiopulmonary resuscitation
CSF . . . . cerebrospinal fluid
CV . . . . cardiovascular
CVA . . . . cerebrovascular accident
CVP . . . . central venous pressure
D_5W . . . . dextrose 5% in water
DNA . . . . deoxyribonucleic acid
ECG . . . . electrocardiogram
EEG . . . . electroencephalogram
EENT . . . . . . eyes, ears, nose, throat
FDA . . . . Food and Drug Administration
g . . . . gram
G . . . . gauge
GI . . . . gastrointestinal
GFR . . . . glomerular filtration rate
GU . . . . genitourinary
G6PD . . . . . glucose-6-phosphate dehydrogenase
H_1 . . . . histamine$_1$
H_2 . . . . histamine$_2$
h.s. . . . . at bedtime
ID . . . . intradermal
I.M. . . . . intramuscular
IPPB . . . . intermittent positive-pressure breathing
IU . . . . international unit
I.V. . . . . intravenous
kg . . . . kilogram
L . . . . liter
M . . . . molar
m^2 . . . . square meter
MAO . . . . . . monoamine oxidase
mcg or μg . . microgram
mEq . . . . . . milliequivalent
mg . . . . milligram
MI . . . . myocardial infarction
ml . . . . milliliter
mm^3 . . . . . . cubic millimeter
Na . . . . sodium
ng . . . . nanogram (millimicrogram)
NSAID . . . . . nonsteroidal anti-inflammatory drug
OTC . . . . over the counter
PABA . . . . . . para-aminobenzoic acid
P.O. . . . . by mouth
P.R. . . . . by rectum
p.r.n. . . . . . . as needed
PSVT . . . . . . paroxysmal supraventricular tachycardia
PT . . . . prothrombin time
q . . . . every
q.d. . . . . every day
q.i.d. . . . . . . four times daily
RBC . . . . red blood cell
RDA . . . . recommended daily allowance
REM . . . . rapid eye movement
RNA . . . . ribonucleic acid
RSV . . . . respiratory syncytial virus
SA . . . . sinoatrial
S.C. . . . . subcutaneous
SGOT . . . . . . serum glutamic oxaloacetic transaminase
SGPT . . . . . . serum glutamic pyruvic transaminase
SHBG . . . . . . sex hormone-binding globulin
SIADH . . . . . syndrome of inappropriate antidiuretic hormone
S.L. . . . . sublingual
TCA . . . . tricyclic antidepressant
TIA . . . . transient ischemic attack
t.i.d. . . . . . . three times daily
USP . . . . United States Pharmacopeia
UTI . . . . urinary tract infection
WBC . . . . . . white blood cell

acebutolol hydrochloride Monitan†, Sectral

General
Classification: antihypertensive, antiarrhythmic (beta-adrenergic blocking agent). **Pregnancy risk category:** B.

Mechanism of action
Decreases heart rate and myocardial contractility.

Indications and dosage
- Treatment of hypertension. **Adults:** 400 mg P.O. as a single daily dosage or divided b.i.d. Patients may receive as much as 1,200 mg daily.
- Ventricular arrhythmias. **Adults:** 400 mg P.O. daily divided b.i.d. Dosage is then increased to provide an adequate clinical response. Usual dosage is 600 to 1,200 mg daily.

Adverse reactions
CNS: *fatigue,* headache, dizziness, insomnia. **CV:** chest pain, edema, bradycardia, ***CHF,*** *hypotension.* **GI:** nausea, constipation, diarrhea, dyspepsia. **Metabolic:** hypoglycemia without tachycardia. **Respiratory:** dyspnea, ***bronchospasm.*** **Skin:** rash. **Other:** fever.

Interactions
Digitalis glycosides: excessive bradycardia and increased depressant effect on myocardium. Use together cautiously. **Indomethacin:** decreased antihypertensive effect. Monitor blood pressure and adjust dosage. **Insulin, oral antidiabetic agents:** can alter dosage requirements in previously stabilized diabetic patients. Observe patient carefully.

Nursing diagnoses
- High risk for injury related to the patient's underlying condition.
- Fatigue related to acebutolol-induced adverse CNS reaction.
- Knowledge deficit related to acebutolol therapy.

Nursing interventions
- *Contraindicated* in persistently severe bradycardia, second- and third-degree heart block, overt cardiac failure, and cardiogenic shock.
- *Use cautiously* in patients with cardiac failure.
- Acebutolol is a cardioselective beta blocker similar to metoprolol. Use with caution in patients with bronchospastic diseases such as asthma and emphysema.
- Dosage should be reduced in patients with decreased renal function.
- Elderly patients may require lower acebutolol doses. For such patients, dosage should not exceed 800 mg daily.
- Always check patient's apical pulse before giving this drug; if slower than 60 beats/minute, hold drug and call doctor.
- Acebutolol may mask the signs of hyperthyroidism and hyperglycemia and may potentiate insulin-induced hypoglycemia.
- Before surgery, notify anesthesiologist if patient is receiving this drug.
- Do not discontinue abruptly; can exacerbate angina and MI.
- Teach patient about his disease and therapy. Explain the importance of taking this drug as prescribed, even when he's feeling well. Tell patient not to discontinue drug suddenly, but to call the doctor, if unpleasant adverse reactions occur.
- Instruct patient to check with doctor or pharmacist before taking OTC medications.

Q

R

acetaminophen

Datril ◇, Liquiprin ◇, Panadol ◇, Rounox† ◇, Tylenol ◇

General

Classification: nonnarcotic analgesic, antipyretic (para-aminophenol derivative). **Pregnancy risk category:** B.

Mechanism of action

Produces analgesia by blocking generation of pain impulses, probably by inhibition of prostaglandin synthesis or inhibition of the synthesis or action of other substances that sensitize pain receptors to mechanical or chemical stimulation. It relieves fever by central action in the hypothalamic heat-regulating center.

Indications and dosage

• Mild pain or fever. **Adults and children over 11 years:** 325 to 650 mg P.O. or P.R. q 4 hours; or 1 g q.i.d. p.r.n. Maximum dosage should not exceed 4 g daily. Dosage for long-term therapy should not exceed 2.6 g daily. **Children 11 years:** 480 mg/dose. **Children 9 to 10 years:** 400 mg/dose. **Children 6 to 8 years:** 320 mg/dose. **Children 4 to 5 years:** 240 mg/dose. **Children 2 to 3 years:** 160 mg/dose. **Children 12 to 23 months:** 120 mg/dose. **Children 4 to 11 months:** 80 mg/dose. **Children up to 3 months:** 40 mg/dose.

Adverse reactions

Hepatic: ***severe liver damage with toxic doses.***
Skin: rash, urticaria.

Interactions

Barbiturates, carbamazepine, hydantoins, rifampin, sulfinpyrazone: high doses or long-term use of these drugs may enhance the hepatotoxic effects of acetaminophen. Avoid concomitant use. **Caffeine:** may enhance analgesic effects of acetaminophen. **Diflunisal:** increases acetaminophen blood levels. Don't use together. **Ethanol:** increased risk of hepatic damage. **Warfarin:** increased hypoprothrombinemic effect with chronic acetaminophen use. **Zidovudine:** conflicting evidence suggests possible impaired zidovudine metabolism. Monitor patient closely.

Nursing diagnoses

• Pain related to the patient's underlying condition.
• High risk for injury related to acetaminophen-induced liver damage with toxic doses.
• Knowledge deficit related to acetaminophen therapy.

Nursing interventions

• *Contraindicated* for repeated use in anemia, renal or hepatic disease.
• *Use cautiously* in patients with a history of chronic alcohol abuse because hepatotoxicity has occurred at therapeutic doses. Limit daily intake to 2 g.
• Consult a doctor before administering this drug to children under age 2.
• This drug is for short-term use only. Tell patients to consult a doctor if administering to children for more than 5 days or adults for more than 10 days.
• Has no significant anti-inflammatory effect.
• Should not be used for self-medication of marked fever (over 103.1° F [39.5° C]), fever persisting longer than 3 days, or recurrent fever unless directed by doctor.
• Warn patient that high doses or unsupervised chronic use can cause hepatic damage.
• Many nonprescription products contain acetaminophen. Be aware of this when calculating total daily dosages.
• Recommend the liquid form for children and for all patients who have difficulty swallowing.
• Acetaminophen crosses the placenta, but is apparently safe for short-term use at therapeutic doses during pregnancy. It is routinely used during all stages of pregnancy for the treatment of pain and fever.
• Acetaminophen may interfere with certain laboratory tests for urinary 5-hydroxyindoleacetic acid. It may also produce false-positive decreases in blood glucose levels in home monitoring systems using Chemstrip bG, Dextrostix, or Visidex II.

acetazolamide

Acetazolam†, Ak-Zol, Diamox, Storzolamide; Diamox Parenteral, Diamox Sodium†

General

Classification: anticonvulsant, antiglaucoma agent, diuretic (carbonic anhydrase inhibitor).
Pregnancy risk category: C.

Mechanism of action

Blocks action of carbonic anhydrase, promoting renal excretion of sodium, potassium, bicarbonate, and water. Reduces aqueous humor secretion, lowering intraocular pressure. As an anticonvulsant, may inhibit carbonic anhydrase in CNS, resulting in increased carbon dioxide tension and diminishing neuronal discharge.

Indications and dosage

- Narrow-angle glaucoma. **Adults:** 250 mg P.O. q 4 hours; or 250 mg P.O., I.M., or I.V. b.i.d. for short-term therapy.
- Open-angle glaucoma. **Adults:** 250 mg to 1 g P.O., I.M., or I.V. daily divided q.i.d.
- Edema in CHF. **Adults:** 250 to 375 mg P.O., I.M., or I.V. daily in a.m.
- Adjunctive treatment of myoclonic, refractory generalized tonic-clonic, absence, or mixed seizures. **Adults:** 375 mg to 1 g P.O., I.M., or I.V. daily. Alternatively, use sustained-release capsules 250 to 500 mg P.O. daily or b.i.d. Initial dosage when used with other anticonvulsants usually is 250 mg daily.

Adverse reactions

Blood: ***aplastic anemia,*** hemolytic anemia, leukopenia. **CNS:** drowsiness, paresthesia, confusion. **EENT:** transient myopia. **GI:** nausea, vomiting, anorexia. **GU:** crystalluria, renal calculi, hematuria. **Metabolic:** hyperchloremic acidosis, hypokalemia, asymptomatic hyperuricemia. **Skin:** rash. **Local:** *pain at injection site,* sterile abscesses.

Interactions

None significant.

Nursing diagnoses

- Fluid volume excess related to the patient's underlying condition.
- Altered urinary elimination related to diuretic action (frequency, urgency) of drug.
- Knowledge deficit related to acetazolamide therapy.

Nursing interventions

- *Contraindicated* in long-term therapy for chronic noncongestive narrow-angle glaucoma and in hyponatremia or hypokalemia, renal or hepatic disease or dysfunction, adrenal gland failure, or hyperchloremic acidosis.
- *Use cautiously* in patients with respiratory acidosis, emphysema, or chronic pulmonary disease and in those receiving other diuretics.
- Monitor intake and output and electrolytes, especially serum potassium. When used in diuretic therapy, consult with doctor and dietitian to provide high-potassium diet.
- Weigh patient daily. Rapid or excessive fluid loss causes weight loss and hypotension.
- Elderly patients are especially susceptible to excessive diuresis.
- Diuretic effect is decreased when acidosis occurs but can be reestablished by withdrawing drug for several days and then restarting or by using intermittent administration schedules.
- Reconstitute 500-mg vial with at least 5 ml sterile water for injection. Use within 24 hours of reconstitution.
- I.M. injection may be painful because of alkalinity of solution.
- *I.V. use:* Administer direct I.V. using a 21G or 23G needle. Inject 100 to 500 mg/minute into a large vein. Intermittent or continuous infusion is not recommended.
- May cause false-positive urine protein tests by alkalinizing the urine.
- To make an oral liquid: soften 1 tablet in 2 teaspoonfuls of very warm water and add 2 teaspoonfuls honey or syrup (chocolate or cherry). Don't use fruit juice.

O

acetohexamide Dimelor†, Dymelor

General

Classification: antidiabetic agent (sulfonylurea). **Pregnancy risk category:** D.

Mechanism of action

Stimulates insulin release from the pancreatic beta cells and reduces glucose output by the liver. An extrapancreatic effect increases peripheral sensitivity to insulin.

Indications and dosage

- Adjunct to diet to lower blood glucose of non-insulin-dependent (type II) diabetes mellitus patients. **Adults:** initially, 250 mg P.O. daily before breakfast; may increase dosage q 5 to 7 days (by 250 to 500 mg) p.r.n. to maximum of 1.5 g daily, divided b.i.d. to t.i.d., before meals.
- Replacement of insulin therapy. **Adults:** if insulin dosage is less than 20 units daily, insulin may be stopped and oral therapy started with 250 mg P.O. daily before breakfast, increased as above if needed. If insulin dosage is 20 to 40 units daily, start oral therapy with 250 mg daily before breakfast, while reducing insulin dosage 25% to 30% daily or every other day, depending on response to oral therapy.

Adverse reactions

GI: nausea, heartburn, vomiting. **Metabolic:** sodium loss, ***hypoglycemia.*** **Skin:** rash, pruritus, facial flushing. **Other:** ***hypersensitivity reactions.***

Interactions

Anabolic steroids, chloramphenicol, clofibrate, guanethidine, MAO inhibitors, phenylbutazone, salicylates, sulfonamides: increased hypoglycemic activity. Monitor blood glucose level. **Beta blockers, clonidine:** prolonged hypoglycemic effect and masked symptoms of hypoglycemia. Use together cautiously. **Corticosteroids, glucagon, rifampin, thiazide diuretics:** decreased hypoglycemic response. Monitor blood glucose level. **Hydantoins:** increased blood levels of hydantoins. **Oral anticoagulants:** increased hypoglycemic activity or enhanced anticoagulant effect. Monitor blood glucose level and prothrombin time.

Nursing diagnoses

- Altered nutrition: More than body requirements, related to patient's inability to release sufficient insulin to maintain normal blood glucose levels.
- High risk for injury related to acetohexamide-induced hypoglycemia.
- Knowledge deficit related to acetohexamide therapy.

Nursing interventions

- *Contraindicated* in type I (insulin-dependent) diabetes; diabetes adequately controlled by diet; and type II (non-insulin-dependent) diabetes complicated by ketosis, acidosis, diabetic coma, Raynaud's disease, gangrene, renal or hepatic impairment, or thyroid or other endocrine dysfunction. Also, don't use during pregnancy or breast-feeding.
- *Use cautiously* in patients with sulfonamide hypersensitivity.
- Instruct patient about nature of disease; importance of following therapeutic regimen, adhering to specific diet, weight reduction, exercise, and personal hygiene programs, and avoiding infection; self-monitoring of blood glucose level; and recognition of hypoglycemia and hyperglycemia.
- Make sure patient understands that therapy relieves symptoms but doesn't cure the disease.
- Patient transferring from insulin therapy to an oral antidiabetic requires blood glucose monitoring at least t.i.d. before meals. Patient may require hospitalization during transition.
- During periods of increased stress, such as infection, fever, surgery, or trauma, patient may require insulin therapy. Monitor patient closely for hyperglycemia in these situations.
- Advise patient to avoid large intake of alcohol; disulfiram-like reaction is possible.
- Patient should not take other medications, including OTC drugs, without first asking doctor.

N

General

Classification: antipsychotic (phenothiazine). **Pregnancy risk category:** C.

Mechanism of action

Blocks postsynaptic dopamine receptors in the brain. A piperazine phenothiazine.

Indications and dosage

• Psychotic disorders. **Adults:** initially, 20 mg P.O. t.i.d. or q.i.d. Daily dosage ranges from 40 to 80 mg in outpatients, 80 to 120 mg in hospitalized patients, and up to 600 mg daily in severe psychotic states.

Adverse reactions

Blood: transient leukopenia, ***agranulocytosis.*** **CNS:** *extrapyramidal reactions, tardive dyskinesia,* sedation, pseudoparkinsonism, EEG changes, dizziness. **CV:** *orthostatic hypotension,* tachycardia, ECG changes. **EENT:** ocular changes, *blurred vision.* **GI:** *dry mouth, constipation.* **GU:** *urine retention,* menstrual irregularities, gynecomastia, inhibited ejaculation. **Hepatic:** cholestatic jaundice, abnormal liver function tests. **Metabolic:** weight gain, increased appetite, hyperprolactinemia. **Skin:** *mild photosensitivity,* dermal allergic reactions. **Other:** rarely, ***neuroleptic malignant syndrome*** (fever, tachycardia, tachypnea, profuse diaphoresis). **After abrupt withdrawal of long-term therapy:** gastritis, vomiting, dizziness, tremor, feeling of warmth or cold, sweating, tachycardia, insomnia.

Interactions

Alcohol, other CNS depressants: increased CNS depression. Avoid concomitant use. **Antacids:** inhibit absorption of oral phenothiazines. Separate antacid and phenothiazine doses by 2 hours. **Anticholinergics:** decreased anticholinergic effect. **Barbiturates:** may decrease phenothiazine effect.

Nursing diagnoses

• Altered health maintenance related to patient's underlying condition.
• Impaired physical mobility related to extrapyramidal effects of adverse drug reactions.
• Knowledge deficit related to acetophenazine therapy.

Nursing interventions

• *Contraindicated* in CNS depression, bone marrow suppression, subcortical damage, and coma; with spinal or epidural anesthetic; or with adrenergic blockers.
• *Use cautiously* in elderly or debilitated patients; in hepatic disease, arteriosclerosis or cardiovascular disease (may cause sudden drop in blood pressure), exposure to extreme heat or cold (including antipyretic therapy), respiratory disorders, hypocalcemia, or seizure disorders (may lower seizure threshold), severe reactions to insulin or electroconvulsive therapy, suspected brain tumor or intestinal obstruction, glaucoma, or prostatic hypertrophy.
• Tardive dyskinesia may occur after prolonged use. It may not appear until months or years later and may disappear spontaneously or persist for life despite discontinuation of drug.
• Acute dystonic reactions may be treated with I.V. diphenhydramine.
• Neuroleptic malignant syndrome is rare, but frequently fatal. It is not necessarily related to length of drug use or type of neuroleptic; over 60% of affected patients are men. Watch for symptoms.
• Hold dose and notify doctor if patient develops symptoms of blood dyscrasias (fever, sore throat, infection, cellulitis, weakness), persistent (longer than a few hours) extrapyramidal reactions, or any such reaction during pregnancy.
• A 20-mg dose equals 100 mg chlorpromazine.
• Tell patient to use sunscreen and wear protective clothing to avoid photosensitivity reactions.
• Obtain baseline measures of blood pressure before therapy and monitor routinely. Watch for orthostatic hypotension. Advise patient to get up slowly.
• Do not withdraw drug abruptly unless required by severe adverse reactions.
• Patient may take medication at bedtime to facilitate sleep and decrease sedation during daytime.

General

Classification: mucolytic agent, antidote for acetominophen overdose (amino acid). **Pregnancy risk category:** B.

Mechanism of action

Increases production of respiratory tract fluids to help liquefy and reduce the viscosity of tenacious secretions. Also restores liver stores of glutathione in the treatment of acetaminophen toxicity.

Indications and dosage

- Pneumonia, bronchitis, tuberculosis, cystic fibrosis, emphysema, atelectasis (adjunct), complications of thoracic surgery and CV surgery. **Adults and children:** 1 to 2 ml 10% to 20% by direct instillation into trachea as often as every hour; or 3 to 5 ml 20% (6 to 10 ml 10%) by mouthpiece t.i.d. or q.i.d.
- Acetaminophen toxicity. **Adults and children:** 140 mg/kg P.O. initially, followed by 70 mg/kg q 4 hours for 17 doses. Alternatively, administer 300 mg/kg by I.V. infusion as follows: initially, dilute 150 mg/kg in up to 200 ml dextrose 5% in water (D_5W) and infuse over 15 minutes. Follow with a second infusion of 50 mg/kg diluted in 500 ml D_5W over 4 hours. Finally, give 100 mg/kg diluted in 1,000 ml D_5W and infuse over 16 hours.

Adverse reactions

EENT: *rhinorrhea, hemoptysis.* **GI:** *stomatitis, nausea, vomiting.* **Other:** ***bronchospasm*** *(especially in asthmatics).*

Interactions

Activated charcoal: don't use together in treating acetaminophen toxicity. Limits acetylcysteine's effectiveness. **Oxytetracycline, tetracycline, erythromycin lactobionate, amphotericin B, ampicillin, iodized oil, chymotrypsin, trypsin, and hydrogen peroxide:** Incompatible. Administer separately.

Nursing diagnoses

- Ineffective airway clearance related to the patient's underlying condition.
- Altered oral mucous membrane related to acetylcysteine-induced stomatitis.
- Knowledge deficit related to acetylcysteine therapy.

Nursing interventions

- *Use cautiously* in asthma or severe respiratory insufficiency and in elderly or debilitated patients.
- Use plastic, glass, stainless steel, or another nonreactive metal when administering by nebulization. Hand-bulb nebulizers are not recommended because output is too small and particle size too large.
- After opening, store in refrigerator; use within 96 hours.
- Monitor cough type and frequency. For maximum effect, instruct patient to clear his airway by coughing before aerosol administration.
- Acetylcysteine is administered for treatment of acetaminophen overdose within 24 hours after ingestion. Treatment should not be delayed for results of acetaminophen blood levels.
- When used orally to treat acetaminophen overdose, dilute oral doses with cola, fruit juice, or water before administering. Dilute the 20% solution to a concentration of 5% (add 3 ml diluent to each ml acetylcysteine). If patient vomits within 1 hour of administration of loading or maintenance dose, repeat dose.

H

I

General

Classification: antiviral. **Pregnancy risk category:** C.

Mechanism of action

Becomes incorporated into viral DNA and inhibits viral multiplication.

Indications and dosage

• Treatment of initial and recurrent episodes of mucocutaneous herpes simplex virus (HSV-1 and HSV-2) infections in immunocompromised patients; severe initial episodes of herpes genitalis in patients not immunocompromised. **Adults and children over 11 years:** 5 mg/kg, given at a constant rate over a period of 1 hour by I.V. infusion q 8 hours for 7 days (5 days for herpes genitalis). **Children under 12 years:** 250 mg/m², given at a constant rate over a period of 1 hour by I.V. infusion q 8 hours for 7 days (5 days for herpes genitalis).
• Treatment of initial genital herpes. **Adults:** 200 mg P.O. q 4 hours while awake (a total of 5 capsules daily). Treatment should continue for 10 days.
• Intermittent therapy for recurrent genital herpes. **Adults:** Same as for initial genital herpes. Initiate therapy at the first sign of recurrence.
• Chronic suppressive therapy for recurrent genital herpes. **Adults:** 200 mg P.O. t.i.d. or 400 mg b.i.d. for 6 to 12 months.
• Chicken pox. **Adults and children:** 20 mg/kg P.O. q.i.d. for 5 days. Start therapy as soon as symptoms appear.

Adverse reactions

CNS: (associated with I.V. dosage) *headache, encephalopathic changes (lethargy, obtundation, tremor, confusion, hallucinations, agitation,* ***seizures, coma****).* **CV:** hypotension. **GI:** *nausea, vomiting,* diarrhea. **GU:** *transient elevations of serum creatinine levels,* hematuria. **Skin:** rash, itching. **Local:** *inflammation, vesicular eruptions and phlebitis at injection site.*

Interactions

Probenecid: increased acyclovir blood levels. Monitor for possible toxicity. **Zidovudine:** may cause drowsiness or lethargy. Use together cautiously.

Nursing diagnoses

• High risk for injury related to ineffectiveness of acyclovir to eradicate the infection.
• High risk for fluid volume deficit related to adverse GI reactions to oral acyclovir.
• Knowledge deficit related to acyclovir therapy.

Nursing interventions

• Some clinicians consider acyclovir therapy of marginal benefit for chicken pox because the disease is usually self-limiting. However, acyclovir may be more beneficial in adolescents than in young children.
• Teach patient that drug is effective in managing the disease but does not eliminate or cure it and will not prevent spread of infection to others.
• Urge patient to recognize the early symptoms of herpes infection (such as tingling, itching, or pain) so he can take acyclovir before the infection fully develops.
• **I.V. use:** Infusion must be administered over at least 1 hour to prevent renal tubular damage. Bolus injection, dehydration (decreased urine output), preexisting renal disease, and the concomitant use of other nephrotoxic drugs increase the risk of renal toxicity.
• Concentrated solutions (10 mg/ml or more) may be associated with a higher incidence of phlebitis.
• Don't administer I.V. form topically, intramuscularly, orally, subcutaneously, or ophthalmically.
• Notify doctor if serum creatinine level does not return to normal within a few days. He may increase hydration, adjust dose, or discontinue acyclovir.
• Encephalopathic changes are more likely in patients with neurologic disorders or in those who have had neurologic reactions to cytotoxic drugs.
• Patient must be adequately hydrated during acyclovir infusion.

F

G

adenosine

Adenocard

General

Classification: antiarrhythmic (nucleoside).
Pregnancy risk category: C.

Mechanism of action

A naturally occurring nucleoside. In the heart, it acts on the AV node to slow conduction and inhibit reentry pathways.

Indications and dosage

- Conversion of PSVT to sinus rhythm. **Adults:** 6 mg I.V. by rapid bolus injection (1 to 2 seconds). If PSVT not eliminated in 1 to 2 minutes, give 12 mg by rapid I.V. push. Repeat 12-mg dose if necessary. Single doses over 12 mg not recommended.

Adverse reactions

CNS: apprehension, back pain, blurred vision, burning sensation, dizziness, heaviness in arms, light-headedness, neck pain, numbness, tingling in arms. **CV:** chest pain, *facial flushing,* headache, hypotension, palpitations, sweating. **GI:** metallic taste, nausea. **Respiratory:** *chest pressure, dyspnea, shortness of breath,* hyperventilation. **Other:** *tightness in throat, groin pressure.*

Interactions

Carbamazepine: higher degrees of heart block may occur. **Dipyridamole:** may potentiate the drug's effects. Smaller doses may be necessary. **Methylxanthines:** antagonism of the drug's effects. Patients receiving theophylline or caffeine may require higher doses or not respond to adenosine therapy.

Nursing diagnoses

- Decreased cardiac output related to ineffectiveness of adenosine therapy.
- Altered protection related to adenosine-induced proarrhythmias.
- Knowledge deficit related to adenosine therapy.

Nursing interventions

- *Contraindicated* in patients with atrial flutter, atrial fibrillation, and ventricular tachycardia because drug is ineffective in the treatment of these arrhythmias. Because adenosine decreases conduction through the AV node, it may produce a transient first-, second-, or third-degree heart block. For this reason, it is contraindicated in patients with second- or third-degree heart block or sick sinus syndrome, unless the patient has an artificial pacemaker. Because the drug has a very short half-life, these effects are usually transient; however, patients who develop significant heart block after a dose of adenosine should not receive additional doses.
- In clinical trials, more than half of the patients exhibited new arrhythmias when adenosine was used to convert to normal sinus rhythm. The arrhythmias are usually transient, but may include sinus bradycardia or tachycardia, premature atrial contractions, various degrees of AV block, premature ventricular contractions, and skipped beats.
- Inhaled adenosine will cause bronchoconstriction in asthmatic patients. Asthma attacks have not been reported, but the potential for bronchoconstriction exists.
- Adenosine may also be useful for the treatment of PSVT associated with accessory bypass tracts.
- There is experimental evidence that high concentrations of adenosine may induce chromosomal damage. The clinical significance of this property is not known.
- **I.V. use:** Rapid I.V. injection is necessary for drug action. Administer directly into a vein if possible; if an I.V. line is used, employ the most proximal port and follow with a rapid saline flush to ensure that the drug reaches the systemic circulation quickly.
- Check solution for crystals, which may occur if solution is cold. If crystals are visible, gently warm solution to room temperature. Do not use solutions that aren't clear.
- Because it contains no preservatives, unused drug should be discarded.

E

General

Classification: bronchodilator (adrenergic). **Pregnancy risk category:** C.

Mechanism of action

Relaxes bronchial and uterine smooth muscle by acting on $beta_2$-adrenergic receptors.

Indications and dosage

• Prevention and treatment of bronchospasm in patients with reversible obstructive airway disease. **Adults and children over 13 years:** 1 to 2 inhalations q 4 to 6 hours. More frequent administration or a greater number of inhalations is not recommended. Or 2 to 4 mg P.O. t.i.d. or q.i.d. (sulfate). Maximum dosage is 8 mg q.i.d. Or 4 to 8 mg extended-release tablets q 12 hours (sulfate). Maximum dosage is 16 mg b.i.d. **Children 6 to 13 years:** 2 mg (1 teaspoonful) P.O. t.i.d. or q.i.d. (sulfate). **Children 2 to 5 years:** 0.1 mg/kg P.O. t.i.d., not to exceed 2 mg (1 teaspoonful) t.i.d. **Adults over 65 years:** 2 mg P.O. t.i.d. or q.i.d.
• Prevention of exercise-induced asthma. **Adults:** 2 inhalations 15 minutes before exercise.

Adverse reactions

CNS: *tremor, nervousness,* dizziness, insomnia, headache. **CV:** tachycardia, palpitations, hypertension. **EENT:** drying and irritation of nose and throat (with inhaled form). **GI:** heartburn, nausea, vomiting. **Other:** muscle cramps, hypokalemia (with high doses).

Interactions

CNS stimulants: increased CNS stimulation. Avoid concomitant use. **Levodopa:** risk of cardiac arrhythmias. Monitor closely. **MAO inhibitors, tricyclic antidepressants:** increased adverse CV effects. **Propranolol and other beta blockers:** mutual antagonism. Monitor patient carefully.

Nursing diagnoses

• Ineffective airway clearance related to patient's underlying condition.
• High risk for injury related to albuterol-induced adverse reactions.
• Knowledge deficit related to albuterol therapy.

Nursing interventions

• Warn patient about the possibility of paradoxical bronchospasm. If this occurs, the drug should be discontinued immediately.
• Patients may use tablets and aerosol concomitantly. Monitor closely for toxicity.
• Albuterol reportedly produces less cardiac stimulation than other sympathomimetics, especially isoproterenol.
• Teach patient how to perform oral inhalation correctly. Give the following instructions for using a metered-dose inhaler: Clear nasal passages and throat. Breathe out, expelling as much air from lungs as possible. Place mouthpiece well into mouth as dose from inhaler is released, and inhale deeply. Hold breath for several seconds, remove mouthpiece, and exhale slowly.
• If more than one inhalation is ordered, the patient should wait at least 2 minutes before repeating the procedure for a second dose.
• Tell patient who is also using a steroid inhaler to use the bronchodilator first, then wait about 5 minutes before using the steroid. This allows the bronchodilator to open air passages for maximum effectiveness.
• Pleasant-tasting syrup may be taken by children as young as age 2. Contains no alcohol or sugar.

D

General

Classification: analgesic, anesthetic (opioid). **Pregnancy risk category:** B (D for prolonged use or use of high doses at term). **Controlled substance schedule:** II.

Mechanism of action

Binds with opiate receptors at many sites in the CNS (brain, brain stem, and spinal cord), altering perception of and emotional response to pain.

Indications and dosage

- Primary anesthetic. **Adults:** initially, 130 to 245 mcg/kg I.V., then 0.5 to 1.5 mcg/kg/minute I.V.
- Adjunct to general anesthetic. **Adults:** initially, 8 to 50 mcg/kg I.V., then give increments of 3 to 15 mcg/kg I.V.

Adverse reactions

CNS: blurred vision, *confusion*. **CV:** hypotension, hypertension, bradycardia, tachycardia. **GI:** nausea, vomiting. **Skin:** itching. **Other:** ***chest wall rigidity,*** intraoperative muscle movement, ***respiratory depression,*** hypercapnia.

Interactions

Alcohol, CNS depressants: additive effects. Use together cautiously.

Nursing diagnoses

- Decreased cardiac output related to adverse cardiac effects of therapy.
- Ineffective breathing pattern related to alfentanil-induced respiratory depression.
- Knowledge deficit related to alfentanil therapy.

Nursing interventions

- *Contraindicated* in patients with hypersensitivity to the drug or other opiate analgesics.
- *Use cautiously* in patients with head injury, pulmonary disease, or decreased respiratory reserve.
- Should be administered only by persons specifically trained in the use of I.V. anesthetics.
- As a primary anesthetic, alfentanil may be prescribed for induction of anesthesia for general surgery requiring endotracheal intubation and medical ventilation.
- **I.V. use:** Discontinue infusion at least 10 to 15 minutes before the end of surgery.
- Keep narcotic antagonist (naloxone) and resuscitative equipment available when giving drug I.V.
- To administer small volumes of alfentanil accurately, use a tuberculin syringe.
- Reduce dose in elderly and debilitated patients.
- Periodically monitor postoperative vital signs and bladder function. Because drug decreases both rate and depth of respirations, monitoring of arterial oxygen saturation may aid in assessing respiratory depression.

allopurinol

Lopurin, Zyloprim

General

Classification: antigout (xanthine oxidase inhibitor). **Pregnancy risk category:** C.

Mechanism of action

Reduces uric acid production by inhibiting the biochemical reactions preceding its formation.

Indications and dosage

- Gout, primary or secondary to hyperuricemia; secondary to diseases such as acute or chronic leukemia, polycythemia vera, multiple myeloma, and psoriasis. Dosage varies with disease severity; divide doses larger than 300 mg. **Adults:** mild gout, 200 to 300 mg P.O. daily; severe gout, 400 to 600 mg P.O. daily.
- Impaired renal function. **Adults:** 200 mg P.O. daily if creatinine clearance is 10 to 20 ml/minute; 100 mg P.O. daily, if less than 10 ml/minute; 100 mg P.O. more than 24 hours apart, if less than 3 ml/minute.
- Prevention of acute gout attacks. **Adults:** 100 mg P.O. daily; increase at weekly intervals by 100 mg without exceeding maximum dose (800 mg) until serum uric acid falls to 6 mg/100 ml or less.
- Prevention of uric acid nephropathy during cancer chemotherapy. **Adults:** 600 to 800 mg P.O. daily for 2 to 3 days.
- Recurrent calcium oxalate calculi. **Adults:** 200 to 300 mg P.O. daily in single or divided doses.

Adverse reactions

Blood: ***agranulocytosis,*** anemia, ***aplastic anemia.*** **CNS:** drowsiness, headache. **EENT:** cataracts, retinopathy. **GI:** nausea, vomiting, diarrhea, abdominal pain. **Hepatic:** altered liver function studies, ***hepatitis.*** **Skin:** *rash, usually maculopapular;* ***exfoliative,*** urticarial, and purpuric lesions; ***erythema multiforme;*** severe furunculosis of nose; ichthyosis, ***toxic epidermal necrolysis.***

Interactions

Alcohol, diazoxide, diuretics, mecamylamine, pyrazinamide: increased serum acid concentration. Adjust dosage of allopurinol. **Amoxicillin, ampicillin, bacampicillin:** increased possibility of skin rash. Avoid concomitant use. **Anticoagulants:** potentiation of anticoagulant effect. **Antineoplastic agents:** increased potential for bone marrow suppression. **Chlorpropamide:** possible increased hypoglycemic effect. Avoid concomitant use. **Ethacrynic acid, thiazide diuretics:** increased risk of allopurinol toxicity. **Uricosuric agents:** additive effect. May be used to therapeutic advantage. **Urinary acidifying agents (ammonium chloride, ascorbic acid, potassium or sodium phosphate):** may increase possibility of kidney stone formation. **Xanthines:** increased serum theophylline. Adjust theophylline dosage.

Nursing diagnoses

- Pain (joint) related to patient's underlying condition.
- High risk for infection related to allopurinol-induced agranulocytosis.
- Knowledge deficit related to allopurinol therapy.

Nursing interventions

- *Contraindicated* in idiopathic hemochromatosis.
- *Use cautiously* in cataracts and hepatic or renal disease.
- Discontinue at first sign of rash, which may precede severe hypersensitivity reaction. Tell patient to report all adverse reactions immediately. Skin rash is more common in patients taking diuretics and in those with renal disorders.
- Monitor intake and output; daily urine output of at least 2 liters and maintenance of neutral or slightly alkaline urine are desirable. Patient should be encouraged to drink plenty of fluids.
- If renal insufficiency exists at any time during treatment, allopurinol dosage should be reduced.
- Optimal benefits of treatment may require 2 to 6 weeks of therapy. Because acute gout attacks may occur during this time, concurrent use of colchicine may be prescribed prophylactically.
- Allopurinol may provoke amoxicillin or ampicillin-induced rash weeks after discontinuation.

Index

General

Classification: anxiolytic (benzodiazepine). **Pregnancy risk category:** D. **Controlled substance schedule:** IV.

Mechanism of action

Depresses the CNS at the limbic and subcortical levels of the brain.

Indications and dosage

• Anxiety and tension. **Adults:** usual starting dose is 0.25 to 0.5 mg P.O. t.i.d. Maximum total daily dosage is 4 mg in divided doses. In elderly or debilitated patients, usual starting dose is 0.25 mg b.i.d. or t.i.d.

Adverse reactions

CNS: *drowsiness, light-headedness,* headache, confusion, hostility. **CV:** transient hypotension, tachycardia. **GI:** nausea, vomiting, constipation, discomfort, dry mouth.

Interactions

Alcohol, other CNS depressants: increased CNS depression. Avoid concomitant use. **Cigarette smoking:** increased clearance of benzodiazepines. Monitor for lack of effect. **Cimetidine:** increased sedation. Monitor carefully. **Digoxin:** benzodiazepines may increase serum levels of digoxin, increasing risk of toxicity. Monitor closely. **Tricyclic antidepressants:** increased plasma levels of tricyclic antidepressants. Monitor for toxicity.

Nursing diagnoses

• Anxiety related to the patient's underlying condition.
• High risk for injury related to alprazolam-induced CNS reactions.
• Knowledge deficit related to alprazolam therapy.

Nursing interventions

• *Contraindicated* in acute narrow-angle glaucoma, psychoses, or anxiety-free psychiatric disorders.
• *Use cautiously* in patients with hepatic or renal disease and in elderly or debilitated patients.
• Reduce dosage in elderly or debilitated patients because they may be more susceptible to the adverse CNS effects of the drug.
• Do not withdraw drug abruptly after long-term use. Withdrawal symptoms may occur. Abuse or addiction is possible.
• Warn patient not to combine drug with alcohol or other depressants and also to avoid hazardous activities that require alertness and psychomotor coordination until CNS effects are known.
• Drug should not be prescribed for everyday stress or for long-term use (more than 4 months).
• Warn patient not to increase dosage or discontinue drug without doctor's approval.
• Alprazolam is more rapidly metabolized and excreted than most of the other benzodiazepines and has a lower incidence of lethargy than other drugs of this class.
• May also be effective for treatment of depression.
• Periodic hepatic, renal, and hematopoietic function studies should be performed in patients receiving repeated or prolonged therapy.
• If alprazolam overdose occurs, flumazenil (a specific benzodiazepine antagonist) may be useful. The duration of action of alprazolam is longer than that of flumazenil, and resedation is possible.

General
Classification: antiviral (thymidine derivative). **Pregnancy risk category:** C.

Mechanism of action
Prevents replication of the human immunodeficiency virus (HIV) by inhibiting the enzyme reverse transcriptase.

Indications and dosage
• Patients with AIDS or advanced AIDS-related complex (ARC) who have a history of *Pneumocystis carinii* pneumonia or a CD4 lymphocyte count below 200 cells/mm^3. **Adults:** initially, 200 mg P.O. q 4 hours around the clock for 1 month, then 100 mg P.O. q 4 hours around the clock. **Children:** dosage is individualized and will vary according to investigational drug treatment protocol. Early studies have employed doses between 0.9 and 1.4 mg/kg/hour by continuous I.V. infusion; others have used 100 mg/m^2 I.V. or P.O. q 6 hours.
• Postexposure prophylaxis. **Adults:** dosage will vary according to study protocol, but most studies use 200 mg P.O. q 4 hours around the clock for 6 to 8 weeks. Some investigators attempt to initiate therapy within 1 hour of exposure.
• Asymptomatic HIV infection. **Adults:** 100 mg P.O. q 4 hours while awake (500 mg daily). **Children 3 months to 12 years:** 180 mg/m^2 P.O. q 6 hours (720 mg/m^2/day) not to exceed 200 mg q 6 hours.

Adverse reactions
Blood: ***severe bone marrow depression (resulting in anemia), granulocytopenia, thrombocytopenia.*** **CNS:** *headache, malaise,* agitation, restlessness, insomnia, confusion, anxiety. **GI:** *nausea,* anorexia. **Skin:** *rash,* itching. **Other:** myalgia.

Interactions
Acyclovir: possible seizures, lethargy, and fatigue. Use together cautiously. **Co-trimoxazole, acetaminophen, aspirin, indomethacin:** may impair hepatic metabolism of zidovudine, increasing the drug's toxicity. **Other cytotoxic drugs:** additive adverse effects on the bone marrow. Avoid concomitant use. **Pentamidine, dapsone, flucytosine, amphotericin B:** increased risk of nephrotoxicity and bone marrow suppression. Monitor closely. **Probenecid:** may decrease the renal clearance of zidovudine. Avoid concomitant use.

Nursing diagnoses
• High risk for injury related to ineffectiveness of zidovudine to prevent or eradicate the infection.
• Noncompliance (medication administration) related to prolonged therapy.
• Knowledge deficit related to zidovudine therapy.

Nursing interventions
• Advise patient that he may need blood transfusions during treatment with zidovudine, which frequently causes a low RBC count by suppressing the bone marrow.
• Frequent monitoring of blood studies (every 2 weeks) is recommended to detect anemia or granulocytopenia. Patients may require dosage reduction or temporary discontinuation of the drug.
• Remind patients that they *must* comply with the every-4-hour dosage schedule. Suggest ways to avoid missing doses, such as use of alarm clocks.
• Warn patients not to take any other drugs for AIDS (especially street drugs) unless their doctors have approved them. Some purported AIDS cures may interfere with zidovudine's effectiveness.
• Health-care workers who consider zidovudine prophylaxis following occupational exposure (after needlestick injury, for example) should understand that animal and human studies are insufficient to judge the drug's safety or efficacy. These persons should consider the potential toxicity of the drug, as well as their risk of acquiring HIV from occupational exposure. Some doctors don't advocate using zidovudine for this purpose.
• **I.V. use:** Dilute before administration following manufacturer's instructions. Avoid rapid infusion or bolus injection. Adding mixture to biological or colloidal fluids (for example, blood products, protein solutions) is not recommended.
• Also known as AZT.

General
Classification: thrombolytic (enzyme). **Pregnancy risk category:** C.

Mechanism of action
Binds to fibrin in a thrombus, converting plasminogen to plasmin, which initiates local fibrinolysis.

Indications and dosage
- Lysis of thrombi obstructing coronary arteries in acute MI. **Adults:** 100 mg I.V. infused over 3 hours: 60 mg in first hour, then 20 mg/hour for 2 hours. Smaller adults (65 kg or less) should receive a dose of 1.25 mg/kg; then 20% of the total dose per hour for 2 hours.
- Management of acute massive pulmonary embolism. **Adults:** 100 mg I.V. infusion over 2 hours. Begin heparin at the end of the infusion when the partial thromboplastin time or thrombin time returns to twice normal or less.

Adverse reactions
Blood: ***severe, spontaneous bleeding (cerebral, retroperitoneal, GU, GI).*** **CNS:** ***cerebral hemorrhage,*** fever. **CV:** hypotension, arrhythmias. **GI:** nausea, vomiting. **Local:** bleeding at puncture sites. **Other:** hypersensitivity, urticaria.

Interactions
Aspirin, dipyridamole, heparin, coumarin anticoagulants: increased risk of bleeding. Monitor patient carefully.

Nursing diagnoses
- Altered cardiopulmonary tissue perfusion related to underlying condition.
- High risk for injury related to the adverse effects of alteplase.
- Knowledge deficit related to alteplase therapy.

Nursing interventions
- *Contraindicated* in active internal bleeding, intracranial neoplasm, arteriovenous malformation, aneurysm, and severe uncontrolled hypertension and in patients with a history of CVA, intraspinal or intracranial trauma or surgery within 2 months, or known bleeding diathesis.
- *Use cautiously* in patients with recent major surgery, organ biopsy, trauma (including CPR), and GI or GU bleeding; in pregnancy and first 10 days postpartum; in patients with cerebrovascular disease or hypertension; mitral stenosis, atrial fibrillation, or other conditions that may lead to left heart thrombus; acute pericarditis or subacute bacterial endocarditis; and septic thrombophlebitis; patients age 75 and older; in patients with diabetic hemorrhagic retinopathy; and in those receiving anticoagulants.
- Also known as recombinant tissue plasminogen activator and t-PA.
- Do not exceed dose of 100 mg. Higher doses are associated with an increased incidence of intracranial bleeding.
- Coronary thrombolysis is associated with arrhythmias induced by reperfusion of ischemic myocardium. Such arrhythmias are not different from those associated with MI. Have antiarrhythmics readily available and carefully monitor the ECG.
- Successful recanalization of occluded coronary arteries and improvement of heart function are time-dependent phenomena and require initiation of treatment with alteplase as soon as possible after the onset of symptoms.
- Carefully monitor patient for signs of internal bleeding and frequently check all puncture sites; bleeding is the most common adverse effect. Avoid invasive procedures during thrombolytic therapy.
- Heparin therapy is frequently initiated after treatment with alteplase to decrease the risk of rethrombosis.
- Drug may be administered as reconstituted (1 mg/ml) or diluted with equal volume of 0.9% sodium chloride or D_5W to make a 0.5 mg/ml solution.
- Reconstitute alteplase solution immediately before use, and administer it within 8 hours. The drug may be temporarily stored at 35° to 86° F (1.7° to 30° C), and it is stable for 8 hours at room temperature. Discard any solution unused after that time because it contains no preservatives.

General

Classification: antiviral (synthetic pyrimidine nucleoside analogue). **Pregnancy risk category:** C.

Mechanism of action

Enzymes in cell convert zalcitabine to its active metabolite, dideoxycytidine 5′-triphosphate (ddCTP), which inhibits replication of human immunodeficiency virus (HIV) by blocking viral DNA synthesis.

Indications and dosage

• Advanced HIV infection (CD4+ T-cell count below 300 cells/mm³) in patients with significant clinical or immunologic deterioration. **Adults 30 kg and over:** 0.75 mg P.O. q 8 hours. Must be taken with zidovudine 200 mg P.O. q 8 hours.

• Dosage adjustment in patients with renal failure. **Adults:** Patients with a creatinine clearance above 40 ml/minute/1.73 m² should receive the usual dose; 10 to 40 ml/minute/1.73 m², the usual dose q 12 hours; below 10 ml/minute/1.73 m², the usual dose q 24 hours.

Adverse reactions

CNS: *peripheral neuropathy,* headache. **EENT:** pharyngitis. **GI:** nausea, vomiting, diarrhea, abdominal pain, anorexia, constipation, stomatitis. **Skin:** pruritus; night sweats; erythematous, maculopapular, or follicular rash. **Other:** myalgia, arthralgia, fatigue, fever, rigors, chest pain, weight increase, ***pancreatitis.***

Interactions

Aminoglycosides, amphotericin B, foscarnet, and other drugs that may impair renal function: increased risk of nephrotoxicity. Avoid concomitant use. **Chloramphenicol, cisplatin, dapsone, disulfiram, ethionamide, glutethimide, gold salts, hydralazine, iodoquinol, isoniazid, metronidazole, nitrofurantoin, phenytoin, ribavirin, vincristine, and other drugs that can cause peripheral neuropathy:** increased risk of peripheral neuropathy. Avoid concomitant use. **Pentamidine:** increased risk of pancreatitis. Avoid concomitant use.

Nursing diagnoses

• High risk for injury related to ineffectiveness of zalcitabine to prevent or eradicate the infection.
• Noncompliance (medication administration) related to prolonged therapy.
• Knowledge deficit related to zalcitabine.

Nursing interventions

• *Use with extreme caution* in patients with preexisting peripheral neuropathy; no data exist regarding toxicity of zalcitabine in these patients.
• *Use cautiously* in patients with renal and hepatic impairment. Drug regimen (zalcitabine plus zidovudine) may exacerbate hepatic dysfunction in patients with preexisting liver impairment.
• Use cautiously in patients with a history of pancreatitis. Rarely, pancreatitis has been fatal in patients receiving zalcitabine. In patients receiving zalcitabine as the only treatment (monotherapy), incidence of pancreatitis was less than 1%.
• Peripheral neuropathy, characterized by numbness and burning in the extremities, is the major toxicity of the drug. It may or may not be reversible.
• If patient experiences symptoms that resemble peripheral neuropathy, drug should be discontinued if symptoms are bilateral and persist beyond 72 hours. If symptoms persist or worsen beyond 1 week, drug should be permanently discontinued. However, if all findings relevant to peripheral neuropathy have resolved to minor symptoms, the drug may be reintroduced at 0.375 mg P.O. q 8 hours.
• If zalcitabine is discontinued because of toxicity, the patient should resume the recommended dose for zidovudine monotherapy (100 mg q 4 hours).

General

Classification: antineoplastic (s-triazine derivative). **Pregnancy risk category:** D.

Mechanism of action

Unknown. Structurally similar to the alkylating agent triethylenemelamine but not an alkylating agent. However, metabolism is known to be important for antitumor activity; metabolites of the drug are known alkylating agents.

Indications and dosage

• Palliative treatment of patients with persistent or recurrent ovarian cancer after first-line therapy with cisplatin or alkylating agent-based combination therapy. **Adults:** 260 mg/m² P.O. daily in four divided doses with meals and h.s. for 14 or 21 consecutive days in a 28-day cycle.

Adverse reactions

Blood: ***leukopenia, thrombocytopenia, anemia.*** **CNS:** *sensory neuropathy*, anorexia, ataxia, paresthesia, hyporeflexia, fatigue, ***seizures.*** **GI:** *nausea and vomiting.* **Skin:** alopecia, erythematous maculopapular eczema. **Other:** increased serum creatinine and BUN levels.

Interactions

Cimetidine: may increase the half-life and toxicity of altretamine. Monitor closely for toxicity. **MAO inhibitors:** severe orthostatic hypotension. Avoid concomitant use.

Nursing diagnoses

• High risk for fluid volume deficit related to drug-induced adverse reactions.
• High risk for infection related to drug-induced adverse reactions.
• Knowledge deficit related to altretamine therapy.

Nursing interventions

• *Contraindicated* in patients hypersensitive to the drug and in patients with preexisting bone marrow depression or severe neurologic toxicity. However, patients with preexisting cisplatin neuropathies caused by high-dose cisplatin therapy have been successfully treated with altretamine. Carefully monitor these patients for worsening neurologic function.
• Also known as as hexamethylmelamine and HMM.
• Continuous high-dose daily treatment with altretamine is associated with a higher incidence of mild to moderate neurotoxicity. It appears to be reversible when therapy is discontinued.
• Discontinue the drug temporarily for at least 14 days if laboratory tests show a platelet count below 75,000/mm³, WBC count below 2,000/mm³, or granulocyte count below 1,000/mm³. Also discontinue temporarily if the patient experiences severe GI distress that is unresponsive to symptomatic treatment or develops signs of progressive neuropathy. Drug should be discontinued if neurologic symptoms fail to stabilize.
• Unconfirmed reports suggest that the severity and incidence of neurotoxicity may be decreased by concomitant administration of pyridoxine.
• A careful neurologic assessment should be performed before each course of therapy.
• Monitor CBC and platelet count before each course of therapy and monthly thereafter. Altretamine causes a mild to moderate dose-related myelosuppression. Nadirs of leukocyte and platelet counts are reached by 3 to 4 weeks. Normal counts are regained by 6 weeks. Be sure that the patient understands that the drug may cause fetal harm and advise patient to avoid pregnancy.
• Continuous daily administration of this drug is associated with nausea and vomiting, which is usually treatable with antiemetics. If nausea and vomiting is severe, dosage reduction or temporary discontinuation of the drug may be necessary.

General

Classification: anticoagulant (coumarin derivative). **Pregnancy risk category:** D.

Mechanism of action

Inhibits vitamin K-dependent activation of clotting factors II, VII, IX, and X.

Indications and dosage

• Pulmonary emboli; emboli associated with deep vein thrombosis, MI, rheumatic heart disease with heart valve damage, prosthetic heart valves, atrial arrhythmias. **Adults:** 10 to 15 mg P.O. for 3 days, then dosage based on daily PTs. Usual maintenance dosage is 2 to 10 mg daily. Alternative regimen: initially, 40 to 60 mg P.O. as a single dose, or 20 to 30 mg for elderly patients; then 2 to 10 mg daily based on PT determinations. Drug is also available I.V.

Adverse reactions

Blood: ***hemorrhage (excessive dosage),*** eosinophilia, leukopenia. **GI:** paralytic ileus, intestinal obstruction, diarrhea, vomiting, cramps, nausea. **GU:** excessive uterine bleeding. **Skin:** dermatitis, urticaria, *rash,* necrosis, gangrene, alopecia. **Other:** *fever,* hepatitis, jaundice.

Interactions

Acetaminophen: increased bleeding with chronic use with acetaminophen. Monitor carefully. **Amiodarone, cephalosporins, chloramphenicol, ciprofloxacin, clofibrate, diflunisal, thyroid drugs, heparin, anabolic steroids, cimetidine, disulfiram, glucagon, methimazole, metronidazole, propylthiouracil, sulindac, sulfinpyrazone, sulfonamides, vitamin E:** increased PT. Monitor for bleeding. Reduce warfarin dosage if needed. **Barbiturates:** inhibition of hypoprothrombinemic effect of anticoagulants. If barbiturates are withdrawn, reduce anticoagulant dose; inhibition may last weeks after barbiturate is withdrawn, but fatal hemorrhage can occur when inhibition disappears. **Cholestyramine:** decreased response when used too close together. Give 6 hours after oral anticoagulants. **Glutethimide, chloral hydrate, triclofos sodium:** increased or decreased PT. Avoid use or monitor closely. **Griseofulvin, ethchlorvynol, carbamazepine, paraldehyde, rifampin:** decreased PT with reduced anticoagulant effect. Monitor closely. **Hydantoins:** increased serum levels of hydantoins. Monitor closely. **Indomethacin, mefenamic acid, oxyphenbutazone, phenylbutazone, salicylates:** increased PT; ulcerogenic effects. Don't use together. **Sulfonylureas (oral antidiabetic agents):** increased hypoglycemic response. Monitor blood glucose levels.

Nursing diagnoses

• Altered cardiopulmonary and peripheral tissue perfusion related to the patient's condition.
• High risk for injury related to the adverse effects of warfarin sodium.
• Knowledge deficit related to warfarin sodium.

Nursing interventions

• *Contraindicated* in bleeding or hemorrhagic tendencies resulting from open wounds, visceral cancer, GI ulcers, severe hepatic or renal disease, severe uncontrolled hypertension, subacute bacterial endocarditis, polycythemia vera, and vitamin K deficiency and after recent operations in eye, brain, or spinal cord.
• *Use cautiously* in diverticulitis, colitis, mild or moderate hypertension, mild or moderate hepatic or renal disease; lactation; presence of drainage tubes; regional or lumbar block anesthesia; or in any condition increasing risk of hemorrhage.
• Observe breast-feeding infants of mothers on drug for unexpected bleeding.
• Stress patient compliance with prescribed dosage and follow-up appointments.
• Regularly inspect patient for bleeding gums, bruises on arms or legs, petechiae, nosebleeds, melena, tarry stools, hematuria, hematemesis.
• Warn patient to avoid OTC products containing salicylates or drugs that interact with warfarin.

General

Classification: antacid, hypophosphatemia agent (inorganic aluminum salt). **Pregnancy risk category:** C.

Mechanism of action

Reduces total acid load in the GI tract and elevates gastric pH to reduce pepsin activity. Also strengthens the gastric mucosal barrier and increases esophageal sphincter tone.

Indications and dosage

• As antacid. **Adults:** suspension: 5 to 10 ml P.O., p.r.n. Extra-strength suspension: 2.5 to 5 ml, p.r.n. Tablets or capsules: 1 to 2, p.r.n.
• Prevention of formation of urinary phosphate stones (with low-phosphate diet). **Adults:** suspension: 15 to 30 ml in water or juice P.O. 1 hour after meals and h.s.; 5 to 15 ml extra-strength suspension in water or juice 1 hour after meals and h.s.; 2 to 6 tablets or capsules 1 hour after meals and h.s.

Adverse reactions

GI: anorexia, *constipation,* intestinal obstruction.
Metabolic: hypophosphatemia.

Interactions

Allopurinol, antibiotics (including quinolones and tetracyclines), diflunisal, digoxin, iron, isoniazid, penicillamine, phenothiazines, quinidine: decreased pharmacologic effect; absorption may be impaired. Administer separately.

Nursing diagnoses

• Pain related to gastric hyperacidity.
• Constipation related to aluminum carbonate-induced adverse reactions.
• Knowledge deficit related to aluminum carbonate therapy.

Nursing interventions

• *Use cautiously* in elderly patients, especially those with decreased GI motility (those receiving antidiarrheals, antispasmodics, or anticholinergics), dehydration, fluid restriction, chronic renal disease, and suspected intestinal obstruction.
• Record amount and consistency of stools. Manage constipation with laxatives or stool softeners; alternate with magnesium-containing antacids (if patient does not have renal disease).
• Shake suspension well; give with small amount of water or fruit juice to ensure passage to stomach. When administering through nasogastric tube, be sure tube is placed correctly and is patent; follow antacid with water to clear tube.
• Watch long-term high-dose use in patient on restricted sodium intake.
• Warn patient not to take aluminum carbonate indiscriminately and not to switch antacids without doctor's advice.
• Because drug contains aluminum, may be used in renal failure to help control hyperphosphatemia. Binds to phosphate in GI tract.
• Monitor serum phosphate.
• Watch for symptoms of hypophosphatemia with prolonged use (anorexia, malaise, muscle weakness); can also lead to resorption of calcium and bone demineralization.
• May cause enteric-coated drugs to be released prematurely in stomach. Separate doses by 1 hour.

General

Classification: antineoplastic (vinca alkaloid).
Pregnancy risk category: D.

Mechanism of action

Arrests mitosis in metaphase, blocking cell division.

Indications and dosage

- Acute lymphoblastic and other leukemias, Hodgkin's disease, non-Hodgkin's lymphoma, lymphosarcoma, reticulum cell sarcoma, neuroblastoma, rhabdomyosarcoma, Wilms' tumor, Ewing's sarcoma, osteogenic and other sarcomas, lung and breast cancer. **Adults:** 0.4 to 1.4 mg/m² I.V. weekly. **Children over 10 kg:** 1.5 to 2 mg/m² I.V. weekly. **Children 10 kg and under:** initially, 0.05 mg/kg I.V. weekly. Maximum single dosage (adults and children) is 2 mg.

Adverse reactions

Blood: rapidly reversible mild anemia and leukopenia. **CNS:** *peripheral neuropathy,* sensory loss, *loss of deep tendon reflexes, paresthesia, wristdrop and footdrop,* ataxia, cranial nerve palsies (headache, *jaw pain,* hoarseness, vocal cord paralysis, visual disturbances), *muscle weakness and cramps,* depression, agitation, insomnia; some neurotoxicities may be permanent. **CV:** hypotension. **EENT:** diplopia, optic and extraocular neuropathy, ptosis. **GI:** diarrhea, *constipation, cramps,* ileus that mimics surgical abdomen, *nausea, vomiting,* anorexia, *stomatitis,* weight loss, dysphagia, ***intestinal necrosis.*** **GU:** urine retention, SIADH. **Local:** severe local reaction when extravasated, *phlebitis,* cellulitis. **Other:** ***acute bronchospasm,*** *reversible alopecia (up to 71% of patients),* fever.

Interactions

Asparaginase: decreased hepatic clearance of vincristine. **Calcium channel blockers:** enhanced vincristine accumulation in cells. **Digoxin:** decreased digoxin effects. Monitor serum digoxin. **Mitomycin:** possibly increased frequency of bronchospasm and acute pulmonary reactions.

Nursing diagnoses

- High risk for fluid volume deficit related to adverse drug reactions.
- Body image disturbance related to adverse drug reactions.
- Knowledge deficit related to vincristine therapy.

Nursing interventions

- *Contraindicated* in hypersensitivity to the drug. Don't administer to those receiving radiation therapy through ports that include the liver.
- *Use cautiously* in jaundice or hepatic dysfunction, neuromuscular disease, infection, and with other neurotoxic drugs.
- After administering, monitor for life-threatening acute bronchospasm reaction. If this occurs, notify doctor immediately.
- Monitor for hyperuricemia, especially in patients with leukemia or lymphoma. Maintain good hydration. Allopurinol may be ordered to prevent uric acid nephropathy.
- Neurotoxicity is dose-related and usually reversible; don't give drug more than once a week.
- **I.V. use:** Give directly into vein or tubing of running I.V. slowly over 1 minute, or in 50-ml D_5W or 0.9% sodium chloride solution infused over 15 minutes. If drug infiltrates, stop infusion immediately. Apply ice packs on and off every 2 hours for 24 hours.
- Check for depression of Achilles tendon reflex, numbness, tingling, footdrop or wristdrop, difficulty walking (including walking on heels), ataxia, and slapping gait. Support walking patient.
- Monitor bowel function. Give stool softener, laxative, or water before dosing. Constipation may be an early sign of neurotoxicity.
- Warn patient that reversible alopecia may occur.
- Be extremely careful about doses. Don't confuse vincristine with vinblastine or vindesine.
- 5-mg vials are for multiple-dose use only. Don't administer entire vial as a single dose.

aluminum hydroxide

AlternaGEL ◇, Alu-Cap ◇, Alu-Tab ◇, Amphojel ◇, Dialume ◇, Nephrox ◇

General

Classification: antacid, hypophosphatemia agent, adsorbent (aluminum salt). **Pregnancy risk category:** C.

Mechanism of action

Reduces total acid load in the GI tract and elevates gastric pH to reduce pepsin activity. Also strengthens the gastric mucosal barrier and increases esophageal sphincter tone.

Indications and dosage

- Antacid. **Adults:** 5 to 10 ml oral suspension or 600 mg P.O. 1 hour after meals and h.s.; or 300- or 600-mg tablet, chewed before swallowing, taken with milk or water five or six times daily after meals and h.s.; or one to three 475 or 500 mg capsules 1 hour after meals and h.s. (maximum nine capsules/day).
- Hyperphosphatemia in renal failure. **Adults:** 500 mg to 2 g P.O. b.i.d. to q.i.d.

Adverse reactions

GI: anorexia, *constipation,* intestinal obstruction.
Metabolic: hypophosphatemia.

Interactions

Allopurinol, antibiotics (including quinolones and tetracyclines), diflunisal, digoxin, iron, isoniazid, penicillamine, phenothiazines, quinidine: decreased pharmacologic effect because absorption may be impaired. Administer at separate times.

Nursing diagnoses

- Pain related to gastric hyperacidity.
- Constipation related to binding effect of aluminum hydroxide.
- Knowledge deficit related to aluminum hydroxide therapy.

Nursing interventions

- *Use cautiously* in elderly patients, especially those with decreased GI motility (those receiving antidiarrheals, antispasmodics, or anticholinergics), dehydration, fluid restriction, chronic renal disease, and suspected intestinal obstruction.
- Record amount and consistency of stools. Manage constipation with laxatives or stool softeners; alternate with magnesium-containing antacids (if patient does not have renal disease).
- Shake suspension well; give with small amount of milk or water to ensure passage to stomach. When administering through nasogastric tube, make sure tube is placed correctly and is patent. After instilling antacid, flush tube with water.
- Watch long-term high-dose use in patient on restricted sodium intake.
- Warn patient not to take aluminum hydroxide indiscriminately or switch antacids without doctor's advice.
- Because it contains aluminum, may be used in renal failure to help control hyperphosphatemia. Binds to phosphate in the GI tract.
- Monitor serum phosphate.
- Watch for symptoms of hypophosphatemia with prolonged use (anorexia, malaise, and muscle weakness); can also lead to reabsorption of calcium and bone demineralization.
- May cause enteric-coated drugs to be released prematurely in stomach. Separate doses by 1 hour.

General

Classification: antineoplastic (vinca alkaloid).
Pregnancy risk category: D.

Mechanism of action

Arrests mitosis in metaphase, blocking cell division.

Indications and dosage

• Breast or testicular cancer, Hodgkin's and non-Hodgkin's lymphomas, choriocarcinoma, lymphosarcoma, neuroblastoma, mycosis fungoides, Kaposi's sarcoma, histiocytosis. **Adults:** 0.1 mg/kg or 3.7 mg/m^2 I.V. weekly or q 2 weeks. May be increased to maximum dosage of 0.5 mg/kg or 18.5 mg/m^2 I.V. weekly according to response. Dosage should not be repeated if WBC less than 4,000/mm^3. **Children:** initial dose 2.5 mg/m^2 I.V. Increase dose by 1.25 mg/m^2 until leukocytes are below 3,000/mm^3 or a tumor response is seen. Maximum dose is 7.5 mg/m^2.

Adverse reactions

Blood: ***anemia, leukopenia*** (nadir days 4 to 10 and lasts another 7 to 14 days), ***thrombocytopenia.*** **CNS:** depression, *paresthesia, peripheral neuropathy and neuritis, numbness, loss of deep tendon reflexes, muscle pain and weakness,* ***seizures,*** headache. **CV:** hypertension. **EENT:** pharyngitis. **GI:** *nausea, vomiting, stomatitis,* ulcer and bleeding, *constipation, ileus, anorexia, weight loss,* abdominal pain. **GU:** oligospermia, aspermia, urine retention. **Skin:** dermatitis, vesiculation. **Local:** *irritation, phlebitis,* cellulitis, necrosis if I.V. extravasates. **Other:** ***acute bronchospasm,*** reversible alopecia, *pain in tumor site,* low fever.

Interactions

Mitomycin: increased risk of bronchospasm and shortness of breath. **Phenytoin:** decreased plasma phenytoin levels.

Nursing diagnoses

• High risk for impaired skin integrity related to adverse drug reactions.
• Body image disturbance related to adverse drug reactions.
• Knowledge deficit related to vinblastine therapy.

Nursing interventions

• *Contraindicated* in severe leukopenia or bacterial infection.
• *Use cautiously* in jaundice or hepatic dysfunction.
• Don't inject into a limb with compromised circulation.
• Decrease dose by 50% if bilirubin levels are greater than 3 mg/100 ml.
• After administering, monitor for life-threatening acute bronchospasm reaction. If this occurs, notify doctor immediately.
• Give antiemetic before administering to reduce nausea.
• Stop drug if patient develops stomatitis.
• Assess bowel activity. Give laxatives as needed. May use stool softeners prophylactically.
• Don't repeat dosage more frequently than every 7 days or severe leukopenia will develop.
• Assess for numbness and tingling in hands and feet. Assess gait for early evidence of footdrop.
• **I.V. use:** inject directly into vein or tubing of running I.V. over 1 minute, or give in a 50-ml D_5W or 0.9% sodium chloride solution infused over 15 minutes. If extravasation occurs, stop infusion immediately. Manufacturer recommends that moderate heat be applied to the area of leakage. Local injection of hyaluronidase may help disperse the drug. Some clinicians prefer to apply ice packs on and off every 2 hours for 24 hours, with local injection of hydrocortisone or 0.9% sodium chloride.
• Warn patient that alopecia may occur but is usually reversible.
• Reconstitute 10-mg vial with 10 ml of sodium chloride injection or sterile water. This yields 1 mg/ml.
• Don't confuse vinblastine with vincristine or the investigational agent vindesine.
• Follow institutional policy to reduce risks associated with preparation of parenteral form.

aluminum phosphate

Phosphaljel ◇

General

Classification: antacid (aluminum salt). **Pregnancy risk category:** C.

Mechanism of action

Provides supplemental phosphate.

Indications and dosage

• To reduce fecal elimination of phosphorus. **Adults:** 15 to 30 ml undiluted P.O. q 2 hours between meals and h.s.

Adverse reactions

GI: *constipation,* intestinal obstruction.

Interactions

Ciprofloxacin, other quinolone antibiotics, tetracyclines: decreased antibiotic effect. Separate administration times.

Nursing diagnoses

• Pain related to gastric hyperacidity.
• Constipation related to aluminum phosphate-induced adverse reactions.
• Knowledge deficit related to aluminum phosphate therapy.

Nursing interventions

• *Use cautiously* in elderly patients, especially those with decreased GI motility (those receiving antidiarrheals, antispasmodics, or anticholinergics), dehydration, fluid restriction, chronic renal disease, and suspected intestinal obstruction.
• Record amount and consistency of stools. Manage constipation with laxatives or stool softeners; alternate with magnesium-containing antacids (if patient does not have renal disease).
• Shake well; give alone or with small amount of milk or water. When administering through nasogastric tube, make sure tube is placed correctly and is patent; after instilling, flush tube with water to facilitate passage to stomach and maintain tube patency.
• Watch long-term high-dose use in patient on restricted sodium intake.
• Warn patient not to take aluminum phosphate indiscriminately and not to switch antacids without doctor's advice.
• Can reverse hypophosphatemia induced by aluminum hydroxide.
• May cause enteric-coated drugs to be released prematurely in stomach. Separate doses by 1 hour.

General
Classification: antiviral (purine nucleoside). **Pregnancy risk category:** C.

Mechanism of action
Becomes incorporated into viral DNA and inhibits viral multiplication.

Indications and dosage
- Herpes simplex virus encephalitis. **Adults and children** (including neonates): 15 mg/kg I.V. daily for 10 days. Slowly infuse the total daily dose by I.V. infusion at a constant rate over 12- to 24-hour period. Avoid rapid or bolus injection.
- Herpes zoster in immunosuppressed patients. **Adults:** 10 mg/kg I.V. daily for 5 days.

Adverse reactions
Blood: anemia, neutropenia, thrombocytopenia. **CNS:** tremor, dizziness, hallucinations, confusion, psychosis, ataxia. **GI:** *anorexia, nausea,* vomiting, diarrhea. **Hepatic:** elevated AST, bilirubin. **Skin:** pruritus, rash. **Local:** pain at injection site. **Other:** weight loss.

Interactions
Allopurinol: concurrent therapy reduces metabolism of vidarabine and increases risk of adverse CNS effects.

Nursing diagnoses
- High risk for injury related to ineffectiveness of vidarabine to eradicate the infection.
- High risk for fluid volume deficit related to vidarabine-induced adverse GI reactions.
- Knowledge deficit related to vidarabine therapy.

Nursing interventions
- Can reduce mortality caused by herpes simplex virus encephalitis from about 70% to 28%. Vidarabine is not effective against other viruses.
- Monitor hematologic tests, such as hemoglobin, hematocrit, WBC count, and platelet count during therapy. Also monitor renal and liver function studies.
- Patient with impaired renal function may need dosage adjustment.
- **I.V. use:** Use with a 0.45-micron (or smaller) I.V. filter. Any I.V. solution is suitable as a diluent. Must be diluted to a concentration of less than 0.5 mg/ml. Because vidarabine is not highly soluble, each milligram of drug requires 2.2 ml of I.V. solution to solubilize; the maximum concentration is 450 mg/liter. Dilute just before using, and use within 48 hours.
- Don't give I.M. or S.C. because of low solubility and poor absorption. Because large volumes of solution must be administered, monitor patient for fluid overload.

General

Classification: antiviral, antiparkinsonian agent (synthetic cyclic primary amine). **Pregnancy risk category:** C.

Mechanism of action

Interferes with influenza A virus penetration into susceptible cells. Its action in the treatment of parkinsonism is unknown.

Indications and dosage

- Prophylaxis or symptomatic treatment of influenza type A virus, respiratory tract illnesses. **Adults to 64 years and children 10 years and over:** 200 mg P.O. daily in a single dose or divided b.i.d. **Children 1 to 9 years:** 4.4 to 8.8 mg/kg P.O. daily, as a single dose or divided b.i.d. or t.i.d. Don't exceed 150 mg daily. **Adults over 64 years:** 100 mg P.O. once daily.

  Treatment should continue for 24 to 48 hours after symptoms disappear. Prophylaxis should start as soon as possible after initial exposure and continue for at least 10 days. May continue prophylactic treatment up to 90 days for repeated or suspected exposures if influenza vaccine unavailable. If used with influenza vaccine, continue dose for 2 to 3 weeks until protection from vaccine develops.
- Treatment of drug-induced extrapyramidal reactions. **Adults:** 100 mg P.O. b.i.d., up to 300 mg daily in divided doses. Patient may benefit from as much as 400 mg daily, but dosages over 200 mg must be closely supervised.
- Treatment of idiopathic parkinsonism, parkinsonian syndrome. **Adults:** 100 mg P.O. b.i.d.; in patients who are seriously ill or receiving other antiparkinsonian drugs, 100 mg daily for at least 1 week, then 100 mg b.i.d., p.r.n.

Adverse reactions

CNS: depression, fatigue, confusion, dizziness, psychosis, hallucinations, anxiety, *irritability*, ataxia, *insomnia*, weakness, headache, light-headedness, difficulty concentrating. **CV:** peripheral edema, orthostatic hypotension, ***CHF***. **GI:** anorexia, nausea, constipation, vomiting, dry mouth. **GU:** urine retention. **Skin:** *livedo reticularis* (with prolonged use).

Interactions

Anticholinergics: increased adverse anticholinergic effects. Use together cautiously. **Triamterene, hydrochlorothiazide:** increased levels of amantadine. Use together cautiously.

Nursing diagnoses

- High risk for injury related to ineffectiveness of amantadine to eradicate the infection.
- High risk for fluid volume deficit related to adverse GI reactions to amantadine.
- Knowledge deficit related to amantadine therapy.

Nursing interventions

- *Use cautiously* in seizure disorders, CHF, peripheral edema, hepatic disease, mental illness, eczematoid rash, renal impairment, orthostatic hypotension, and CV disease and in elderly patients. Dosage may need to be adjusted in patients with renal failure.
- For best absorption, drug should be taken after meals.
- Instruct patient to report adverse reactions, especially dizziness, depression, anxiety, nausea, and urine retention, to the doctor.
- Elderly patients are more susceptible to neurologic adverse effects. Taking the drug in two daily doses rather than in a single dose may reduce their incidence.
- If orthostatic hypotension occurs, instruct patient not to stand or change positions too quickly.
- If insomnia occurs, dose should be taken several hours before bedtime.
- When prescribed for parkinsonism, warn patient against discontinuing drug abruptly since this might precipitate a parkinsonian crisis.

General

Classification: antianginal, anthypertensive, antiarrhythmic (calcium channel blocker). **Pregnancy risk category:** C.

Mechanism of action

Inhibits calcium ion influx across cardiac and smooth muscle cells, thus decreasing myocardial contractility and oxygen demand, and dilating coronary arteries and arterioles.

Indications and dosage

- Prinzmetal's or variant angina and classic chronic, stable angina pectoris; chronic atrial fibrillation. **Adults:** starting dose is 80 mg P.O. t.i.d. or q.i.d. Dosage may be increased at weekly intervals up to 480 mg daily, if needed.
- Treatment of supraventricular arrhythmias. **Adults:** 0.075 to 0.15 mg/kg (5 to 10 mg) I.V. push over 2 minutes with ECG and blood pressure monitoring. Repeat dose in 30 minutes if no response. **Children 1 to 15 years:** 0.1 to 0.3 mg/kg as I.V. bolus over 2 minutes. **Children under 1 year:** 0.1 to 0.2 mg/kg as I.V. bolus over 2 minutes under continuous ECG monitoring. Dose can be repeated in 30 minutes if no response.
- Migraine headache prophylaxis. **Adults:** 80 mg P.O. q.i.d.
- Treatment of hypertension. **Adults:** 240-mg sustained-release tablet once daily in the morning. If response is not adequate, may give an additional half tablet in the evening or one tablet q 12 hours. Alternatively, may give 80-mg immediate-release tablet t.i.d. or q.i.d.

Adverse reactions

CNS: dizziness, headache, fatigue. **CV:** *transient hypotension,* ***CHF,*** bradycardia, AV block, ***ventricular asystole,*** peripheral edema. **GI:** *constipation,* nausea (primarily from oral form). **Hepatic:** elevated liver enzymes.

Interactions

Carbamazepine, digitalis glycosides: verapamil may increase the serum levels of these drugs. Monitor for toxicity. **Lithium:** verapamil may decrease serum lithium levels. Monitor closely. **Propranolol (and other beta blockers, including ophthalmic timolol), disopyramide, flecainide:** may cause heart failure. Use together cautiously. **Quinidine, antihypertensives:** may result in hypotension. Monitor blood pressure. **Rifampin:** may decrease oral bioavailability of verapamil. Monitor for lack of effect.

Nursing diagnoses

- Pain related to ineffectiveness of verapamil therapy.
- Altered cerebral tissue perfusion related to adverse reactions to verapamil therapy.
- Knowledge deficit related to verapamil.

Nursing interventions

- *Contraindicated* in hypersensitivity to the drug and in advanced heart failure, AV block, severe left ventricular dysfunction, cardiogenic shock, sinus node disease, and severe hypotension.
- *Use cautiously* in elderly patients; in MI followed by coronary occlusion, sick sinus syndrome, impaired AV conduction, heart failure with atrial tachyarrhythmia; and in hepatic or renal disease; and in patients with a history of CHF, especially if given with a beta-adrenergic blocker.
- All patients receiving I.V. verapamil should be on a cardiac monitor. Monitor the R-R interval.
- Patients with severely compromised cardiac function or those receiving beta blockers should receive lower doses of verapamil and should be monitored closely. Don't administer I.V. beta blockers at the same time as I.V. verapamil.
- Notify doctor if signs of CHF occur.
- Nitroglycerin may be taken as needed when anginal symptoms are acute.
- Monitor blood pressure at start of therapy and during dosage adjustments. Assist patient with ambulation because dizziness may occur. Monitor liver function during prolonged treatment.
- Encourage patient to increase fluid and fiber intake to combat constipation.

General

Classification: antimyasthenic agent (cholinesterase inhibitor). **Pregnancy risk category:** C.

Mechanism of action

Inhibits the destruction of acetylcholine released from the parasympathetic and somatic efferent nerves. Acetylcholine accumulates, promoting increased stimulation of the receptor.

Indications and dosage

- Symptomatic treatment of myasthenia gravis in patients who cannot take neostigmine bromide or pyridostigmine bromide. **Adults:** 5 to 25 mg P.O. t.i.d. to q.i.d. Starting dose usually is 5 mg P.O. t.i.d. to q.i.d. Increase gradually and adjust at 1- to 2-day intervals to avoid drug accumulation and overdosage. Usual dosage range is 15 to 100 mg daily, but some patients may require as much as 75 mg two to four times a day.

Adverse reactions

CNS: headache, dizziness, muscle weakness, incoordination, ***seizures,*** mental confusion, jitters, sweating. **CV:** bradycardia, hypotension. **EENT:** miosis, blurred vision. **GI:** *nausea, vomiting, diarrhea, abdominal cramps,* increased salivation. **GU:** urinary frequency, incontinence. **Other:** ***bronchospasm,*** *muscle cramps,* ***bronchoconstriction,*** increased bronchial secretions, ***respiratory paralysis.***

Interactions

Aminoglycosides, anesthetics, atropine, corticosteroids, magnesium, procainamide, quinidine: may impair drug effect. **Mecamylamine, other ganglionic blockers:** increased toxicity. Avoid concomitant use.

Nursing diagnoses

- Altered health maintenance related to underlying condition.
- Urinary retention related to adverse drug reactions.
- Knowledge deficit related to ambenonium therapy.

Nursing interventions

- *Contraindicated* in obstruction of intestine or urinary tract, bradycardia, or hypotension.
- *Use with extreme caution* in bronchial asthma.
- *Use cautiously* in epilepsy, recent coronary occlusion, vagotonia, hyperthyroidism, cardiac arrhythmias, and peptic ulcer.
- Avoid large doses in patients with decreased GI motility or megacolon.
- Discontinue all other cholinergics before administering this drug.
- Watch patient very closely for adverse reactions, particularly if total dosage is greater than 200 mg daily. Adverse reactions may indicate drug toxicity. Notify doctor immediately if they develop.
- Monitor and document vital signs frequently, being especially careful to check respirations. Have atropine injection available and be prepared to give atropine 0.5 mg subcutaneously or slow I.V. push as ordered, and provide respiratory support.
- If muscle weakness is severe, doctor must determine if this is caused by drug toxicity or exacerbation of myasthenia gravis. A test dose of edrophonium I.V. will aggravate drug-induced weakness but will temporarily relieve weakness that results from the disease.
- Weakness occurring 30 to 60 minutes after taking dose is a warning sign of drug toxicity.
- Observe and record the patient's variations in muscle strength. Show him how to do it himself.
- Explain to patient that this drug will relieve symptoms of ptosis, double vision, difficulty in chewing and swallowing, and trunk and limb weakness. Stress the importance of taking this drug exactly as ordered and that he may have to take this drug for the rest of his life.
- Seek approval when indicated for hospitalized patient to have bedside supply of tablets to take himself. Patients with long-standing disease often insist on this.
- Give with milk or food to produce fewer muscarinic adverse reactions.

General

Classification: antidiuretic (posterior pituitary hormone). **Pregnancy risk category:** B.

Mechanism of action

Increases the permeability of the renal tubular epithelium to adenosine monophosphate and water; the epithelium promotes reabsorption of water and produces a concentrated urine (antidiuretic hormone effect).

Indications and dosage

- Nonnephrogenic, nonpsychogenic diabetes insipidus. **Adults:** 5 to 10 units I.M. or S.C. b.i.d. to q.i.d., p.r.n.; or intranasally (aqueous solution used as spray or applied to cotton balls) in individualized doses, based on response. **Children:** 2.5 to 10 units I.M. or S.C. b.i.d. to q.i.d., p.r.n.; or intranasally (aqueous) in individualized doses.
- Postoperative abdominal distention. **Adults:** 5 units (aqueous) I.M. initially, then q 3 to 4 hours, increasing dose to 10 units, if needed. Reduce dosage proportionately for children.
- Expelling of gas before abdominal X-ray. **Adults:** inject 10 units S.C. at 2 hours, then again at 30 minutes before X-ray. Enema before first dose may also help to eliminate gas.
- Upper GI tract hemorrhage. **Adults:** 0.2 to 0.4 units/minute by intra-arterial injection.

Adverse reactions

CNS: tremor, dizziness, headache. **CV:** angina in patients with vascular disease, vasoconstriction. Large doses may cause hypertension, electrocardiographic changes. (With intra-arterial infusion: ***bradycardia, cardiac arrhythmias, pulmonary edema.***) **GI:** abdominal cramps, nausea, vomiting, diarrhea, intestinal hyperactivity. **GU:** uterine cramps, anuria. **Skin:** circumoral pallor. **Other:** water intoxication (drowsiness, listlessness, headache, confusion, weight gain), hypersensitivity reactions (urticaria, angioneurotic edema, bronchoconstriction, fever, rash, wheezing, dyspnea, ***anaphylaxis***), sweating.

Interactions

Carbamazepine, chlorpropamide, clofibrate: increased antidiuretic response. Use together cautiously. **Demeclocycline, lithium, norepinephrine:** reduced antidiuretic activity. Use together cautiously.

Nursing diagnoses

- Fluid volume deficit related to a compromised regulatory system causing excretion of large volumes of urine.
- Pain related to vasopressin-induced angina in patients with vascular disease.
- Knowledge deficit related to vasopressin therapy.

Nursing interventions

- *Contraindicated* in chronic nephritis with nitrogen retention. Use cautiously in children, elderly persons, pregnant women, and in patients with epilepsy, migraine, asthma, cardiovascular disease, or fluid overload.
- Never inject during first stage of labor; may cause ruptured uterus.
- Monitor specific gravity of urine and intake and output to aid evaluation of drug effectiveness.
- Rotate injection sites to prevent tissue damage.
- Give with 1 to 2 glasses of water to reduce adverse reactions and to improve therapeutic response.
- To prevent possible seizures, coma, and death, observe patient closely for early signs of water intoxication.
- May be used for transient polyuria resulting from antidiuretic hormone deficiency related to neurosurgery or head injury.
- Monitor blood pressure twice daily. Watch for excessively elevated blood pressure or lack of response to drug, which may be indicated by hypotension.

General

Classification: aminoglycoside (antibiotic). **Pregnancy risk category:** D.

Mechanism of action

Inhibits protein synthesis by binding directly to the 30S ribosomal subunit. Generally bactericidal.

Indications and dosage

- Serious infections caused by sensitive *Pseudomonas aeruginosa, Escherichia coli, Proteus, Klebsiella, Serratia, Enterobacter, Acinetobacter, Providencia, Citrobacter,* and *Staphylococcus.* **Adults and children with normal renal function:** 15 mg/kg/day divided q 8 to 12 hours I.M. or I.V. infusion. May be given by direct I.V. push. **Neonates with normal renal function:** initially, 10 mg/kg I.M. or I.V. infusion, then 7.5 mg/kg q 12 hours I.M. or I.V.
- Meningitis. **Adults:** systemic therapy as above; or 20 mg intrathecally or intraventricularly daily. **Children:** systemic therapy as above; or 1 to 2 mg intrathecally daily.
- Uncomplicated urinary tract infections. **Adults:** 250 mg I.M. or I.V. b.i.d. **Adults with impaired renal function:** initially, 7.5 mg/kg. Subsequent doses and frequency determined by blood amikacin levels and renal function studies.

Adverse reactions

CNS: headache, lethargy, ***neuromuscular blockade.*** **EENT:** *ototoxicity.* **GU:** *nephrotoxicity (oliguria, proteinuria, decreased creatinine clearance, increased BUN and serum creatinine levels).* **Other:** ***hypersensitivity reactions, hepatic necrosis.***

Interactions

Cephalothin: increased nephrotoxicity. Use together cautiously. **Dimenhydrinate:** may mask symptoms of ototoxicity. Use cautiously. **General anesthetics, neuromuscular blockers:** may potentiate neuromuscular blockade. **I.V. loop diuretics (such as furosemide):** increased ototoxicity. Use cautiously. **Other aminoglycosides, amphotericin B, cisplatin, methoxyflurane:** increases nephrotoxicity. Use together cautiously. **Parenteral penicillins (such as ticarcillin):** amikacin inactivation in vitro. Don't mix together in I.V.

Nursing diagnoses

- High risk for injury related to ineffectiveness of amikacin to eradicate the infection.
- Altered urinary elimination related to amikacin-induced nephrotoxicity.
- Knowledge deficit related to amikacin therapy.

Nursing interventions

- *Use cautiously* in impaired renal function, in neonates and infants, and in elderly patients.
- Obtain specimen for culture and sensitivity tests before first dose. Begin therapy pending test results. Therapy usually lasts 7 to 10 days. If no response after 3 to 5 days, doctor may stop therapy and order new specimens for culture and sensitivity.
- Weigh patient and obtain baseline renal function studies before therapy begins.
- Monitor renal function and notify doctor of signs of decreasing renal function.
- Patient should be well hydrated to minimize chemical irritation of the renal tubules.
- Evaluate patient's hearing before and during therapy. Notify doctor if patient complains of tinnitus, vertigo, or hearing loss (symptoms of ototoxicity).
- Watch for superinfection (continued fever and other signs of new infections), especially of upper respiratory tract.
- Peak blood levels that are above 35 mcg/ml and trough levels that are above 10 mcg/ml may be associated with higher incidence of toxicity.
- **I.V. use:** After I.V. infusion, flush line with 0.9% sodium chloride solution or D_5W.
- Draw blood to measure peak amikacin level 1 hour after I.M. injection and 30 minutes to 1 hour after infusion ends; for trough levels, draw blood just before next dose. Don't collect blood in a heparinized tube because heparin is incompatible with aminoglycosides.
- Potency of drug is not affected if solution turns light yellow.

vancomycin hydrochloride

Vancocin, Vancoled

General

Classification: antibiotic (glycopeptide). **Pregnancy risk category:** C.

Mechanism of action

Hinders bacterial cell wall synthesis, damaging the bacterial plasma membrane and making the cell more vulnerable to osmotic pressure.

Indications and dosage

- Severe staphylococcal infections when other antibiotics ineffective or contraindicated. **Adults:** 500 mg I.V. q 6 hours, or 1 g q 12 hours. **Children:** 40 mg/kg I.V. daily, divided q 6 hours. **Neonates:** 10 mg/kg I.V. daily, divided q 6 to 12 hours.
- Antibiotic-associated pseudomembranous and staphylococcal enterocolitis. **Adults:** 125 to 500 mg P.O. q 6 hours for 7 to 10 days. **Children:** 40 mg/kg P.O. daily, divided q 6 hours. Maximum daily dosage is 2 g.
- Endocarditis prophylaxis for dental procedures. **Adults:** 1 g I.V. slowly over 1 hour, starting 1 hour before procedure.

Adverse reactions

Blood: transient eosinophilia, leukopenia. **EENT:** tinnitus, ototoxicity. **GI:** nausea. **GU:** nephrotoxicity. **Skin:** "red-neck" syndrome with rapid I.V. infusion (maculopapular rash on face, neck, trunk, and extremities). **Local:** pain or thrombophlebitis with I.V. administration, necrosis. **Other:** chills, fever, ***anaphylaxis***, superinfection.

Interactions

Aminoglycosides, amphotericin B, cisplatin, pentamidine: increased risk of nephrotoxicity. Monitor closely.

Nursing diagnoses

- High risk for injury related to ineffectiveness of vancomycin to eradicate the infection.
- Sensory/perceptual alterations (auditory) related to vancomycin-induced ototoxicity.
- Knowledge deficit related to vancomycin.

Nursing interventions

- *Use cautiously* in patients receiving other neurotoxic, nephrotoxic, or ototoxic drugs; in patients over 60 years, and in those with impaired hepatic or renal function, preexisting hearing loss, or allergies to other antibiotics. Patients with renal dysfunction require adjustment of dosage or dosing interval.
- Obtain specimen for culture and sensitivity tests before first dose. Therapy may begin pending results.
- Tell patient to take medication exactly as directed, even after he feels better, and to take entire amount prescribed. Treat staphylococcal endocarditis for at least 4 weeks.
- Do not give drug I.M.
- **I.V. use:** For I.V. infusion, dilute in 200 ml sodium chloride injection or 5% glucose solution and infuse over 60 minutes. Check site daily for phlebitis and irritation. Report pain at infusion site. Avoid extravasation. Severe irritation and necrosis can result.
- Refrigerate I.V. solution after reconstitution and use within 96 hours.
- Monitor patient carefully for "red-neck" syndrome. Stop infusion and report this reaction promptly.
- Patients should have hearing tests before and during prolonged therapy.
- Tell patient to stop drug immediately and report adverse reactions, especially fullness or ringing in ears.
- Monitor renal function (BUN, serum creatinine, urinalysis, creatinine clearance, and urine output) before and during therapy. Also monitor for signs of superinfection.
- Oral preparation stable for 2 weeks if refrigerated.

amiloride hydrochloride Midamor

General

Classification: diuretic, antihypertensive (potassium-sparing diuretic). **Pregnancy risk category:** B.

Mechanism of action

Inhibits sodium reabsorption and potassium excretion by direct action on the distal tubule.

Indications and dosage

• Hypertension; edema associated with CHF, usually in patients who are also taking thiazide or other potassium-wasting diuretics. **Adults:** usual dosage is 5 mg P.O. daily. Dosage may be increased to 20 mg daily, if necessary.

Adverse reactions

CNS: *headache,* weakness, dizziness. **CV:** orthostatic hypotension. **GI:** *nausea, anorexia, diarrhea, vomiting,* abdominal pain, constipation. **GU:** impotence. **Metabolic:** hyperkalemia.

Interactions

ACE inhibitors, potassium-sparing diuretics, potassium supplements: possible hyperkalemia. Avoid concomitant use. **NSAIDs:** decreased diuretic effectiveness. Avoid concomitant use.

Nursing diagnoses

• Fluid volume excess related to the patient's underlying condition as evidenced by edema.
• High risk for injury related to hyperkalemia caused by amiloride therapy.
• Knowledge deficit related to amiloride therapy.

Nursing interventions

• *Contraindicated* in patients with elevated serum potassium level (greater than 5.5 mEq/liter). Don't administer to patients receiving other potassium-sparing diuretics, such as spironolactone and triamterene. Also contraindicated in anuria and acute or chronic renal insufficiency because potassium retention is increased.
• Risk of hyperkalemia is greater when a potassium-wasting drug is not taken concurrently. When amiloride is taken this way, be sure to monitor daily potassium.
• Discontinue immediately if potassium level exceeds 6.5 mEq/liter.
• Advise patient to avoid sudden posture changes and rise slowly to avoid orthostatic hypotension.
• Warn patient to avoid excessive ingestion of potassium-rich foods or potassium-containing salt substitutes. Concomitant potassium supplement can lead to serious hyperkalemia.
• Administer amiloride with meals to prevent nausea.

General

Classification: anticonvulsant (carboxylic acid derivative). **Pregnancy risk category:** D.

Mechanism of action

Increases brain levels of gamma-aminobutyric acid, which transmits inhibitory nerve impulses in the CNS.

Indications and dosage

• Simple and complex absence seizures, mixed seizure types (including absence seizures), investigationally in generalized tonic-clonic seizures. **Adults and children:** initially, 15 mg/kg P.O. daily divided b.i.d. or t.i.d.; then increase by 5 to 10 mg/kg daily at weekly intervals up to maximum of 60 mg/kg daily, divided b.i.d. or t.i.d. Delayed-release tablets and capsules (divalproex sodium) are usually administered b.i.d.

Adverse reactions

Because drug usually used in combination with other anticonvulsants, adverse reactions reported may not be caused by valproic acid alone.
Blood: inhibited platelet aggregation, thrombocytopenia, increased bleeding time. **CNS:** *sedation,* emotional upset, depression, psychosis, aggression, hyperactivity, behavioral deterioration, muscle weakness, tremor. **EENT:** stomatitis. **GI:** *nausea, vomiting,* indigestion, diarrhea, abdominal cramps, constipation, increased appetite and weight gain, *anorexia,* ***pancreatitis.*** (*Note:* there is a lower incidence of GI effects with divalproex sodium.) **Hepatic:** *elevated enzymes,* ***toxic hepatitis.*** **Metabolic:** *elevated serum ammonia.* **Other:** alopecia.

Interactions

Antacids, aspirin: May cause valproic acid toxicity. Use together cautiously and monitor blood levels. **Phenobarbital:** increased phenobarbital levels. **Phenytoin:** increased or decreased phenytoin levels.

Nursing diagnoses

• High risk for injury related to patient's underlying seizure disorder.
• Altered protection related to drug-induced bleeding.
• Knowledge deficit related to drug therapy.

Nursing interventions

• *Contraindicated* in hepatic dysfunction.
• *Use cautiously* in children under 2 years; in children with congenital metabolic disorders or mental retardation; in patients with organic brain disease; and in those taking multiple anticonvulsants.
• Tell patient not to discontinue the drug suddenly. Call doctor at once if adverse reactions develop.
• Obtain liver function studies, platelet counts, and PT before starting drug and periodically thereafter.
• Serious or fatal hepatotoxicity may follow nonspecific symptoms, such as malaise, fever, and lethargy.
• Warn patient to avoid activities that require alertness and good psychomotor coordination until CNS effects of the drug are known.
• May give drug with food or milk to reduce adverse GI reactions. Advise against chewing capsules; causes irritation of mouth and throat.
• May need to reduce dosage if tremor occurs.
• May produce false-positive test results for ketones in urine.
• Available as good-tasting red syrup (valproate sodium). Keep out of reach of children.
• Syrup is more rapidly absorbed. Peak effect within 15 minutes.
• Syrup shouldn't be mixed with carbonated beverages; may be irritating to mouth and throat.
• Don't administer syrup to patients who need sodium restriction. Check with doctor.
• Valproic acid has been used investigationally to prevent recurrent febrile seizures in children.

General

Classification: antineoplastic (antiadrenal hormone). **Pregnancy risk category:** D.

Mechanism of action

Blocks conversion of cholesterol to delta-5-pregnenolone in the adrenal cortex, inhibiting the synthesis of glucocorticoids, mineralocorticoids, and other steroids.

Indications and dosage

• Suppression of adrenal function in Cushing's syndrome and adrenal cancer; metastatic breast cancer; prostate cancer. **Adults:** initially, 250 mg P.O. b.i.d. or t.i.d. for 14 days. Maintenance dosage is 250 mg q.i.d. at 6-hour intervals. Dosage may be increased in increments of 250 mg daily q 1 to 2 weeks to a maximum daily dosage of 2 g.

Adverse reactions

Blood: transient leukopenia, ***agranulocytosis.*** **CNS:** *drowsiness,* headache, dizziness. **CV:** hypotension, tachycardia. **Endocrine:** adrenal insufficiency, masculinization, hirsutism. **GI:** nausea, anorexia. **Skin:** *morbilliform skin rash,* pruritus, urticaria. **Other:** fever, myalgia.

Interactions

Alcohol: may potentiate the effects of aminoglutethimide. **Dexamethasone, medroxyprogesterone:** aminoglutethimide increases hepatic metabolism of these agents. **Oral anticoagulants:** decreased anticoagulant effect.

Nursing diagnoses

• High risk for injury related to drug-induced drowsiness.
• High risk for impaired skin integrity related to drug-induced rash.
• Knowledge deficit related to aminoglutethimide therapy.

Nursing interventions

• *Contraindicated* in patients with hypersensitivity to the drug.
• May cause adrenal hypofunction, especially under stressful conditions, such as surgery, trauma, or acute illness. Patients may need mineralocorticoid supplements to treat hyponatremia and orthostatic hypotension. Glucocorticoid replacement may also be necessary, especially in patients with breast cancer. Monitor such patients carefully.
• Monitor blood pressure frequently. Advise patient to stand up slowly to minimize orthostatic hypotension.
• May cause a decrease in thyroid hormone production. Monitor thyroid function studies.
• Perform baseline hematologic studies and monitor CBC periodically.
• Warn patient to watch for signs of infection (fever, sore throat, fatigue) and bleeding (easy bruising, nosebleeds, bleeding gums, melena). Take temperature daily.
• Warn patient that drug can cause drowsiness and dizziness. Advise him to avoid activities that require alertness and good psychomotor coordination until CNS effects of the drug are known.
• Tell patient to report if skin rash persists for more than 8 days. Reassure patient that drowsiness, nausea, and loss of appetite will diminish within 2 weeks after start of aminoglutethimide therapy. However, if these symptoms persist, tell patient to notify doctor.

General
Classification: throbolytic enzyme. **Pregnancy risk category:** B.

Mechanism of action
Activates plasminogen by directly cleaving peptide bonds at two different sites.

Indications and dosage
• Lysis of acute massive pulmonary emboli and lysis of pulmonary emboli accompanied by unstable hemodynamics. **Adults:** for I.V. infusion only by constant infusion pump that will deliver a total volume of 195 ml. Priming dose: 4,400 IU/kg of urokinase-0.9% sodium chloride solution admixture given over 10 minutes. Follow with 4,400 IU/kg hourly for 12 to 24 hours. Total volume not to exceed 200 ml. Follow therapy with continuous I.V. infusion of heparin, then oral anticoagulants.
• Coronary artery thrombosis. **Adults:** following a bolus dose of heparin ranging from 2,500 to 10,000 units, infuse 6,000 IU/minute of urokinase into the occluded artery for up to 2 hours. Average total dosage is 500,000 IU.
• Venous catheter occlusion. **Adults:** Instill 5,000 IU into occluded line, wait 5 minutes, then aspirate. Repeat aspiration attempts q 5 minutes for 30 minutes. If not patent after 30 minutes, cap line and let urokinase work for 30 to 60 minutes before aspirating. May require second instillation.

Adverse reactions
Blood: ***bleeding,*** low hematocrit. **Local:** phlebitis at injection site. **Other:** hypersensitivity, musculoskeletal pain, bronchospasm, ***anaphylaxis.***

Interactions
Anticoagulants: increased risk of bleeding. Monitor closely. **Aspirin, dipyridamole, indomethacin, phenylbutazone, other drugs affecting platelet activity:** increased risk of bleeding.

Nursing diagnoses
• Altered cardiopulmonary tissue perfusion related to the patient's underlying condition.
• Fluid volume deficit related to the adverse effects of urokinase.
• Knowledge deficit related to urokinase therapy.

Nursing interventions
• *Contraindicated* in ulcerative wounds, active internal bleeding, and cerebrovascular accident; aneurysm; arteriovenous malformation; known bleeding diathesis, recent trauma with possible internal injuries; visceral or intracranial malignancy; pregnancy and first 10 days postpartum; ulcerative colitis; diverticulitis; severe hypertension; acute or chronic hepatic or renal insufficiency; uncontrolled hypocoagulation; chronic pulmonary disease with cavitation; subacute bacterial endocarditis or rheumatic valvular disease; and recent cerebral embolism, thrombosis, or hemorrhage. Also contraindicated within 10 days after intra-arterial diagnostic procedure or any surgery (liver or kidney biopsy, lumbar puncture, thoracentesis, paracentesis, or extensive or multiple cutdowns); intracranial or intraspinal surgery in the past 2 months; and I.M. injections and other invasive procedures during therapy.
• Maintain the involved extremity in straight alignment to prevent bleeding from infusion site. Monitor pulses, color, and sensation of extremities every hour and vital signs.
• **I.V. use:** Add 5 ml sterile water for injection to vial. Dilute further with 0.9% sodium chloride or D_5W solution before infusion. Total volume of fluid given not to exceed 200 ml.
• Monitor patient for bleeding every 15 minutes for the first hour, every 30 minutes for the second through eighth hours, then once every shift. Pretreatment with drugs affecting platelets places patient at high risk of bleeding.
• Have typed and crossmatched RBCs, whole blood, and aminocaproic acid available to treat bleeding and corticosteroids to treat allergic reactions.
• Keep venipuncture sites to a minimum; use pressure dressing for at least 15 minutes.
• Bruising more likely during therapy; avoid unnecessary handling of patient. Bed rails should be padded.

General

Classification: bronchodilator (xanthine derivative). **Pregnancy risk category:** C.

Mechanism of action

Inhibits phosphodiesterase, the enzyme that degrades cyclic AMP. Results in relaxation of smooth muscle of the bronchial airways and pulmonary blood vessels.

Indications and dosage

• Symptomatic relief of bronchospasm. **Patients not receiving theophylline:** 6 mg/kg (equivalent to 4.7 mg/kg anhydrous theophylline) I.V. slowly (25 mg/minute), then maintenance infusion. **Adults (nonsmokers):** 0.7 mg/kg/hour for 12 hours; then 0.5 mg/kg/hour. **Otherwise healthy adult smokers:** 1 mg/kg/hour for 12 hours; then 0.8 mg/kg/hour. **Older patients and adults with cor pulmonale:** 0.6 mg/kg/hour for 12 hours; then 0.3 mg/kg/hour. **Adults with CHF or liver disease:** 0.5 mg/kg/hour for 12 hours; then 0.1 to 0.2 mg/kg/hour. **Children 9 to 16 years:** 1 mg/kg/hour for 12 hours; then 0.8 mg/kg/hour. **Children 6 months to 9 years:** 1.2 mg/kg/hour for 12 hours; then 1 mg/kg/hour.

• Chronic bronchial asthma. **Adults:** 600 to 1,600 mg P.O. daily divided t.i.d. or q.i.d. **Children:** 12 mg/kg P.O. daily divided t.i.d. or q.i.d.

Adverse reactions

CNS: *nervousness, restlessness, dizziness, insomnia,* light-headedness, ***seizures,*** muscle twitching. **CV:** *palpitations, sinus tachycardia,* extrasystoles, marked hypotension, increase in respiratory rate. **GI:** *nausea, vomiting, anorexia,* dyspepsia, diarrhea. **Skin:** urticaria.

Interactions

Adenosine: decreased antiarrhythmic effectiveness. **Alkali-sensitive drugs:** reduced activity. Do not add to I.V. fluids containing aminophylline. **Barbiturates, carbamazepine, nicotine, phenytoin, rifampin:** enhanced metabolism and decreased theophylline blood levels. Monitor for decreased aminophylline effect. **Beta-adrenergic blockers:** antagonism. Propranolol and nadolol, especially, may cause bronchospasm in sensitive patients. Use together cautiously. **Cimetidine, influenza virus vaccine, macrolide antibiotics, oral contraceptives, quinolone antibiotics:** decreased hepatic clearance of theophylline; elevated theophylline levels.

Nursing diagnoses

• Ineffective airway clearance related to patient's underlying condition.
• High risk for fluid volume deficit related to aminophylline-induced GI adverse reactions.
• Knowledge deficit related to aminophylline therapy.

Nursing interventions

• *Contraindicated* in hypersensitivity to xanthine compounds and in preexisting cardiac arrhythmias, especially tachyarrhythmias.
• *Use cautiously* in young children; in elderly patients with CHF or other cardiac or circulatory impairment, cor pulmonale, or hepatic disease; in active peptic ulcer, because drug may increase volume and acidity of gastric secretions; and in hyperthyroidism or diabetes mellitus.
• Individuals metabolize xanthines at different rates. Adjust dosage by monitoring response, tolerance, pulmonary function, and serum theophylline levels. Theophylline concentrations should range from 10 to 20 mcg/ml; toxicity has been reported with levels above 20 mcg/ml.
• Before giving loading dose, check that patient has not had recent theophylline therapy.
• Warn patient that OTC remedies may contain ephedrine combined with theophylline salts; excess CNS stimulation may result. Tell him to check with his doctor before taking *any* other medications.
• If patient experiences urticaria, he may still tolerate other theophylline preparations. Urticaria may be caused by the ethylene diamine salt.

General

Classification: osmotic diuretic (carbonic acid salt). **Pregnancy risk category:** C.

Mechanism of action

Increases the osmotic pressure of glomerular filtrate, inhibiting tubular reabsorption of water and electrolytes. Also elevates blood plasma osmolality, resulting in enhanced flow of water into extracellular fluid.

Indications and dosage

• Intracranial or intraocular pressure. **Adults:** 1 to 1.5 g/kg as a 30% solution by slow I.V. infusion over 1 to 2.5 hours. **Children over 2 years:** 0.5 to 1.5 g/kg slow I.V. infusion. **Children under 2 years:** as little as 0.1 g/kg slow I.V. infusion. Maximum rate is 4 ml/minute.

Maximum adult daily dosage is 120 g. To prepare 135 ml 30% solution, mix contents of 40-g vial of urea with 105 ml dextrose 5% or 10% in water or 10% invert sugar in water. Each ml of 30% solution provides 300 mg urea.

Adverse reactions

CNS: *headache.* **CV:** tachycardia, CHF, *pulmonary edema.* **GI:** *nausea, vomiting.* **Metabolic:** sodium and potassium depletion. **Local:** irritation or necrotic sloughing may occur with extravasation.

Interactions

None significant.

Nursing diagnoses

• Fluid volume excess related to the patient's underlying condition as evidenced by edema.
• Altered urinary elimination related to diuretic therapy.
• Knowledge deficit related to urea therapy.

Nursing interventions

• *Contraindicated* in severely impaired renal function, marked dehydration, frank hepatic failure, or active intracranial bleeding.
• *Use cautiously* in pregnancy, lactation, cardiac disease, hepatic impairment, and sickle cell disease with CNS involvement.
• **I.V. use:** Avoid rapid I.V. infusion; may cause hemolysis or increased capillary bleeding. Avoid extravasation; may cause reactions ranging from mild irritation to necrosis.
• Use freshly reconstituted urea only for I.V. infusion; solution becomes ammonia upon standing.
• Use drug within minutes of reconstitution.
• Don't infuse into leg veins; may cause phlebitis or thrombosis, especially in elderly patients.
• Watch for hyponatremia or hypokalemia (muscle weakness, lethargy); may indicate electrolyte depletion before serum levels are reduced.
• Maintain adequate hydration; monitor blood pressure, intake and output, and serum electrolytes.
• Assess breath sounds for crackles, indicating pulmonary edema.
• In renal disease, monitor BUN.
• Indwelling urethral catheter should be used in comatose patients to ensure bladder emptying. Use an hourly urometer collection bag for accurate evaluation of diuresis.
• If satisfactory diuresis does not occur in 6 to 12 hours, urea should be discontinued and renal function reevaluated.

General

Classification: antiarrhythmic (benzofuran derivative). **Pregnancy risk category:** C.

Mechanism of action

A class III antiarrhythmic that prolongs the refractory period and action potential duration, and decreases repolarization.

Indications and dosage

• Ventricular and supraventricular arrhythmias, including recurrent supraventricular tachycardia (Wolff-Parkinson-White syndrome), atrial fibrillation, and ventricular tachycardia refractory to other antiarrhythmics. **Adults:** give loading dose of 800 to 1,600 mg P.O. daily for 1 to 3 weeks until initial therapeutic response occurs. Maintenance dosage is 200 to 600 mg P.O. daily.

Adverse reactions

CNS: peripheral neuropathy, extrapyramidal symptoms, headache, *malaise, fatigue.* **CV:** bradycardia, hypotension, ***arrhythmias, CHF.*** **EENT:** *corneal microdeposits,* visual disturbances. **Endocrine:** hypothyroidism, hyperthyroidism, gynecomastia. **GI:** *nausea, vomiting,* constipation. **Hepatic:** *altered liver enzymes,* hepatic dysfunction. **Respiratory:** ***severe pulmonary toxicity (pneumonitis, alveolitis).*** **Skin:** *photosensitivity,* blue-gray skin pigmentation. **Other:** muscle weakness.

Interactions

Antiarrhythmic agents: amiodarone may induce torsades de pointes; may also reduce the hepatic or renal clearance of flecainide, procainamide, and quinidine. **Antihypertensives:** increased hypotensive effect. **Beta blockers, calcium channel blockers:** increased cardiac depressant effects; may potentiate slowing of sinus node and AV conduction. **Digitalis glycosides:** increased serum digoxin levels. **Phenytoin:** phenytoin metabolism may be decreased. **Warfarin:** increased anticoagulant effect.

Nursing diagnoses

• Decreased cardiac output related to ineffectiveness of amiodarone therapy.
• Impaired gas exchange related to amiodarone-induced pulmonary toxicity.
• Knowledge deficit related to amiodarone.

Nursing interventions

• *Use with extreme caution* in patients receiving class I antiarrhythmics.
• *Use cautiously* in preexisting bradycardia or sinus node disease; conduction disturbances; severely depressed ventricular function; cardiomegaly.
• **I.V. use:** The loading dose is 5 to 10 mg/kg by I.V. infusion via a central line, followed by an I.V. infusion of 10 mg/kg/day for 3 to 5 days.
• Most patients treated show corneal microdeposits upon slit-lamp ophthalmologic examination. Onset of this effect is from 1 to 4 months after beginning amiodarone therapy. To minimize, recommend instillation of methylcellulose ophthalmic solution during amiodarone therapy.
• Monitor carefully for pulmonary toxicity, which can be fatal. Incidence increases in patients receiving more than 400 mg/day.
• Monitor for symptoms of pneumonitis – exertional dyspnea, nonproductive cough, and pleuritic chest pain. Monitor pulmonary function tests and chest X-ray.
• Monitor blood pressure and heart rate and rhythm frequently. Continuous ECG monitoring should be performed during initiation and alteration of dosage.
• Monitor hepatic and thyroid function tests. Also monitor serum electrolytes, particularly potassium and magnesium levels.
• Monitor for burning or tingling skin followed by erythema and possible skin blistering.
• Divide oral loading dose into three equal doses and give with meals to decrease GI intolerance. Maintenance dosage may be given once daily, but may be divided into two doses taken with meals if GI intolerance occurs.

General

Classification: antineoplastic (alkylating agent).
Pregnancy risk category: X.

Mechanism of action

Cross-links strands of cellular DNA and interferes with RNA transcription, causing an imbalance of growth that leads to cell death. Cell cycle-nonspecific.

Indications and dosage

• Chronic lymphocytic and myelocytic leukemia; Hodgkin's disease; non-Hodgkin's lymphomas of the histiocytic and lymphocytic types; reticulum cell sarcoma; lymphomas; mycosis fungoides; polycythemia vera; cancer of ovaries, cervix, and lungs.
Adults: 1 to 2 mg P.O. daily for 3 months or until desired response or toxicity reached; maintenance dosage is 1 mg daily for 3 out of 4 weeks until optimum response or relapse; or 3 to 5 mg P.O. for 7 days not to exceed total dosage of 0.5 mg/kg, then 1 mg daily until response, then 1 mg daily 3 out of 4 weeks.

Adverse reactions

Blood: bone marrow suppression, delayed 2 to 4 weeks; ***thrombocytopenia; leukopenia; anemia.*** **CNS:** irritability, nervousness, mental cloudiness, and depression. **GI:** *nausea, vomiting, diarrhea, epigastric distress,* abdominal pain, anorexia. **Metabolic:** hyperuricemia. **Skin:** pruritus, dermatitis, hyperpigmentation, alopecia.

Interactions

None significant.

Nursing diagnoses

• High risk for infection related to immunosuppressant effects of uracil mustard.
• Altered nutrition: Less than body requirements, related to adverse GI effects as evidenced by nausea and vomiting.
• Knowledge deficit related to uracil mustard therapy.

Nursing interventions

• *Contraindicated* in hypersensitivity to the drug and in aplastic anemia, thrombocytopenia, or leukopenia.
• *Use cautiously.* Dosage modification may be required in patients with bone marrow suppression.
• Some commercially available capsules contain tartrazine dye, which may provoke allergic reactions in certain individuals. This reaction is rare but is more likely to occur in aspirin-sensitive persons.
• Give at bedtime to reduce nausea.
• Warn patient to watch for signs of infection (fever, sore throat, fatigue) and bleeding (easy bruising, nosebleeds, bleeding gums, melena). Take temperature daily.
• Monitor platelet count. Check CBC once or twice weekly for 4 weeks; then 4 weeks after stopping drug.
• To prevent hyperuricemia and resulting uric acid nephropathy, allopurinol may be used with adequate hydration. Monitor serum uric acid.
• Avoid all I.M. injections when platelets are below 100,000/mm^3.
• Anticoagulants and aspirin products should be used cautiously. Watch closely for signs of bleeding. Instruct patient to avoid OTC products containing aspirin.
• Therapeutic effects are often accompanied by toxicity.

amitriptyline hydrochloride

Amitril, Apo-Amitriptyline†, Elavil, Endep, Levate†

General

Classification: antidepressant (tricyclic antidepressant). **Pregnancy risk category:** D.

Mechanism of action

Increases the amount of norepinephrine or serotonin, or both, in the CNS by blocking their reuptake by the presynaptic neurons. This allows these neurotransmitters to accumulate.

Indications and dosage

• Treatment of depression. **Adults:** 50 to 100 mg P.O. h.s., increasing to 200 mg daily; maximum dosage is 300 mg daily if needed; or 20 to 30 mg I.M. q.i.d. Alternatively, the entire dosage can be given at bedtime. **Elderly patients and adolescents:** 30 mg P.O. daily in divided doses. May be increased to 150 mg.

Adverse reactions

CNS: *drowsiness, dizziness,* excitation, tremors, weakness, confusion, headache, nervousness, EEG alterations, seizures, extrapyramidal reactions. **CV:** *orthostatic hypotension, tachycardia, ECG changes,* hypertension. **EENT:** *blurred vision,* tinnitus, mydriasis. **GI:** *dry mouth, constipation,* nausea, vomiting, anorexia, paralytic ileus. **GU:** *urine retention.* **Skin:** rash, urticaria, photosensitivity. **Other:** *sweating,* allergy. **After abrupt withdrawal of long-term therapy:** nausea, headache, malaise.

Interactions

Alcohol, other depressants: additive effects. **Barbiturates:** decreased TCA blood levels. **Cimetidine, methylphenidate:** increase TCA blood levels. **Epinephrine, norepinephrine:** increase hypertensive effect. Use with caution. **MAO inhibitors:** may cause severe excitation, hyperpyrexia, or seizures, usually with high dosage.

Nursing diagnoses

• Ineffective individual coping related to the patient's underlying condition.
• High risk for injury related to adverse CNS reactions to amitriptyline.
• Knowledge deficit related to amitriptyline therapy.

Nursing interventions

• *Contraindicated* during acute recovery phase of myocardial infarction, in patients with history of seizure disorders, and in prostatic hypertrophy.
• *Use cautiously* in suicidal patients; in patients with urine retention, narrow-angle glaucoma, increased intraocular pressure, cardiovascular disease, impaired hepatic function, or hyperthyroidism; and in patients receiving thyroid medications, electroshock therapy, or elective surgery.
• Reduce dosage in elderly or debilitated persons and adolescents.
• Do not withdraw drug abruptly.
• Warn patient to avoid activities that require alertness and good psychomotor coordination until CNS effects of the drug are known. Drowsiness and dizziness usually subside after first few weeks. Has strong anticholinergic effects; one of the most sedating TCAs.
• Whenever possible, patient should take full dose at bedtime. Warn patient about the possibility of morning orthostatic hypotension.
• Check for urine retention and constipation. Increase fluids to lessen constipation. Suggest stool softener or high-fiber diet, if needed.
• Expect delay of 2 weeks or more before noticeable effect. Full effect may take 4 weeks or more.
• Advise the patient not to take *any* other drugs without first consulting the doctor.
• Hypertensive episodes have occurred during surgery in patients receiving TCAs, so they should be discontinued several days before surgery.
• Some patients may experience photosensitivity reactions. Advise patient to use a sunscreen, wear protective clothing, and avoid prolonged exposure to strong sunlight.
• Has been used to treat intractable hiccups, chronic severe pain, and patients with eating disorders (bulimia or anorexia nervosa). Dosage is highly variable and individualized.

General

Classification: skeletal muscle relaxant (nondepolarizing neuromuscular blocker). **Pregnancy risk category:** C.

Mechanism of action

Prevents acetylcholine from binding to the receptors on the muscle end plate, thus blocking depolarization.

Indications and dosage

- Adjunct to anesthesia to induce skeletal muscle relaxation; facilitate intubation, orthopedic manipulations. *Dosage depends on anesthetic used, individual needs, and response. Dosages listed are representative and must be adjusted.* **Adults:** 1 unit/kg or 0.15 mg/kg I.V. slowly over 60 to 90 seconds. Average, initially, 40 to 60 units I.V. May give 20 to 30 units in 3 to 5 minutes. For longer procedures, give 20 units, p.r.n. **Children:** 1 unit/kg or 0.15 mg/kg.
- Assistance with mechanical ventilation. **Adults and children:** initially, 0.0165 mg/kg I.V. (average 1 mg or 7 units), then adjust subsequent doses to patient's response.
- Lessening of muscle contractions in pharmacologically or electrically induced seizures. **Adults and children:** 1 unit/kg or 0.15 mg/kg slowly over 60 to 90 seconds. Initial dose is 20 units (3 mg) less than calculated dose.

Adverse reactions

CV: hypotension, circulatory depression. **Other:** profound and prolonged muscle relaxation, ***respiratory depression or apnea,*** hypersensitivity, idiosyncrasy, residual muscle weakness, increased salivation, ***bronchospasm.***

Interactions

Aminoglycoside antibiotics, polymyxin antibiotics, general anesthetics: potentiated neuromuscular blockade. Use cautiously during surgical and postoperative periods. **Quinidine:** prolonged neuromuscular blockade. Use together with caution. Monitor closely. **Thiazide diuretics, furosemide, ethacrynic acid, amphotericin B, propranolol, methotrimeprazine, narcotic analgesics:** potentiated neuromuscular blockade. Use with extreme caution during surgical and postoperative periods.

Nursing diagnoses

- Ineffective breathing pattern related to the patient's underlying condition.
- Impaired verbal communication related to drug-induced paralysis.
- Knowledge deficit related to tubocurarine.

Nursing interventions

- *Contraindicated* in patients for whom histamine release is a hazard (asthmatics) and in neonates.
- *Use cautiously* in elderly or debilitated patients; in hepatic or pulmonary impairment, respiratory depression, myasthenia gravis, myasthenic syndrome of lung cancer or bronchogenic carcinoma, dehydration, thyroid disorders, collagen diseases, porphyria, electrolyte disturbances, fractures, muscle spasms, and cesarean section.
- Tubocurarine should be used only by personnel experienced in airway management. Keep airway clear. Have emergency respiratory support equipment on hand.
- Give sedatives or general anesthetics before giving tubocurarine. Allow succinylcholine effects to subside before giving tubocurarine.
- Monitor baseline electrolyte determinations.
- Once recovery starts, reverse blockade with an anticholinesterase agent (such as neostigmine or edrophonium). Usually given with an anticholinergic (such as atropine).
- Monitor respirations closely until patient is fully recovered from neuromuscular blockade, as evidenced by tests of muscle strength (hand grip, head lift, and ability to cough).
- Check vital signs every 15 minutes. Notify doctor at once of changes. Measure intake and output.
- Don't mix with barbiturates (forms precipitate).
- Give deep I.M. in deltoid muscle.

General

Classification: antianginal, antihypertensive (calcium channel blocker). **Pregnancy risk category:** C.

Mechanism of action

Inhibits calcium ion influx across cardiac and smooth muscle cells, thus decreasing myocardial contractility and oxygen demand and dilating coronary arteries and arterioles.

Indications and dosage

• Chronic stable angina; vasospastic angina (Prinzmetal's or variant angina). **Adults:** initially, 10 mg P.O. daily. Small, frail, or elderly patients or patients with hepatic insufficiency should begin therapy at 5 mg daily. Most patients require 10 mg daily for adequate therapy.
• Hypertension. **Adults:** initially, 5 mg P.O. daily. Small, frail, or elderly patients, patients currently receiving other antihypertensive drugs, or patients with hepatic insufficiency should begin therapy at 2.5 mg daily. Adjust dosage according to the patient's response and tolerance. Maximum dosage is 10 mg daily.

Adverse reactions

CNS: *headache,* fatigue, somnolence. **CV:** *edema,* dizziness, flushing, palpitation. **GI:** nausea, abdominal pain.

Interactions

Beta blockers, digoxin, peripheral vasodilators: increased risk of hypotension. Avoid concomitant use.

Nursing diagnoses

• Pain related to the ineffectiveness of amlodipine therapy.
• High risk for injury related to amlodipine-induced adverse reactions.
• Knowledge deficit related to amlodipine therapy.

Nursing interventions

• *Contraindicated* in patients with hypersensitivity to the drug or in patients with second- or third-degree atrioventricular block.
• *Use cautiously* in patients with severe aortic stenosis and in patients with CHF.
• Also use cautiously and in reduced dosage in patients with severe hepatic disease because drug is metabolized by the liver.
• Dosage adjustments are not necessary in patients with renal failure because the drug is eliminated primarily by the liver. Monitor liver function studies during prolonged treatment.
• Monitor the patient, especially one with severe obstructive coronary artery disease, for an increase in the frequency, duration, or severity of angina or even acute MI after the initiation of amlodipine therapy or at the time of dosage increase.
• Assess the patient's angina before initiating therapy.
• Tell the patient to take sublingual nitroglycerin as needed when anginal symptoms are acute.
• Notify the doctor if signs of CHF, such as peripheral edema or shortness of breath, occur.
• Keep emergency equipment and drugs readily available to treat any arrhythmias.
• Monitor the patient's blood pressure frequently at initiation and during therapy. Because drug-induced vasodilation develops gradually, acute hypotension is rare.
• Be sure that the patient understands his disease. He should continue taking the drug, even when he's feeling better, and check with the doctor or pharmacist before taking other medications, including OTC drugs.
• Warn the patient to avoid any potentially hazardous activities that require alertness if adverse CNS reactions occur.
• Tell the patient to schedule activities to allow adequate rest.
• Tell the patient that amlodipine may be taken without regard to meals.
• Obtain an order for a mild analgesic if headache occurs.

General

Classification: systemic alkalinizer (sodium-free organic amine). **Pregnancy risk category:** C.

Mechanism of action

Combines with hydrogen ions and associated acid anions; the resulting salts are excreted.

Indications and dosage

- Metabolic acidosis (associated with cardiac bypass surgery or with cardiac arrest). **Adults:** dosage depends on bicarbonate deficit. Calculate as follows: each ml of 0.3 M tromethamine solution required = weight in kg × bicarbonate deficit (mEq/liter). Additional therapy based on serial determinations of existing bicarbonate deficit. **Children:** calculate dosage as above. Give slowly over 3 to 6 hours. Additional therapy based on degree of acidosis. Total 24-hour dosage should not exceed 33 to 40 ml/kg.

Adverse reactions

CNS: ***respiratory depression.*** **Metabolic:** hypoglycemia, ***hyperkalemia*** (with decreased urine output). **Local:** venospasm; I.V. thrombosis; inflammation, necrosis, and sloughing if extravasation occurs.

Interactions

None significant.

Nursing diagnoses

- High risk for injury related to acid-base imbalance.
- Altered protection related to tromethamine-induced hypoglycemia or hyperkalemia.
- Knowledge deficit related to tromethamine therapy.

Nursing interventions

- *Contraindicated* in anuria, uremia, chronic respiratory acidosis, or pregnancy (except in acute, life-threatening situations).
- *Use cautiously* in renal disease and poor urine output. Monitor ECG and serum potassium in these patients.
- To prevent blood pH from rising above normal, adjust dosage carefully.
- **I.V. use:** Give slowly through large needle (18G to 20G) into largest antecubital vein or by indwelling I.V. catheter.
- Measure blood pH; carbon dioxide tension; bicarbonate, glucose, and electrolyte levels before, during, and after therapy.
- When giving drug to patient with associated respiratory acidosis, mechanical ventilation should be readily available.
- Except in life-threatening situations, do not use longer than 1 day.
- If extravasation occurs, infiltrate area with 1% procaine and hyaluronidase 150 units; may reduce vasospasm and dilute remaining drug in local area.

General

Classification: acidifying agent, expectorant (acid-forming salt). **Pregnancy risk category:** B.

Mechanism of action

Increases free hydrogen ion (H^+) concentration. Also acts as an expectorant by causing reflex stimulation of bronchial mucous glands.

Indications and dosage

- Metabolic alkalosis; chloride replacement. **Adults and children:** I.V. dose (in mEq) is equal to the serum chloride deficit (in mEq/ml) multiplied by the extracellular fluid volume (estimated as 20% of the body weight in kilograms). One-half the calculated volume should be given, then patient should be reassessed.
- As an acidifying agent. **Adults:** 4 to 12 g P.O. daily in divided doses. **Children:** 75 mg/kg P.O. daily in four divided doses.
- As expectorant. **Adults:** 250 to 500 mg P.O. q 2 to 4 hours.

Adverse reactions

Adverse reactions usually result from ammonia toxicity or too-rapid I.V. administration.

CNS: headache, confusion, progressive drowsiness, excitement alternating with ***coma,*** hyperventilation, ***calcium-deficient tetany,*** twitching, hyperreflexia, EEG abnormalities. **CV:** bradycardia. **GI:** (with oral dose) *gastric irritation, nausea, vomiting,* thirst, anorexia, retching. **GU:** glycosuria. **Metabolic:** ***acidosis, hyperchloremia, hypokalemia,*** hyperglycemia. **Skin:** rash, pallor. **Local:** pain at injection site. **Other:** irregular respirations with periods of apnea.

Interactions

Spironolactone: systemic acidosis. Use together cautiously.

Nursing diagnoses

- High risk for injury related to acid-base imbalance.
- Altered protection related to ammonium chloride overdose.
- Knowledge deficit related to ammonium chloride therapy.

Nursing interventions

- *Contraindicated* in severe hepatic or renal dysfunction.
- *Use cautiously* in pulmonary insufficiency or cardiac edema and in infants.
- **I.V. use:** Dilute concentrated form (26.75%) before administration. Add 100 to 200 mEq (20 to 40 ml of the 26.75% solution) to 500 or 1,000 ml of 0.9% sodium chloride injection. Administer via infusion pump not exceeding 5 ml/minute in adults.
- Give oral form after meals to decrease adverse GI reactions. Enteric-coated tablets may also minimize GI symptoms but are absorbed erratically.
- Do not administer drug with milk or other alkaline solutions because they are not compatible.
- Determine CO_2-combining power and serum electrolyte levels before and during therapy to prevent acidosis.
- Monitor urine pH and output. Diuresis is normal for first 2 days.
- Monitor rate and depth of respirations frequently.
- When using as an expectorant, give with full glass of water.

General
Classification: antihistamine, H_1-receptor antagonist (alkylamine). **Pregnancy risk category:** C.

Mechanism of action
Competes with histamine for H_1-receptor sites on effector cells. Prevents but does not reverse histamine-mediated responses.

Indications and dosage
• Colds and allergy symptoms. **Adults:** 2.5 mg P.O. q 4 to 6 hours. Maximum dosage is 10 mg/day. **Children over 6 years:** 1.25 mg P.O. q 4 to 6 hours. Maximum dosage is 5 mg/day. **Children 4 to 6 years:** 0.9 mg P.O. q 4 to 6 hours. Maximum dosage is 3.75 mg/day. **Children 2 to 4 years:** 0.6 mg P.O. q 4 to 6 hours. Maximum dosage is 2.5 mg/day. **Children 4 months to 2 years:** 0.3 mg P.O. q 4 to 6 hours. Maximum dosage is 1.25 mg/day.

Note: Children under 12 years should use only as directed by a doctor.

Adverse reactions
CNS: (especially in elderly patients) *drowsiness,* dizziness, confusion, restlessness, insomnia, *stimulation.* **GI:** anorexia, diarrhea or constipation, nausea, vomiting, *dry mouth.* **GU:** urinary frequency, urine retention. **Skin:** urticaria, rash.

Interactions
CNS depressants: increased sedation. **MAO inhibitors:** increased anticholinergic effects. Don't use together.

Nursing diagnoses
• Ineffective airway clearance related to the patient's underlying condition.
• High risk for injury related to adverse CNS reactions to triprolidine.
• Knowledge deficit related to triprolidine therapy.

Nursing interventions
• *Contraindicated* in acute asthma attacks.
• *Use cautiously* in elderly patients and in increased intraocular pressure, hyperthyroidism, cardiovascular or renal disease, hypertension, diabetes mellitus, bronchial asthma, urine retention, prostatic hypertrophy, bladder-neck obstruction, and stenosing peptic ulcers.
• Warn patient against drinking alcoholic beverages during therapy and against driving or other activities that require alertness until CNS response to drug is determined.
• Reduce GI distress by giving with food or milk.
• Coffee or tea may reduce drowsiness. Sugarless gum or sour hard candy, or ice chips may relieve dry mouth.
• Warn patient to stop taking drug 4 days before allergy skin tests to preserve accuracy of tests.
• Antihistamines are not recommended for use by women who are breast-feeding because small amounts of drug are excreted in breast milk.

General

Classification: sedative-hypnotic, anticonvulsant (barbiturate). **Pregnancy risk category:** B. **Controlled substance schedule**: II.

Mechanism of action

Probably interferes with transmission of impulses from the thalamus to the cortex of the brain.

Indications and dosage

- Sedation. **Adults:** 50 mg P.O. b.i.d. or t.i.d. **Children:** 3 to 6 mg/kg P.O. daily in four equally divided doses.
- Insomnia. **Adults:** 50 to 200 mg P.O. or deep I.M. h.s. (sodium); I.M. injection not to exceed 5 ml in any one site. Maximum dosage is 500 mg. **Children:** 3 to 5 mg/kg deep I.M. h.s.; I.M. injection not to exceed 5 ml in any one site.
- Preanesthetic sedation. **Adults and children:** 200 mg P.O. or I.M. (sodium) 1 to 2 hours before surgery.
- Manic reactions, as an adjunct in psychotherapy, anticonvulsant. **Adults and children over 6 years:** 65 to 500 mg slow I.V. (sodium); not to exceed 100 mg/minute. Maximum dose is 1 g. **Children under 6 years:** 3 to 5 mg/kg slow I.V. or I.M.

Adverse reactions

CNS: *drowsiness, lethargy, hangover,* paradoxical excitement. **GI:** nausea, vomiting. **Skin:** rash, urticaria. **Local:** pain, irritation, sterile abscess at injection site. **Other:** ***Stevens-Johnson syndrome, angioedema,*** exacerbation of porphyria.

Interactions

Alcohol or other CNS depressants, including narcotic analgesics: excessive CNS and respiratory depression. **Griseofulvin:** decreased absorption of griseofulvin. **MAO inhibitors:** inhibit metabolism of barbiturates; may cause prolonged CNS depression. Reduce barbiturate dosage. **Oral anticoagulants, estrogens and oral contraceptives, doxycycline, corticosteroids:** amobarbital may enhance the metabolism of these drugs. Monitor for decreased effect. **Rifampin:** may decrease barbiturate levels.

Nursing diagnoses

- Sleep pattern disturbance related to underlying patient problem.
- High risk for trauma related to adverse CNS reactions caused by amobarbital.
- Knowledge deficit related to amobarbital therapy.

Nursing interventions

- *Contraindicated* in uncontrolled severe pain, respiratory disease with dyspnea or obstruction, hypersensitivity to barbiturates, previous addiction to sedatives, or porphyria.
- *Use cautiously* in hepatic or renal impairment.
- Elderly patients are more sensitive to the drug's adverse CNS effects. Assess mental status before and after initiating therapy.
- **I.V. use:** Reserve I.V. injection for emergency treatment. Give under close supervision. Have emergency resuscitation equipment readily available. Administer slowly I.V.; do not exceed 100 mg/minute.
- I.V. administration may cause severe respiratory depression, laryngospasm, or hypotension.
- Local tissue reactions and pain at the injection site have been noted with I.V. use. Assess patency of I.V. site before and during administration.
- Administer I.M. injection deeply. Superficial injection may cause pain, sterile abscess, and sloughing.
- Long-term high dosage may cause drug dependence and severe withdrawal symptoms. Withdraw barbiturates gradually.
- Watch for signs of barbiturate toxicity: coma, pupillary constriction, cyanosis, clammy skin, and hypotension. Overdose can be fatal.
- Observe for signs of hematologic toxicity, such as easy bruising or bleeding, or signs of infection.
- Skin eruptions may precede potentially fatal reactions to barbiturate therapy. Discontinue drug when skin reactions occur. In some patients, high fever, stomatitis, headache, or rhinitis may precede skin reactions.

General

Classification: antihistamine, H_1-receptor antagonist (ethylenediamine-derived antihistamine). **Pregnancy risk category:** B.

Mechanism of action

Competes with histamine for H_1-receptor sites on effector cells. Prevents but does not reverse histamine-mediated responses.

Indications and dosage

• Rhinitis, allergy symptoms. **Adults:** 25 to 50 mg P.O. q 4 to 6 hours; or (timed-release) 100 mg b.i.d. or t.i.d. Maximum dosage is 600 mg daily. **Children:** 5 mg/kg P.O. daily in four to six divided doses. Maximum dosage is 300 mg daily.

Adverse reactions

CNS: (especially in elderly patients) *drowsiness,* dizziness, confusion, restlessness, tremors, irritability, insomnia. **CV:** palpitations. **GI:** anorexia, diarrhea or constipation, *nausea, vomiting, dry mouth.* **GU:** urinary frequency, urine retention. **Skin:** urticaria, rash. **Other:** thick bronchial secretions.

Interactions

CNS depressants: increased sedation. Use together cautiously. **MAO inhibitors:** increased anticholinergic effects. Don't use together.

Nursing diagnoses

• Ineffective airway clearance related to patient's underlying condition.
• High risk for fluid volume deficit related to adverse GI effects of tripelennamine.
• Knowledge deficit related to tripelennamine therapy.

Nursing interventions

• *Contraindicated* in acute asthmatic attacks.
• *Use cautiously* in elderly patients, and in increased intraocular pressure, hyperthyroidism, CV or renal disease, hypertension, bronchial asthma, urine retention, prostatic hypertrophy, bladder-neck obstruction, and stenosing peptic ulcers.
• Warn patient against drinking alcoholic beverages during therapy and against driving or other activities that require alertness until CNS response to drug is determined.
• Reduce GI distress by giving with food or milk.
• Coffee or tea may reduce drowsiness. Sugarless gum or sour hard candy, or ice chips may relieve dry mouth.
• If tolerance develops, another antihistamine may be substituted.
• Warn patient to stop taking drug 4 days before allergy skin tests to preserve accuracy of tests.
• Antihistamines are not recommended for use by women who are breast-feeding because small amounts of drug are excreted in breast milk.

General

Classification: tricyclic antidepressant (dibenzoxapine). **Pregnancy risk category:** C.

Mechanism of action

Increases the amount of norepinephrine or serotonin, or both, in the CNS by blocking their reuptake by the presynaptic neurons, allowing these neurotransmitters to accumulate.

Indications and dosage

• Treatment of depression. **Adults:** initial dose 50 mg P.O. t.i.d. May increase to 100 mg t.i.d. on third day of treatment. Increase above 300 mg daily only if 300 mg daily has been ineffective during a trial period of at least 2 weeks. When effective dosage is established, entire dosage (not exceeding 300 mg) may be given h.s. Maximum dosage is 600 mg in hospitalized patients.

Adverse reactions

CNS: *drowsiness, dizziness,* excitation, tremor, weakness, confusion, headache, nervousness, *tardive dyskinesia* (especially in elderly women), EEG changes, ***seizures,*** extrapyramidal reactions. **CV:** *orthostatic hypotension, tachycardia, ECG changes,* hypertension. **EENT:** *blurred vision,* tinnitus, mydriasis. **GI:** *dry mouth, constipation,* nausea, vomiting, anorexia, paralytic ileus. **GU:** ***urine retention, acute renal failure (with overdose).*** **Skin:** rash, urticaria, photosensitivity. **Other:** *sweating;* weight gain and craving for sweets; allergy; rarely, ***neuroleptic malignant syndrome*** (high fever, tachycardia, tachypnea, profuse diaphoresis). **After abrupt withdrawal of long-term therapy:** nausea, headache, malaise. (Does not indicate addiction.)

Interactions

Barbiturates: decrease TCA blood levels. Monitor for decreased antidepressant effect. **Cimetidine:** may increase amoxapine serum levels. Monitor for increased adverse effects. **Epinephrine, norepinephrine:** increase hypertensive effect. Use with caution. **MAO inhibitors:** may cause severe excitation, hyperpyrexia, or seizures, usually with high dose. **Methylphenidate:** increases TCA blood levels. Monitor for enhanced antidepressant effect.

Nursing diagnoses

• Ineffective individual coping related to the patient's underlying condition.
• High risk for injury related to amoxapine-induced adverse reactions.
• Knowledge deficit related to amoxapine therapy.

Nursing interventions

• *Contraindicated* in acute recovery phase of MI, in patients with history of seizure disorders, and in prostatic hypertrophy.
• *Use cautiously* in patients who are suicide risks; in urine retention, narrow-angle glaucoma, increased intraocular pressure, CV disease, impaired hepatic function, or hyperthyroidism; and in patients receiving thyroid medications, electroshock therapy, or elective surgery.
• Whenever possible, patient should take full dose at bedtime.
• Monitor for signs and symptoms of tardive dyskinesia, especially in elderly women.
• Reduce dosage in elderly or debilitated persons and adolescents.
• Do not withdraw drug abruptly.
• If psychotic signs increase, reduce dosage. Record mood changes. Allow minimum supply of tablets to lessen suicide risk.
• Expect delay of 2 weeks or more before noticeable effect. Full effect may take 4 weeks or more.
• Check for urine retention and constipation. Increase fluids to lessen constipation. Suggest stool softener, if needed.
• Because hypertensive episodes have occurred during surgery in patients receiving TCAs, discontinue these drugs several days before surgery.
• Amoxapine therapy has been associated with neuroleptic malignant syndrome, a rare but life-threatening syndrome usually seen with phenothiazines. Discontinue drug immediately and institute appropriate therapy if symptoms occur.

General
Classification: antidepressant (tricyclic). **Pregnancy risk category:** C.

Mechanism of action
Increases the amount of norepinephrine or serotonin, or both, in the CNS by blocking their reuptake by the presynaptic neurons. This allows these neurotransmitters to accumulate.

Indications and dosage
• Treatment of depression. **Adults:** 75 mg P.O. daily in divided doses, increased to 200 mg daily. Dosages over 300 mg daily not recommended.
• Enuresis. **Children over 6 years:** initial dosage 25 mg P.O. 1 hour before bedtime; if no response, increase dosage to 50 mg in children under 12 years, and to 75 mg in children over 12 years.

Adverse reactions
CNS: *drowsiness, dizziness,* excitation, tremors, weakness, confusion, headache, nervousness, EEG changes, ***seizures,*** extrapyramidal reactions. **CV:** *orthostatic hypotension, tachycardia, ECG changes,* hypertension. **EENT:** *blurred vision,* tinnitus, mydriasis. **GI:** *dry mouth, constipation,* nausea, vomiting, anorexia, paralytic ileus. **GU:** *urine retention.* **Skin:** rash, urticaria, photosensitivity. **Other:** *sweating,* allergy. **After abrupt withdrawal of long-term therapy:** nausea, headache, malaise. (Does not indicate addiction.)

Interactions
Barbiturates: decrease TCA blood levels. Monitor for decreased antidepressant effect. **Cimetidine:** may increase trimipramine serum levels. Monitor for increased adverse reactions. **Epinephrine, norepinephrine:** increase hypertensive effect. Use with caution. **MAO inhibitors:** may cause severe excitation, hyperpyrexia, or seizures (usually with high dose). Use together cautiously. **Methylphenidate:** increases TCA blood levels. Monitor for enhanced antidepressant effects.

Nursing diagnoses
• Ineffective individual coping related to the patient's underlying condition.
• High risk for injury related to adverse reactions to trimipramine.
• Knowledge deficit related to trimipramine therapy.

Nursing interventions
• *Contraindicated* during acute recovery phase of myocardial infarction; in patients with prostatic hypertrophy, seizure disorders, and suicidal ideation; and in those receiving electroshock therapy, thyroid drugs, or elective surgery.
• *Use with extreme caution* in CV disease, urine retention, narrow-angle glaucoma or increased intraocular pressure, thyroid disease, blood dyscrasia, or impaired hepatic function.
• Dry mouth may be relieved with sugarless hard candy or gum. Saliva substitutes may be necessary.
• Check for urine retention and constipation. Increase fluids to lessen constipation or suggest stool softener.
• Reduce dosage in elderly or debilitated persons and adolescents.
• Don't withdraw drug abruptly.
• Watch for increased psychotic signs; reduce dosage if they occur. Record mood changes. Watch for suicidal tendencies. Allow only minimum supply of tablets to lessen suicide risk.
• Warn patient to avoid activities requiring alertness until CNS response is determined. Drowsiness and dizziness usually subside after a few weeks.
• Don't combine with alcohol or other depressants.
• Full effect may take 4 weeks or more.
• Effectiveness in enuresis may decrease over time.
• To avoid daytime sedation, patient should take full dose at bedtime if possible. Warn patient about possible morning orthostatic hypotension.
• Because hypertensive episodes have occurred during surgery in patients receiving TCAs, discontinue trimipramine several days before surgery.
• Advise patient to protect himself from sunlight.

amoxicillin/clavulanate potassium

Augmentin, Clavulin†

General

Classification: antibiotic (aminopenicillin). **Pregnancy risk category:** B.

Mechanism of action

Prevents bacterial cell wall synthesis during active replication. Clavulanic acid increases amoxicillin effectiveness by deactivating beta lactamases, which destroy amoxicillin.

Indications and dosage

• Lower respiratory infections, otitis media, sinusitis, skin and skin structure infections, and urinary tract infections caused by susceptible strains of gram-positive and gram-negative organisms. **Adults:** 250 mg (based on the amoxicillin component) P.O. q 8 hours. For more severe infections, 500 mg q 8 hours. **Children:** 20 to 40 mg/kg (based on the amoxicillin component) P.O. daily given in divided doses q 8 hours.

Adverse reactions

Blood: anemia, thrombocytopenia, thrombocytopenic purpura, eosinophilia, leukopenia. **GI:** *nausea,* vomiting, *diarrhea.* **Other:** hypersensitivity (erythematous maculopapular rash, urticaria, ***anaphylaxis***), overgrowth of nonsusceptible organisms.

Interactions

Allopurinol: increased incidence of skin rash. **Probenecid:** increases blood levels of amoxicillin, other penicillins. Probenecid may be used for this purpose.

Nursing diagnoses

• High risk for injury related to ineffectiveness of amoxicillin to eradicate the infection.
• High risk for fluid volume deficit related to amoxicillin-induced adverse GI reactions.
• Knowledge deficit related to drug therapy.

Nursing interventions

• *Use cautiously* in patients with other drug allergies, especially to cephalosporins (possible cross-allergenicity), and in mononucleosis (high incidence of maculopapular rash).
• Before giving, ask patient about any allergic reactions to penicillin. However, a negative history doesn't rule out future penicillin allergy.
• Obtain specimen for culture and sensitivity tests before first dose. Therapy may begin pending test results.
• Tell patient to take drug exactly as prescribed, even after he feels better. Patient should take entire quantity prescribed.
• Give with food to prevent GI distress.
• With large doses and prolonged therapy, bacterial and fungal superinfection may occur, especially in elderly, debilitated, or immunosuppressed patients. Close observation is essential.
• Both "250" and "500" tablets contain the same amount of clavulanic acid (125 mg); two "250" tablets aren't equivalent to one "500" tablet.
• Particularly useful in clinical settings with high prevalence of amoxicillin-resistant organisms.
• Give amoxicillin/clavulanate potassium at least 1 hour before bacteriostatic antibiotics.

General

Classification: antibiotic (synthetic folate antagonist). **Pregnancy risk category:** C.

Mechanism of action

Interferes with the action of dihydrofolate reductase, inhibiting bacterial synthesis of folic acid.

Indications and dosage

- Treatment of uncomplicated UTIs caused by susceptible strains of *Escherichia coli, Proteus mirabilis, Klebsiella,* and *Enterobacter*. **Adults:** 100 mg P.O. every 12 hours for 10 days.

Not recommended for children under 12 years.

Adverse reactions

Blood: thrombocytopenia, leukopenia, megaloblastic anemia, methemoglobinemia. **GI:** *epigastric distress, nausea, vomiting,* glossitis. **Skin:** *rash, pruritus,* ***exfoliative dermatitis.*** **Other:** fever.

Interactions

Phenytoin: trimethoprim may decrease phenytoin metabolism and increase serum levels of phenytoin.

Nursing diagnoses

- High risk for injury related to ineffectiveness of trimethoprim to eradicate the infection.
- High risk for fluid volume deficit related to trimethoprim-induced adverse GI reactions.
- Knowledge deficit related to trimethoprim therapy.

Nursing interventions

- *Contraindicated* in documented megaloblastic anemia due to folate deficiency.
- Clinical signs such as sore throat, fever, pallor, or purpura may be early indications of serious blood disorders. CBCs should be done routinely. Prolonged use of trimethoprim at high doses may cause bone marrow suppression.
- *Use cautiously* in patients with impaired hepatic function. Dosage should be decreased in patients with severely impaired renal function.
- Obtain specimen for culture and sensitivity tests before first dose. Therapy may begin pending test results.
- Instruct patient to continue taking the drug, even if he feels better, and to take entire amount prescribed.
- Because resistance to trimethoprim develops rapidly when it is used alone, it is usually given in combination with other drugs.

General
Classification: antibiotic (aminopenicillin). **Pregnancy risk category:** B.

Mechanism of action
Bactericidal against microorganisms; inhibits cell wall synthesis during active multiplication. Bacteria resist amoxicillin by producing penicillinases—enzymes that hydrolyze amoxicillin.

Indications and dosage
- Systemic infections, acute and chronic urinary tract infections caused by susceptible strains of gram-positive and gram-negative organisms. **Adults:** 750 mg to 1.5 g P.O. daily in divided doses given q 8 hours. **Children:** 20 to 40 mg/kg P.O. daily in divided doses given q 8 hours.
- Uncomplicated gonorrhea. **Adults:** 3 g P.O. with 1 g probenecid given as a single dose.
- Uncomplicated urinary tract infections caused by susceptible organisms. **Adults:** 3 g P.O. given as a single dose.

Adverse reactions
Blood: anemia, thrombocytopenia, thrombocytopenic purpura, eosinophilia, leukopenia. **GI:** *nausea,* vomiting, *diarrhea.* **Other:** hypersensitivity (erythematous maculopapular rash, urticaria, ***anaphylaxis),*** overgrowth of nonsusceptible organisms.

Interactions
Allopurinol: increased incidence of skin rash. **Probenecid:** increases blood levels of amoxicillin and other penicillins. Probenecid may be used for this purpose.

Nursing diagnoses
- High risk for injury related to ineffectiveness of amoxicillin to eradicate the infection.
- High risk for fluid volume deficit related to amoxicillin-induced adverse GI reactions.
- Knowledge deficit related to amoxicillin therapy.

Nursing interventions
- *Use cautiously* in patients with other drug allergies, especially to cephalosporins (possible cross-allergenicity), and in mononucleosis (high incidence of maculopapular rash).
- Obtain specimen for culture and sensitivity tests before first dose. Therapy may begin pending test results.
- Before giving amoxicillin, ask patient if he's had any allergic reactions to penicillin. However, a negative history of penicillin allergy is no guarantee against a future allergic reaction.
- Tell patient to take medication exactly as prescribed, even after he feels better. Entire quantity prescribed should be taken.
- Give with food to prevent GI distress.
- With large doses and prolonged therapy, bacterial and fungal superinfections may occur, especially in elderly, debilitated, or immunosuppressed patients. Close observation is essential.
- Warn patient never to use leftover amoxicillin for a new illness or to share it with family and friends.
- Trimox oral suspension may be stored at room temperature for up to 2 weeks. Be sure to check individual product labels for storage information.
- Tell patient to call the doctor if rash, fever, or chills develop. A rash is the most common allergic reaction. The rash is most common if the patient is also taking allopurinol.
- Urine glucose determinations may be false-positive with copper sulfate tests (Clinitest); glucose enzymatic tests (Clinistix, Tes-Tape) are not affected.
- Give amoxicillin at least 1 hour before bacteriostatic antibiotics.

trimethobenzamide hydrochloride

Tebamide, Tegamide, Ticon, Tigan, Tiject-20

General

Classification: antiemetic (ethanolamine-related antihistamine). **Pregnancy risk category:** C.

Mechanism of action

Acts on the chemoreceptor trigger zone to inhibit nausea and vomiting.

Indications and dosage

• Nausea and vomiting (treatment). **Adults:** 250 mg P.O. t.i.d. or q.i.d.; or 200 mg I.M. or P.R. t.i.d. or q.i.d.

• Postoperative nausea and vomiting (prevention). **Adults:** 200 mg I.M. or P.R. (single dose) before or during surgery; may repeat 3 hours after termination of anesthesia, p.r.n. **Children 13 to 40 kg:** 100 to 200 mg P.O. or P.R. t.i.d. or q.i.d. **Children under 13 kg:** 100 mg P.R. t.i.d. or q.i.d. Limited to prolonged vomiting of known etiology.

Adverse reactions

CNS: *drowsiness,* dizziness (in large doses). **CV:** hypotension. **GI:** diarrhea, exaggeration of preexisting nausea (in large doses). **Hepatic:** *liver toxicity.* **Skin:** skin hypersensitivity reactions. **Local:** pain, stinging, burning, redness, swelling at I.M. injection site. **Other:** antiemetic effect may mask signs of overdosage of toxic agents, or intestinal obstruction, brain tumor, or other conditions.

Interactions

Alcohol, CNS depressants: additive CNS depression. Avoid concomitant use.

Nursing diagnoses

• High risk for fluid volume deficit related to nausea and vomiting.

• Pain related to trimethobenzamide-induced stinging and burning at injection site.

• Knowledge deficit related to trimethobenzamide therapy.

Nursing interventions

• *Contraindicated* in children with viral illness (a possible cause of vomiting in children); may contribute to the development of Reye's syndrome, a potentially fatal acute childhood encephalopathy characterized by fatty degeneration of the liver.

• Suppositories contraindicated in hypersensitivity to benzocaine hydrochloride or similar local anesthetic.

• Stop drug if allergic skin reaction occurs.

• Give I.M. dose by deep injection into upper outer quadrant of gluteal region to reduce pain and local irritation.

• Warn patient of the possibility of drowsiness and dizziness, and caution him against driving or other activities requiring alertness until CNS effects of the drug are known.

• Store suppositories in refrigerator.

• Has little or no value in preventing motion sickness; limited value as antiemetic.

General

Classification: antifungal (macrolide). **Pregnancy risk category:** B.

Mechanism of action

Probably acts by binding to sterols in the fungal cell membrane, altering cell permeability and allowing leakage of intracellular components.

Indications and dosage

- Systemic fungal infections, meningitis. **Adults:** initially, 1 mg in 250 ml of D_5W infused over 2 to 4 hours; or 0.25 mg/kg daily by slow infusion over 6 hours. Increase daily dosage gradually as patient tolerance develops, to maximum 1.5 mg/kg daily. If drug is discontinued for 1 week or more, administration must resume with initial dose and again increase gradually.

  Intrathecal: 25 mcg/0.1 ml diluted with 10 to 20 ml CSF and administered by barbotage two or three times weekly. Initial dose should not exceed 100 mcg.

Adverse reactions

Blood: normochromic, normocytic anemia. **CNS:** peripheral neuropathy; with intrathecal administration—peripheral nerve pain, paresthesia. **CV:** hypotension, ***cardiac arrhythmias, asystole.*** **GI:** *anorexia, weight loss, nausea,* vomiting, dyspepsia, diarrhea, epigastric cramps. **GU:** abnormal renal function with hypokalemia, azotemia, hyposthenuria, hypomagnesemia, renal tubular acidosis, nephrocalcinosis; with large doses—permanent renal impairment, anuria, oliguria. **Local:** burning, stinging, tissue damage with extravasation, *thrombophlebitis,* pain at site of injection. **Other:** arthralgia, myalgia, muscle weakness secondary to hypokalemia, *fever, chills.*

Interactions

Nephrotoxic antibiotics: may cause additive nephrotoxicity. Administer very cautiously.

Nursing diagnoses

- High risk for injury related to ineffectiveness of amphotericin B to eradicate the infection.
- Altered health maintenance related to amphotericin B-induced adverse reactions.
- Knowledge deficit related to amphotericin B therapy.

Nursing interventions

- *Use cautiously* in patients with impaired renal function.
- Use only in hospitalized patients, under close supervision, when diagnosis of potentially fatal fungal infection has been confirmed.
- Fever, shaking chills, and hypotension may appear 1 to 2 hours after start of I.V. infusion and should subside within 4 hours of discontinuation.
- If BUN level exceeds 40 mg/100 ml or if serum creatinine exceeds 3 mg/100 ml, doctor may reduce or stop drug until renal function improves. Stop drug if alkaline phosphatase or bilirubin levels become elevated. Renal damage usually reversible if drug is stopped at first sign of dysfunction.
- In the dry state, store at 35.6° to 46.4° F (2° to 8° C). Reconstitute with 10 ml sterile water only. Mixing with solutions containing sodium chloride, other electrolytes, or bacteriostatic agents, such as benzyl alcohol, causes precipitation (do not use drug).
- Severity of adverse reactions can be reduced by premedication with antipyretics, antihistamines, antiemetics, or small doses of corticosteroids; adding phosphate buffer and heparin to the solution; and alternate-day dose schedule.
- **I.V. use:** Initial test dose: 1 mg added to 50 to 250 ml D_5W and infused over 20 to 30 minutes; patient's pulse rate, respiratory rate, temperature, and blood pressure are monitored for at least 4 hours. Infuse very slowly; rapid infusion may result in CV collapse.
- Administer in distal veins. If veins become thrombosed, doctor may administer every other day.
- Don't mix or piggyback with amphotericin B; antibiotics should be given separately.

General

Classification: antihypertensive (ganglionic blocker). **Pregnancy risk category:** C.

Mechanism of action

Stabilizes postsynaptic membranes.

Indications and dosage

• Lowering blood pressure quickly in hypertensive emergencies; for controlled hypotension during surgery. **Adults:** 500 mg (10 ml) diluted in 500 ml D_5W to yield concentration of 1 mg/ml I.V. Start I.V. drip at 1 to 2 mg/minute and titrate to achieve desired hypotensive response. Range is 0.3 mg to 6 mg/minute.

Adverse reactions

CNS: dilated pupils, *extreme weakness.* **CV:** *severe orthostatic hypotension, tachycardia.* **GI:** anorexia, *nausea, vomiting, dry mouth.* **GU:** urine retention. **Other:** respiratory depression.

Interactions

Anesthetics, diuretics, procainamide: Increased hypotensive effect. Monitor patient closely.

Nursing diagnoses

• High risk for aspiration related to trimethaphan-induced adverse reactions.

• Ineffective breathing pattern related to trimethaphan-induced adverse reactions.

• Knowledge deficit related to trimethaphan therapy.

Nursing interventions

• *Contraindicated* in anemia and respiratory insufficiency.

• *Use cautiously* in arteriosclerosis; cardiac, hepatic, or renal disease; degenerative CNS disorders; Addison's disease; and diabetes and in patients receiving glucocorticoids or other antihypertensives.

• Monitor patient's blood pressure and vital signs continuously.

• Patient should be supine during drug administration. May require elevation of the head of the bed for maximal effect to avoid cerebral anoxia. Do not elevate bed more than 30 degrees.

• Watch closely for respiratory distress, especially if large doses are used. Large doses have caused apnea and respiratory arrest.

• If extreme hypotension occurs, discontinue drug and call doctor. Use phenylephrine or mephentermine to counteract hypotension.

• Patient should receive oxygen therapy during use of this agent.

• Use continuous infusion pump to administer this drug slowly and precisely.

• Discontinue drug before wound closure in surgery to allow blood pressure to return to normal.

General

Classification: antibiotic (aminopenicillin). **Pregnancy risk category:** B.

Mechanism of action

Bactericidal against microorganisms; inhibits cell wall synthesis during active multiplication. Bacteria resist ampicillin by producing penicillinases—enzymes that hydrolyze ampicillin.

Indications and dosage

- Systemic infections, acute and chronic urinary tract infections caused by susceptible strains of gram-positive and gram-negative organisms. **Adults:** 1 to 4 g P.O. daily, divided into doses given q 6 hours; 2 to 12 g I.M. or I.V. (sodium) daily, divided into doses given q 4 to 6 hours. **Children:** 50 to 100 mg/kg P.O. daily, divided into doses given q 6 hours; or 100 to 200 mg/kg I.M. or I.V. daily, divided into doses given q 6 hours.
- Meningitis. **Adults:** 8 to 14 g I.V. daily in divided doses q 3 to 4 hours. **Children:** up to 300 mg/kg I.V. daily in divided doses q 3 to 4 hours.
- Uncomplicated gonorrhea. **Adults:** 3.5 g P.O. with 1 g probenecid given as a single dose.

Adverse reactions

Blood: anemia, thrombocytopenia, thrombocytopenic purpura, eosinophilia, leukopenia. **GI:** *nausea*, vomiting, *diarrhea*, glossitis, stomatitis. **Local:** pain at injection site, vein irritation, thrombophlebitis. **Other:** hypersensitivity (erythematous maculopapular rash, urticaria, ***anaphylaxis***), overgrowth of nonsusceptible organisms.

Interactions

Allopurinol: increased incidence of skin rash. **Probenecid:** increases blood levels of ampicillin and other penicillins. Probenecid may be used for this purpose.

Nursing diagnoses

- High risk for injury related to ineffectiveness of ampicillin to eradicate the infection.
- High risk for fluid volume deficit related to ampicillin-induced adverse GI reactions.
- Knowledge deficit related to ampicillin therapy.

Nursing interventions

- *Use cautiously* in patients with other drug allergies, especially to cephalosporins (possible cross-allergenicity), and in mononucleosis (high incidence of maculopapular rash in those receiving ampicillin).
- Obtain specimen for culture and sensitivity tests before first dose. Therapy may begin pending test results.
- Tell the patient to call the doctor if rash, fever, or chills develop. A rash is the most common allergic reaction. Rash is most common if the patient is also taking allopurinol.
- When given orally, drug may cause GI disturbances. Food may interfere with absorption; give 1 to 2 hours before meals, 2 to 3 hours after.
- Don't give I.M. or I.V. unless infection is severe or patient can't take oral dose.
- Dosage should be altered in patients with impaired renal function.
- Give I.V. intermittently to prevent vein irritation. Change site every 48 hours.
- With large doses or prolonged therapy, bacterial or fungal superinfections may occur, especially in elderly, debilitated, or immunosuppressed patients. Close observation is essential.
- Reconstituted solution is stable for 1 hour. Follow manufacturer's directions for stability data when ampicillin is further diluted for I.V. infusion.
- In pediatric meningitis, may be given concurrently with parenteral chloramphenicol for 24 hours pending cultures.
- Urine glucose determinations may be false-positive with copper sulfate tests; glucose enzymatic tests are not affected.

General

Classification: anticonvulsant (oxazolidinedione derivative). **Pregnancy risk category:** D.

Mechanism of action

Raises the threshold for cortical seizure but does not modify seizure pattern. Decreases projection of focal activity and reduces both repetitive spinal-cord transmission and spike-and-wave patterns of absence (petit mal) seizures.

Indications and dosage

• Refractory absence seizures. **Adults and children over 13 years:** initially, 300 mg P.O. t.i.d. May increase by 300 mg weekly up to 600 mg P.O. q.i.d. **Children:** 13 mg/kg P.O. t.i.d. or 335 mg/m² P.O. t.i.d.; alternatively, give according to age. **Children under 2 years:** 100 mg P.O. t.i.d. **Children 2 to 6 years:** 200 mg P.O. t.i.d. **Children 6 to 13 years:** 300 mg P.O. t.i.d.

Adverse reactions

Blood: ***neutropenia, leukopenia,*** eosinophilia, ***thrombocytopenia, pancytopenia, agranulocytosis, hypoplastic and aplastic anemia.*** **CNS:** *drowsiness,* fatigue, *malaise,* insomnia, dizziness, headache, paresthesias, irritability. **CV:** hypertension, hypotension. **EENT:** *hemeralopia,* diplopia, photophobia, epistaxis, retinal hemorrhage. **GI:** nausea, vomiting, anorexia, abdominal pain, bleeding gums. **GU:** nephrosis, albuminuria, vaginal bleeding. **Hepatic:** abnormal liver function tests. **Skin:** acneiform and morbilliform rash, ***exfoliative dermatitis, erythema multiforme,*** petechiae, alopecia. **Other:** lymphadenopathy, systemic lupus-like syndrome, myasthenia-like syndrome.

Interactions

None significant.

Nursing diagnoses

• High risk for injury related to ineffectiveness of trimethadione to raise seizure threshhold.
• High risk for infection related to trimethadione-induced adverse reactions.
• Knowledge deficit related to trimethadione therapy.

Nursing interventions

• *Contraindicated* in paramethadione and trimethadione hypersensitivity, severe blood dyscrasia, or hepatic dysfunction.
• *Use with extreme caution* in retinal and optic nerve diseases.
• Don't withdraw drug suddenly. Abrupt withdrawal may precipitate absence seizures. Call doctor immediately if adverse reactions develop.
• Check CBC, hepatic function, and urinalysis before starting therapy and monthly thereafter. Drug should be stopped if neutrophil count falls below 2,500/mm³.
• Watch for impending toxicity; may precipitate tonic-clonic seizure.
• Warn patient to report skin rash, alopecia, sore throat, fever, bruises, or epistaxis to doctor immediately.
• Warn patient to avoid activities requiring alertness and good psychomotor coordination until CNS effects of the drug are known.
• Suggest sunglasses if vision blurs in bright light. Notify doctor.
• If scotomata or rash develops, drug should be discontinued.
• May increase risk of tonic-clonic seizures if used alone to treat patients who have mixed types of seizures.
• Has been largely replaced by succinimide derivatives.

General

Classification: antibiotic (aminopenicillin and beta-lacatamase inhibitor). **Pregnancy risk category:** C.

Mechanism of action

Ampicillin inhibits cell wall synthesis during active multiplication. Sulbactam inactivates bacterial beta-lactamase, the enzyme that inactivates ampicillin and provides bacterial resistance to it.

Indications and dosage

- Intra-abdominal, gynecologic, and skin and skin structure infections caused by susceptible strains of bacteria. **Adults:** dosage expressed as total drug (each 1.5-g vial contains 1 g ampicillin sodium and 0.5 g sulbactam sodium): 1.5 to 3 g I.M. or I.V. q 6 hours. Maximum daily dose is 4 g sulbactam (12 g of the combined drugs).

Adverse reactions

Blood: anemia, thrombocytopenia, thrombocytopenic purpura, eosinophilia, leukopenia. **GI:** *nausea,* vomiting, *diarrhea,* glossitis, stomatitis. **Local:** pain at injection site, vein irritation, thrombophlebitis. **Other:** *hypersensitivity (erythematous maculopapular rash, urticaria,* ***anaphylaxis****), overgrowth of nonsusceptible organisms.*

Interactions

Allopurinol: increased incidence of skin rash. **Probenecid:** increased levels of ampicillin. Probenecid may be used for this purpose.

Nursing diagnoses

- High risk for injury related to ineffectiveness of ampicillin to eradicate the infection.
- High risk for fluid volume deficit related to ampicillin-induced adverse GI reactions.
- Knowledge deficit related to ampicillin therapy.

Nursing interventions

- *Use cautiously* in patients with other drug allergies, especially to cephalosporins (possible cross-allergenicity), and in mononucleosis (high incidence of maculopapular rash in those receiving ampicillin).
- Obtain specimen for culture and sensitivity tests before first dose. Therapy may begin pending test results.
- Before giving ampicillin, ask if patient has had any allergic reactions to penicillin. However, a negative history of penicillin allergy is no guarantee against a future allergic reaction.
- **I.V. use:** When preparing I.V. injection, reconstitute powder with any of the following diluents: 0.9% sodium chloride solution, D_5W, lactated Ringer's injection, 1/6 M sodium lactate, and 10% invert sugar. Stability varies with diluent, temperature, and concentration of solution.
- Give I.V. dose by slow injection, or dilute in 50 to 100 ml of a compatible diluent and infuse over 15 to 30 minutes. If permitted, give intermittently to prevent vein irritation. Change site every 48 hours.
- When giving I.V., don't add or mix with other drugs: They might be physically or chemically incompatible.
- When administering I.M., give by deep injection. Drug may be reconstituted with sterile water for injection, or 0.5% or 2% lidocaine hydrochloride injection. Add 3.2 ml to a 1.5-g vial (or 6.4 ml to a 3-g vial) to yield a concentration of 375 mg/ml.
- Dosage should be altered in patients with impaired renal function.
- With large doses and prolonged therapy, bacterial and fungal superinfections may occur, especially in elderly, debilitated, or immunosuppressed patients. Close observation is essential.
- Urine glucose determinations may be false-positive with copper sulfate tests; glucose enzymatic tests are not affected.
- Give drug at least 1 hour before bacteriostatic antibiotics.

General

Classification: antipruritic (phenothiazine-derived antihistamine). **Pregnancy risk category:** C.

Mechanism of action

Competes with histamine for H_1-receptor sites on effector cells. Prevents but does not reverse histamine-mediated responses.

Indications and dosage

- Pruritus. **Adults:** 2.5 mg P.O. q.i.d.; or (timed-release) 5 mg P.O. b.i.d. **Children 3 to 12 years:** 2.5 mg P.O. at bedtime or t.i.d., p.r.n. **Children 6 months to 3 years:** 1.25 mg P.O. h.s. or t.i.d., p.r.n.

Note: Children under 12 years should use only as directed by a doctor.

Adverse reactions

Blood: ***agranulocytosis,*** leukopenia. **CNS:** (especially in elderly patients) drowsiness, dizziness, confusion, headache, restlessness, tremor, irritability, insomnia; (in children) paradoxical excitation. **CV:** hypotension, palpitations, tachycardia. **GI:** anorexia, nausea, vomiting, *dry mouth and throat.* **GU:** urinary frequency, urine retention. **Skin:** urticaria, rash, *photosensitivity.*

Interactions

Alcohol, CNS depressants: increased sedation. Use together cautiously. **Anticholinergics, MAO inhibitors, phenothiazines, TCAs:** increased anticholinergic effect. Don't use together. **Levodopa:** trimeprazine may block levodopa's antiparkinsonian effects. Don't use together. **Lithium:** trimeprazine may decrease GI absorption and enhance renal excretion of lithium. Don't use together.

Nursing diagnoses

- High risk for impaired skin integrity related to pruritus.
- High risk for infection related to trimeprazine-induced agranulocytosis.
- Knowledge deficit related to trimeprazine therapy.

Nursing interventions

- *Contraindicated* in acute asthmatic attacks.
- *Use cautiously* in pulmonary, hepatic, or cardiovascular disease; asthma; hypertension; narrow-angle glaucoma; intestinal obstruction; prostatic hypertrophy; bladder-neck obstruction; seizure disorder; bone-marrow depression; coma; CNS depression; stenosing peptic ulcers; in elderly or debilitated patients; and in acutely ill or dehydrated children.
- Warn patient against drinking alcoholic beverages during therapy and against driving or other activities that require alertness until CNS response to drug is determined.
- Reduce GI distress by giving with food or milk.
- Coffee or tea may reduce drowsiness. Sugarless gum or sour hard candy, or ice chips may relieve dry mouth.
- Warn patient to stop taking drug 4 days before allergy skin tests to preserve accuracy of tests.
- Monitor blood counts during long-term therapy.
- Warn patient about risk of photosensitivity. Recommend use of a sunscreen. If photosensitivity occurs, tell patient to stop taking the drug and call the doctor.
- If patient is scheduled for a myelogram, drug should be discontinued 48 hours before and not resumed until 24 hours after the procedure because of the risk of seizures.
- Antihistamines are not recommended for use by women who are breast-feeding because small amounts of drug are excreted in breast milk.

General

Classification: inotropic, vasodilator (bipyridine derivative). **Pregnancy risk category:** C.

Mechanism of action

Produces inotropic action by increasing cellular levels of cyclic adenosine monophosphate. Produces vasodilation through a direct relaxant effect on vascular smooth muscle.

Indications and dosage

- Short-term management of CHF. **Adults:** initially, 0.75 mg/kg I.V. bolus over 2 to 3 minutes. Then begin maintenance infusion of 5 to 10 mcg/kg/minute. Additional bolus of 0.75 mg/kg may be given 30 minutes after start of therapy. Total daily dosage should not exceed 10 mg/kg.

Adverse reactions

Blood: *thrombocytopenia* (dose dependent). **CV:** *arrhythmias,* hypotension. **GI:** nausea, vomiting, cramps, dyspepsia, diarrhea. **Hepatic:** elevated enzymes, hepatotoxicity (rare). **Local:** burning at injection site. **Other:** hypersensitivity reactions (pericarditis, ascites, myositis, vasculitis, pleuritis).

Interactions

Digitalis glycosides: Enhanced inotropic effect. Beneficial drug interaction. **Disopyramide:** excessive hypotension. Don't administer concurrently.

Nursing diagnoses

- Fluid volume excess related to ineffectiveness of amrinone to relieve CHF.
- Decreased cardiac output related to amrinone-induced arrhythmias.
- Knowledge deficit related to amrinone therapy.

Nursing interventions

- *Contraindicated* in severe aortic or pulmonic valvular disease. Not recommended during acute phase of myocardial infarction.
- *Use cautiously* in idiopathic hypertrophic subaortic stenosis.
- Dosage should be based on clinical response, including assessment of pulmonary artery pressures and cardiac output. Cardiovascular effects begin within 2 to 5 minutes after starting infusion and may last for 30 minutes to 2 hours after infusion is discontinued.
- Amrinone may be added to digitalis glycoside therapy in atrial fibrillation and flutter since it enhances AV conduction and increases ventricular response rate.
- Monitor blood pressure and heart rate throughout the infusion. Slow or stop infusion and notify doctor if patient's blood pressure falls.
- Monitor platelet count. Platelet count below 150,000/mm^3 usually requires a decreased dosage.
- **I.V. use:** Amrinone must be administered with an infusion pump. Administer amrinone as supplied, or dilute in 0.4% or 0.9% sodium chloride solution to a concentration of 1 to 3 mg/ml. Use diluted solution within 24 hours. Don't mix other drugs into this solution.
- Don't dilute with solutions containing dextrose because a slow chemical reaction occurs over 24 hours. However, amrinone can be injected into running dextrose infusions through a Y connector or directly into the tubing.
- Furosemide will form a precipitate with amrinone solutions. Don't mix together.
- Amrinone is primarily prescribed for patients who have not responded to digitalis glycoside, diuretic, or vasodilator therapy.
- Patients with end-stage cardiac disease may receive home treatment with an amrinone drip while awaiting a heart transplant.

General

Classification: adrenocortical steroidogenesis inhibitor (testosterone derivative). **Pregnancy risk category:** X.

Mechanism of action

Reversibly lowers elevated circulating levels of glucocorticoids by inhibiting the enzyme system essential for their production in the adrenal gland.

Indications and dosage

• Adrenal cortical hyperfunction in Cushing's syndrome. **Adults:** 30 mg P.O. q.i.d. initially. May be increased at intervals of 3 to 4 days to maximum of 480 mg daily.

Adverse reactions

CNS: headache. **CV:** *orthostatic hypotension.* **EENT:** burning of oral and nasal membranes. **GI:** *diarrhea, upset stomach,* nausea, flatulence, bloating. **Metabolic:** hyperkalemia. **Skin:** flushing, rash. **Other:** fever, fatigue, hot flashes.

Interactions

Aminoglutethimide, mitotane: may cause severe adrenocortical hypofunction. **Thiazides, loop diuretics:** decreased potassium loss because trilostane inhibits aldosterone production.

Nursing diagnoses

• High risk for fluid volume deficit related to adverse drug reactions.
• High risk for injury related to drug-induced adverse reactions.
• Knowledge deficit related to trilostane therapy.

Nursing interventions

• *Contraindicated* in patients with severe renal or hepatic disease.
• *Use cautiously* in patients who are receiving other drugs that suppress adrenal function.
• Trilostane may prevent normal response to physiologic stressful situation. Therefore, patients who develop a severe illness or need surgery may need to have this drug temporarily discontinued.
• Because the drug may cause orthostatic hypotension by suppressing aldosterone production, monitor blood pressure regularly in all patients.
• Patient should show therapeutic response within 2 weeks. If no response has occurred, the doctor may discontinue the drug.
• Most patients show a therapeutic response at doses below 360 mg/day.
• Trilostane is prescribed when surgery or pituitary radiation is inappropriate or must be delayed. Explain to patient that the drug does not cure the underlying disease.

General
Classification: vasodilator, cyanide poisoning adjunct (nitrate). **Pregnancy risk category:** C.

Mechanism of action
Reduces cardiac oxygen demand by decreasing left ventricular end-diastolic pressure (preload) and systemic vascular resistance (afterload). Also increases blood flow through the collateral coronary vessels. Converts hemoglobin to methemoglobin (which binds cyanide) to treat cyanide poisoning.

Indications and dosage
• Relief of angina pectoris; relief of renal or gallbladder colic. **Adults and children:** 0.2 to 0.3 ml by inhalation (one glass ampule inhaler), p.r.n.
• Antidote for cyanide poisoning. 0.2 or 0.3 ml by inhalation for 30 to 60 seconds q 5 minutes until conscious.

Adverse reactions
Blood: methemoglobinemia. **CNS:** *headache, sometimes with throbbing;* dizziness; weakness. **CV:** *orthostatic hypotension, tachycardia,* flushing, palpitations, fainting. **GI:** nausea, vomiting. **Skin:** cutaneous vasodilation. **Other:** hypersensitivity reactions.

Interactions
None significant.

Nursing diagnoses
• Pain related to the patient's underlying condition.
• High risk for injury related to amyl nitrite-induced adverse reactions.
• Knowledge deficit related to amyl nitrite therapy.

Nursing interventions
• *Contraindicated* in hypersensitivity to nitrites and during acute MI.
• *Use cautiously* in cerebral hemorrhage, hypotension, head injury, or glaucoma.
• Watch for orthostatic hypotension. Have patient sit down and avoid rapid position changes while inhaling drug.
• Wrap ampule in cloth and crush. Hold near patient's nose and mouth so vapor is inhaled.
• Extinguish all cigarettes before use, or ampule may ignite.
• Effective within 30 seconds but has a short duration of action (3 to 5 minutes).
• Keeping the head low, deep breathing, and movement of extremities may help relieve dizziness, syncope, or weakness from orthostatic hypotension.
• Drug is often abused; abusers claim it has aphrodisiac qualities. Street name: "poppers."
• Seldom, if ever, used for treatment of angina because it is expensive and inconvenient and frequently causes adverse reactions.
• Sometimes used to induce changes in heart murmurs. Patient inhales the drug until reflex tachycardia is induced, then discontinues.

General
Classification: antiparkinsonian agent (anticholinergic). **Pregnancy risk category:** C.

Mechanism of action
Blocks central cholinergic receptors, helping to balance cholinergic activity in the basal ganglia.

Indications and dosage
• Drug-induced parkinsonism. **Adults:** 1 mg P.O. 1st day, 2 mg 2nd day, then increase by 2 mg q 3 to 5 days until total of 6 to 10 mg is given daily. Usually given t.i.d. with meals and, if needed, q.i.d. (last dose should be before bedtime) or may switch to extended-release form b.i.d. Postencephalitic parkinsonism may require 12 to 15 mg total daily dosage.

Adverse reactions
Adverse reactions are dose-related. **CNS:** nervousness, dizziness, headache, restlessness, agitation, hallucinations, euphoria, delusion, amnesia. **CV:** tachycardia. **EENT:** blurred vision, mydriasis, increased intraocular pressure. **GI:** constipation, *dry mouth, nausea.* **GU:** urinary hesitancy, urine retention.

Interactions
Amantadine: additive anticholinergic adverse reactions, such as confusion and hallucinations. Reduce dosage before administering amantadine.

Nursing diagnoses
• Impaired physical mobility related to underlying parkinsonism.
• Altered oral mucous membrane related to trihexyphenidyl-induced dry mouth.
• Knowledge deficit related to trihexyphenidyl therapy.

Nursing interventions
• *Use cautiously* in patients with narrow-angle glaucoma; cardiac, hepatic, or renal disorders; hypertension; obstructive disease of the GI and GU tracts; possible prostatic hypertrophy; patients over 60 years; and those with arteriosclerosis or history of drug hypersensitivities. Adverse reactions are usually mild and transient.
• Warn patient to avoid activities requiring alertness until CNS effects of the drug are known.
• Causes nausea if given before meals.
• Relieve dry mouth with cool drinks, ice chips, sugarless gum, or hard candy.
• Patient may develop a tolerance to this drug, so dosage may need to be gradually increased.
• Advise patient to report signs of urinary hesitancy or urine retention.
• Gonioscopic evaluation and close monitoring of intraocular pressure is advised, especially in patients over 40 years.

General

Classification: antimuscarinic, GI antispasmodic (synthetic belladonna alkaloid derivative). **Pregnancy risk category:** C.

Mechanism of action

Competitively blocks acetylcholine, which decreases GI motility and inhibits gastric acid secretion.

Indications and dosage

- Adjunctive treatment of peptic ulcer. **Adults:** 50 mg P.O. t.i.d. To be effective, should be titrated to individual patient's needs.

Adverse reactions

CNS: headache, insomnia, drowsiness, dizziness, *confusion or excitement in elderly patients,* nervousness, weakness. **CV:** *palpitations,* tachycardia. **EENT:** *blurred vision,* mydriasis, increased ocular tension, cycloplegia, photophobia. **GI:** *dry mouth,* dysphagia, heartburn, loss of taste, nausea, vomiting, *paralytic ileus, constipation.* **GU:** *urinary hesitancy, urine retention,* impotence. **Skin:** urticaria, decreased sweating and possible anhidrosis, other dermal manifestations. **Other:** fever, allergic reactions. Overdose may cause curare-like symptoms.

Interactions

Amantadine, antihistamines, antiparkinsonian agents, disopyramide, glutethimide, meperidine, phenothiazines, procainamide, quinidine: additive adverse effects. Avoid concomitant use. **Ketoconazole:** anisotropine may interfere with absorption of ketoconazole. Avoid concomitant use. **Methotrimeprazine:** possible extrapyramidal symptoms. Avoid concomitant use.

Nursing diagnoses

- Pain related to the patient's underlying condition.
- Constipation related to adverse GI reactions to anisotropine.
- Knowledge deficit related to anisotropine therapy.

Nursing interventions

- *Contraindicated* in narrow-angle glaucoma, obstructive uropathy, obstructive disease of the GI tract, severe ulcerative colitis, myasthenia gravis, hypersensitivity to anticholinergics, paralytic ileus, intestinal atony, unstable CV status in acute hemorrhage, or toxic megacolon.
- *Use cautiously* in autonomic neuropathy, hyperthyroidism, coronary artery disease, cardiac arrhythmias, CHF, hypertension, hiatal hernia associated with reflux esophagitis, hepatic or renal disease, and ulcerative colitis or in patients over 40 years because of increased incidence of glaucoma. Also use cautiously in hot or humid environments. Drug-induced heatstroke can develop.
- Give 30 minutes to 1 hour before meals.
- Administer smaller doses to elderly patients.
- Monitor patient's vital signs and urine output carefully.
- Instruct patient to avoid driving and other hazardous activities if he is drowsy or dizzy or has blurred vision; to drink plenty of fluids to help prevent constipation; and to report any skin rash or local eruption.

trifluoperazine hydrochloride

Apo-Trifluoperazine†, Novo-Flurazine†, Solazine†, Stelazine, Suprazine, Terfluzine†

General

Classification: antipsychotic, antiemetic (piperazine-derived phenothiazine). **Pregnancy risk category:** C.

Mechanism of action

Blocks postsynaptic dopamine receptors in the brain.

Indications and dosage

- Anxiety states. **Adults:** 1 to 2 mg P.O. b.i.d.
- Schizophrenia and other psychotic disorders. **Adults:** *outpatients*—1 to 2 mg P.O. b.i.d., up to 4 mg daily; *hospitalized*—2 to 5 mg P.O. b.i.d., increased to 40 mg daily; or 1 to 2 mg I.M. q 4 to 6 hours, p.r.n. **Children 6 to 12 years** (hospitalized or under close supervision): 1 mg P.O. daily or b.i.d., increased to 15 mg daily.

Adverse reactions

Blood: transient leukopenia, ***agranulocytosis.*** **CNS:** *extrapyramidal reactions (high incidence), tardive dyskinesia,* sedation (low incidence), pseudoparkinsonism, EEG changes, dizziness. **CV:** *orthostatic hypotension,* tachycardia, ECG changes. **EENT:** ocular changes, *blurred vision.* **GI:** *dry mouth, constipation.* **GU:** *urine retention,* dark urine, menstrual irregularities, gynecomastia, inhibited ejaculation. **Hepatic:** cholestatic jaundice. **Metabolic:** hyperprolactinemia. **Skin:** *mild photosensitivity,* dermal allergic reactions. **Local:** pain at I.M. injection site, sterile abscess. **Other:** weight gain; increased appetite; ***neuroleptic malignant syndrome*** (rare). **After abrupt withdrawal of long-term therapy:** gastritis, nausea, vomiting, dizziness, tremors, feeling of warmth or cold, sweating, tachycardia, headache, insomnia.

Interactions

Adrenergic blockers, epidural or spinal anesthetics: increased hypotension. Don't use together. **Alcohol, other CNS depressants:** increased CNS depression. Avoid concomitant use. **Antacids:** inhibit absorption of oral phenothiazines. Separate doses by at least 2 hours. **Barbiturates, lithium:** may decrease phenothiazine effect. Observe patient. **Centrally acting antihypertensives:** decreased antihypertensive effect.

Nursing diagnoses

- Altered thought processes related to patient's underlying condition.
- Urinary retention related to adverse drug reaction.
- Knowledge deficit related to trifluoperazine therapy.

Nursing interventions

- *Contraindicated* in coma, CNS depression, bone marrow suppression, and subcortical damage.
- *Use cautiously* in elderly or debilitated patients; in hepatic disease, arteriosclerosis or CV disease, exposure to extreme heat or cold, respiratory disorders, hypocalcemia, seizure disorders, reactions to insulin or electroshock therapy, suspected brain tumor or intestinal obstruction, glaucoma, or prostatic hypertrophy; and in acutely ill or dehydrated children.
- Tardive dyskinesia may occur after prolonged use.
- Watch for symptoms of neuroleptic malignant syndrome, which is rare but frequently fatal.
- Hold dose and notify doctor if patient develops jaundice, symptoms of blood dyscrasia, or persistent extrapyramidal reactions.
- Monitor therapy by bilirubin tests, CBC and liver function tests, and ophthalmic tests.
- Tell patient to protect himself from sunlight.
- Warn against activities requiring alertness until CNS effects of the drug are known. Drowsiness and dizziness usually subside after a few weeks.
- Watch for orthostatic hypotension, especially with I.M. dose. Keep patient supine for 1 hour afterward. Advise changing positions slowly.
- Give deep I.M. only in upper outer quadrant of buttocks. Massage slowly afterward.
- Discard markedly discolored solutions.
- Keep drug off skin and clothes.
- Dilute liquid concentrate just before giving.
- Don't withdraw drug abruptly.

General

Classification: thrombolytic (enzyme). **Pregnancy risk category:** C.

Mechanism of action

Derived from Lys-plasminogen and streptokinase; includes a fibrinolytic enzyme plus activator complex. The activator is temporarily blocked by an anisoyl group; drug is activated in vivo by a nonenzymatic process that removes the anisoyl group.

Indications and dosage

- Lysis of cornary artery thrombi following acute MI. **Adults:** 30 units I.V. over 2 to 5 minutes. Administer by direct injection.

Adverse reactions

Blood: ***bleeding,*** eosinophilia. **CNS:** ***intracranial hemorrhage.*** **CV:** arrhythmias, conduction disorders, hypotension. **EENT:** hemoptysis, gum/mouth hemorrhage. **GI:** ***bleeding.*** **GU:** hematuria. **Skin:** hematomas, urticaria, itching, flushing, delayed (2 weeks after therapy) purpuric rash. **Local:** bleeding at puncture sites. **Other:** ***anaphylactoid reactions (rare).***

Interactions

Heparin, oral anticoagulants, and drugs that alter platelet function: may increase risk of bleeding.

Nursing diagnoses

- Altered cardiopulmonary tissue perfusion related to the patient's underlying condition.
- High risk for injury related to the adverse effects of anistreplase.
- Knowledge deficit related to drug therapy.

Nursing interventions

- *Contraindicated* in active internal bleeding, history of CVA, recent intraspinal and intracranial surgery or trauma, aneurysm, arteriovenous malformation, intracranial neoplasm, uncontrolled hypertension, or known bleeding diathesis.
- *Use cautiously* in patients with recent major surgery, trauma (including CPR), GI or GU bleeding, and cerebrovascular disease or hypertension; mitral stenosis, atrial fibrillation, or other condition that may lead to left heart thrombus; patients with acute pericarditis or subacute bacterial endocarditis; septic thrombophlebitis; in patients 75 years and older; in those with diabetic hemorrhagic retinopathy; in pregnancy and first 10 days postpartum; and in patients receiving anticoagulants.
- Unlike other thrombolytics that must be infused, anistreplase is given by direct injection over 2 to 5 minutes.
- Thrombolytic therapy is associated with the occurrence of reperfusion arrhythmias that may signify successful thrombolysis. These arrhythmias may include sinus bradycardia, accelerated idioventricular rhythm, ventricular tachycardia, or premature ventricular depolarizations. Be prepared to treat bradycardia or ventricular irritability during anistreplase therapy.
- Anistreplase is derived from human plasma. No cases of hepatitis or HIV infection have been reported to date.
- Do not mix the drug with other medications; do not dilute the solution after reconstitution. If the drug is not administered within 30 minutes of reconstituting, discard the vial.
- In vitro coagulation tests will be affected by the presence of anistreplase. This can be attenuated if blood samples are collected in the presence of aprotinin (150 to 200 units/ml).
- Bleeding is the most common adverse reaction and may occur internally and at puncture sites.
- Heparin therapy is frequently initiated after treatment with thrombolytics to decrease the risk of rethrombosis.
- Teach the patient signs of internal bleeding. Tell him to report these immediately. Advise the patient about proper dental care to avoid excessive gum trauma.

General
Classification: diuretic, antihypertensive (thiazide diuretic). **Pregnancy risk category:** D.

Mechanism of action
Increases urine excretion of sodium and water by inhibiting sodium reabsorption in the cortical diluting site of the nephron.

Indications and dosage
• Edema. **Adults:** 1 to 4 mg P.O. daily or in two divided doses. **Children over 6 months:** 0.07 mg/kg (2 mg/m^2) P.O. daily or in two divided doses.
• Hypertension. **Adults:** 2 to 4 mg P.O. daily. **Children over 6 months:** 0.07 mg/kg (2 mg/m^2) P.O. daily or in two divided doses.

Adverse reactions
Blood: ***aplastic anemia, agranulocytosis,*** leukopenia, thrombocytopenia. **CV:** volume depletion and dehydration, orthostatic hypotension. **GI:** anorexia, nausea, pancreatitis. **Hepatic:** hepatic encephalopathy. **Metabolic:** hypokalemia, asymptomatic hyperuricemia, hyperglycemia and impairment of glucose tolerance, fluid and electrolyte imbalances including dilutional hyponatremia and hypochloremia, metabolic alkalosis, hypercalcemia, gout. **Skin:** dermatitis, photosensitivity, rash. **Other:** hypersensitivity reactions, such as pneumonitis and vasculitis.

Interactions
Cholestyramine, colestipol: intestinal absorption of thiazides decreased. Keep doses as separate as possible. **Diazoxide:** increased antihypertensive, hyperglycemic, and hyperuricemic effects. Use together cautiously.

Nursing diagnoses
• Fluid volume excess related to ineffectiveness of trichlormethiazide to relieve edema.
• Altered urinary elimination related to trichlormethiazide therapy.
• Knowledge deficit related to trichlormethiazide therapy.

Nursing interventions
• *Contraindicated* in anuria or hypersensitivity to other thiazides or other sulfonamide-derived drugs.
• *Use cautiously* in severe renal disease and impaired hepatic function.
• Monitor intake and output, weight, blood pressure, and serum electrolytes.
• Patients also on digitalis glycosides have an increased risk of digitalis toxicity from the potassium-depleting effect of this diuretic. Monitor carefully.
• Watch for hypokalemia (muscle weakness and cramps). May use with potassium-sparing diuretic to prevent hypokalemia.
• Consult with doctor and dietitian to provide high-potassium diet. Foods rich in potassium include citrus fruits, tomatoes, bananas, dates, and apricots.
• Monitor serum creatinine and BUN regularly. Not as effective if these levels are more than twice normal.
• Check insulin requirements in patients with diabetes. May treat severe hyperglycemia with oral antidiabetic agents. Monitor blood glucose levels.
• Monitor blood uric acid, especially in patients with a history of gout.
• In hypertension, therapeutic response may be delayed several days.
• Give in a.m. to prevent nocturia.
• Elderly patients are especially susceptible to excessive diuresis.
• Thiazides and thiazide-like diuretics should be stopped before tests for parathyroid function are performed.
• Advise patient to avoid sudden posture changes and rise slowly to avoid orthostatic hypotension.
• Advise patient to use a sunscreen.

General

Classification: nonnarcotic analgesic, anti-inflammatory, antipyretic (salicylate). **Pregnancy risk category:** C (D in 3rd trimester).

Mechanism of action

Produces analgesia by affecting the hypothalamus and by blocking generation of pain impulses. Exerts anti-inflammatory effect by inhibiting prostaglandin synthesis. Relieves fever by acting on the hypothalamic thermoregulatory center; also decreases platelet aggregation (impedes clotting).

Indications and dosage

- Arthritis. **Adults:** 2.6 to 5.4 g P.O. daily in divided doses. **Children:** 90 to 130 mg/kg P.O. daily divided q 4 to 6 hours.
- Mild pain or fever. **Adults:** 325 to 650 mg P.O. or P.R. q 4 hours, p.r.n. **Children:** For mild pain, 65 to 100 mg/kg P.O. or P.R. daily divided q 4 to 6 hours, p.r.n. For fever, 40 to 80 mg/kg P.O. or P.R. daily divided q 6 hours, p.r.n.
- Thromboembolic disorders. **Adults:** 325 to 650 mg P.O. daily or b.i.d.

Adverse reactions

Blood: *prolonged bleeding time.* **EENT:** *tinnitus and hearing loss.* **GI:** *nausea, vomiting, GI distress, occult bleeding.* **Hepatic:** abnormal liver function studies, hepatitis. **Skin:** *rash,* bruising. **Other:** ***hypersensitivity manifested by anaphylaxis or asthma.***

Interactions

Alcohol, steroids, other NSAIDs: increased risk of GI bleeding. **Antacids in high doses (and other urine alkalinizers):** decreased levels of aspirin. **Antihypertensives:** decreased antihypertensive effect; avoid long-term aspirin ingestion. **Corticosteroids:** enhanced aspirin elimination. Monitor for decreased salicylate effect. **Methotrexate:** increased risk of methotrexate toxicity. **NSAIDs, including diflunisal, fenoprofen, ibuprofen, indomethacin, piroxicam, meclofenamate, naproxen:** altered pharmacokinetics of these agents, leading to lowered serum levels and decreased effectiveness. **Oral anticoagulants, heparin:** increased risk of bleeding. **Oral antidiabetic agents:** increased hypoglycemic effect. Monitor closely. **Probenecid, sulfinpyrazone:** decreased uricosuric effect.

Nursing diagnoses

- Pain related to the patient's underlying condition.
- Altered nutrition: Less than body requirements, related to adverse GI reactions to aspirin.
- Knowledge deficit related to aspirin therapy.

Nursing interventions

- *Contraindicated* in GI ulcer, GI bleeding, or bleeding disorders.
- *Use cautiously* in patients with hypoprothrombinemia, renal failure, or vitamin K deficiency and in asthmatics with nasal polyps.
- When used to treat inflammatory conditions, rheumatic fever, and thrombosis, aspirin is administered on a scheduled, not p.r.n., basis.
- Avoid aspirin during pregnancy. The drug may increase risk of hemorrhage in both neonate and mother; may also contribute to congenital heart disease or other malformations.
- Because of epidemiologic association with Reye's syndrome, the CDC recommends that children or teenagers with chicken pox or influenza-like illness should not be given aspirin.
- Therapeutic blood salicylate level in arthritis is 10 to 30 mg/100 ml. Tinnitus may occur at plasma levels of 30 mg/100 ml and above, but this is not a reliable indicator of toxicity, especially in very young patients and those over age 60.
- May cause an increase in serum levels of AST, ALT, alkaline phosphatase, and bilirubin.
- Advise patients receiving prolonged treatment with large doses of aspirin to watch for petechiae, bleeding gums, and signs of GI bleeding and to maintain adequate fluid intake.
- Aspirin may prevent sunburn and treat sunburn pain by preventing manufacture of prostaglandins.
- Aspirin irreversibly inhibits platelet aggregation. If possible, aspirin should be discontinued 5 to 7 days before elective surgery to allow time for the production and release of new platelets.

General

Classification: sedative-hypnotic (benzodiazepine). **Pregnancy risk category:** X. **Controlled substance schedule:** IV.

Mechanism of action

Acts on the limbic system, thalamus, and hypothalamus of the CNS to produce hypnotic effects.

Indications and dosage

• Insomnia. **Adults:** 0.125 to 0.25 mg P.O. h.s. **Adults over 65:** 0.125 mg P.O. h.s.; increase as needed to 0.25 mg P.O. h.s.

Adverse reactions

CNS: *drowsiness, dizziness, headache,* rebound insomnia, amnesia, light-headedness, lack of coordination, mental confusion, depression. **GI:** nausea, vomiting.

Interactions

Alcohol or other CNS depressants, including narcotic analgesics: excessive CNS depression. Use together cautiously. **Cimetidine, erythromycin:** may cause prolonged triazolam blood levels. Monitor for increased sedation.

Nursing diagnoses

• Sleep pattern disturbance related to underlying patient problem.
• High risk for trauma related to adverse CNS reactions to triazolam.
• Knowledge deficit related to triazolam therapy.

Nursing interventions

• *Contraindicated* in patients with hypersensitivity to benzodiazepines.
• *Use cautiously* in impaired hepatic or renal function, mental depression, suicidal tendencies, or history of drug abuse.
• Elderly patients are more sensitive to the drug's adverse CNS effects. Assess mental status before initiating therapy.
• Drug should be used in the lowest effective dose for very short duration (5 to 7 days).
• Take precautions to prevent hoarding or self-overdosing by patients who are depressed, suicidal, or drug-dependent or who have a history of drug abuse.
• Advise caution with hazardous activities requiring mental alertness or physical coordination. Supervise walking; raise bed rails, especially for elderly patients.
• Dependence is possible with long-term use.
• Triazolam is a benzodiazepine compound with similarities to flurazepam. However, it is very short-acting and therefore has less tendency to cause morning drowsiness.
• Faster acting than temazepam, another benzodiazepine derivative.
• Warn patient not to take more than the prescribed amount since overdosage can occur at a total daily dose of 2 mg (or four times the highest recommended amount).
• Tell patient that rebound insomnia may develop for one or two nights after stopping therapy.
• Because of numerous reports of adverse CNS reactions, triazolam has been withdrawn from several foreign markets. An FDA panel recently reviewed the safety and efficacy of the drug; it is currently still available in the United States.
• If triazolam overdose occurs, flumazenil (a specific benzodiazepine antagonist) may be useful. Know that the duration of action of flumazenil is shorter than that of triazolam, and resedation is possible.

General
Classification: antiallergy agent (histamine$_1$ receptor agonist). **Pregnancy risk category:** C.

Mechanism of action
Blocks the effects of histamine at H_1 receptors. Astemizole is a nonsedating antihistamine because its chemical structure prevents entry into the CNS.

Indications and dosage
• Relief of symptoms associated with chronic idiopathic urticaria and seasonal allergic rhinitis. **Adults and children over 12 years:** 10 mg P.O. daily. A loading dose may be given in order to achieve steady-state plasma levels quickly. Begin therapy at 30 mg on the first day, followed by 20 mg on the second day, and 10 mg daily thereafter.

Adverse reactions
CV: arrhythmias (with overdose). **CNS:** headache, nervousness, dizziness, drowsiness. **EENT:** dry mouth, pharyngitis, conjunctivitis. **GI:** nausea, diarrhea, abdominal pain, increased appetite. **Other:** arthralgia, weight gain, cholestatic jaundice.

Interactions
Itraconazole, ketoconazole, or macrolide antibiotics such as erythromycin: risk of serious adverse cardiac reactions. Don't use together.

Nursing diagnoses
• Ineffective airway clearance related to the patient's underlying condition.
• High risk for injury related to astemizole-induced adverse CNS reactions.
• Knowledge deficit related to astemizole therapy.

Nursing interventions
• *Use cautiously* in patients with hepatic or renal disease. Astemizole is not believed to be dialyzable.
• Because of its potential for anticholinergic effects, also use cautiously in patients with lower respiratory diseases (including asthma) because drying effects can increase the risk of bronchial mucus plug formation.
• Be sure the patient understands that this drug should be taken only once a day. If symptoms persist or worsen, he should contact the doctor. He should not increase the dose, because high doses may increase risk of cardiac arrhythmias.
• Instruct patient to take this drug on an empty stomach at least 2 hours after a meal and to avoid eating for at least 1 hour after dosing.
• Warn patient not to increase dosage without consulting the doctor.
• Warn patient to stop taking drug 4 days before allergy skin tests to preserve accuracy of tests.

General

Classification: diuretic (potassium-sparing diuretic). **Pregnancy risk category:** D.

Mechanism of action

Inhibits sodium reabsorption and potassium excretion by direct action on the distal tubule.

Indications and dosage

• Edema. **Adults:** initially, 100 mg P.O. b.i.d. after meals. Total daily dosage should not exceed 300 mg.

Adverse reactions

Blood: megaloblastic anemia related to low folic acid levels. **CNS:** dizziness. **CV:** hypotension. **EENT:** sore throat. **GI:** dry mouth, nausea, vomiting. **Metabolic:** ***hyperkalemia,*** dehydration, hyponatremia, transient elevation in BUN, acidosis. **Skin:** photosensitivity, rash. **Other:** ***anaphylaxis,*** muscle cramps.

Interactions

ACE inhibitors, potassium supplements: increased risk of hyperkalemia. Don't use together. **Indomethacin, NSAIDs:** may enhance the risk of nephrotoxicity. Avoid concomitant use. **Quinidine:** may interfere with some laboratory tests that measure quinidine levels. Inform laboratory that patient is taking triamterene.

Nursing diagnoses

• Fluid volume excess related to sodium and fluid retention.
• High risk for injury related to hyperkalemia due to triamterene therapy.
• Knowledge deficit related to triamterene therapy.

Nursing interventions

• *Contraindicated* in anuria, severe or progressive renal disease or dysfunction, severe hepatic disease, or hyperkalemia.
• *Use cautiously* in impaired hepatic function, diabetes mellitus, pregnancy, or lactation.
• Watch for blood dyscrasias.
• Monitor blood pressure, BUN, and serum electrolytes.
• A potassium-sparing diuretic, useful as an adjunct to other diuretic therapy. Less potent than thiazides and loop diuretics. Usually used with potassium-wasting diuretics. Full effect delayed 2 to 3 days when used alone.
• Warn patients to avoid excessive ingestion of potassium-rich foods or potassium-containing salt substitutes. Concomitant potassium supplement can lead to serious hyperkalemia.
• Give medication after meals to prevent nausea.
• Withdraw gradually to prevent excessive rebound potassium excretion.

General

Classification: antihypertensive, antianginal (beta-adrenergic blocking agent). **Pregnancy risk category:** C.

Mechanism of action

Blocks response to beta stimulation and depresses renin secretion.

Indications and dosage

- Hypertension. **Adults:** 50 mg P.O. daily; dosage may be increased to 100 mg once daily after 7 to 14 days. Dosages greater than 100 mg are unlikely to produce further benefit. Dosage adjustment is necessary in patients with creatinine clearance below 35 ml/minute.
- Angina pectoris. **Adults:** 50 mg P.O. once daily. May increase to 100 mg daily after 7 days for optimal effect. May give as much as 200 mg daily.
- To reduce CV mortality and risk of reinfarction in patients with acute MI. **Adults:** 5 mg I.V. over 5 minutes, followed by another 5 mg I.V. 10 minutes later. After an additional 10 minutes, administer 50 mg P.O., followed by 50 mg in 12 hours. Thereafter, give 100 mg daily (as a single dose or 50 mg b.i.d.) for 7 days.
- To reduce the incidence of supraventricular tachycardia in patients undergoing coronary artery bypass. **Adults:** 50 mg P.O. daily starting 3 days before surgery.

Adverse reactions

CNS: fatigue, lethargy. **CV:** *bradycardia, hypotension, **CHF,*** peripheral vascular disease. **GI:** nausea, vomiting, diarrhea. **Respiratory:** dyspnea, ***bronchospasm.*** **Skin:** rash. **Other:** fever.

Interactions

Antihypertensives: enhanced hypotensive effect. **Digitalis glycosides:** excessive bradycardia and increased depressant effect on myocardium. **Indomethacin:** decrease in antihypertensive effect. Monitor blood pressure and adjust dosage. **Insulin, oral antidiabetic agents:** can alter dosage requirements in previously stabilized diabetics.

Nursing diagnoses

- High risk for injury related to patient's underlying condition.
- Decreased cardiac output related to atenolol-induced adverse CV reactions.
- Knowledge deficit related to atenolol therapy.

Nursing interventions

- *Contraindicated* in sinus bradycardia, greater than first-degree conduction block, and cardiogenic shock.
- *Use cautiously* in cardiac failure.
- Atenolol is a cardioselective beta blocker similar to metoprolol. Although atenolol can be used in patients with bronchospastic diseases such as asthma and emphysema, the drug should still be used cautiously, especially when 100 mg is given. Twice-daily dosing may help minimize risk.
- Dosage should be reduced if patient has renal insufficiency. Patients with a creatinine clearance of 15 to 35 ml/min/1.73 m^2 should receive a maximum of 50 mg daily; if creatinine clearance is less than 15 ml/min/1.73 m^2, the maximum dosage is 50 mg every other day. Hemodialysis patients should receive 50 mg after each dialysis session, but close supervision is mandatory because of the risk of marked decreases in blood pressure.
- Full antihypertensive effect may not appear for 1 to 2 weeks after initiating therapy.
- Always check patient's apical pulse before giving this drug; if slower than 60 beats/minute, hold drug and call doctor.
- Don't discontinue abruptly; can exacerbate angina and MI. Drug should be withdrawn gradually over a 2-week period.
- This drug masks common signs of shock and hypoglycemia. However, atenolol doesn't potentiate insulin-induced hypoglycemia or delay recovery of blood glucose to normal levels.
- Has also been prescribed effectively in treatment of patients with alcohol withdrawal syndrome.

General

Classification: anti-inflammatory, immunosuppressant (glucocorticoid). **Pregnancy risk category:** C.

Mechanism of action

Decreases inflammation by stabilizing leukocyte lysosomal membranes. Also suppresses the immune response, stimulates bone marrow, and influences protein, fat, and carbohydrate metabolism.

Indications and dosage

- Severe inflammation or immunosuppression. **Adults:** 4 to 48 mg P.O. daily divided b.i.d., t.i.d., or q.i.d., or 40 mg I.M. (diacetate or acetonide) weekly; or 5 to 48 mg (diacetate or acetonide) into lesions; or 2 to 40 mg (diacetate or acetonide) into joints and soft tissue; or up to 0.5 mg (hexacetonide) per square inch of affected skin intralesional; or 2 to 20 mg (hexacetonide) intra-articular or intrasynovial into soft tissue or into joint or lesion.
- Steroid-dependent asthma. **Adults:** 2 inhalations t.i.d. to q.i.d. Maximum 16 inhalations daily. **Children 6 to 12 years:** 1 to 2 inhalations t.i.d. to q.i.d. Maximum 12 inhalations daily.

Adverse reactions

Most adverse reactions are dose- or duration-dependent. **CNS:** *euphoria, insomnia,* psychotic behavior, pseudotumor cerebri. **CV:** ***CHF,*** hypertension, edema. **EENT:** cataracts, glaucoma; hoarseness, fungal mouth and throat (inhalation). **GI:** *peptic ulcer,* GI irritation, increased appetite; dry mouth (inhalation). **Metabolic:** hypokalemia, hyperglycemia and carbohydrate intolerance, growth suppression in children. **Skin:** delayed wound healing, acne, various skin eruptions. **Other:** muscle weakness, osteoporosis, pancreatitis, hirsutism, susceptibility to infections. Acute adrenal insufficiency (with increased stress) or abrupt withdrawal after long-term therapy. **Withdrawal symptoms:** rebound inflammation, fatigue, weakness, arthralgia, fever, dizziness, lethargy, depression, fainting, orthostatic hypotension, dyspnea, anorexia, hypoglycemia. ***Sudden withdrawal may be fatal.***

Interactions

Systemic: Barbiturates, phenytoin, rifampin: decreased corticosteroid effect. **NSAIDs, indomethacin, aspirin:** increased risk of GI distress and bleeding. Give together cautiously. **Oral anticoagulants:** altered dosage requirements. Monitor PT. **Potassium-depleting drugs:** enhanced potassium-wasting effects of triamcinolone. Monitor serum potassium levels. **Skin-test antigens:** decreased response. Defer skin testing until therapy is completed. **Vaccines and toxoids:** decreased antibody response and increased risk of neurologic complications. Avoid concomitant use.

Nursing diagnoses

- Impaired tissue integrity related to inflammation from patient's underlying condition.
- High risk for injury related to adverse reactions to triamcinolone.
- Knowledge deficit related to triamcinolone.

Nursing interventions

- *Systemic: contraindicated* in systemic fungal infections, hypersensitivity to the drug, and sulfite sensitivity (injectable form).
- *Systemic: use cautiously* in GI ulceration, renal disease, hypertension, osteoporosis, varicella, vaccinia, exanthema, diabetes mellitus, Cushing's syndrome, thromboembolic disorders, seizures, myasthenia gravis, metastatic cancer, CHF, tuberculosis, ocular herpes simplex, hypoalbuminemia, and emotional instability.
- *Inhalation: contraindicated* in status asthmaticus, asthma controlled by bronchodilators or noncorticosteroids alone, and nonasthmatic bronchial diseases.
- Don't discontinue drug abruptly; monitor patient's status, watching for depression or psychotic episodes and potassium depletion; and teach patient signs of early adrenal insufficiency and cushingoid symptoms.

General
Classification: antiarrhythmic, vagolytic (anticholinergic, belladonna alkaloid). **Pregnancy risk category:** C.

Mechanism of action
Inhibits acetylcholine at the parasympathetic neuroeffector junction, blocking vagal effects on the SA node; this enhances conduction through the AV node and speeds heart rate.

Indications and dosage
- Symptomatic bradycardia, bradyarrhythmia. **Adults:** 0.5 to 1 mg I.V. push; repeat q 5 minutes, to maximum of 2 mg. **Children:** 0.01 mg/kg I.V. dose up to maximum of 0.4 mg; or 0.3 mg/m² dose; may repeat q 4 to 6 hours.
- Antidote for anticholinesterase insecticide poisoning. **Adults:** 2 to 4 mg I.V. repeated q 5 to 10 minutes until muscarinic symptoms disappear or signs of atropine toxicity appear. Severe poisoning may require up to 6 mg q 1 hour. **Children:** 1 mg I.V. or I.M. then 0.5 to 1 mg I.V. or I.M. q 5 to 10 minutes until muscarinic signs disappear or signs of atropine toxicity appear.
- Preoperatively for diminishing secretions and blocking cardiac vagal reflexes. **Adults:** 0.4 to 0.6 mg I.M. 45 to 60 minutes before anesthesia. **Children:** 0.01 mg/kg I.M. up to a maximum dose of 0.4 mg 45 to 60 minutes before anesthesia.
- Adjunctive treatment of peptic ulcer disease; treatment of functional GI disorders such as irritable bowel syndrome. **Adults:** 0.4 to 0.6 mg P.O. q 4 to 6 hours. **Children:** 0.01 mg/kg or 0.3 mg/m² (not to exceed 0.4 mg) q 4 to 6 hours.

Adverse reactions
Blood: leukocytosis. **CNS:** *headache, restlessness,* ataxia, disorientation, hallucinations, delirium, coma, *insomnia, dizziness;* excitement, agitation, and confusion (especially in elderly patients). **CV:** 1 to 2 mg—*tachycardia, palpitations;* greater than 2 mg—***extreme tachycardia, angina.*** **EENT:** 1 mg—*slight mydriasis,* photophobia; 2 mg—*blurred vision, mydriasis.* **GI:** *dry mouth (common even at low doses),* thirst, *constipation,* nausea, vomiting. **GU:** urine retention. **Skin:** hot, flushed skin.

Interactions
Amantadine, glutethimide, meperidine, antiarrhythmics, antiparkinsonian agents, phenothiazines, tricyclic antidepressants: additive anticholinergic effects. **Antacids:** decreased anticholinergic absorption. Separate administration times by at least 1 hour. **Digoxin:** increased digoxin levels if slow dissolving tablets are used. **Ketoconazole, levodopa:** decreased absorption. Avoid concomitant use. **Methotrimeprazine:** may produce extrapyramidal symptoms. **Potassium chloride wax-matrix tablets:** increased risk of mucosal lesions.

Nursing diagnoses
- Decreased cardiac output related to ineffectiveness of atropine therapy.
- Altered protection related to atropine-induced tachycardia.
- Knowledge deficit related to atropine therapy.

Nursing interventions
- *Contraindicated* in narrow-angle glaucoma, obstructive uropathy, obstructive disease of GI tract, myasthenia gravis, paralytic ileus, intestinal atony, unstable CV status in acute hemorrhage, and toxic megacolon.
- *Use cautiously* in Down's syndrome patients because they may be more sensitive to drug.
- Watch for tachycardia in cardiac patients. It may precipitate ventricular fibrillation.
- Other anticholinergic drugs may increase vagal blockage.
- **I.V. use:** Administer by direct I.V. into a large vein or I.V. tubing over at least 1 to 2 minutes.
- When given I.V., atropine may cause paradoxical initial bradycardia, especially when small doses (0.4 to 0.6 mg) are given. This usually disappears within 2 minutes.
- Monitor closely for urine retention in elderly men with benign prostatic hypertrophy.

General

Classification: antidepressant (triazolopyridine). **Pregnancy risk category:** C.

Mechanism of action

Inhibits serotonin uptake in the brain. Not a tricyclic derivative; considered an atypical antidepressant.

Indications and dosage

• Treatment of depression. **Adults:** initial dosage is 150 mg P.O. daily in divided doses, which can be increased by 50 mg daily q 3 to 4 days. Average dosage ranges from 150 mg to 400 mg daily. Maximum dosage is 600 mg.

Adverse reactions

CNS: *drowsiness, dizziness,* nervousness, fatigue, confusion, tremors, weakness. **CV:** orthostatic hypotension, tachycardia. **EENT:** blurred vision, tinnitus. **GI:** dry mouth, constipation, nausea, vomiting, anorexia. **GU:** urine retention, priapism possibly leading to impotence. **Skin:** rash, urticaria. **Other:** sweating.

Interactions

Alcohol, CNS depressants: enhanced CNS depression. Use together cautiously. **Antihypertensives:** added hypotensive effect of trazodone. Antihypertensive dosage may have to be decreased. **Digoxin, phenytoin:** trazodone may increase serum levels of these drugs. Monitor for toxicity. **MAO inhibitors:** No clinical experience. Use together very cautiously.

Nursing diagnoses

• Ineffective individual coping related to the patient's underlying condition.
• High risk for injury related to adverse CNS reactions to trazodone.
• Knowledge deficit related to trazodone therapy.

Nursing interventions

• *Contraindicated* during initial recovery phase of MI and with concurrent administration with electroshock therapy. Drug may be discontinued before surgery.
• *Use cautiously* in cardiac disease and in suicidal patients.
• Priapism is a potential problem in men taking trazodone. Be sure to note if patient complains of prolonged and painful erections. May need surgical intervention.
• Watch for suicidal tendencies and record mood changes. Allow minimum amount of tablets to lessen suicide risk.
• Teach family how to recognize signs of suicidal tendency or ideation.
• Warn patient to avoid activities that require alertness until CNS effects of the drug are known. Drowsiness and dizziness usually subside after the first few weeks.
• Administer after meals or a light snack for optimal absorption and to decrease incidence of dizziness.
• Anticholinergic and adverse cardiac effects are minimal.
• Full effect may take 4 weeks or more.

General

Classification: antirheumatic (gold derivative).
Pregnancy risk category: C.

Mechanism of action

Anti-inflammatory effects in rheumatoid arthritis are probably caused by inhibition of sulfhydryl systems, which alters cellular metabolism. Auranofin may also alter enzyme function and immune response and suppress phagocytic activity.

Indications and dosage

- Rheumatoid arthritis. **Adults:** 6 mg P.O. daily, administered either as 3 mg b.i.d. or 6 mg/day. After 6 months, may be increased to 9 mg/day.

Adverse reactions

Blood: ***thrombocytopenia*** (with or without purpura), ***aplastic anemia, agranulocytosis,*** leukopenia, eosinophilia. **GI:** *diarrhea, abdominal pain, nausea, vomiting, stomatitis,* enterocolitis, anorexia, metallic taste, dyspepsia, flatulence. **GU:** proteinuria, hematuria, nephrotic syndrome, glomerulonephritis. **Hepatic:** jaundice, elevated liver enzymes. **Respiratory:** interstitial pneumonitis. **Skin:** *rash, pruritus, dermatitis,* ***exfoliative dermatitis.***

Interactions

Phenytoin: auranofin may increase phenytoin blood levels. Monitor for toxicity.

Nursing diagnoses

- Pain (arthritic) related to patient's underlying condition.
- High risk for fluid volume deficit related to adverse GI reactions to auranofin.
- Knowledge deficit related to auranofin therapy.

Nursing interventions

- *Contraindicated* in patients with history of necrotizing enterocolitis, pulmonary fibrosis, exfoliative dermatitis, bone marrow aplasia, or severe hematologic disorders.
- *Use cautiously* with other drugs that cause blood dyscrasias. Also use cautiously in patients who have preexisting renal disease, liver disease, inflammatory bowel disease, and skin rash.
- Remind patients to see their doctors on schedule for monthly platelet counts. Auranofin should be discontinued if platelet count falls below 100,000/mm^3, if hemoglobin drops suddenly, if granulocytes are below 1,500/mm^3, and if leukopenia (WBC count below 4,000/mm^3) or eosinophilia (eosinophils greater than 75%) is present.
- Reassure patient that beneficial drug effect may be delayed as long as 3 months. However, if response is inadequate after 3 months and after maximum dose is reached, doctor will probably discontinue auranofin.
- Tell patient to continue taking concomitant drug therapy, such as NSAIDs, if prescribed.
- Regular urinalysis is advisable. If proteinuria or hematuria is detected, discontinue drug because it can produce a nephrotic syndrome or glomerulonephritis.
- Diarrhea is the most common adverse reaction. Tell patient to continue taking this drug if he experiences mild diarrhea; however, if he notes blood in his stool, he should contact his doctor.
- Dermatitis is also common. Advise patient to report any rashes or other skin problems immediately. Pruritus often precedes dermatitis and should be considered a warning of impending skin reactions. Any pruritic skin eruption while a patient is receiving auranofin should be considered a reaction to this drug until proven otherwise. Therapy is stopped until reaction subsides.
- Stomatitis is another common adverse reaction. Tell patient that stomatitis is often preceded by a metallic taste. Advise him to report this symptom to his doctor immediately. Careful oral hygiene is recommended during therapy.
- Auranofin, like injectable gold preparations, should be prescribed only for selected rheumatoid arthritis patients. Warn your patient *not* to give the drug to others.

General

Classification: antidepressant (MAO inhibitor).
Pregnancy risk category: C.

Mechanism of action

Promotes accumulation of neurotransmitters by inhibiting MAO.

Indications and dosage

• Treatment of depression. **Adults:** 10 mg P.O. b.i.d. Increase to maximum of 30 mg daily, if necessary, after 2 weeks. Not recommended for children under 16 years.

Adverse reactions

CNS: *dizziness,* vertigo, headache, overactivity, hyperreflexia, tremors, muscle twitching, mania, jitters, confusion, memory impairment, fatigue. **CV:** *orthostatic hypotension,* ***arrhythmias,*** paradoxical hypertension. **EENT:** blurred vision. **GI:** dry mouth, *anorexia,* nausea, diarrhea, constipation, abdominal pain. **GU:** impotence. **Skin:** rash. **Other:** peripheral edema, sweating, weight changes, chills, altered libido.

Interactions

Alcohol, barbiturates, and other sedatives; narcotics; dextromethorphan; TCAs: use with caution and in reduced dosage. **Amphetamines, antihistamines, ephedrine, levodopa, meperidine, metaraminol, methotrimeprazine, methylphenidate, phenylephrine, phenylpropanolamine, sympathomimetics:** pressor effects of these drugs are enhanced by tranylcypromine. Avoid concomitant use. **Insulin, oral antidiabetic agents:** tranylcypromine may alter requirements of antidiabetic medications.

Nursing diagnoses

• Ineffective individual coping related to the patient's underlying condition.
• High risk for injury related to tranylcypromine-induced dizziness or orthostatic hypotension.
• Knowledge deficit related to tranylcypromine therapy.

Nursing interventions

• *Contraindicated* in severe hepatic or renal impairment; CHF; pheochromocytoma, hypertension, or cardiovascular or cerebrovascular disease; severe or frequent headaches; in patients taking antihypertensives or diuretics; in elderly or debilitated patients; in patients for whom close supervision is not possible; and in hyperactive, agitated, or schizophrenic patients. Also contraindicated with foods containing tryptophan or tyramine; during therapy with other MAO inhibitors (phenelzine, isocarboxazid) or within 7 days of such therapy; and within 7 days of elective surgery requiring general anesthetic, cocaine, or local anesthetic containing sympathomimetic vasoconstrictors.
• *Use cautiously* with antiparkinsonian drugs or spinal anesthetics; in renal disease, diabetes, seizure disorder, Parkinson's disease, and hyperthyroidism; and in those at risk for suicide.
• Warn patients with angina to moderate activities to avoid overexertion.
• Obtain baseline blood pressure readings, CBC, and liver function tests before beginning therapy, and monitor throughout treatment.
• If patient develops symptoms of overdose (palpitations, severe hypotension, or frequent headaches), hold dose and notify doctor.
• Watch for suicidal tendencies.
• Have phentolamine (Regitine) available to combat severe hypertension.
• Warn patient to avoid foods high in tyramine or tryptophan (aged cheese, Chianti wine, beer, chocolate, bananas, salami, bologna) and caffeine.
• Severe effects can occur if MAO inhibitors are taken with OTC cold, hay fever, or diet preparations.
• To prevent orthostatic hypotension, tell patient to get out of bed slowly, sitting up for 1 minute.
• Don't withdraw drug abruptly. Continue precautions for 7 days after stopping drug.
• Expect delay of 2 weeks or more before noticeable effect; 4 weeks or more before full effect.

General

Classification: antirheumatic (gold derivative).
Pregnancy risk category: C.

Mechanism of action

Anti-inflammatory effects in rheumatoid arthritis are probably caused by inhibition of sulfhydryl systems, which alters cellular metabolism. Gold salts may also alter enzyme function and immune response and suppress phagocytic activity.

Indications and dosage

• Rheumatoid arthritis. **Adults:** Drug is given once weekly by I.M. injection. For the first dose, give 10 mg I.M., followed by 25 mg I.M. as a single dose for weeks 2 and 3. If tolerated, increase to 50 mg by week 4. Continue once weekly injections of 50 mg until a cumulative dose of 800 mg to 1g has been administered (usually 18 to 22 weeks). If the patient has improved and there are no signs of toxicity, decrease frequency to once every 3 or 4 weeks. If the patient hasn't improved, reevaluated the need for gold therapy. Never give more than 50 mg weekly. **Children age 6 to 12 years:** Givc one-fourth of the adult dosage, based upon the above schedule. Maximum single dose is 25 mg.

Adverse reactions

Adverse reactions to gold are potentially severe and life-threatening. **Blood:** ***thrombocytopenia, aplastic anemia, agranulocytosis,*** leukopenia, eosinophilia. **CNS:** *dizziness,* syncope, sweating. **CV:** bradycardia, hypotension. **EENT:** corneal gold deposition, corneal ulcers. **GI:** *metallic taste, stomatitis,* difficulty swallowing, nausea, vomiting. **GU:** albuminuria, proteinuria, ***nephrotic syndrome,*** nephritis, acute tubular necrosis. **Hepatic:** hepatitis, jaundice. **Skin:** *rash, pruritus, and dermatitis in 20% of patients. (If drug not stopped, may lead to fatal* ***exfoliative dermatitis.****)* **Other:** ***anaphylaxis, angioneurotic edema.***

Interactions

Phenytoin: may increase phenytoin blood levels.

Nursing diagnoses

• Pain (joint) related to patient's underlying condition.
• Altered oral mucous membrane related to aurothioglucose-induced adverse reactions.
• Knowledge deficit related to aurothioglucose therapy.

Nursing interventions

• *Contraindicated* in severe uncontrollable diabetes, renal disease, hepatic dysfunction, hypertension, heart failure, systemic lupus erythematosus, Sjögren's syndrome, and skin rash.
• *Use cautiously* with other drugs that cause blood dyscrasias.
• Usually reserved for rheumatoid arthritis that has not responded adequately to salicylates, rest, and physical therapy.
• Administer all gold salts I.M., preferably intragluteally.
• Observe patient for 15 minutes after administration because of possible anaphylactoid reaction.
• Inform patient that benefits of therapy may not appear for 3 to 4 months or longer.
• Patient should remain recumbent for 10 minutes after injection.
• CBC, including platelet count, should be performed before every second injection.
• Dermatitis is the most common adverse reaction. Pruritus often precedes dermatitis and should be considered a warning of impending skin reactions. Therapy is stopped until reaction subsides.
• Stomatitis is the second most common adverse reaction to gold therapy. Advise patient that stomatitis is often preceded by a metallic taste.
• Platelet counts should be performed if patient develops purpura or ecchymoses.
• Serious adverse reactions are usually treated with high-dose corticosteroids such as prednisone, 40 to 100 mg P.O. daily in divided doses.

tolmetin sodium

Tolectin, Tolectin DS

General

Classification: nonnarcotic analgesic, antipyretic, anti-inflammatory (NSAID). **Pregnancy risk category:** B (D in 3rd trimester).

Mechanism of action

Produces anti-inflammatory, analgesic, and antipyretic effects, possibly through inhibition of prostaglandin synthesis.

Indications and dosage

- Rheumatoid arthritis, osteoarthritis, gout, dysmenorrhea, juvenile rheumatoid arthritis. **Adults:** 400 mg P.O. t.i.d. or q.i.d. Maximum dosage is 2 g daily. **Children 2 years or over:** 15 to 30 mg/kg P.O. daily in divided doses.

Adverse reactions

Blood: prolonged bleeding time. **CNS:** headache, dizziness, drowsiness. **GI:** *epigastric distress,* ***peptic ulceration,*** *occult blood loss, nausea.* **GU:** ***nephrotoxicity,*** pseudoproteinuria. **Skin:** rash, urticaria, pruritus. **Other:** sodium retention, edema.

Interactions

Oral anticoagulants: increased risk of bleeding. Monitor patient closely.

Nursing diagnoses

- Pain related to the patient's underlying condition.
- Impaired tissue integrity related to peptic ulceration, a possible adverse reaction to therapy.
- Knowledge deficit related to tolmetin therapy.

Nursing interventions

- *Contraindicated* in patients with hypersensitivity to the drug, other NSAIDs, or aspirin.
- *Use cautiously* in cardiac and renal disease, GI bleeding, and history of peptic ulcer disease.
- Serious GI toxicity can occur at any time in patients taking chronic NSAID therapy. Teach patient signs and symptoms of GI bleeding and tell him to report these immediately.
- Tell patient to notify doctor immediately if any visual or hearing changes occur. During prolonged therapy, patients should have regular eye examinations, hearing tests, CBCs, and renal function tests to monitor for toxicity.
- Give with food, milk, or antacids to reduce adverse GI reactions.
- Tell patient therapeutic effect should begin within 1 week, but full effect may be delayed 2 to 4 weeks.
- Prolonged therapy requires periodic eye examinations and liver and renal function studies.
- Tolmetin may interfere with certain tests for urinary proteins; it does not interfere with dye-impregnated reagent strips.
- Because of their antipyretic and anti-inflammatory actions, NSAIDs may mask the signs and symptoms of infection.

General

Classification: antiallergy agent (piperidine antihistamine). **Pregnancy risk category:** B.

Mechanism of action

Competes with histamine for H_1-receptor sites on effector cells. Prevents but does not reverse histamine-mediated responses.

Indications and dosage

- Rhinitis, allergy symptoms, chronic urticaria. **Adults:** 1 to 2 mg P.O. b.i.d. Maximum dosage is 4 mg daily. Not intended for children under 12.

Adverse reactions

Blood: thrombocytopenia. **CNS:** (especially in elderly patients) *drowsiness, dizziness,* vertigo, disturbed coordination. **CV:** hypotension, palpitations. **GI:** anorexia, nausea, vomiting, *dry mouth and throat,* epigastric distress. **GU:** urine retention. **Skin:** urticaria, rash. **Other:** thick bronchial secretions.

Interactions

CNS depressants: increased sedation. Use together cautiously. **MAO inhibitors:** increased anticholinergic effects. Don't use together.

Nursing diagnoses

- Ineffective airway clearance related to the patient's underlying condition.
- High risk for injury related to azatadine-induced adverse CNS reactions.
- Knowledge deficit related to azatadine therapy.

Nursing interventions

- *Contraindicated* in acute asthmatic attacks.
- *Use cautiously* in elderly patients and in increased intraocular pressure, hyperthyroidism, CV or renal disease, hypertension, bronchial asthma, urine retention, prostatic hypertrophy, bladder-neck obstruction, and stenosing peptic ulcers.
- Warn patient against drinking alcoholic beverages during therapy and against activities that require alertness until CNS response to drug is determined.
- Reduce GI distress by giving with food or milk.
- Coffee or tea may reduce drowsiness. Sugarless gum, sour hard candy, or ice chips may relieve dry mouth.
- If tolerance develops, another antihistamine may be substituted.
- Warn patient to stop taking drug 4 days before allergy skin tests to preserve accuracy of tests.
- Monitor blood counts during long-term therapy; watch for signs of blood dyscrasias.
- Antihistamines are not recommended for use by women who are breast-feeding because small amounts of drug are excreted in breast milk.

General

Classification: antidiabetic agent (sulfonylurea).
Pregnancy risk category: C.

Mechanism of action

Stimulates insulin release from the pancreatic beta cells and reduces glucose output by the liver. An extrapancreatic effect increases peripheral sensitivity to insulin.

Indications and dosage

- Stable, maturity-onset (Type II) nonketotic diabetes mellitus uncontrolled by diet alone and previously untreated. **Adults:** initially, 1 to 2 g P.O. daily as single dose or divided b.i.d. to t.i.d. May adjust dosage to maximum of 3 g daily.
- Change from insulin to oral therapy. **Adults:** if insulin dosage is under 20 units daily, insulin may be stopped and oral therapy started at 1 to 2 g P.O. daily. If insulin dosage is 20 to 40 units daily, insulin is reduced 30% to 50% and oral therapy started as above. If insulin dosage is over 40 units daily, insulin is decreased 20% and oral therapy started as above. Further reductions based on patient's response to oral therapy.

Adverse reactions

GI: nausea, heartburn. **Metabolic:** ***hypoglycemia, dilutional hyponatremia.*** **Skin:** rash, pruritus, facial flushing. **Other:** ***hypersensitivity reactions.***

Interactions

Alcohol: with moderate to large intake, possible disulfiram reaction. Avoid concomitant use. **Anabolic steroids, chloramphenicol, clofibrate, guanethidine, MAO inhibitors, phenylbutazone, salicylates, sulfonamides:** increased hypoglycemic activity. Monitor blood glucose level. **Beta blockers, clonidine:** prolonged hypoglycemic effect and masked symptoms of hypoglycemia. Use together cautiously. **Corticosteroids, glucagon, rifampin, thiazide diuretics:** decreased hypoglycemic response. Monitor blood glucose level. **Hydantoins:** increased blood levels of hydantoins. Monitor blood levels closely. **Oral anticoagulants:** increased hypoglycemic activity or enhanced anticoagulant effect. Monitor blood glucose and PT.

Nursing diagnoses

- Altered nutrition: More than body requirements, related to inability to produce sufficient insulin to maintain normal blood glucose levels.
- High risk for injury related to tolbutamide-induced hypoglycemia.
- Knowledge deficit related to tolbutamide therapy.

Nursing interventions

- *Contraindicated* for treating type I diabetes (insulin-dependent); diabetes adequately controlled by diet; and type II diabetes (non-insulin-dependent) complicated by fever, ketosis, acidosis, coma, major surgery, severe trauma, Raynaud's disease, renal or hepatic impairment, or thyroid or other endocrine dysfunction; and during pregnancy or breast-feeding.
- *Use cautiously* in patients with sulfonamide hypersensitivity.
- Instruct patient about nature of disease; importance of following therapeutic regimen, adhering to specific diet, weight reduction, exercise, and personal hygiene program, and avoiding infection; how and when to perform self-monitoring of blood glucose level; and recognition of hypoglycemia and hyperglycemia.
- Patient transferring from another oral sulfonylurea antidiabetic drug usually needs no transition period.
- Patient transferring from insulin therapy to an oral hypoglycemic should test for blood glucose at least t.i.d. before meals. Hospitalization may be required during the transition.
- Teach patient not to change drug dosage without the doctor's approval and to report abnormal blood or urine glucose tests.
- Advise patient to check with doctor before taking any other medication, including OTC drugs.

azathioprine Imuran

General
Classification: immunosupressive (purine agonist). **Pregnancy risk category:** D.

Mechanism of action
Inhibits purine synthesis.

Indications and dosage
- Immunosuppression in renal transplants. **Adults and children:** initially, 3 to 5 mg/kg P.O. or I.V. (sodium) daily usually beginning on the day of transplantation. Maintain at 1 to 3 mg/kg daily (dosage varies considerably according to patient response).
- Treatment of severe, refractory rheumatoid arthritis. **Adults:** initially, 1 mg/kg P.O. taken as a single dose or as two doses. If patient response is not satisfactory after 6 to 8 weeks, dosage may be increased by 0.5 mg/kg daily (up to a maximum of 2.5 mg/kg daily) at 4-week intervals.

Adverse reactions
Blood: ***leukopenia, bone marrow suppression,*** anemia, ***pancytopenia, thrombocytopenia.*** **GI:** nausea, vomiting, anorexia, ***pancreatitis,*** steatorrhea, mouth ulceration, esophagitis. **Hepatic:** ***hepatotoxicity,*** jaundice. **Skin:** rash. **Other:** ***immunosuppression (possibly profound),*** arthralgia, muscle wasting, alopecia.

Interactions
Allopurinol: impaired inactivation of azathioprine. Decrease azathioprine dose to ¼ or ⅓ normal dose. **Nondepolarizing neuromuscular blocking agents:** azathioprine may reverse the neuromuscular blockade.

Nursing diagnoses
- Altered protection related to the threat of organ rejection.
- High risk for infection related to azathioprine-induced immunosuppression.
- Knowledge deficit related to azathioprine therapy.

Nursing interventions
- *Contraindicated* in patients with hypersensitivity to the drug.
- *Use cautiously* in hepatic or renal dysfunction.
- Watch for clay-colored stools, dark urine, pruritus, and yellow skin and sclera and for increased alkaline phosphatase, bilirubin, AST, and ALT levels.
- In renal homotransplants, start drug 1 to 5 days before surgery.
- Hemoglobin, WBC, and platelet counts should be done at least once monthly; more often at beginning of treatment. Drug should be stopped immediately when WBC count is less than 3,000/mm^3, to prevent irreversible bone marrow suppression.
- Azathioprine is a potent immunosuppressive. Warn patient to report even mild infections (colds, fever, sore throat, and malaise).
- **I.V. use:** Only for patients unable to tolerate oral medications. Reconstitute 100-mg vial with 10 ml of sterile water for injection. Visually inspect for particles before giving. Drug may be administered by direct I.V. injection or further diluted in 0.9% sodium chloride solution or D_5W and infused over 30 to 60 minutes.
- Instruct patient to avoid conception during therapy and for 4 months after stopping therapy.
- Warn patient that some thinning of hair is possible.
- Avoid I.M. injections of any drugs in patients with severely depressed platelet counts (thrombocytopenia) to prevent bleeding.
- Therapeutic response usually occurs within 8 weeks. When used for refractory rheumatoid arthritis, inform patient that it may take up to 12 weeks to be effective.

General

Classification: antihypertensive (peripheral vasodilator, alpha-adrenergic blocker). **Pregnancy risk category:** C.

Mechanism of action

Direct-acting vasodilator. May have some alpha-receptor blocking effects.

Indications and dosage

• Persistent pulmonary hypertension of the newborn. **Neonates:** initially, 1 to 2 mg/kg I.V. over 10 minutes, followed by infusion of 1 to 2 mg/kg/hour.
• Peripheral vasospastic disorders. **Adults:** 10 to 50 mg I.M. or I.V. q.i.d.

Adverse reactions

CV: ***arrhythmias,*** anginal pain, *hypertension, flushing,* transient postural vertigo, palpitations, *orthostatic hypotension.* **GI:** *nausea, vomiting, diarrhea, epigastric discomfort, exacerbation of peptic ulcer.* **Local:** burning at injection site. **Other:** weakness, paradoxical response in seriously damaged limbs, increased pilomotor activity, tingling, chilliness, apprehension, pulmonary hemorrhage.

Interactions

Ethyl alcohol: possible disulfiram reaction from accumulation of acetaldehyde. Use together cautiously. **Vasopressors (epinephrine, norepinephrine):** may cause a paradoxical fall in blood pressure.

Nursing diagnoses

• Altered cardiopulmonary tissue perfusion related to the patient's underlying condition.
• High risk for injury related to adverse drug reaction.
• Knowledge deficit related to tolazoline therapy.

Nursing interventions

• *Contraindicated* in coronary artery disease or active peptic ulcer, or following CVA.
• *Use cautiously* in patients with history of peptic ulcer disease, gastritis, or known or suspected mitral stenosis.
• **I.V. use:** Response to treatment of persistent pulmonary hypertension of the newborn should be evident within 30 minutes. There is little information regarding infusions lasting longer than 48 hours.
• Keep patient warm during parenteral administration to increase response.
• Patient should be supine during infusion.
• Appearance of flushing usually indicates maximum tolerable dose.
• Monitor vital signs. Watch especially for blood pressure changes and arrhythmias.
• Instruct patient to avoid sudden posture changes to minimize risks of orthostatic hypotension.
• Instruct patient to avoid alcohol; chills and flushing may occur.
• Warn patient against exposure to cold, which can aggravate tissue damage.
• Often used to distinguish between functional (vasospastic) and organic (obstructive) forms of peripheral vascular disease.

General

Classification: macrolide antibiotic (erythromycin derivative). **Pregnancy risk category:** B.

Mechanism of action

Binds to the 50S subunit of bacterial ribosomes, blocking protein synthesis. Bacteriostatic or bactericidal, depending on concentration.

Indications and dosage

• Acute bacterial exacerbations of COPD caused by *Haemophilus influenzae, Moraxella (Branhamella) catarrhalis,* or *Streptococcus pneumoniae;* mild community-acquired pneumonia caused by *H. influenzae* or *S. pneumoniae;* uncomplicated skin and skin structure infections caused by *Staphylococcus aureus, Streptococcus pyogenes,* or *S. agalactiae;* second-line therapy of pharyngitis or tonsillitis caused by *S. pyogenes.* **Adults and adolescents 16 years and over:** initially, 500 mg P.O. as a single dose on day 1, followed by 250 mg daily on days 2 through 5. Total dose is 1.5 g.
• Nongonococcal urethritis or cervicitis caused by *Chlamydia trachomatis.* **Adults and adolescents 16 years and over:** 1 g P.O. as a single dose.

Adverse reactions

CNS: dizziness, vertigo, headache, fatigue, somnolence. **CV:** palpitations, chest pain. **GI:** *nausea, vomiting, diarrhea, abdominal pain,* dyspepsia, flatulence, melena, cholestatic jaundice. **GU:** monilia, vaginitis, nephritis. **Skin:** rash, photosensitivity. **Other:** angioedema, pseudomembranous colitis.

Interactions

Aluminum- and magnesium-containing antacids: lower peak plasma levels of azithromycin. Separate administration times by at least 2 hours. **Theophylline:** other macrolides may increase plasma theophylline levels; effect of azithromycin is unknown. Monitor theophylline levels carefully. **Warfarin:** other macrolides may increase prothrombin time (PT); effect of azithromycin is unknown. Monitor PT carefully.

Nursing diagnoses

• High risk for injury related to ineffectiveness of azithromycin to eradicate the infection.
• High risk for fluid volume deficit related to azithromycin-induced adverse GI reactions.
• Knowledge deficit related to azithromycin therapy.

Nursing interventions

• *Contraindicated* in patients with hypersensitivity to erythromycin or other macrolides. Do not use azithromycin to treat gonorrhea or syphilis; moderate-to-severe pneumonia in patients for whom outpatient oral therapy is inappropriate; nosocomial infections; known or suspected bacteremia; conditions requiring hospitalization; elderly or debilitated patients; or immunocompromised patients (for example, those with cancer or AIDS).
• *Use cautiously* in patients with impaired hepatic function.
• Obtain culture and sensitivity tests before first dose. Therapy can begin before results are obtained.
• Administer 1 hour before or 2 hours after a meal, and do not administer with antacids. Remind patient that the drug should always be taken on an empty stomach because food or antacids will decrease absorption.
• May cause overgrowth of nonsusceptible bacteria or fungi. Monitor for signs and symptoms of superinfection.
• Tell patient to take all of the medication prescribed, even after he feels better.

General

Classification: antidiabetic agent (sulfonylurea). **Pregnancy risk category:** C.

Mechanism of action

Stimulates insulin release from the pancreatic beta cells and reduces glucose output by the liver. An extrapancreatic effect increases peripheral sensitivity to insulin.

Indications and dosage

- Adjunct to diet to lower the blood glucose in patients with non-insulin-dependent diabetes mellitus (type II). **Adults:** initially, 100 mg P.O. daily with breakfast if fasting blood sugar (FBS) is under 200 mg/dl; or 250 mg if FBS is over 200 mg/dl. May adjust dosage at weekly intervals by 100 to 250 mg. Maximum dosage is 500 mg b.i.d. before meals. **Adults over 65:** 100 mg P.O. once daily.
- Change from insulin to oral therapy. **Adults:** if insulin dosage is under 20 units daily, insulin may be stopped and oral therapy started at 100 mg P.O. daily with breakfast. If insulin dosage is 20 to 40 units daily, insulin may be stopped and oral therapy started at 250 mg P.O. daily with breakfast. If insulin dosage is over 40 units daily, decrease insulin 50% and start oral therapy at 250 mg P.O. daily with breakfast. Increase dosages as above.

Adverse reactions

GI: nausea, vomiting. **Metabolic:** ***hypoglycemia.*** **Skin:** rash, urticaria, facial flushing. **Other:** ***hypersensitivity reactions.***

Interactions

Alcohol: with moderate to large intake, possible disulfiram-like reaction. Avoid concomitant use. **Anabolic steroids, chloramphenicol, clofibrate, guanethidine, MAO inhibitors, phenylbutazone, salicylates, sulfonamides:** increased hypoglycemic activity. Monitor blood glucose level. **Beta blockers, clonidine:** prolonged hypoglycemic effect and masked symptoms of hypoglycemia. Use together cautiously. **Corticosteroids, glucagon, rifampin, thiazide diuretics:** decreased hypoglycemic response. Monitor blood glucose level. **Hydantoins:** increased blood levels of hydantoins. Monitor blood levels closely. **Oral anticoagulants:** increased hypoglycemic activity or enhanced anticoagulant effect. Monitor blood glucose and prothrombin time.

Nursing diagnoses

- Altered nutrition: More than body requirements, related to the patient's inability to release sufficient insulin to maintain normal blood glucose levels.
- High risk for injury related to tolazamide-induced hypoglycemia.
- Knowledge deficit related to tolazamide therapy.

Nursing interventions

- *Contraindicated* for treating type I diabetes (insulin-dependent); diabetes adequately controlled by diet; and type II diabetes (non-insulin-dependent) complicated by fever, ketosis, acidosis, coma, major surgery, severe trauma, Raynaud's disease, renal or hepatic impairment, or thyroid or other endocrine dysfunction; and during pregnancy or breast-feeding.
- *Use cautiously* in sulfonamide hypersensitivity and in elderly, debilitated, or malnourished patients.
- Instruct patient about nature of disease; importance of following therapeutic regimen, adhering to specific diet, weight reduction, exercise, and personal hygiene programs, and avoiding infection; how and when to perform self-monitoring of blood glucose level; and recognition of hypoglycemia and hyperglycemia.
- Patient transferring from another oral sulfonylurea antidiabetic drug usually needs no transition period. Patient transferring from insulin therapy to an oral antidiabetic agent should test for blood glucose at least t.i.d. before meals. Hospitalization may be required during the transition.
- Teach patient not to change drug dosage without the doctor's orders and to report abnormal blood or urine glucose tests.
- Advise patient to carry a medical identification bracelet identifying him as a diabetic patient.

aztreonam Azactam

General
Classification: antibiotic (monobactam). **Pregnancy risk category:** B.

Mechanism of action
Bactericidal; inhibits bacterial cell wall synthesis, ultimately causing cell wall destruction.

Indications and dosage
• Treatment of urinary tract infections, lower respiratory tract infections, septicemia, skin and skin structure infections, intra-abdominal infections, surgical infections, and gynecologic infections caused by various aerobic organisms. **Adults:** 500 mg to 2 g I.V. or I.M. q 8 to 12 hours. For severe systemic or life-threatening infections, 2 g q 6 to 8 hours may be given. Maximum dosage is 8 g daily.

Adverse reactions
Blood: neutropenia, anemia. **CNS:** ***seizures,*** headache, insomnia. **CV:** hypotension. **GI:** diarrhea, nausea, vomiting. **Hepatic:** transient elevations of AST and ALT. **Local:** thrombophlebitis at I.V. site, discomfort and swelling at I.M. injection site. **Other:** hypersensitivity, ***anaphylaxis,*** altered taste, halitosis, rash.

Interactions
Furosemide, probenecid: increased serum aztreonam levels. Avoid concomitant use.

Nursing diagnoses
• High risk for injury related to ineffectiveness of aztreonam to eradicate the infection.
• High risk for fluid volume deficit related to adverse GI reactions to aztreonam.
• Knowledge deficit related to aztreonam therapy.

Nursing interventions
• *Use cautiously* in elderly patients and in impaired renal function.
• Aztreonam is the first commercially available member of a newer antibiotic family, the monobactams. Its effectiveness against gram-negative organisms is comparable to that of the aminoglycoside antibiotics, without the ototoxicity or nephrotoxicity usually associated with aminoglycosides.
• Aztreonam is a narrow-spectrum antibiotic, effective solely against gram-negative organisms. Because it is ineffective against gram-positive and anaerobic organisms, aztreonam must be used with other antibiotics for immediate treatment of life-threatening illnesses.
• Patients who are allergic to penicillins or cephalosporins may not be allergic to aztreonam since there is no cross-allergenicity. However, closely monitor patients who have had an immediate hypersensitivity reaction to these antibiotics.
• **I.V. use:** To administer a bolus of aztreonam, inject drug slowly (over 3 to 5 minutes) directly into a vein or I.V. tubing. Give infusions over 20 minutes to 1 hour.
• I.M. injections should be given deep into a large muscle mass, such as the upper outer quadrant of the gluteus maximus or the lateral part of the thigh. Doses greater than 1 g should be given I.V.
• Obtain specimen for culture and sensitivity tests before first dose. Therapy may begin pending test results.
• Watch for superinfection (fever or other signs of new infection).

General

Classification: antiarrhythmic (local amide anesthetic). **Pregnancy risk category:** C.

Mechanism of action

A class Ib antiarrhythmic that depresses phase 0 and shortens the action potential. All class I drugs have membrane stabilizing effects.

Indications and dosage

• Suppression of symptomatic ventricular arrhythmias, including frequent premature ventricular contractions and ventricular tachycardia. **Adults:** initially, 400 mg P.O. q 8 hours. Usual dosage is between 1,200 and 1,800 mg daily in three divided doses.

Adverse reactions

Blood: ***blood dyscrasias, including aplastic anemia.*** **CNS:** *light-headedness, tremor,* restlessness, paresthesia, confusion, dizziness. **CV:** hypotension, ***new or worsened arrhythmias, CHF.*** **EENT:** blurred vision. **GI:** *nausea, vomiting, epigastric pain,* constipation, diarrhea, anorexia. **Hepatic:** hepatitis. **Respiratory:** ***respiratory arrest,*** pulmonary fibrosis, pneumonitis, ***pulmonary edema.*** **Skin:** rash.

Interactions

Beta blockers: decreased myocardial contractility; increased CNS toxicity.

Nursing diagnoses

• Decreased cardiac output related to ineffectiveness of tocainide therapy.
• Altered protection related to tocainide-induced proarrhythmias.
• Knowledge deficit related to tocainide therapy.

Nursing interventions

• *Contraindicated* in patients with hypersensitivity to lidocaine or other amide-type local anesthetics and in patients with second- or third-degree AV block in the absence of a ventricular pacemaker.
• *Use cautiously* in CHF or diminished cardiac reserve and in hepatic or renal impairment. These patients may often be treated effectively with a lower dose.
• Therapeutic blood levels range from 4 to 10 mcg/ml.
• Adverse reactions are generally mild, transient, and reversible by reducing dosage. GI reactions can be minimized by taking the drug with food.
• Dizziness and falling are more likely to occur in elderly patients.
• Monitor patient for tremor, which may indicate approaching maximum dose.
• Considered by cardiologists as an "oral lidocaine." May ease transition from I.V. lidocaine to oral antiarrhythmic therapy. Monitor patient carefully during this transition period.

bacampicillin hydrochloride

Penglobe†, Spectrobid

General

Classification: antibiotic (aminopenicillin). **Pregnancy risk category:** B.

Mechanism of action

Converted to ampicillin in vivo; each mg of bacampicillin yields 623 to 727 mcg ampicillin. It is bactericidal against microorganisms by inhibiting cell wall synthesis during active multiplication. Bacteria resist bacampicillin by producing penicillinases—enzymes that hydrolyze its active form (ampicillin).

Indications and dosage

• Upper respiratory tract infections due to streptococci, pneumococci, staphylococci, and *Haemophilus influenzae;* urinary tract infections due to *Escherichia coli, Proteus mirabilis,* and *Enterococcus faecalis;* skin infections due to streptococci and susceptible staphylococci. **Adults:** 400 mg P.O. q 12 hours. **Children weighing more than 25 kg:** 25 mg/kg/day P.O. in divided doses q 12 hours.
• Lower respiratory tract or other severe infections. **Adults:** 800 mg P.O. q 12 hours. **Children weighing more than 25 kg:** 50 mg/kg/day P.O. in divided doses q 12 hours.
• Gonorrhea. **Adults:** 1.6 g plus 1 g probenecid given as a single dose. Children's dosage has not been established.

Adverse reactions

Blood: anemia, thrombocytopenia, thrombocytopenic purpura, eosinophilia, leukopenia. **GI:** *nausea,* vomiting, *diarrhea,* glossitis, stomatitis. **Other:** hypersensitivity (*erythematous maculopapular rash,* urticaria, ***anaphylaxis***), overgrowth of nonsusceptible organisms.

Interactions

Allopurinol: increased incidence of skin rash. **Probenecid:** increases blood levels of bacampicillin or other penicillins. Probenecid may be used for this purpose.

Nursing diagnoses

• High risk for injury related to ineffectiveness of bacampicillin to eradicate the infection.
• High risk for fluid volume deficit related to bacampicillin-induced adverse GI reactions.
• Knowledge deficit related to bacampicillin therapy.

Nursing interventions

• *Use cautiously* in patients with other drug allergies, especially to cephalosporins (possible cross-allergenicity), and in mononucleosis. This drug, like ampicillin, is linked to a high incidence of maculopapular rash.
• Obtain specimen for culture and sensitivity tests before first dose. Therapy may begin pending test results.
• Before giving bacampicillin, ask patient if he's had any previous allergic reactions to penicillin. However, a negative history of penicillin allergy is no guarantee against a future allergic reaction.
• Bacampicillin is especially formulated to produce high blood levels of antibiotic when administered twice daily.
• Diarrhea may occur less frequently with bacampicillin than with ampicillin.
• Tell patient to take medication even after he feels better. Entire quantity prescribed should be taken.
• Tell patient to call the doctor if rash, fever, or chills develop. A rash is the most common allergic reaction.
• With large doses and prolonged therapy, bacterial or fungal superinfections may occur, especially in elderly, debilitated, or immunosuppressed patients. Monitor closely.
• Unlike ampicillin, bacampicillin tablets may be taken with meals without fear of diminished drug absorption. Give with food to prevent GI distress. However, bacampicillin suspension should be taken on an empty stomach.
• Administer bacampicillin at least 1 hour before bacteriostatic antibiotics.

General

Classification: antibiotic (aminoglycoside). **Pregnancy risk category:** D.

Mechanism of action

Bactericidal; inhibits protein synthesis by binding directly to the 30S ribosomal subunit.

Indications and dosage

- Serious infections caused by sensitive strains of *Escherichia coli, Proteus, Klebsiella, Enterobacter, Serratia, Staphylococcus aureus, Pseudomonas, Citrobacter, Providencia.* **Adults and children with normal renal function:** 3 mg/kg I.M. or I.V. daily divided q 8 hours. Up to 5 mg/kg I.M. or I.V. daily divided q 6 to 8 hours for life-threatening infections. **Neonates under 1 week:** up to 4 mg/kg I.M. or I.V. daily divided q 12 hours. For I.V. use, dilute in 50 to 100 ml 0.9% sodium chloride solution or D_5W for adults and in less volume for children. Infuse over 20 to 60 minutes. **Patients with impaired renal function:** initial dose is same as for those with normal renal function. Subsequent doses and frequency determined by renal function and serum concentrations of tobramycin.

Adverse reactions

CNS: headache, lethargy, ***neuromuscular blockade.***
EENT: *ototoxicity (tinnitus, vertigo, hearing loss).*
GU: *nephrotoxicity (cells or casts in the urine, oliguria, proteinuria, decreased creatinine clearance, increased BUN and serum creatinine levels).* **Other:** ***hypersensitivity reactions.***

Interactions

Cephalothin: increase nephrotoxicity. Use together cautiously. **Dimenhydrinate:** may mask symptoms of ototoxicity. Use with caution. **General anesthetics, neuromuscular blocking agents:** may potentiate neuromuscular blockade. **I.V. loop diuretics (such as furosemide):** increase ototoxicity. Use cautiously. **Other aminoglycosides, amphotericin B, cisplatin, methoxyflurane:** increases nephrotoxicity. Use together cautiously. **Parenteral penicillins:** tobramycin inactivation in vitro. Don't combine in I.V.

Nursing diagnoses

- High risk for injury related to ineffectiveness of tobramycin to eradicate the infection.
- Altered urinary elimination related to tobramycin-induced nephrotoxicity.
- Knowledge deficit related to tobramycin therapy.

Nursing interventions

- *Use cautiously* in impaired renal function and in elderly patients.
- Obtain specimen for culture and sensitivity tests before first dose. Therapy may begin pending test results.
- Weigh patient and obtain baseline renal function studies before starting therapy.
- Usual duration of therapy is 7 to 10 days.
- Monitor renal function (output, specific gravity, urinalysis, BUN and creatinine levels, and creatinine clearance). Notify doctor of signs of decreasing renal function.
- Patient should be well hydrated during therapy.
- Evaluate patient's hearing before and during therapy. Notify doctor if patient complains of tinnitus, vertigo, or hearing loss.
- Watch for superinfection (continued fever and other signs of new infections).
- **I.V. use:** Dilute in 50 to 100 ml 0.9% sodium chloride or D_5W for adults and in less volume for children. Infuse over 20 to 60 minutes. After I.V. infusion, flush line with 0.9% sodium chloride or D_5W.
- Peak blood levels over 12 mcg/ml and trough levels above 2 mcg/ml may be associated with increased incidence of toxicity.
- Draw blood for peak tobramycin level 1 hour after I.M. injection and 30 minutes to 1 hour after infusion ends; draw blood for trough level just before next dose. Don't collect blood in a heparinized tube; heparin is incompatible.

bacitracin

Baciguent◇

General

Classification: topical antibiotic (polypeptide).
Pregnancy risk category: C.

Mechanism of action

Hinders bacterial cell wall synthesis, damaging the bacterial plasma membrane and making the cell more vulnerable to osmotic pressure.

Indications and dosage

• Topical infections, impetigo, abrasions, cuts, and minor burns or wounds. **Adults and children:** apply thin film b.i.d. or t.i.d. or more often, depending on severity of condition.

Adverse reactions

CV: hypotension. **Skin:** stinging, rashes, and other allergic reactions; itching, burning, swelling of lips or face. **Other:** *possible systemic adverse reactions when used over large areas for prolonged periods: potentially nephrotoxic and ototoxic; allergic reactions;* tightness in chest.

Interactions

None significant.

Nursing diagnoses

• Impaired skin integrity related to patient's underlying condition.
• Altered urinary elimination related to bacitracin-induced nephrotoxicity.
• Knowledge deficit related to bacitracin therapy.

Nursing interventions

• *Contraindicated* for use in the external ear canal if the eardrum is perforated.
• *Use cautiously* in patient with known allergic reaction to neomycin.
• Obtain baseline renal function studies before starting therapy. Monitor daily during therapy. Notify doctor of any change.
• Consider alternative treatment for burns that cover more than 20% of the patient's body surface area, especially if patient suffers impaired renal function.
• Prolonged therapy may result in overgrowth of nonsusceptible organisms, especially *Candida albicans.*

General
Classification: antihypertensive (beta-adrenergic blocker). **Pregnancy risk category:** C.

Mechanism of action
Blocks response to beta stimulation and depresses renin secretion.

Indications and dosage
• Hypertension. **Adults:** initially, 10 mg P.O. b.i.d. Usual daily maintenance dosage is 20 to 40 mg. Maximum daily dosage is 60 mg. Drug is used either alone or in combination with diuretics.
• MI (long-term prophylaxis in patients who have survived acute phase). **Adults:** Recommended dosage is 10 mg P.O. b.i.d.
• Migraine headache prophylaxis. **Adults:** initially, 20 mg P.O. daily as a single dose or in divided doses b.i.d. Increase dosage to maximum 30 mg daily as needed and tolerated. Discontinue treatment if no response after 6 to 8 weeks treatment at maximum dosage.
• Prophylaxis of angina pectoris. **Adults:** dosage is highly individualized; dosages of 15 to 45 mg P.O. daily in three or four divided doses have been used. Dosage is adjusted to maintain clinical response and keep patient's resting heart rate at 55 to 60 beats/minute.

Adverse reactions
CNS: fatigue, lethargy, vivid dreams. **CV:** *bradycardia, hypotension,* ***CHF,*** peripheral vascular disease. **GI:** nausea, vomiting, diarrhea. **Metabolic:** hypoglycemia without tachycardia. **Respiratory:** dyspnea, ***bronchospasm.*** Skin: rash. **Other:** *increased airway resistance,* fever.

Interactions
Digitalis glycosides: excessive bradycardia and increased depressant effect on myocardium. Use together cautiously. **Indomethacin:** decreased antihypertensive effect. Monitor blood pressure and adjust dosage. **Insulin, oral antidiabetic agents:** can alter requirements for these drugs in previously stabilized diabetic patients. Monitor for hypoglycemia.

Nursing diagnoses
• Altered tissue perfusion (renal, cerebral, cardiopulmonary, peripheral) related to the patient's underlying condition.
• Decreased cardiac output related to adverse CV reactions to timolol.
• Knowledge deficit related to timolol therapy.

Nursing interventions
• *Contraindicated* in diabetes mellitus, asthma, allergic rhinitis; during ethyl ether anesthesia; in sinus bradycardia and heart block greater than first degree; in cardiogenic shock; and in right ventricular failure secondary to pulmonary hypertension.
• *Use cautiously* in CHF; hepatic, renal, or respiratory disease; and in patients taking other antihypertensives.
• Always check patient's apical pulse rate before giving this drug. If you detect extremes in pulse rates, withhold medication and call the doctor immediately.
• Monitor blood pressure frequently.
• Teach patient about his disease and therapy. Explain the importance of taking drug as prescribed, even when he's feeling well. Tell patient not to discontinue drug suddenly because this can exacerbate angina and MI. Tell patient to call doctor if unpleasant adverse reactions occur.
• Instruct patient to check with doctor or pharmacist before taking OTC medications.
• This drug masks common signs of shock and hypoglycemia.
• Warn patient who is taking drug for hypertension not to increase the dose without first consulting the doctor. At least 7 days should elapse between increases in dosage.
• Do not discontinue drug abruptly. Reduce dosage gradually over 1 to 2 weeks.

General

Classification: skeletal muscle relaxant (chlorophenyl derivative). **Pregnancy risk category:** C.

Mechanism of action

Reduces transmission of impulses from the spinal cord to skeletal muscle.

Indications and dosage

• Spasticity in multiple sclerosis, spinal cord injury. **Adults:** 5 mg P.O. t.i.d. for 3 days, 10 mg t.i.d. for next 3 days, 15 mg t.i.d. for next 3 days, and 20 mg t.i.d. for next 3 days. Increase up to maximum of 80 mg daily.

• Severe spasticity in patients who don't respond to or can't tolerate oral baclofen therapy. *Screening phase:* **Adults:** After a test dose (1 ml of a 50-mcg/ml dilution administered intrathecally by barbotage over 1 minute or more), drug is administered by an implantable infusion pump. Significantly decreased severity or frequency of muscle spasm or reduced muscle tone should be evident within 8 hours. If response inadequate, give a second screening dose of 75 mcg/1.5 ml 24 hours after the first. If still inadequate, a final test dose of 100 mcg/2 ml may be given 24 hours later. *Maintenance therapy:* **Adults:** titrate initial dosage based on the screening dose that elicited an adequate response. Double this effective dose and administer over 24 hours. If screening dose efficacy maintained for 12 hours or more, don't double the dose. After the first 24 hours, increase the dose slowly as needed and tolerated by 10% to 40% daily. Maintenance dosages have ranged from 12 mcg to 1,500 mcg daily; however, experience with dosages over 1,000 mcg daily is limited. Most patients need 300 to 800 mcg daily.

Adverse reactions

CNS: *drowsiness, dizziness,* headache, *weakness, fatigue,* confusion, insomnia, dysarthria, ***seizures.*** **CV:** hypotension. **EENT:** nasal congestion, blurred vision. **GI:** *nausea,* constipation. **GU:** urinary frequency. **Hepatic:** increased AST and alkaline phosphatase. **Metabolic:** hyperglycemia. **Skin:** rash, pruritus. **Other:** ankle edema, excessive perspiration, weight gain.

Interactions

Alcohol, CNS depressants: increased CNS depression. Avoid concomitant use.

Nursing diagnoses

• Pain related to the patient's underlying condition.
• Injury related to high risk for drug-induced drowsiness.
• Knowledge deficit related to baclofen therapy.

Nursing interventions

• Orally administered drug shouldn't be used to treat muscle spasm caused by rheumatic disorders, cerebral palsy, Parkinson's disease, or CVA because efficacy hasn't been established. Don't administer intrathecal injection by I.V., I.M., S.C., or epidural route.
• *Use cautiously* in patients with impaired renal function or seizure disorder or when spasticity is used to maintain motor function.
• Tell patient to avoid activities that require alertness until CNS effects of the drug are known.
• Watch for increased incidence of seizures in patients with seizure disorder.
• Watch for sensitivity reactions, such as fever, skin eruptions, and respiratory distress.
• Don't withdraw abruptly after long-term use unless required by severe adverse reactions; may precipitate hallucinations or rebound spasticity.
• Treatment of oral overdosage is supportive only; don't induce emesis or use a respiratory stimulant in obtunded patients.
• Limited experience with long-term intrathecal use suggests that about 10% of patients may develop tolerance to the drug. In some cases, this may be treated by hospitalizing the patient and slowly withdrawing the drug over a 2-week period.
• Used investigationally for treatment of unstable bladder.

General

Classification: antibiotic (extended spectrum penicillin combined with beta-lactamase inhibitor). **Pregnancy risk category:** B.

Mechanism of action

Ticarcillin is an extended-spectrum penicillin that inhibits cell wall synthesis during active bacterial replication. Clavulanic acid increases ticarcillin's effectiveness by inactivating beta lactamases, which destroy ticarcillin.

Indications and dosage

• Infections of the lower respiratory tract, urinary tract, bones and joints, skin and skin structure, and septicemia when caused by beta-lactamase-producing strains of bacteria or by ticarcillin-susceptible organisms. **Adults:** 1 vial (ticarcillin 3 g and clavulanate potassium 0.1 g) administered by I.V. infusion q 4 to 6 hours.

Adverse reactions

Blood: leukopenia, neutropenia, eosinophilia, *thrombocytopenia,* hemolytic anemia. **CNS:** seizures, neuromuscular excitability. **GI:** nausea, diarrhea. **Metabolic:** *hypokalemia.* **Local:** pain at injection site, vein irritation, phlebitis. **Other:** hypersensitivity (rash, pruritus, urticaria, chills, fever, edema, ***anaphylaxis***), overgrowth of nonsusceptible organisms.

Interactions

Aminoglycoside antibiotics (such as gentamicin and tobramycin): chemically incompatible. Don't mix together in I.V. **Probenecid:** increases blood levels of ticarcillin. Probenecid may be used for this purpose.

Nursing diagnoses

• High risk for injury related to ineffectiveness of ticarcillin/clavulanate to eradicate the infection.
• Altered protection related to ticarcillin/clavulanate-induced allergic reaction.
• Knowledge deficit related to ticarcillin/clavulanate therapy.

Nursing interventions

• *Use cautiously* in patients with other drug allergies, especially to cephalosporins (possible cross-allergenicity), and in impaired renal function, hemorrhagic conditions, hypokalemia, or sodium restrictions.
• Obtain specimen for culture and sensitivity tests before first dose. Therapy may begin pending test results.
• Before giving Timentin, ask patient if he's had any allergic reactions to penicillin. However, a negative history of penicillin allergy is no guarantee against a future allergic reaction.
• Dosage should be decreased in patients with impaired renal functions.
• With large doses and prolonged therapy, bacterial and fungal superinfections may occur, especially in elderly, debilitated, or immunosuppressed patients. Close observation is essential.
• Check CBC and platelets frequently. Drug may cause thrombocytopenia.
• Monitor serum potassium.
• **I.V. use:** Administer by I.V. infusion over 30 minutes. Don't give by I.V. push or I.M.
• Particularly useful in clinical settings with a high prevalence of ticarcillin-resistant organisms.
• Give drug at least 1 hour before bacteriostatic antibiotics.

beclomethasone dipropionate Beclovent, Vanceril

General
Classification: anti-inflammatory, antiasthmatic (glucocorticoid). **Pregnancy risk category:** C.

Mechanism of action
Decreases inflammation, mainly by stabilizing leukocyte lysosomal membranes. Also suppresses immune response, stimulates bone marrow; influences protein, fat, carbohydrate metabolism.

Indications and dosage
• Steroid-dependent asthma. **Adults:** 2 to 4 inhalations t.i.d. or q.i.d. Maximum dosage is 20 inhalations daily. **Children 6 to 12 years:** 1 to 2 inhalations t.i.d. or q.i.d. Maximum dosage is 10 inhalations daily.

Adverse reactions
EENT: hoarseness, fungal infections of mouth and throat, throat irritation. **GI:** dry mouth.

Interactions
None significant.

Nursing diagnoses
• Ineffective airway clearance related to the patient's underlying condition.
• Altered oral mucous membrane related to drug-induced fungal infections.
• Knowledge deficit related to beclomethasone therapy.

Nursing interventions
• *Contraindicated* in status asthmaticus. Not for use in asthma controlled by bronchodilators or other noncorticosteroids alone or for nonasthmatic bronchial diseases. Also contraindicated in patients hypersensitive to any component of the formulation (fluorocarbons, oleic acid) and in patients with systemic fungal infections.
• Oral glucocorticoid therapy should be tapered slowly. Acute adrenal insufficiency and death have occurred in asthmatics who changed abruptly from oral corticosteroids to beclomethasone. Be sure patient reports symptoms associated with corticosteroid withdrawal (fatigue, weakness, arthralgia, orthostatic hypotension, and dyspnea).
• Periodic measurement of growth and development may be necessary during high-dose or prolonged therapy in children.
• During times of stress (trauma, surgery, or infection), systemic corticosteroids may be needed to prevent adrenal insufficiency in previously steroid-dependent patients.
• Instruct patient to carry a card indicating his need for supplemental systemic glucocorticoids during stress.
• Patient requiring bronchodilator should use it several minutes before beclomethasone.
• Tell patient to allow 1 minute to elapse before taking subsequent puffs of medication and to hold breath for a few seconds to enhance action of drug.
• Inform patient that drug doesn't relieve emergency asthma attacks.
• Instruct patient to contact doctor if he notices a decreased response or if symptoms don't improve within 3 weeks of initiating therapy. Dose may have to be adjusted. Patient shouldn't exceed recommended dose on his own.
• Patient can prevent oral fungal infections by gargling or rinsing mouth with water after each use of the inhaler. However, tell patient not to swallow the water. Check mucous membranes frequently for signs of fungal infection.
• Tell patient to keep inhaler clean and unobstructed. Wash with warm water; dry thoroughly.
• A spacer device may help ensure delivery of proper medication dose.
• Tell patient that before using medication or when carrying canister, to gently warm the canister to room temperature by keeping it in his pocket. If the canister is cold, the proper dose of medication may not be delivered.

General
Classification: antibiotic (extended-spectrum penicillin, alpha-carboxypenicillin). **Pregnancy risk category:** B.

Mechanism of action
Bactericidal; inhibits cell-wall synthesis during active multiplication. Bacteria resist penicillins by producing penicillinases—enzymes that convert penicillin to inactive penicilloic acid.

Indications and dosage
• Severe systemic infections caused by susceptible strains of gram-positive and especially gram-negative organisms (including *Pseudomonas, Proteus*). **Adults:** 18 g I.V. or I.M. daily, divided into doses given q 4 to 6 hours. **Children:** 200 to 300 mg/kg I.V. or I.M. daily, divided into doses given q 4 to 6 hours.

Adverse reactions
Blood: leukopenia, neutropenia, eosinophilia, *thrombocytopenia,* hemolytic anemia. **CNS:** seizures, neuromuscular excitability. **GI:** nausea, diarrhea. **Metabolic:** *hypokalemia.* **Local:** pain at injection site, vein irritation, phlebitis. **Other:** hypersensitivity (rash, pruritus, urticaria, chills, fever, edema, ***anaphylaxis***), overgrowth of nonsusceptible organisms.

Interactions
Aminoglycoside antibiotics (such as gentamicin and tobramycin): chemically incompatible. Don't mix together in I.V. **Probenecid:** increases blood levels of ticarcillin and other penicillins. Probenecid may be used for this purpose.

Nursing diagnoses
• High risk for injury related to ineffectiveness of ticarcillin to eradicate the infection.
• Fluid volume excess related to administration of the drug.
• Knowledge deficit related to ticarcillin therapy.

Nursing interventions
• *Use cautiously* in other drug allergies, especially to cephalosporins (possible cross-allergenicity), and in impaired renal function, hemorrhagic conditions, hypokalemia, or sodium restrictions (contains 5.2 mEq sodium/g).
• Obtain specimen for culture and sensitivity tests before first dose. Therapy may begin pending test results.
• Before giving ticarcillin, ask patient if he's had any allergic reactions to penicillin. However, a negative history of penicillin allergy is no guarantee against a future allergic reaction.
• Reduce dosage in patients with impaired renal functions.
• Check CBC and platelets frequently. Drug may cause thrombocytopenia.
• If patient has high blood level of this drug, he may develop seizures. Institute seizure precautions.
• **I.V. use:** When giving I.V., mix with D_5W or other suitable I.V. fluids. Give I.V. intermittently to prevent vein irritation. Change site every 48 hours.
• Administer deep I.M. into large muscle mass.
• Almost always used with another antibiotic, such as gentamicin.
• With large doses and prolonged therapy, bacterial and fungal superinfections may occur, especially in elderly, debilitated, or immunosuppressed patients. Close observation is essential.
• Monitor serum potassium.
• Give ticarcillin at least 1 hour before bacteriostatic antibiotics.

General

Classification: antihypertensive (ACE inhibitor).
Pregnancy risk category: C (X in 2nd and 3rd trimesters).

Mechanism of action

Benazepril and its active metabolite, benazeprilat, inhibit ACE, preventing conversion of angiotensin I to angiotensin II, reducing sodium and water retention and lowering blood pressure.

Indications and dosage

• Hypertension. **Adults:** initially, 10 mg daily. Titrate dosage as needed and tolerated; most patients take 20 to 40 mg daily in one or two doses.

Adverse reactions

CNS: headache, dizziness, light-headedness, anxiety, amnesia, ***seizures,*** depression, insomnia, nervousness, neuralgia, neuropathy, paresthesia, somnolence, tremor, vertigo. **CV:** symptomatic hypotension, syncope, angina, arrhythmia, chest pain, palpitations, ***MI.*** **EENT:** epistaxis. **GI:** nausea, vomiting, abdominal pain, anorexia, constipation, diarrhea, dry mouth, dyspepsia, dysphagia, gastroenteritis, increased salivation. **Respiratory:** dry, persistent, tickling, nonproductive cough; dyspnea. **Skin:** rash, dermatitis, pruritus, photosensitivity, purpura. **Other:** angioedema, arthralgia, arthritis, edema, impotence, increased sweating, myalgia, weight gain, asthenia.

Interactions

Diuretics, other antihypertensives: risk of excessive hypotension. Discontinue diuretic or lower dose of benazepril as needed. **Lithium:** possible increased serum lithium levels, lithium toxicity. **Potassium-sparing diuretics, potassium supplements, sodium substitutes containing potassium:** risk of hyperkalemia. Avoid concomitant use.

Nursing diagnoses

• High risk for injury related to the patient's underlying condition.
• Altered protection related to benazepril-induced blood disorder or renal dysfunction.
• Knowledge deficit related to benazepril therapy.

Nursing interventions

• *Contraindicated* in patients with hypersensitivity to ACE inhibitors or with history of angioneurotic edema.
• *Use cautiously* in patients with impaired renal or hepatic function and in diabetes mellitus.
• Blood pressure measurements should be made when drug levels are at peak (2 to 6 hours after dosing) and at trough (just before a dose) to verify adequate blood pressure control.
• Excessive hypotension can occur when drug is given with diuretics. If possible, diuretic therapy should be discontinued 2 to 3 days before starting benazepril to decrease potential for excessive hypotensive response. If benazepril does not adequately control blood pressure, diuretic may be reinstituted with care. If the diuretic cannot be discontinued, initiate benazepril therapy at 5 mg P.O. daily.
• Assess renal and hepatic function before and periodically throughout therapy. Also monitor CBC and serum potassium levels.
• Tell patient to take drug on an empty stomach because meals, particularly high-fat meals, can impair absorption.
• Tell patient to stop taking drug and notify doctor if any signs or symptoms of angioedema occur: swelling of face, eyes, lips, tongue, or difficulty in breathing.
• Inadequate fluid intake, vomiting, diarrhea, and excessive perspiration can lead to light-headedness and syncope. Tell patient to use caution in hot weather and during periods of exercise.
• Tell patient to avoid sodium substitutes; they contain potassium and can cause hyperkalemia.

General

Classification: thyroid-stimulating hormone (anterior pituitary hormone). **Pregnancy risk category:** C.

Mechanism of action

Stimulates the uptake of radioactive iodine in patients with thyroid carcinoma. Also promotes thyroid hormone production by the anterior pituitary.

Indications and dosage

- Diagnosis of thyroid cancer remnant with ^{131}I after surgery. **Adults:** 10 IU I.M. or S.C. for 3 to 7 days.
- Differential diagnosis of primary and secondary hypothyroidism. **Adults:** 10 IU I.M. or S.C. for 1 to 3 days.
- In PBI or ^{131}I uptake determinations for differential diagnosis of subclinical hypothyroidism or low thyroid reserve. **Adults:** 10 IU I.M. or S.C.
- Therapy for thyroid carcinoma (local or metastatic) with ^{131}I. **Adults:** 10 IU I.M. or S.C. for 3 to 8 days.
- Determination of thyroid status of patient receiving thyroid hormone. **Adults:** 10 units I.M. or S.C. for 1 to 3 days.

Adverse reactions

CNS: headache. **CV:** *tachycardia,* atrial fibrillation, angina pectoris, ***CHF,*** hypotension. **GI:** nausea, vomiting. **Other:** thyroid hyperplasia (large doses), fever, menstrual irregularities, allergic reactions (postinjection flare, urticaria, ***anaphylaxis***).

Interactions

Antidiabetic agents: change in serum glucose levels. Monitor blood glucose levels. Adjust dosage if necessary. **Oral anticoagulants:** change in PT. Monitor; adjust dosage if necessary. **Sympathomimetics such as epinephrine:** increased risk of coronary insufficiency. Monitor closely.

Nursing diagnoses

- High risk for activity intolerance related to patient's underlying condition.
- Ineffective breathing pattern related to thyrotropin-induced anaphylaxis.
- Knowledge deficit related to thyrotropin therapy.

Nursing interventions

- *Contraindicated* in hypersensitivity to the drug, and in coronary thrombosis and untreated Addison's disease.
- *Use cautiously* in angina pectoris, CHF, hypopituitarism, and adrenocortical suppression.
- May cause thyroid hyperplasia.
- Diagnostic use: to identify subclinical hypothyroidism or low thyroid reserve, to evaluate need for thyroid hormone therapy, to distinguish between primary and secondary hypothyroidism, and to detect thyroid remnants and metastasis of thyroid carcinoma.
- Three-day dosage schedule may be used in long-standing pituitary myxedema or with prolonged use of thyroid medication.

bendroflumethiazide

Naturetin

General

Classification: diuretic, antihypertensive (thiazide diuretic). **Pregnancy risk category:** B.

Mechanism of action

Increases urine excretion of sodium and water by inhibiting sodium reabsorption in the cortical diluting site of the ascending loop of Henle.

Indications and dosage

- Edema, hypertension. **Adults:** 5 to 20 mg P.O. daily or divided b.i.d. **Children:** initially, 0.1 to 0.4 mg/kg (3 to 12 mg/m^2) P.O. daily or divided b.i.d. *Maintenance:* 0.05 to 0.1 mg/kg (1.5 to 3 mg/m^2) P.O. daily or divided b.i.d.

Adverse reactions

Blood: ***aplastic anemia, agranulocytosis,*** leukopenia, thrombocytopenia. **CV:** volume depletion and dehydration, orthostatic hypotension. **GI:** anorexia, nausea, pancreatitis. **Hepatic:** hepatic encephalopathy. **Metabolic:** hypokalemia, asymptomatic hyperuricemia, hyperglycemia and impairment of glucose tolerance, fluid and electrolyte imbalances including dilutional hyponatremia and hypochloremia, metabolic alkalosis, hypercalcemia, gout. **Skin:** dermatitis, photosensitivity, rash. **Other:** hypersensitivity reactions, such as pneumonitis and vasculitis.

Interactions

Cholestyramine, colestipol: intestinal absorption of thiazides decreased. Keep doses as separate as possible. **Diazoxide:** increased antihypertensive, hyperglycemic, and hyperuricemic effects. Use together cautiously. **NSAIDs:** may decrease diuretic effectiveness. Avoid concomitant use.

Nursing diagnoses

- Fluid volume excess related to ineffectiveness of bendroflumethiazide to relieve edema.
- Altered urinary elimination related to bendroflumethiazide therapy.
- Knowledge deficit related to bendroflumethiazide therapy.

Nursing interventions

- *Contraindicated* in anuria or hypersensitivity to other thiazides or other sulfonamide-derived drugs.
- *Use cautiously* in severe renal disease and impaired hepatic function.
- Monitor intake and output, weight, and serum electrolytes regularly. Monitor serum creatinine and BUN regularly. Not as effective if these are more than twice normal.
- Consult with doctor and dietitian to provide high-potassium diet. Watch for signs of hypokalemia (for example, muscle weakness and cramps). Patients taking digitalis glycosides have an increased risk of digitalis toxicity from potassium-depleting adverse effect of this diuretic. May be used with potassium-sparing diuretic to prevent potassium loss.
- Monitor blood glucose levels. Check insulin requirements in patients with diabetes. May treat severe hyperglycemia with oral antidiabetic agents.
- Monitor blood uric acid, especially in patients with a history of gout.
- Elderly patients are especially susceptible to excessive diuresis.
- Give in a.m. to prevent nocturia.
- In hypertension, therapeutic response may be delayed several days.
- Thiazides and thiazide-like diuretics should be discontinued before tests for parathyroid function are performed.
- Advise patient to avoid sudden posture changes and rise slowly to avoid orthostatic hypotension.
- Advise patient to use a sunscreen.

General

Classification: thyroid replacement (thyroid hormone). **Pregnancy risk category:** A.

Mechanism of action

Stimulates the metabolism of all body tissues by accelerating the rate of cellular oxidation.

Indications and dosage

• Hypothyroidism. **Adults:** initially, 60 mg P.O. daily, increased by 60 mg q 30 days until desired response. Usual maintenance dosage is 60 to 180 mg daily, as a single dose. **Adults over 65 years:** 7.5 to 15 mg P.O. daily; dosage is doubled at 6- to 8-week intervals.
• Myxedema. **Adults:** 16 mg P.O. daily. May double dosage q 2 weeks to maximum 120 mg.
• Cretinism and juvenile hypothyroidism. **Children 1 year and older:** dosage may approach adult dosage (60 to 180 mg P.O.) daily, depending on response. **Children 4 to 12 months:** 30 to 60 mg P.O. daily. **Children 1 to 4 months:** initially, 15 to 30 mg P.O. daily, increased at 2-week intervals. Usual maintenance dosage is 30 to 45 mg daily.

Adverse reactions

Adverse reactions of thyroid hormones are extensions of their pharmacologic properties and reflect patient sensitivity to them.

CNS: *hyperirritability, nervousness, insomnia,* twitching, tremor, headache. **CV:** increased cardiac output, *tachycardia,* ***arrhythmias,*** angina pectoris, increased blood pressure, ***cardiac decompensation and collapse.*** **GI:** diarrhea, abdominal cramps, vomiting. **Other:** weight loss, heat intolerance, hyperhidrosis, menstrual irregularities; in infants and children—accelerated rate of bone maturation.

Interactions

Antidiabetic agents: change in serum glucose levels. Monitor blood glucose levels. Adjust dosage if necessary. **Cholestyramine:** thyroid absorption impaired. Separate doses by 4 to 5 hours. **I.V. phenytoin:** free thyroid released. Monitor for tachycardia. **Oral anticoagulants:** change in PT. Monitor; adjust dosage if necessary. **Sympathomimetics such as epinephrine:** increased risk of coronary insufficiency. Monitor closely.

Nursing diagnoses

• High risk for activity intolerance related to the patient's underlying condition.
• Altered cardiopulmonary tissue perfusion related to drug-induced angina pectoris.
• Knowledge deficit related to drug therapy.

Nursing interventions

• *Contraindicated* in MI, thyrotoxicosis (except with antithyroid drugs), or uncorrected adrenal insufficiency (thyroid hormones increase tissue demand for adrenocortical hormone and may cause acute adrenal crisis).
• *Use with extreme caution* in angina pectoris, hypertension, or other CV disorders; renal insufficiency; and ischemic states.
• *Use cautiously* in myxedema; these patients are unusually sensitive to thyroid hormone.
• In patients with coronary artery disease, observe carefully for possible coronary insufficiency.
• Potentially dangerous; not indicated to relieve vague symptoms, such as sluggishness, irritability, depression, and ill-defined pains; to treat obesity in euthyroid persons; to treat metabolic insufficiency not associated with thyroid insufficiency; or to treat menstrual disorders or male infertility, unless caused by hypothyroidism.
• Tell patient to take thyroid hormones at same time each day (in morning to prevent insomnia).
• Advise patient not to change product brands.
• Warn patient to tell doctor at once if chest pain, palpitations, sweating, nervousness, or other signs of overdosage occur or if any signs of aggravated cardiovascular disease develop (chest pain, dyspnea, and tachycardia).

General
Classification: nonnarcotic antitussive (local anesthetic). **Pregnancy risk category:** C.

Mechanism of action
Suppresses the cough reflex by direct action on the cough center in the medulla (brain). Also has local anesthetic action.

Indications and dosage
- Nonproductive cough. **Adults and children over 10 years:** 100 mg P.O. t.i.d.; up to 600 mg daily. **Children under 10 years:** 8 mg/kg P.O. in three to six divided doses.

Adverse reactions
CNS: dizziness, drowsiness, headache. **EENT:** nasal congestion, sensation of burning in eyes. **GI:** nausea, constipation. **Skin:** rash. **Other:** chills.

Interactions
None significant.

Nursing diagnoses
- Ineffective airway clearance related to underlying condition producing nonproductive cough.
- High risk for injury related to adverse CNS reactions to benzonatate.
- Knowledge deficit related to benzonatate therapy.

Nursing interventions
- *Contraindicated* in patients with hypersensitivity to the drug.
- Patient should not chew capsules or dissolve in mouth; mouth or airway anesthesia may result, and concomitant CNS stimulation may cause restlessness, tremor, and possibly seizures.
- Don't use when cough is valuable as diagnostic sign or is beneficial (as after thoracic surgery).
- Monitor cough type and frequency.
- Use with percussion and chest vibration.
- Maintain fluid intake to help liquefy sputum.

General

Classification: thyroid replacement (thyroid hormone). **Pregnancy risk category:** A.

Mechanism of action

Stimulates the metabolism of all body tissues by accelerating the rate of cellular oxidation.

Indications and dosage

- Cretinism and juvenile hypothyroidism. **Children 1 year and older:** dosage may approach adult dosage (60 to 180 mg P.O. daily), depending on response. **Children 4 to 12 months:** 60 to 80 mg P.O. daily. **Children 1 to 4 months:** initially, 15 to 30 mg P.O. daily, increased at 2-week intervals. Usual maintenance dosage is 30 to 45 mg P.O. daily.
- Hypothyroidism or myxedema. **Adults:** initially, 15 to 30 mg P.O. daily, increased by 15 to 30 mg at 2-week intervals until desired response. Usual maintenance dosage is 60 to 180 mg P.O. daily, as a single dose. **Adults over 65 years:** initially, 7.5 to 15 mg P.O. daily; dosage is doubled at 6- to 8-week intervals until desired response is obtained.

Adverse reactions

Adverse reactions of thyroid hormones are extensions of their pharmacologic properties and reflect patient sensitivity to them.

CNS: hyperirritability, *nervousness, insomnia,* twitching, *tremors,* headache. **CV:** increased cardiac output, *tachycardia,* ***arrhythmias,*** angina pectoris, increased blood pressure, ***cardiac decompensation and collapse.*** **GI:** diarrhea, abdominal cramps, vomiting. **Other:** weight loss, heat intolerance, hyperhidrosis, menstrual irregularities; in infants and children—accelerated rate of bone maturation.

Interactions

Antidiabetic agents: change in serum glucose levels. Monitor blood glucose levels. Adjust dosage if necessary. **Cholestyramine and colestipol:** thyroglobulin absorption impaired. Separate doses by 4 to 5 hours. **I.V. phenytoin:** free thyroid released. Monitor for tachycardia. **Oral anticoagulants:** change in PT. Monitor PT. Adjust dosage if necessary. **Sympathomimetics such as epinephrine:** increased risk of coronary insufficiency. Monitor closely.

Nursing diagnoses

- High risk for activity intolerance related to the patient's underlying condition.
- Altered cardiopulmonary tissue perfusion related to thyroglobulin-induced angina pectoris.
- Knowledge deficit related to thyroglobulin.

Nursing interventions

- *Contraindicated* in MI, thyrotoxicosis (except with antithyroid drugs), or uncorrected adrenal insufficiency (thyroid hormones increase tissue demand for adrenocortical hormone and may cause acute adrenal crisis).
- *Use with extreme caution* in angina pectoris, hypertension, or other CV disorders; renal insufficiency; and ischemic states.
- *Use cautiously* in myxedema; these patients are unusually sensitive to thyroid hormone.
- Potentially dangerous; not indicated to relieve vague symptoms (sluggishness, irritability, depression, and ill-defined pains); to treat obesity in euthyroid persons; to treat metabolic insufficiency not associated with thyroid insufficiency; or to treat menstrual disorders or male infertility, unless associated with hypothyroidism.
- In patients with coronary artery diseases, observe carefully for coronary insufficiency.
- Tell patient to take thyroid hormones at the same time each day, preferably in the morning.
- Warn patient to tell doctor at once if chest pain, palpitations, sweating, nervousness, or other signs of overdosage occur or if chest pain, dyspnea, or tachycardia develop.
- Advise patient not to change product brands.
- Suggest morning dosage to prevent insomnia.
- Monitor pulse and blood pressure.

General

Classification: antiemetic (benzoquinolizine derivative). **Pregnancy risk category:** C.

Mechanism of action

Acts on the chemoreceptor trigger zone to inhibit nausea and vomiting.

Indications and dosage

- Nausea and vomiting associated with anesthesia and surgery. **Adults:** 50 mg I.M. (0.5 mg/kg to 1 mg/kg). May repeat in 1 hour, and thereafter q 3 to 4 hours, p.r.n.; or 25 mg (0.2 mg/kg to 0.4 mg/kg) I.V. as single dose, administered slowly (25 mg/minute).

Adverse reactions

CNS: *drowsiness,* fatigue, insomnia, restlessness, headache, excitation, tremor, twitching, dizziness. **CV:** sudden rise in blood pressure and transient arrhythmias (premature atrial and ventricular contractions, atrial fibrillation) after I.V. administration; hypertension; hypotension. **EENT:** salivation, blurred vision. **GI:** anorexia, nausea, dry mouth. **Skin:** urticaria, rash. **Other:** muscle weakness, flushing, hiccups, sweating, chills, fever. May mask symptoms of ototoxicity, brain tumor, or intestinal obstruction.

Interactions

Alcohol, CNS depressants: enhanced CNS depression. Avoid concomitant use.

Nursing diagnoses

- High risk for aspiration related to nausea and vomiting induced by anesthesia and surgery.
- Altered cardiopulmonary tissue perfusion related to benzquinamide-induced cardiac arrhythmias.
- Knowledge deficit related to benzquinamide therapy.

Nursing interventions

- *Contraindicated* for I.V. use in CV disease and within 15 minutes of preanesthetic or CV drugs.
- Give I.M. injections in large muscle mass. Use deltoid area only if well developed. Be sure to aspirate syringe for I.M. injection to avoid inadvertent I.V. injection.
- **I.V. use:** Give I.V. dose slowly (25 mg/minute).
- Reconstituted solution is stable for 14 days at room temperature. Store dry powder and reconstituted solution in a light-resistant container.
- Precipitation occurs if reconstituted with 0.9% sodium chloride injection. Use bacteriostatic water for injection instead.
- Monitor blood pressure frequently.
- Excellent alternative if prochlorperazine is contraindicated.

thiothixene Navane

General
Classification: antipsychotic (thioxanthine).
Pregnancy risk category: C.

Mechanism of action
Blocks postsynaptic dopamine receptors in the brain.

Indications and dosage
• Acute agitation. **Adults:** 4 mg I.M. (hydrochloride) b.i.d. to q.i.d. Maximum dosage is 30 mg daily. Change to P.O. as soon as possible.
• Mild to moderate psychosis. **Adults:** initially, 2 mg P.O. t.i.d., increased gradually to 15 mg daily.
• Severe psychosis. **Adults:** initially, 5 mg P.O. b.i.d., increased gradually to 15 to 30 mg daily. Maximum recommended daily dose is 60 mg. Not recommended in children under 12 years.

Adverse reactions
Blood: transient leukopenia, ***agranulocytosis.*** **CNS:** *extrapyramidal reactions (high incidence), tardive dyskinesia,* sedation (low incidence), pseudoparkinsonism, EEG changes, dizziness. **CV:** *orthostatic hypotension,* tachycardia, ECG changes. **EENT:** ocular changes, *blurred vision.* **GI:** *dry mouth, constipation.* **GU:** *urine retention,* dark urine, menstrual irregularities, gynecomastia, inhibited ejaculation. **Hepatic:** cholestatic jaundice. **Metabolic:** hyperprolactinemia. **Skin:** *mild photosensitivity,* dermal allergic reactions. **Local:** pain at I.M. injection site, sterile abscess. **Other:** weight gain; increased appetite; ***neuroleptic malignant syndrome*** (rare). **After abrupt withdrawal of long-term therapy:** gastritis, nausea, vomiting, dizziness, tremors, feeling of warmth or cold, sweating, tachycardia, headache, insomnia.

Interactions
Adrenergic blockers, epidural or spinal anesthetics: increased hypotension. Avoid concomitant use. **Alcohol, other CNS depressants:** increased CNS depression. Avoid concomitant use.

Nursing diagnoses
• Altered thought processes related to patient's underlying condition.
• Urinary retention related to adverse drug reaction.
• Knowledge deficit related to thiothixene therapy.

Nursing interventions
• *Contraindicated* in convulsive seizures, circulatory collapse, coma, CNS depression, blood dyscrasia, bone marrow suppression, alcohol withdrawal, akathisia or restlessness, and subcortical damage.
• *Use cautiously* in elderly or debilitated patients and in patients with hepatic or CV disease, exposure to extreme heat or cold, prolonged exposure to sunlight, respiratory disorders, hypocalcemia, severe reactions to insulin or electroshock therapy, suspected brain tumor or intestinal obstruction, glaucoma, and prostatic hypertrophy.
• Tardive dyskinesia may occur after prolonged use.
• Watch for symptoms of neuroleptic malignant syndrome, which is rare but frequently fatal.
• Hold dose and notify doctor if patient develops jaundice, symptoms of blood dyscrasias, and persistent extrapyramidal reactions.
• Monitor bilirubin tests, CBC and liver function tests, and ophthalmic tests (long-term use).
• Have patient report urine retention or constipation.
• Tell patient to protect himself from sunlight.
• Warn against activities requiring alertness until CNS effects of the drug are known. Drowsiness and dizziness usually subside after a few weeks.
• Watch for orthostatic hypotension, especially after I.M. dose. Keep patient supine position for 1 hour afterward. Advise changing position slowly.
• Give I.M. only in upper outer quadrant of buttocks or midlateral thigh. Massage slowly afterward to prevent sterile abscess.
• Discard markedly discolored solutions.
• Keep drug off skin and clothes.
• Dilute liquid concentrate just before giving.
• Don't withdraw drug abruptly.

General
Classification: diuretic, antihypertensive (thiazide diuretic). **Pregnancy risk category:** D.

Mechanism of action
Increases urine excretion of sodium and water by inhibiting sodium reabsorption in the cortical diluting site of the nephron.

Indications and dosage
- Edema, hypertension. **Adults:** 50 to 200 mg P.O. daily or in divided doses. **Children:** 1 to 4 mg/kg P.O. t.i.d.

Adverse reactions
Blood: ***aplastic anemia, agranulocytosis,*** leukopenia, thrombocytopenia. **CV:** volume depletion and dehydration, orthostatic hypotension. **GI:** anorexia, nausea, pancreatitis. **Hepatic:** hepatic encephalopathy. **Metabolic:** hypokalemia, asymptomatic hyperuricemia, hyperglycemia and impairment of glucose tolerance, fluid and electrolyte imbalances including dilutional hyponatremia and hypochloremia, metabolic alkalosis, hypercalcemia, gout. **Skin:** dermatitis, photosensitivity, rash. **Other:** hypersensitivity reactions, such as pneumonitis and vasculitis.

Interactions
Cholestyramine, colestipol: intestinal absorption of thiazides decreased. Keep doses as separate as possible. **Diazoxide:** increased antihypertensive, hyperglycemic, and hyperuricemic effects. Use together cautiously. **Digitalis glycosides:** increased risk of toxicity from potassium-depleting effect. Use with potassium-sparing diuretic to prevent potassium loss. **NSAIDs:** may decrease diuretic effectiveness. Avoid concomitant use.

Nursing diagnoses
- Fluid volume excess related to ineffectiveness of benzthiazide to relieve edema.
- Altered urinary elimination related to benzthiazide therapy.
- Knowledge deficit related to benzthiazide therapy.

Nursing interventions
- *Contraindicated* in anuria, hypersensitivity to other thiazides, or other sulfonamide-derived drugs.
- *Use cautiously* in severe renal disease and impaired hepatic function.
- Monitor intake and output, weight, and serum electrolytes regularly. Consult with doctor and dietitian to provide high-potassium diet. Watch for signs of hypokalemia.
- Monitor serum creatinine and BUN regularly. Not as effective if these levels are more than twice normal.
- Monitor blood glucose levels. Check insulin requirements in diabetic patients. May treat severe hyperglycemia with oral antidiabetic agents.
- Monitor blood uric acid level, especially in patients with a history of gout.
- Give in a.m. to prevent nocturia.
- Elderly patients are especially susceptible to excessive diuresis.
- In hypertension, therapeutic response may be delayed several days.
- Thiazides and thiazide-like diuretics should be discontinued before tests for parathyroid function are performed.
- Advise patient to avoid sudden posture changes and rise slowly to avoid orthostatic hypotension.
- Advise patient to use a sunscreen.

thioridazine hydrochloride

Apo-Thioridazine†, Mellaril*, Mellaril-S, Novoridazine†, PMS Thioridazine†

General
Classification: antipsychotic (phenothiazine).
Pregnancy risk category: C.

Mechanism of action
Blocks postsynaptic dopamine receptors in the brain.

Indications and dosage
• Psychosis. **Adults:** initially, 25 to 100 mg P.O. t.i.d., with gradual increases up to 800 mg daily in divided doses, if needed. Dosage varies. **Adults over 65 years:** initial dose, 25 mg P.O. t.i.d.
• Depressive neurosis, alcohol withdrawal, dementia in geriatric patients, behavioral problems in children. **Adults:** initially, 25 mg P.O. t.i.d. Maintenance dosage is 20 to 200 mg daily. **Children over 2 years:** 0.5 to 3 mg/kg P.O. daily in divided doses.

Adverse reactions
Blood: transient leukopenia, ***agranulocytosis.*** **CNS:** extrapyramidal reactions (low incidence), *tardive dyskinesia, sedation (high incidence),* EEG changes, dizziness. **CV:** *orthostatic hypotension,* tachycardia, ECG changes. **EENT:** *ocular changes, blurred vision,* pigmentary retinopathy. **GI:** *dry mouth, constipation.* **GU:** urine retention, dark urine, menstrual irregularities, gynecomastia, inhibited ejaculation. **Hepatic:** cholestatic jaundice. **Metabolic:** hyperprolactinemia. **Skin:** *mild photosensitivity,* dermal allergic reactions. **Other:** weight gain, increased appetite, ***neuroleptic malignant syndrome*** (rare). **After abrupt withdrawal of long-term therapy:** gastritis, nausea, vomiting, dizziness, tremors, feeling of warmth or cold, sweating, tachycardia, headache, insomnia.

Interactions
Adrenergic blockers, epidural or spinal anesthetics: excessive hypotension. Avoid concomitant use. **Alcohol, other CNS depressants:** increased CNS depression. Avoid concomitant use. **Antacids:** inhibit absorption of oral thioridazine. Separate doses by at least 2 hours. **Barbiturates, lithium:** may decrease phenothiazine effect. Observe patient. **Centrally acting antihypertensives:** decreased antihypertensive effect.

Nursing diagnoses
• Altered thought processes related to patient's underlying condition.
• Urinary retention related to adverse drug reaction.
• Knowledge deficit related to thioridazine therapy.

Nursing interventions
• *Contraindicated* in coma, CNS depression, bone marrow suppression, hypertensive or hypotensive cardiac disease, or subcortical damage.
• *Use cautiously* in elderly or debilitated patients; in hepatic disease, arteriosclerosis or CV disease, exposure to extreme heat or cold, respiratory disorders, hypocalcemia, seizure disorders, severe reactions to insulin or electroshock therapy, suspected brain tumor or intestinal obstruction, glaucoma, or prostatic hyperplasia; and in acutely ill or dehydrated children.
• Tardive dyskinesia may occur after prolonged use.
• Neuroleptic malignant syndrome is rare, but commonly fatal. Watch for symptoms.
• Hold dose and notify doctor if patient develops jaundice, symptoms of blood dyscrasias, or persistent extrapyramidal reactions. Notify doctor if patient reports blurred vision.
• Monitor therapy by bilirubin tests, CBC, liver function tests, and ophthalmic tests.
• Tell patient that drug may discolor the urine.
• Tell patient to protect himself from sunlight.
• Warn against activities requiring alertness or coordination until CNS response to drug is known.
• Watch for orthostatic hypotension, especially with parenteral administration.
• Keep drug off skin to prevent contact dermatitis.
• Note different concentrations of liquid forms.
• Don't withdraw drug abruptly.

benztropine mesylate

Apo-Benztropine†, Bensylate†, Cogentin

General

Classification: antiparkinsonian agent (anticholinergic). **Pregnancy risk category:** C.

Mechanism of action

Blocks central cholinergic receptors, helping to balance cholinergic activity in the basal ganglia.

Indications and dosage

- Acute dystonic reaction. **Adults:** 1 to 2 mg I.V. or I.M. followed by 1 to 2 mg P.O. b.i.d. to prevent recurrence.
- Parkinsonism. **Adults:** 0.5 to 6 mg P.O. daily. Initial dose is 0.5 mg to 1 mg. Increase 0.5 mg q 5 to 6 days. Adjust dosage to meet individual requirements. Usual dose is 1 to 2 mg per day.

Adverse reactions

Some adverse reactions may be due to pending atropine-like toxicity and are dose-related.

CNS: disorientation, restlessness, irritability, incoherence, hallucinations, headache, sedation, depression, muscular weakness. **CV:** palpitations, tachycardia, paradoxical bradycardia. **EENT:** dilated pupils, blurred vision, photophobia, difficulty swallowing. **GI:** *constipation, dry mouth,* nausea, vomiting, epigastric distress. **GU:** urinary hesitancy, urine retention. **Skin:** warming, dryness, flushing.

Interactions

Amantadine, phenothiazines, tricyclic antidepressants: additive anticholinergic adverse reactions, such as confusion and hallucinations. Reduce dosage before administering amantadine.

Nursing diagnoses

- Impaired physical mobility related to underlying parkinsonism.
- Altered oral mucous membrane related to dry mouth, an adverse reaction to drug therapy.
- Knowledge deficit related to benztropine therapy.

Nursing interventions

- *Contraindicated* in narrow-angle glaucoma.
- *Use cautiously* in prostatic hypertrophy and tendency to tachycardia and in elderly or debilitated patients; produces atropine-like adverse reactions and may aggravate tardive dyskinesia.
- Monitor vital signs carefully. Watch closely for adverse reactions, especially in elderly or debilitated patients. Call doctor promptly.
- Never discontinue this drug abruptly. Dosage must be reduced gradually.
- Warn patient to avoid activities that require alertness until CNS effects of the drug are known. If patient is to receive single daily dose, give at bedtime.
- Explain that drug may take 2 to 3 days to exert full effect.
- **I.V. use:** rarely used because of small difference in onset as compared to I.M. route.
- Advise patient to report signs of urinary hesitancy or urine retention.
- Watch for intermittent constipation, distention, and abdominal pain; may be onset of paralytic ileus.
- To help prevent GI distress, administer after meals.
- Advise patient to limit activities during hot weather because drug-induced anhidrosis may result in hyperthermia.

General

Classification: antineoplastic (antimetabolite).
Pregnancy risk category: D.

Mechanism of action

Inhibits purine synthesis.

Indications and dosage

- Acute leukemia, chronic myelogenous leukemia. **Adults and children:** initially, 2 mg/kg daily P.O. (usually calculated to nearest 20 mg). If necessary, dose is then increased gradually to 3 mg/kg daily as tolerated.

Adverse reactions

Blood: ***leukopenia, anemia, thrombocytopenia*** (occurs slowly over 2 to 4 weeks). **GI:** nausea, vomiting, stomatitis, diarrhea, anorexia. **Hepatic:** ***hepatotoxicity,*** jaundice. **Metabolic:** hyperuricemia.

Interactions

Myelosuppressive drugs: increased risk of toxicity, especially myelosuppression and bleeding. Use together cautiously.

Nursing diagnoses

- Altered protection related to thioguanine-induced myelosuppression and immunosuppression.
- Altered oral mucous membrane related to thioguanine-induced stomatitis.
- Knowledge deficit related to thioguanine therapy.

Nursing interventions

- *Contraindicated* in patients whose disease has shown resistance to the drug.
- *Use cautiously* and with dosage modification in patients with renal or hepatic dysfunction.
- Stop drug if hepatotoxicity or hepatic tenderness occurs. Watch for jaundice; may be reversible if drug is stopped promptly.
- Monitor CBC daily during induction, then weekly during maintenance therapy.
- Monitor serum uric acid.
- Sometimes ordered as 6-thioguanine. The numeral 6 is part of drug name and does not signify dosage units.
- Avoid all I.M. injections when platelet count is below 100,000/mm^3.

bepridil hydrochloride Vascor

General

Classification: antianginal (calcium channel blocker). **Pregnancy risk category:** C.

Mechanism of action

Inhibits calcium ion influx across cardiac and smooth muscle cells, decreasing myocardial contractility and oxygen demand and dilating coronary arteries and peripheral arterioles.

Indications and dosage

• Treatment of chronic stable angina in patients intolerant of or unresponsive to other agents. **Adults:** initially, 200 mg P.O. daily. After 10 days, increase dosage based on response. Maintenance dosage in most patients is 300 mg/day. Maximum daily dosage is 400 mg.

Adverse reactions

Blood: ***agranulocytosis.*** **CNS:** dizziness. **CV:** edema, flushing, palpitations, tachycardia, ***ventricular arrhythmias.*** **GI:** nausea, diarrhea. **Skin:** rash. **Other:** dyspnea.

Interactions

Beta blockers: possible severe hypotension. Avoid concurrent use. **Digitalis glycosides:** may exaggerate AV node conduction. Use with caution. **Potassium-wasting diuretics**: potential hypokalemia, increasing risk of ventricular arrhythmias. **Quinidine, procainamide, tricylic antidepressants:** additive prolongation of QT interval. Avoid concurrent administration.

Nursing diagnoses

• Pain related to ineffectiveness of bepridil therapy.
• Altered protection related to bepridil-induced ventricular arrhythmia.
• Knowledge deficit related to bepridil therapy.

Nursing interventions

• *Contraindicated* in patients with hypersensitivity to the drug.
• *Use cautiously* in patients with CHF, especially if combined with a beta-adrenergic blocking agent.
• Not considered a primary agent because the drug has been associated with severe ventricular arrhythmias, including torsades de pointes; also associated with agranulocytosis.
• Elderly patients may require more frequent monitoring to prevent adverse reactions.
• Tell patient to promptly report any unusual bruising or bleeding or any persistent infections (including sore throat, fever, or malaise).

thiethylperazine maleate

Norzine, Torecan**

General

Classification: antiemetic, antivertigo agent (phenothiazine derivative). **Pregnancy risk category:** C.

Mechanism of action

Acts on the chemoreceptor trigger zone to inhibit nausea and vomiting.

Indications and dosage

• Nausea and vomiting. **Adults:** 10 mg P.O., I.M., or P.R. daily, b.i.d., or t.i.d.

Adverse reactions

Blood: *transient leukopenia,* ***agranulocytosis.*** **CNS:** *extrapyramidal reactions (high incidence),* sedation (low incidence), pseudoparkinsonism, EEG changes, dizziness. **CV:** *orthostatic hypotension,* tachycardia, ECG changes. **EENT:** *ocular changes, blurred vision.* **GI:** *dry mouth, constipation.* **GU:** *urine retention,* dark urine, menstrual irregularities, gynecomastia, inhibited ejaculation. **Hepatic:** *cholestatic jaundice.* **Metabolic:** hyperprolactinemia. **Skin:** *mild photosensitivity,* dermal allergic reactions. **Other:** weight gain, increased appetite.

Interactions

Antacids: inhibited absorption of oral phenothiazines. Separate antacid and phenothiazine administration by at least 2 hours. **Anticholinergics, including antidepressants and antiparkinsonian agents:** increased anticholinergic activity, aggravated parkinsonian symptoms. Use together cautiously. **Barbiturates:** may decrease phenothiazine effect. Monitor for decreased antiemetic effect.

Nursing diagnoses

• High risk for fluid volume deficit related to vomiting.
• Sensory/perceptual alterations (visual) related to thiethylperazine-induced ocular changes and blurred vision.
• Knowledge deficit related to thiethylperazine therapy.

Nursing interventions

• *Contraindicated* in severe CNS depression, hepatic disease, coma, or phenothiazine hypersensitivity.
• Don't give I.V. May cause severe hypotension.
• For nausea and vomiting associated with anesthesia and surgery, give deep I.M. injection on or shortly before terminating anesthesia.
• Possibly effective in dizziness; not effective in motion sickness.
• Use only when vomiting can't be controlled by other measures or when only a few doses are required.
• Warn patient about hypotension. Advise him to stay in bed for 1 hour after receiving the drug.
• Store suppositories tightly covered and at temperatures below 77° F (25° C).
• If drug gets on skin, wash off at once to prevent contact dermatitis.

General

Classification: anti-inflammatory agent (glucocorticoid). **Pregnancy risk category:** C.

Mechanism of action

Decreases inflammation by stabilizing leukocyte lysosomal membranes. Also suppresses immune response, stimulates bone marrow, and influences protein, fat, and carbohydrate metabolism.

Indications and dosage

- Severe inflammation or immunosuppression. **Adults:** 0.6 to 7.2 mg P.O. daily; or 0.5 to 9 mg (sodium phosphate) I.M., I.V. daily into joint or soft tissue; or 1.5 to 12 mg (acetate-sodium phosphate suspension) into joint or soft tissue q 1 to 2 weeks, p.r.n.
- Prevention of neonatal respiratory distress syndrome. **Adults (pregnant women):** 12 mg I.M. (acetate-sodium phosphate suspension) 36 to 48 hours before delivery. Repeat in 24 hours.

Adverse reactions

CNS: *euphoria, insomnia,* psychotic behavior, pseudotumor cerebri. **CV:** ***CHF,*** hypertension, edema. **EENT:** cataracts, glaucoma. **GI:** *peptic ulcer,* GI irritation, increased appetite. **Metabolic:** possible hypokalemia, hyperglycemia and carbohydrate intolerance, growth suppression in children. **Skin:** delayed wound healing, acne, various skin eruptions. **Other:** muscle weakness, osteoporosis, pancreatitis, hirsutism, susceptibility to infections. Acute adrenal insufficiency may follow increased stress (infection, surgery, or trauma) or abrupt withdrawal after long-term therapy. **Withdrawal symptoms:** rebound inflammation, fatigue, weakness, arthralgia, fever, dizziness, lethargy, depression, fainting, orthostatic hypotension, dyspnea, anorexia, hypoglycemia. ***Sudden withdrawal may be fatal.***

Interactions

Barbiturates, phenytoin, rifampin: decreased corticosteroid effect. **Indomethacin, other NSAIDs, aspirin:** increased risk of GI distress and bleeding. **Oral anticoagulants:** altered dosage requirements. Monitor PT closely. **Potassium-depleting drugs such as thiazide diuretics:** enhanced potassium-wasting effects of betamethasone. **Skin-test antigens:** decreased response. Defer skin testing until therapy is completed. **Vaccines and toxoids:** decreased antibody response and increased risk of neurologic complications.

Nursing diagnoses

- Impaired tissue integrity related to the patient's underlying condition.
- High risk for injury related to betamethasone-induced adverse reactions.
- Knowledge deficit related to betamethasone therapy.

Nursing interventions

- *Contraindicated* in systemic fungal infections.
- *Use cautiously* in patients with GI ulceration or renal disease, hypertension, osteoporosis, varicella, vaccinia, exanthema, diabetes mellitus, Cushing's syndrome, thromboembolic disorders, seizures, myasthenia gravis, CHF, tuberculosis, ocular herpes simplex, hypoalbuminemia, emotional instability, and psychotic tendencies.
- Don't use for alternate-day therapy.
- Adrenal suppression may last up to 1 year after drug is stopped. Gradually reduce drug dosage after long-term therapy. Tell patient not to stop drug abruptly or without doctor's consent. Be sure patient reports symptoms associated with corticosteroid withdrawal.
- To prevent muscle atrophy, give I.M. injection deeply. Rotate injection sites.
- Monitor blood glucose and serum potassium regularly. Diabetic patients may require adjustments in insulin dosage.
- Watch for additional potassium depletion from diuretics and amphotericin B. Potassium supplements may be necessary for patients receiving long-term therapy.

General

Classification: anthelmintic (benzimidazole).
Pregnancy risk category: C.

Mechanism of action

Unknown.

Indications and dosage

• Cutaneous infestations with larva migrans (creeping eruption). **Adults and children:** 25 mg/kg P.O. b.i.d. for 2 to 5 days. Maximum 3 g daily. If lesions persist after 2 days, repeat course.
– Pinworm: **Adults and children:** 25 mg/kg P.O. in two doses daily for 1 day; repeat in 7 days.
– Roundworm, threadworm, whipworm: **Adults and children:** 25 mg/kg P.O. in two doses daily for 2 successive days.
– Trichinosis: **Adults and children:** 25 mg/kg P.O. in two doses daily for 2 to 4 successive days.

Adverse reactions

CNS: impaired mental alertness, impaired physical coordination, *drowsiness, fatigue,* giddiness, *headache,* dizziness. **CV:** *hypotension.* **GI:** *anorexia, nausea, vomiting,* diarrhea, epigastric distress. **Skin:** *rash, pruritus,* ***erythema multiforme.*** **Other:** lymphadenopathy, fever, flushing, chills.

Interactions

None significant.

Nursing diagnoses

• Altered health maintenance related to ineffectiveness of thiabendazole.
• High risk for fluid volume deficit related to adverse GI reactions to thiabendazole.
• Knowledge deficit related to thiabendazole therapy.

Nursing interventions

• *Use cautiously* in hepatic or renal dysfunction, severe malnutrition, and anemia and in patients who are vomiting. Supportive therapy indicated for anemic, dehydrated, or malnourished patients. In children under 15 kg, weigh benefits against risks.
• Administer after meals. For oral suspension, shake before measuring dose. For tablets, advise patient to chew before swallowing.
• No dietary restrictions, laxatives, or enemas are necessary.
• Treat all family members.
• Emphasize the need for good personal hygiene. To avoid reinfection, patient should wash perianal area daily, change undergarments and bedclothes daily, and wash hands and clean fingernails before meals and after bowel movements.

General

Classification: antihypertensive (beta-adrenergic blocker). **Pregnancy risk category:** C.

Mechanism of action

Decreases blood pressure, probably by slowing heart rate and decreasing cardiac output.

Indications and dosage

• Management of hypertension (used alone or with other antihypertensives). **Adults:** initially, 10 mg P.O. once daily. After 7 to 14 days, full antihypertensive effect should be seen. If necessary, may double dosage to 20 mg once daily.

Adverse reactions

CV: bradycardia, chest pain, hypotension, worsening of angina, peripheral vascular insufficiency, ***CHF,*** edema, syncope, postural hypotension, conduction disturbances. **CNS:** dizziness, fatigue, headache, lethargy, anxiety. **GI:** flatulence, constipation, nausea, diarrhea, dry mouth, vomiting, anorexia. **Respiratory:** dyspnea, wheezing, ***bronchospasm.*** **Skin:** rash.

Interactions

Calcium channel blockers: increased risk of hypotension, left ventricular failure, and AV conduction disturbances. I.V. calcium antagonists should be used with caution. **General anesthetics:** increased hypotensive effects. Observe carefully for excessive hypotension, bradycardia, or orthostatic hypotension. **Lidocaine:** may increase the effects of lidocaine. **Reserpine, catecholamine-depleting drugs:** may have an additive effect when administered with betatolol.

Nursing diagnoses

• High risk for injury related to patient's underlying condition.
• Decreased cardiac output related to betaxolol-induced adverse CV reactions.
• Knowledge deficit related to betaxolol therapy.

Nursing interventions

• *Contraindicated* in patients with severe bradycardia, greater than first-degree heart block, cardiogenic shock, or uncontrolled CHF.
• *Use cautiously* in patients with CHF controlled by digitalis glycosides and diuretics because beta-adrenergic blockers do not block the inotropic effects of digitalis glycosides.
• Note that asymptomatic patients with a history of CHF may exhibit signs of cardiac decompensation with beta blocker therapy.
• Patients with bronchospastic disease (including asthma, chronic bronchitis, emphysema) should avoid beta blocker therapy because some $beta_2$-receptor antagonism may be associated with cardioselective agents such as betaxolol. However, some clinicians will use betatolol in such patients if the patients cannot tolerate other antihypertensives.
• Patients with unrecognized coronary artery disease may exhibit signs of angina pectoris upon withdrawal of the drug.
• Beta blockade may inhibit glycogenolysis and signs and symptoms of hypoglycemia.
• Betaxolol may mask tachycardia associated with hyperthyroidism. In patients with suspected thyrotoxicosis, therapy should be withdrawn gradually to avoid thyroid storm.
• The anesthesiologist should be advised that the patient is receiving a beta blocker so that isoproterenol or dobutamine is made readily available for reversal of the cardiac effects of the drug.
• Withdrawal of therapy before surgery is controversial. Some clinicians advocate withdrawal to prevent any impairment of cardiac responsiveness to reflex stimuli and decreased responsiveness to administration of catecholamines.
• Emphasize the importance of promptly reporting shortness of breath or difficulty breathing, unusually fast heartbeat, cough, or fatigue with exertion.

General

Classification: bronchodilator (xanthine derivative). **Pregnancy risk category:** C.

Mechanism of action

Inhibits phosphodiesterase, the enzyme that degrades cAMP, resulting in relaxation of smooth muscle of the bronchial airways and pulmonary blood vessels.

Indications and dosage

• Prophylaxis and symptomatic relief of bronchial asthma, bronchospasm of chronic bronchitis and emphysema. **Adults:** 6 mg/kg P.O. followed by 2 to 3 mg/kg q 4 hours for two doses. Maintenance dosage is 1 to 3 mg/kg q 8 to 12 hours. **Children 9 to 16 years:** 6 mg/kg P.O. followed by 3 mg/kg q 4 hours for 3 doses. Maintenance dosage is 3 mg/kg q 6 hours. **Children 6 months to 9 years:** 6 mg/kg P.O. followed by 4 mg/kg q 4 hours for three doses. Maintenance dosage is 4 mg/kg q 6 hours. *Note:* Most oral timed-release forms are given q 8 to 12 hours, but some products may be given q 24 hours.

Alternatively, give drug by I.V. infusion. **Loading dose:** 4.7 mg/kg I.V. slowly; then maintenance infusion. **Adults (nonsmokers):** 0.55 mg/kg/hour for 12 hours; then 0.39 mg/kg/hour. **Otherwise healthy adult smokers:** 0.79 mg/kg/hour for 12 hours; then 0.63 mg/kg/hour. **Older adults with cor pulmonale:** 0.47 mg/kg/hour for 12 hours; then 0.24 mg/kg/hour. **Adults with CHF or liver disease:** 0.38 mg/kg/hour for 12 hours; then 0.08 to 0.16 mg/kg/hour. **Children 9 to 16 years:** 0.79 mg/kg/hour for 12 hours; then 0.63 mg/kg/hour. **Children 6 months to 9 years:** 0.95 mg/kg/hour for 12 hours; then 0.79 mg/kg/hour. Switch to oral theophylline as soon as patient shows adequate improvement.

• Symptomatic relief of bronchospasm in patients currently receiving theophylline. **Adults and children:** each 0.5 mg/kg I.V. or P.O. (loading dose) will increase plasma levels by 1 mcg/ml.

• Adjunctive treatment of neonatal apnea. **Neonates:** 5 mg/kg I.V. as a loading dose, followed by 2 mg/kg/day in two or three divided doses.

Adverse reactions

CNS: *restlessness, dizziness,* headache, *insomnia,* light-headedness, *seizures,* muscle twitching. **CV:** *palpitations, sinus tachycardia,* extrasystoles, flushing, marked hypotension, increase in respiratory rate. **GI:** *nausea, vomiting, anorexia,* bitter aftertaste, dyspepsia, heavy feeling in stomach, diarrhea. **Skin:** urticaria.

Interactions

Adenosine: decreased antiarrhythmic effectiveness. May need higher doses of adenosine. **Barbiturates, carbamazepine, nicotine, phenytoin, rifampin:** enhanced metabolism and decreased theophylline blood levels. Monitor for decreased effect. **Beta-adrenergic blockers:** antagonism; may cause bronchospasms in sensitive patients. Use together cautiously. **Cimetidine, influenza virus vaccine, macrolide antibiotics, oral contraceptives, quinolone antibiotics:** elevated theophylline levels. Monitor for signs of toxicity.

Nursing diagnoses

• Ineffective airway clearance related to patient's underlying condition.
• Fluid volume deficit related to theophylline-induced vomiting.
• Knowledge deficit related to theophylline therapy.

Nursing interventions

• *Contraindicated* in hypersensitivity to xanthine compounds and in preexisting arrhythmias.
• *Use cautiously* in hypothyroidism, peptic ulcer, or diabetes mellitus; in elderly patients with CHF or other circulatory disorders, cor pulmonale, or renal or hepatic disease; and in young children. Reduced dosage may be necessary for this group.
• Monitor vital signs and intake and output.
• Tell patient to check with doctor or pharmacist before taking *any* other medications.
• Be careful not to confuse sustained-release dosage forms with standard-release dosage forms.

bethanechol chloride

Duvoid, Myotonachol, Urabeth, Urecholine

General

Classification: urinary and GI tract stimulant (cholinergic agonist). **Pregnancy risk category:** C.

Mechanism of action

Binds to cholinergic (muscarinic) receptors, mimicking the action of acetylcholine.

Indications and dosage

- Acute postoperative and postpartum nonobstructive (functional) urine retention, neurogenic atony of urinary bladder with retention, abdominal distention, megacolon, or reflux esophagitis caused by low esophageal sphincter pressure. **Adults:** 10 to 30 mg P.O. b.i.d. to q.i.d. Or 2.5 to 10 mg S.C. When used for urine retention, some patients may require 50 to 100 mg P.O. per dose (use with extreme caution). Test dose is 2.5 mg S.C. repeated at 15- to 30-minute intervals to total of four doses to determine minimal effective dose; use minimal effective dose q 6 to 8 hours.

Adverse reactions

CNS: headache, malaise. **CV:** bradycardia, hypotension, ***cardiac arrest,*** reflex tachycardia. **EENT:** lacrimation, miosis. **GI:** *abdominal cramps, diarrhea,* salivation, nausea, vomiting, belching, borborygmus, esophageal spasms. **GU:** urinary urgency. **Skin:** flushing, sweating. **Other:** ***bronchoconstriction,*** increased bronchial secretions.

Interactions

Atropine, anticholinergic agents, procainamide, quinidine: may reverse cholinergic effects. Observe for lack of drug effect. **Cholinergic agonists, anticholinergic agents:** may cause additive effects, or increase toxicity. Avoid concomitant use. **Ganglionic blockers:** may cause hypotension. Avoid concomitant use.

Nursing diagnoses

- Altered urinary elimination related to patient's underlying condition.
- Ineffective breathing pattern related to adverse drug reactions.
- Knowledge deficit related to bethanechol therapy.

Nursing interventions

- *Contraindicated* in patients with uncertain strength or integrity of bladder wall; when increased muscular activity of GI or urinary tract is harmful; in mechanical obstructions of GI or urinary tract; and in hyperthyroidism, peptic ulcer, latent or active bronchial asthma, cardiac or coronary artery disease, vagotonia, seizure disorder, Parkinson's disease, bradycardia, COPD, and hypotension.
- *Use cautiously* in hypertension, vasomotor instability, peritonitis, and other acute inflammatory conditions of GI tract.
- *Never* give I.M. or I.V.; could cause circulatory collapse, hypotension, severe abdominal cramping, bloody diarrhea, shock, or cardiac arrest.
- Watch closely for adverse reactions that may indicate drug toxicity, especially with S.C. administration.
- Stop all other cholinergics before giving this drug.
- Monitor vital signs frequently, especially respirations. Always have atropine injection and respiratory support readily available.
- When used to prevent abdominal distention and GI distress, the doctor may also order a rectal tube inserted to help passage of gas.
- Poor and variable oral absorption requires larger oral doses. Oral and S.C. doses are *not* interchangeable.
- Bethanechol increases pancreatic secretion, raising serum levels of amylase and lipase. Because drug causes a spasm in the sphincter of Oddi, it may raise serum bilirubin and AST levels and increase sulfobromophthalein retention.

General
Classification: antibiotic (tetracycline). **Pregnancy risk category:** D.

Mechanism of action
Inhibits protein synthesis by binding to the 30S ribosomal subunit (bacteriostatic).

Indications and dosage
• Infections caused by sensitive gram-negative and gram-positive organisms, rickettsiae, *Mycoplasma,* and *Chlamydia;* trachoma. **Adults:** 250 to 500 mg P.O. q 6 hours; 250 mg I.M. daily or 150 mg I.M. q 12 hours; or 250 to 500 mg I.V. q 8 to 12 hours (I.M. and I.V. hydrochloride salt only). **Children over 8 years:** 25 to 50 mg/kg P.O. daily, divided q 6 hours; 15 to 25 mg/kg daily (maximum 250 mg) I.M. single dose or divided q 8 to 12 hours; or 10 to 20 mg/kg I.V. daily, divided q 12 hours.
• Uncomplicated urethral, endocervical, or rectal infection caused by *Chlamydia trachomatis.* **Adults:** 500 mg P.O. q.i.d. for at least 7 days.
• Brucellosis. **Adults:** 500 mg P.O. q 6 hours for 3 weeks with streptomycin 1 g I.M. q 12 hours week 1 and daily week 2.
• Gonorrhea in patients sensitive to penicillin. **Adults:** initially, 1.5 g P.O., then 500 mg q 6 hours for a total dose of 9 g.
• Syphilis in patients sensitive to penicillin.

Adults: 30 to 40 g P.O. total in equally divided doses over 10 to 15 days.
• Acne. **Adults and adolescents:** initially, 250 mg P.O. q 6 hours, then 125 to 500 mg P.O. daily or every other day.
• Shigellosis. **Adults:** 2.5 g P.O. in single dose.

Adverse reactions
Blood: neutropenia, eosinophilia. **CNS:** dizziness, headache, ***intracranial hypertension.*** **CV:** pericarditis. **EENT:** sore throat, glossitis, dysphagia. **GI:** anorexia, *epigastric distress, nausea,* vomiting, *diarrhea,* stomatitis, enterocolitis, inflammatory lesions in anogenital region. **Hepatic:** ***hepatotoxicity*** with large doses given I.V. **Metabolic:** *increased BUN.* **Skin:** maculopapular and erythematous rashes, urticaria, photosensitivity, increased pigmentation. **Local:** *irritation after I.M. injection, thrombophlebitis.*

Interactions
Antacids (including sodium bicarbonate) and laxatives containing aluminum, magnesium, or calcium; food, milk, or other dairy products: decrease antibiotic absorption. Give antibiotic 1 hour before or 2 hours after any of the above. **Ferrous sulfate and other iron products, zinc:** decrease antibiotic absorption. Give tetracyclines 3 hours after or 2 hours before giving iron. **Lithium carbonate:** may alter serum lithium levels. **Methoxyflurane:** may cause severe nephrotoxicity. **Oral contraceptives:** decreased contraceptive effectiveness and increased risk of breakthrough bleeding.

Nursing diagnoses
• Altered protection related to ineffectiveness of tetracycline in eradicating the infection.
• High risk for infection related to development of superinfection caused by tetracycline therapy.
• Knowledge deficit related to tetracycline therapy.

Nursing interventions
• *Use with extreme caution* in renal or hepatic impairment. Use during the last half of pregnancy and in children under 8 years may cause permanent discoloration of teeth, enamel defects, and retardation of bone growth.
• Obtain specimen for culture and sensitivity tests before first dose. Give before results are known.
• Tell patient to take each dose with a full glass of water on an empty stomach 1 hour before or 2 hours after meals and 1 hour before bedtime.
• Patient may develop thrombophlebitis with I.V. administration. Avoid extravasation.
• Check expiration date. Use of outdated tetracycline may cause Fanconi's syndrome.
• Monitor for bacterial and fungal superinfection.
• Warn patient to avoid direct sunlight and ultraviolet light and to use a sunscreen.
• Don't mix tetracycline with any I.V. additive.

biperiden

Akineton; Akineton Lactate

General

Classification: antiparkinsonian agent (anticholinergic). **Pregnancy risk category:** C.

Mechanism of action

Blocks central cholinergic receptors, helping to balance cholinergic activity in the basal ganglia.

Indications and dosage

- Extrapyramidal disorders. **Adults:** 2 to 6 mg P.O. daily, b.i.d., or t.i.d., depending on severity. Usual dose is 2 mg daily, or 2 mg I.M. or I.V. (lactate) q half hour, not to exceed four doses or 8 mg total daily.
- Parkinsonism. **Adults:** 2 mg P.O. t.i.d. to q.i.d. Some patients may require as much as 16 mg/day.

Adverse reactions

Adverse reactions are dose-related and may resemble atropine toxicity.

CNS: disorientation, euphoria, restlessness, irritability, incoherence, dizziness, increased tremor. **CV:** transient postural hypotension (with parenteral use). **EENT:** blurred vision. **GI:** *constipation, dry mouth,* nausea, vomiting, epigastric distress. **GU:** urinary hesitancy, urine retention.

Interactions

Phenothiazines, tricyclic antidepressants: excessive CNS anticholinergic effects.

Nursing diagnoses

- Impaired physical mobility related to underlying parkinsonism or other extrapyramidal disorders.
- High risk for injury related to biperiden's adverse effect on the CNS.
- Knowledge deficit related to biperiden therapy.

Nursing interventions

- *Use cautiously* in prostatism, cardiac arrhythmias, narrow-angle glaucoma, and seizure disorder.
- Monitor vital signs carefully. Watch closely for adverse reactions, especially in elderly or debilitated patients. Call doctor promptly.
- Give oral doses with or after meals to decrease adverse GI reactions.
- When giving parenterally, keep patient in a supine position. Parenteral administration may cause transient postural hypotension and coordination disturbances.
- **I.V. use:** Administer very slowly.
- Because of possible dizziness, help patient when he gets out of bed.
- Tolerance may develop, requiring increased dosage.
- In severe parkinsonism, tremor may increase as spasticity is relieved.
- Warn patient to avoid activities that require alertness until CNS effects of the drug are known.
- Advise patient to report signs of urinary hesitancy or urine retention.
- Relieve dry mouth with cool drinks, ice chips, sugarless gum, or hard candy.

tetanus toxoid

General
Classification: tetanus prophylaxis agent (toxoid).
Pregnancy risk category: C.

Mechanism of action
Promotes immunity to tetanus by inducing production of antitoxin.

Indications and dosage
• Primary immunization. **Adults and children:** 0.5 ml (adsorbed) I.M. 4 to 6 weeks apart for two doses, then third dose 1 year after the second. Or 0.5 ml (fluid) I.M. or S.C. 4 to 8 weeks apart for three doses, then fourth dose of 0.5 ml 6 to 12 months after third dose. Booster is 0.5 ml I.M. at 10-year intervals.

Adverse reactions
Systemic: slight fever, chills, malaise, aches and pains, flushing, urticaria, pruritus, tachycardia, hypotension, ***anaphylaxis.*** **Local:** erythema, induration, nodule.

Interactions
Chloramphenicol: may interfere with response to tetanus toxoid.

Nursing diagnoses
• Altered protection related to lack of immunity to tetanus.
• Ineffective breathing pattern related to vaccine-induced anaphylaxis.
• Knowledge deficit related to tetanus toxoid.

Nursing interventions
• *Contraindicated* in immunosuppression and immunoglobulin abnormalities. Defer in acute illness and polio outbreaks, except in emergencies.
• For prevention, not treatment, of tetanus infections.
• Determine date of last tetanus immunization.
• Don't use hot or cold compresses; may increase severity of local reaction.
• Obtain history of allergies and reaction to immunization.
• Keep epinephrine 1:1,000 available.
• Adsorbed form produces longer duration of immunity and must only be administered I.M. Fluid form provides quicker booster effect in patients actively immunized previously; it may be given I.M. or S.C.
• Don't confuse this drug with human tetanus immune globulin.

bisacodyl

Bisacolax† ◊, Bisco-Lax** ◊, Dulcolax ◊, Fleet Bisacodyl ◊, Laxit† ◊

General

Classification: stimulant laxative (diphenylmethane derivative). **Pregnancy risk category:** C.

Mechanism of action

Increases peristalsis by direct effect on the smooth muscle of the intestine. Thought either to irritate the musculature or to stimulate the colonic intramural plexus. Also promotes fluid accumulation in the colon and small intestine.

Indications and dosage

- Chronic constipation; preparation for delivery, surgery, or rectal or bowel examination. **Adults:** 10 to 15 mg P.O. in evening or before breakfast. Up to 30 mg may be used for thorough evacuation needed for examinations or surgery. **Children 6 years and older:** 5 to 10 mg P.O. **Adults and children over 2 years:** 10 mg P.R. **Children under 2 years:** 5 mg P.R.

Adverse reactions

CNS: muscle weakness in excessive use. **GI:** *nausea, vomiting, abdominal cramps,* diarrhea with high doses, *burning sensation in rectum with suppositories.* **Metabolic:** alkalosis, hypokalemia, tetany, protein-losing enteropathy in excessive use, fluid and electrolyte imbalance. **Other:** laxative dependence in long-term or excessive use.

Interactions

Antacids: Don't give within 1 hour of milk or antacid intake.

Nursing diagnoses

- Constipation related to interruption of normal pattern of elimination characterized by infrequent or absent stools.
- Pain related to bisacodyl-induced abdominal cramps.
- Knowledge deficit related to bisacodyl therapy.

Nursing interventions

- *Contraindicated* in patients with abdominal pain, nausea, vomiting, or other symptoms of appendicitis or acute surgical abdomen or in rectal fissures or ulcerated hemorrhoids.
- Tell patient to swallow enteric-coated tablet whole to avoid GI irritation. Begins to act 6 to 12 hours after oral administration.
- Soft, formed stool usually produced 15 to 60 minutes after rectal administration. Time administration of drug so as not to interfere with scheduled activities or sleep.
- Tablets and suppositories may be used together to clean colon before and after surgery and before barium enema.
- Insert suppository as high as possible into the rectum, and try to position the suppository against the rectal wall. Avoid embedding within fecal material because this may delay the onset of action.
- Use for short-term treatment, and discourage excessive use.
- Before giving for constipation, determine if patient has adequate fluid intake, exercise, and diet. Tell him that dietary sources of bulk include bran and other cereals, fresh fruit, and vegetables.
- Store tablets and suppositories at temperature below 86° F (30° C).
- Tell patient to report adverse effects to the doctor.

General

Classification: tetanus prophylaxis agent (serum).
Pregnancy risk category: C.

Mechanism of action

Provides passive immunity to tetanus.

Indications and dosage

• Tetanus exposure. **Adults and children:** 250 to 500 units I.M.
• Tetanus treatment. **Adults and children:** single doses of 3,000 to 6,000 units I.M. have been used. Optimal dosage schedules have not been established. Don't give at same site as toxoid.

Adverse reactions

Local: pain, stiffness, erythema. **Other:** slight fever, allergy, ***anaphylaxis.***

Interactions

None significant.

Nursing diagnoses

• High risk for infection related to the patient's underlying condition.
• High risk for injury related to ineffectiveness of human tetanus immune globulin in eradicating the infection.
• Knowledge deficit related to human tetanus immune globulin therapy.

Nursing interventions

• Use tetanus immune globulin only if wound is over 24 hours old or patient has had less than two previous tetanus toxoid injections.
• Obtain history of injury, tetanus immunizations, last tetanus toxoid injection, allergies, and reaction to immunizations.
• Thoroughly cleanse and remove all foreign matter from wound.
• Antibodies remain at effective levels for 3 weeks or longer, which is several times the duration of antitoxin-induced antibodies. Protects the patient for the incubation period of most tetanus cases.
• Human tetanus immune globulin is not a substitute for tetanus toxoid, which should be given at the same time to produce active immunization.
• Inject into the deltoid muscle for adults and children 3 years and older and into the anterolateral aspect of the thigh in neonates and children under 3 years.
• Don't confuse this drug with tetanus toxoid.

General

Classification: antidiarrheal (adsorbent). **Pregnancy risk category:** C (D in 3rd trimester).

Mechanism of action

Has a mild water-binding capacity; also may adsorb toxins and provide protective coating for mucosa.

Indications and dosage

- Mild, nonspecific diarrhea. **Adults:** 30 ml or 2 tablets P.O. q ½ to 1 hour up to a maximum of eight doses and for no longer than 2 days. **Children 9 to 12 years:** 20 ml or 1 tablet P.O. **Children 6 to 9 years:** 10 ml or ⅔ tablet P.O. **Children 3 to 6 years:** 5 ml or ⅓ tablet P.O.
- Prevention and treatment of traveler's diarrhea (turista). **Adults:** prophylactically, 60 ml P.O. q.i.d. during the first 2 weeks of travel. During acute illness, 30 to 60 ml P.O. q 30 minutes for a total of eight doses. Alternatively, 2 tablets P.O. q.i.d. for up to 3 weeks.

Adverse reactions

GI: temporary darkening of tongue and stools. **Other:** salicylism (high doses).

Interactions

Aspirin, other salicylates: risk of salicylate toxicity. Monitor closely. **Oral anticoagulants, oral antidiabetic agents:** theoretical risk of increased effects of these agents after high doses of bismuth subsalicylate. Monitor patient closely. **Probenecid:** theoretical risk of decreased uricosuric effects after high doses of bismuth subsalicylate. Monitor patient closely. **Tetracycline:** decreased tetracycline absorption if taken together. Separate administration times by at least 2 hours.

Nursing diagnoses

- Diarrhea related to interruption of normal pattern of elimination characterized by frequent loose stools.
- Sensory/perceptual alterations (auditory) related to bismuth subsalicylate-induced salicylism.
- Knowledge deficit related to bismuth subsalicylate therapy.

Nursing interventions

- *Use cautiously* in patients already taking aspirin. Discontinue if tinnitus occurs.
- Warn patient that bismuth subsalicylate contains a large amount of salicylate (each tablet provides 102 mg salicylate; the regular strength liquid provides 130 mg/15 ml, and the extra strength liquid yields 230 mg/15 ml).
- Tell patient to call doctor if diarrhea persists for more than 2 days or is accompanied by high fever.
- Avoid use before GI radiologic procedures because bismuth is a radiopaque and may interfere with X-rays.
- Consult with doctor before giving bismuth subsalicylate to children or teenagers during or after recovery from the flu or chicken pox.
- Instruct patient to chew tablets well. Liquid should be shaken well before measuring dose.
- Both liquid and tablet forms are effective against traveler's diarrhea; tablets are more convenient to carry.
- Has been used investigationally to treat peptic ulcers, especially when ulcers are associated with *Helicobacter pylori* infection.

General

Classification: androgen replacement, antineoplastic (androgen). **Pregnancy risk category:** X. **Controlled substance schedule:** III.

Mechanism of action

Stimulates target tissues to develop normally in androgen-deficient men. Exerts inhibitory effects on breast cancers.

Indications and dosage

- Eunuchism, eunuchoidism, deficiency after castration and male climacteric. **Men:** 10 to 25 mg (base) I.M. 2 to 5 times weekly, or 200 to 400 mg (cypionate or enanthate) I.M. q 4 weeks, or 10 to 25 mg (propionate) I.M. 2 to 4 times weekly.
- Oligospermia. **Men:** 100 to 200 mg (cypionate or enanthate) I.M. q 4 to 6 weeks for development and maintenance of testicular function.
- Postpartum breast engorgement. **Women:** 25 to 50 mg (base or propionate) I.M. daily for 3 to 4 days.
- Metastatic breast cancer. **Women:** 50 to 100 mg (propionate) I.M. 3 times weekly, or 200 to 400 mg (cypionate or enanthate) I.M. q 2 to 4 weeks.
- Postmenopausal or primary osteoporosis. **Adults:** 200 to 400 mg (enanthate) I.M. q 4 weeks.
- Breast cancer in women 1 to 5 years postmenopausal. **Women:** 100 mg (base or propionate) I.M. 3 times weekly.

Adverse reactions

Androgenic: in women—*acne, edema, oily skin, weight gain, hirsutism, hoarseness,* clitoral enlargement, decreased or increased libido. In men—prepubertal: premature epiphyseal closure, *acne,* priapism, *growth of body and facial hair,* phallic enlargement; postpubertal: testicular atrophy, oligospermia, decreased ejaculatory volume, impotence, gynecomastia, epididymitis. **CV:** edema. **GI:** gastroenteritis, nausea, vomiting, constipation, diarrhea, change in appetite. **GU:** bladder irritability. **Hepatic:** reversible jaundice. **Hypoestrogenic:** in women—flushing; sweating; vaginitis with itching, drying, burning, or bleeding; menstrual irregularities. **Local:** pain at injection site, induration, irritation and sloughing with pellet implantation, edema. **Other:** hypercalcemia.

Interactions

Antidiabetic agents: altered dosage requirements. Monitor blood glucose levels in diabetics. **Hepatotoxic medications:** increased risk of hepatotoxicity. Monitor closely. **Oral anticoagulants:** altered dosage requirements. Monitor prothrombin time.

Nursing diagnoses

- Sexual dysfunction related to the patient's hormonal deficiency.
- Body image disturbance related to adverse androgenic reactions associated with testosterone.
- Knowledge deficit related to drug therapy.

Nursing interventions

- *Contraindicated* in women of childbearing age (may masculinize female infant); in elderly, asthenic men; in hypercalcemia; cardiac, hepatic, or renal decompensation; prostatic or breast cancer in males; benign prostatic hyperplasia with obstruction; conditions aggravated by fluid retention; hypertension; in pregnancy; in breast-feeding women; and in premature infants.
- *Use cautiously* in MI or coronary artery disease and in prepubertal males.
- Tell patient to use effective nonhormonal contraceptive.
- Perform periodic liver function tests.
- Therapeutic response in breast cancer is usually apparent within 3 months. Stop therapy if signs of disease progression appear. Report signs of hypercalcemia; indicates progression of bone metastasis.
- Instruct men to report priapism, reduced ejaculatory volume, and gynecomastia. Withdraw drug if these occur. Report signs of virilization in females; reevaluate treatment. Monitor prepubertal males by X-ray for rate of bone maturation.

General
Classification: antihypertensive (beta-selective adrenergic blocker). **Pregnancy risk category:** C.

Mechanism of action
Blocks cardiac (beta$_1$-) adrenergic receptors, decreasing heart rate, cardiac output, and blood pressure.

Indications and dosage
- Hypertension. **Adults:** initially, 5 mg P.O. once daily. If response is inadequate, increase to 10 mg daily. Maximum recommended dose is 20 mg daily.

Adverse reactions
CNS: asthenia, fatigue, dizziness, headache, hypoesthesia, vivid dreams, depression, insomnia. **CV:** bradycardia, peripheral edema, chest pain. **EENT:** cough, pharyngitis, rhinitis, sinusitis. **GI:** dry mouth, diarrhea, nausea, vomiting. **Respiratory:** dyspnea, upper respiratory infection. **Other:** arthralgia.

Interactions
Indomethacin: decreased antihypertensive effect. Monitor blood pressure and adjust dosage.

Nursing diagnoses
- Altered tissue perfusion (renal, cerebral, cardiopulmonary, and peripheral) related to the patient's underlying condition.
- High risk for injury related to adverse reactions to bisoprolol.
- Knowledge deficit related to bisoprolol therapy.

Nursing interventions
- *Contraindicated* in patients with hypersensitivity to the drug and in patients with cardiogenic shock, overt cardiac failure, marked sinus bradycardia, and second- or third-degree AV block.
- *Use cautiously* in patients with bronchospastic disease. In general, these patients should avoid beta-adrenergic blockers because blockade of pulmonary beta$_2$-receptors may result in worsening of symptoms. Although considered a beta$_1$-adrenergic blocker, bisoprolol blocks beta$_2$-adrenergic receptors in higher doses (20 mg daily or more).
- Also use cautiously in patients with diabetes, peripheral vascular disease, thyroid disease, and history of heart failure.
- Patients with renal or hepatic dysfunction should start therapy at 2.5 mg daily.
- Patients who cannot tolerate or do not respond to other antihypertensive medications may be given bisoprolol in low doses, starting at 2.5 mg daily.
- Beta blockers may mask some of the manifestations of hypoglycemia, such as tachycardia. Nonselective beta blockers can potentiate insulin-induced hypoglycemia and delay the recovery of serum glucose levels. Warn diabetic patients to closely monitor blood glucose levels.
- Monitor blood pressure frequently.
- Teach patient about his disease and therapy. Explain the importance of taking this drug as prescribed, even when he's feeling better. Tell patient not to discontinue this drug suddenly because doing so can exacerbate angina and MI. Drug must be withdrawn gradually over 1 to 2 weeks. Instruct patient to call doctor if unpleasant adverse reactions occur.
- Instruct patient to check with doctor or pharmacist before taking OTC medications.

testolactone

Teslac

General
Classification: antineoplastic (androgen). **Pregnancy risk category:** C. **Controlled substance schedule:** III.

Mechanism of action
Changes the tumor's hormonal environment and alters the neoplastic process.

Indications and dosage
- Advanced postmenopausal breast cancer. **Women:** 250 mg P.O. q.i.d.

Adverse reactions
CNS: paresthesia, peripheral neuropathy. **CV:** increased blood pressure, edema. **GI:** nausea, vomiting, diarrhea. **Metabolic:** hypercalcemia. **Other:** alopecia.

Interactions
Oral anticoagulants: increased pharmacologic effects. Monitor carefully.

Nursing diagnoses
- Body image disturbance related to adverse drug reactions.
- High risk for fluid volume deficit related to adverse reactions.
- Knowledge deficit related to testolactone therapy.

Nursing interventions
- *Contraindicated* in male breast cancer and not recommended for premenopausal women.
- Adequate trial is 3 months. Reassure patient that therapeutic response isn't immediate.
- Monitor fluids and electrolytes, especially calcium.
- Immobilized patients are prone to hypercalcemia. Exercise may prevent it. Force fluids to aid calcium excretion.
- Drug causes less virilization than testosterone.
- Higher-than-recommended doses do not increase incidence of remission.

General

Classification: bronchodilator (beta$_2$-adrenergic agonist). **Pregnancy risk category:** C.

Mechanism of action

Relaxes bronchial smooth muscle by acting on beta$_2$-adrenergic receptors.

Indications and dosage

- Prevention and treatment of bronchial asthma and bronchospasm. **Adults and children over 12 years:** To treat bronchospasm, two inhalations at an interval of at least 1 to 3 minutes followed by a third inhalation, if needed. To prevent bronchospasm, two inhalations q 8 hours. In either case, dose should never exceed three inhalations q 6 hours or two inhalations q 4 hours.

Adverse reactions

CNS: *tremor,* nervousness, headache, dizziness, light-headedness. **CV:** palpitations, chest discomfort, tachycardia. **EENT:** throat irritation, cough. **GI:** nausea. **Other:** dyspnea, *hypersensitivity.*

Interactions

None significant.

Nursing diagnoses

- Ineffective airway clearance related to the patient's underlying condition.
- High risk for injury related to adverse effects of bitolterol therapy.
- Knowledge deficit related to use of bitolterol therapy.

Nursing interventions

- *Contraindicated* in patients with hypersensitivity to the drug.
- *Use cautiously* in ischemic heart disease or hypertension, hyperthyroidism, diabetes mellitus, cardiac arrhythmias, and seizure disorders.
- Monitor blood pressure regularly.
- Advise patients not to exceed recommended dosages. Too frequent use may cause tachycardia.
- Remind patients that beneficial effects last for up to 8 hours, longer than most other similar bronchodilators.
- Know that bitolterol has rapid onset of action (about 3 to 4 minutes). Peak effect occurs in 30 to 60 minutes.
- Teach patient to perform oral inhalation correctly. Give the following instructions for using a metered-dose inhaler:
  - Clear nasal passages and throat.
  - Breathe out, expelling as much air from lungs as possible.
  - Place mouthpiece well into mouth as dose from inhaler is released, and inhale deeply.
  - Hold breath for several seconds, remove mouthpiece, and exhale slowly.
- If more than one inhalation is ordered, the patient should wait at least 2 minutes before repeating the procedure for a second dose.
- Tell patient who is also using a steroid inhaler to use the bronchodilator first, then wait about 5 minutes before using the steroid. This allows the bronchodilator to open air passages for maximum effectiveness.

General

Classification: antihistamine, H_1-receptor antagonist (butyrophenone derivative). **Pregnancy risk category:** C.

Mechanism of action

Competes with histamine for H_1-receptor sites on effector cells. Prevents but does not reverse histamine-mediated responses.

Indications and dosage

- Rhinitis, allergy symptoms. **Adults and children over 12 years:** 60 mg P.O. b.i.d. **Children 6 to 12 years:** 30 to 60 mg P.O. b.i.d. **Children 3 to 5 years:** 15 mg P.O. b.i.d.

Adverse reactions

CNS: fatigue, dizziness, *headache,* sedation. **CV:** ***arrhythmias*** (with overdose). **GI:** abdominal distress, nausea. **EENT:** dry throat and mouth, nasal stuffiness. **Other:** alopecia, cholestatic jaundice.

Interactions

Cimetidine, ciprofloxacin, itraconazole, ketoconazole, macrolide antibiotics (erythromycin, troleandomycin): decreased hepatic metabolism of terfenadine, leading to increased serum levels and risk of serious arrhythmias. Avoid concomitant use.

Nursing diagnoses

- Ineffective airway clearance related to the patient's underlying condition.
- Pain related to terfenadine-induced headache.
- Knowledge deficit related to terfenadine therapy.

Nursing interventions

- *Contraindicated* in patients with hypersensitivity to terfenadine and in those taking the antifungal agents itraconazole or ketoconazole or macrolide antibiotic.
- May cause a mild anticholinergic drying effect in patients with lower airway disease such as asthma. Keep patients well hydrated.
- Instruct patients not to exceed prescribed dose. In the event of an overdose, monitor patient for arrhythmias.
- Does not cause the degree of drowsiness and sedation associated with other antihistamines because drug does not cross blood-brain barrier; its anticholinergic and antiserotonin effects are mild.
- Tablets must be broken for children's dosages.

General

Classification: antiarrhythmic (adrenergic blocker).
Pregnancy risk category: C.

Mechanism of action

Initially causes transient adrenergic stimulation through release of norepinephrine. Depletion of norepinephrine causes adrenergic blocking, prolonging repolarization and refractory period.

Indications and dosage

• Ventricular fibrillation. **Adults:** 5 mg/kg by I.V. push over 1 minute. If necessary, increase dose to 10 mg/kg and repeat q 15 to 30 minutes until 30 mg/kg have been given. **Children:** safety and efficacy not yet established; some clinicians use 2 to 5 mg/kg I.M. as single dose, or 5 mg/kg I.V. followed by 10 mg/kg I.V. if fibrillation persists.
• Other ventricular arrhythmias. **Adults:** initially, 500 mg diluted in 50 ml D_5W or 0.9% sodium chloride solution and infused over more than 8 minutes at 5 to 10 mg/kg. Dose may be repeated in 1 to 2 hours. Repeat q 6 to 8 hours. *I.V. maintenance*— **Adults:** infused in 500 ml D_5W or 0.9% sodium chloride solution at 1 to 2 mg/minute. *I.M. injection*— **Adults:** 5 to 10 mg/kg undiluted. Repeat in 1 to 2 hours if needed. Thereafter, repeat q 6 to 8 hours.

Adverse reactions

CNS: *vertigo, dizziness, light-headedness, syncope.* **CV:** *severe hypotension, bradycardia,* anginal pain, transient arrhythmias, transient hypertension. **GI:** severe nausea, vomiting (with rapid infusion).

Interactions

All antihypertensives: may potentiate hypotension. **Other antiarrhythmics:** additive or antagonistic antiarrhythmic effects.

Nursing diagnoses

• Decreased cardiac output related to ineffectiveness of bretylium therapy.
• Altered cerebral tissue perfusion related to bretylium-induced severe hypotension.
• Knowledge deficit related to bretylium therapy.

Nursing interventions

• *Contraindicated* with use of the commercially available preparation mixed in D_5W in patients who are hypersensitive to corn or corn products.
• *Use cautiously* in patients with fixed cardiac output, aortic stenosis, and pulmonary hypertension to avoid severe and sudden drop in blood pressure.
• Avoid initiating bretylium therapy concomitantly with digitalis glycoside therapy. Do not use in digitalized patients unless the arrhythmia is life-threatening, not caused by digitalis glycoside therapy, and is unresponsive to other drugs.
• Monitor blood pressure and heart rate and rhythm continuously. If supine systolic blood pressure falls below 75 mm Hg, notify doctor; he may order norepinephrine, dopamine, or volume expanders to raise blood pressure.
• The initial release of norepinephrine caused by bretylium may induce transient hypertension and arrhythmias. Monitor patient closely.
• Keep patient in the supine position until tolerance to hypotension develops. Tell patient to avoid sudden postural changes.
• Know that bretylium is to be used with other cardiopulmonary resuscitation measures, such as countershock, epinephrine, sodium bicarbonate, and lidocaine.
• Avoid subtherapeutic doses (less than 5 mg/kg) because such doses may cause hypotension.
• Decrease dosage in renal impairment.
• Monitor carefully if pressor amines (sympathomimetics) are given to correct hypotension because bretylium potentiates pressor amines.
• Ineffective for atrial arrhythmias.
• Has been used investigationally to treat hypertension.

General

Classification: bronchodilator, tocolytic (beta-adrenergic agonist). **Pregnancy risk category:** B.

Mechanism of action

Relaxes bronchial smooth muscle by acting on $beta_2$-adrenergic receptors. Also relaxes uterine muscle.

Indications and dosage

- Relief of bronchospasm in patients with reversible obstructive airway disease. **Adults and children over 11 years:** 2 inhalations separated by a 60-second interval, repeated q 4 to 6 hours. May also administer 2.5 to 5 mg P.O. or 0.25 mg q 8 hours S.C.
- Treatment of premature labor. **Women:** 0.01 mg/minute by I.V. infusion. Increase by 0.005 mg q 10 minutes up to 0.025 mg/minute or until contractions cease. Or give 0.25 mg S.C. hourly until contractions cease. Maintenance dosage is 5 mg P.O. q 4 hours for 48 hours, then 5 mg q 6 hours.

Adverse reactions

CNS: *nervousness, tremors, headache,* drowsiness, sweating. **CV:** palpitations, increased heart rate. **EENT:** drying and irritation of nose and throat (with inhaled form). **GI:** vomiting, nausea. **Other:** hypokalemia (with high doses).

Interactions

CNS stimulants: increased CNS stimulation. Avoid concomitant use. **Digitalis glycosides, levodopa, halogenated inhalational anesthetics, cyclopropane:** increased risk of arrhythmias. Monitor closely. **Levodopa:** increased risk of arrhythmias. Avoid concomitant use. **MAO inhibitors:** when given with sympathomimetics, may cause severe hypertension (hypertensive crisis). Don't use together. **Propranolol and other beta blockers:** blocked bronchodilating effects of terbutaline.

Nursing diagnoses

- Ineffective airway clearance related to patient's underlying condition.
- High risk for injury related to adverse CNS reactions to terbutaline.
- Knowledge deficit related to terbutaline therapy.

Nursing interventions

- *Contraindicated* in patients with hypersensitivity to the drug; in patients with tachyarrhythmias, tachycardia caused by digitalis toxicity, narrow-angle glaucoma, or shock.
- *Use cautiously* in patients with diabetes, hypertension, hyperthyroidism, severe cardiac disease, or cardiac arrhythmias.
- Make sure patient and his family understand why drug is necessary.
- Give S.C. injections in lateral deltoid area.
- Tolerance may develop with prolonged use.
- Warn patient about the possibility of paradoxical bronchospasm. If it occurs, stop drug immediately.
- Patient may use tablets and aerosol concomitantly. Monitor closely for toxicity.
- Teach patient to perform oral inhalation correctly. Give the following instructions for using a metered-dose inhaler:
  - Clear nasal passages and throat.
  - Breathe out, expelling as much air from lungs as possible.
  - Place mouthpiece well into mouth as dose from inhaler is released, and inhale deeply.
  - Hold breath for several seconds, remove mouthpiece, and exhale slowly.
- If more than one inhalation is ordered, tell patient to wait at least 2 minutes before repeating the procedure for a second dose.
- Tell patient who is also using a steroid inhaler to use the bronchodilator first, then wait about 5 minutes before using the steroid inhaler.
- Use for preterm labor is unlabeled. If used for this indication, monitor neonates for hypoglycemia.

General

Classification: antiparkinsonian (semisynthetic ergot alkaloid). **Pregnancy risk category:** C.

Mechanism of action

Inhibits secretion of prolactin. It acts as a dopamine-receptor agonist by activating postsynaptic dopamine receptors.

Indications and dosage

- Treatment of amenorrhea and galactorrhea associated with hyperprolactinemia; treatment of female infertility. **Women:** 1.25 to 2.5 mg P.O. daily. Increase dosage by 2.5 mg daily at 3- to 7-day intervals. Safety and efficacy of doses greater than 100 mg daily not yet established.
- Prevention of postpartum lactation. **Women:** 2.5 mg P.O. b.i.d. with meals for up to 21 days.
- Treatment of Parkinson's disease. **Adults:** 1.25 mg P.O. b.i.d. with meals. Dosage may be increased q 14 to 28 days, up to 100 mg daily. Usually given with levodopa or levodopa-carbidopa combination.
- Treatment of acromegaly. **Adults:** 1.25 to 2.5 mg P.O. for 3 days. An additional 1.25 to 2.5 mg may be added q 3 to 7 days.

Adverse reactions

CNS: confusion, hallucinations, uncontrolled body movements, *dizziness, headache,* fatigue, mania, insomnia, depression. **CV:** *hypotension,* syncope. **EENT:** nasal congestion, tinnitus, blurred vision. **GI:** *nausea,* vomiting, *abdominal cramps,* constipation, diarrhea. **GU:** urine retention, urinary frequency. **Other:** ***pulmonary infiltration and pleural effusion,*** coolness and pallor of fingers and toes.

Interactions

Antihypertensive drugs: increased hypotensive effects. Adjust antihypertensive dosage. **Haloperidol, loxapine, phenothiazines, methyldopa, metoclopramide, MAO inhibitors, reserpine:** may interfere with bromocriptine's effects. **Levodopa:** additive effects. Adjust dosage of levodopa. **Oral contraceptives, estrogens, progestins:** interfere with effects of bromocriptine.

Nursing diagnoses

- Impaired physical mobility related to Parkinson's disease.
- High risk for injury related to adverse CNS or cardiovascular effects of drug therapy.
- Knowledge deficit related to bromocriptine therapy.

Nursing interventions

- *Contraindicated* in hypersensitivity to ergot derivatives.
- *Use cautiously* in preexisting psychiatric disorders.
- Patient should be examined carefully for pituitary tumor (Forbes-Albright syndrome). Use of bromocriptine will not affect tumor size although it may alleviate associated amenorrhea or galactorrhea.
- Know that bromocriptine may lead to early postpartum conception. Test for pregnancy every 4 weeks or whenever period is missed after menses are reinitiated.
- Baseline and periodic evaluations of cardiac, hepatic, renal, and hematopoietic function are recommended during prolonged therapy.
- Patients with impaired renal function may require dosage adjustments.
- Monitor blood pressure closely in women who receive bromocriptine for suppression of postpartum lactation. In such patients, transient hypotension is common; hypertension, seizures, and stroke have also been reported.
- Incidence of adverse reactions is high (about 68%), and nausea is the most common adverse reaction. Recurrence rates when used to treat amenorrhea or galactorrhea associated with hyperprolactinemia are also high (from 70% to 80%).
- Advise the patient that it may take 8 weeks or longer for menses to be reinstated and galactorrhea suppressed.
- Patient may experience mild to moderate rebound breast secretion, congestion, or engorgement when therapy is discontinued.

terazosin hydrochloride Hytrin

General
Classification: antihypertensive (selective $alpha_1$-adrenergic blocker). **Pregnancy risk category:** C.

Mechanism of action
Decreases blood pressure by vasodilation produced in response to blockade of $alpha_1$-adrenergic receptors.

Indications and dosage
- Hypertension. **Adults:** initial dose is 1 mg P.O. h.s., gradually increased according to patient response. Usual dosage range is 1 to 5 mg daily. Maximum recommended dosage is 20 mg/day.

Adverse reactions
CNS: asthenia, *dizziness,* headache, nervousness, paresthesia, somnolence, decreased libido. **CV:** *palpitations,* postural hypotension, tachycardia, *peripheral edema.* **EENT:** *nasal congestion,* sinusitis, blurred vision. **GI:** *nausea.* **Respiratory:** dyspnea. **Other:** back pain, muscle pain, weight gain, impotence.

Interactions
Antihypertensives: excessive hypotension. Use together cautiously.

Nursing diagnoses
- Altered tissue perfusion (renal, cerebral, cardiopulmonary, peripheral) related to the patient's underlying condition.
- High risk for injury related to adverse reactions.
- Knowledge deficit related to terazosin therapy.

Nursing interventions
- Do not exceed initial dose of 1 mg.
- Instruct patient to avoid hazardous activities that require mental alertness (such as driving or operating heavy machinery) for 12 hours after the first dose.
- If terazosin is discontinued for several days, patient will need to be retitrated using initial dosing regimen (1 mg P.O. at bedtime).
- Teach patient about his disease and therapy. Explain the importance of taking this drug as prescribed, even when he's feeling well. Tell outpatient not to discontinue drug suddenly, but to call the doctor if unpleasant adverse reactions occur.
- Instruct patient to check with doctor or pharmacist before taking OTC medications.

General
Classification: antihistamine (alkylamine H_1-receptor antagonist). **Pregnancy risk category:** C.

Mechanism of action
Competes with histamine for H_1-receptor sites on effector cells. Prevents but does not reverse histamine-mediated responses.

Indications and dosage
• Rhinitis, allergy symptoms. **Adults:** 4 to 8 mg P.O. t.i.d. or q.i.d.; or 8 to 12 mg timed-release P.O. b.i.d. or t.i.d.; or 5 to 20 mg q 6 to 12 hours I.M., I.V., or S.C. Maximum dosage is 40 mg daily. **Children over 6 years:** 2 to 4 mg P.O. t.i.d. or q.i.d.; or 8 to 12 mg timed-release q 12 hours; or 0.5 mg/kg I.M., I.V., or S.C. daily divided t.i.d. or q.i.d. **Children under 6 years:** 0.5 mg/kg P.O., I.M., I.V., or S.C. daily divided t.i.d. or q.i.d. *Note:* Children under 12 years should use only as directed by a doctor.

Adverse reactions
Blood: thrombocytopenia, ***agranulocytosis.*** **CNS:** (especially in elderly patients) dizziness, tremors, irritability, insomnia, *drowsiness, stimulation.* **CV:** hypotension, palpitations. **GI:** anorexia, nausea, vomiting, *dry mouth and throat.* **GU:** urine retention. **Skin:** urticaria, rash. **After parenteral administration:** local reaction, sweating, syncope.

Interactions
CNS depressants: increased sedation. Use together cautiously. **MAO inhibitors:** increased anticholinergic effects. Don't use together.

Nursing diagnoses
• Altered protection related to allergy symptoms.
• Hyperthermia related to potential brompheniramine-induced agranulocytosis.
• Knowledge deficit related to brompheniramine therapy.

Nursing interventions
• *Contraindicated* in acute asthmatic attacks.
• *Use cautiously* in elderly patients, breast-feeding women, and in patients with increased intraocular pressure, hyperthyroidism, cardiovascular or renal disease, hypertension, bronchial asthma, urine retention, prostatic hypertrophy, bladder-neck obstruction, and stenosing peptic ulcers.
• Warn patient against drinking alcohol during therapy and against activities that require alertness until adverse CNS effects are known; however, brompheniramine causes less drowsiness than some other antihistamines.
• Reduce GI distress by giving with food or milk.
• If tolerance develops, another antihistamine may be substituted.
• Warn patient to stop taking drug 4 days before allergy skin tests to preserve accuracy of tests.
• **I.V. use:** Injectable form containing 10 mg/ml can be given diluted or undiluted very slowly. The 100 mg/ml injection should not be given I.V.
• Monitor blood count during long-term therapy; observe for signs of blood dyscrasia.
• Antihistamines are not recommended for use by women who are breast-feeding because small amounts of drug are excreted in breast milk.

General

Classification: sedative-hypnotic (benzodiazepine). **Pregnancy risk category:** X. **Controlled substance schedule:** IV.

Mechanism of action

Acts on the limbic system, thalamus, and hypothalamus of the CNS to produce hypnotic effects.

Indications and dosage

• Insomnia. **Adults:** 15 to 30 mg P.O. h.s. **Adults over 65 years:** 15 mg P.O. h.s.

Adverse reactions

CNS: *drowsiness, dizziness, lethargy,* disturbed coordination, daytime sedation, confusion. **GI:** anorexia, diarrhea.

Interactions

Alcohol or CNS depressants, including narcotic analgesics: increased CNS depression. Use together cautiously.

Nursing diagnoses

• Sleep pattern disturbance related to underlying patient problem.
• High risk for trauma related to adverse CNS reactions to temazepam.
• Knowledge deficit related to temazepam therapy.

Nursing interventions

• *Use cautiously* in impaired hepatic or renal function, mental depression, suicidal tendencies, and history of drug abuse. Also use cautiously and in low end of dosage range in elderly or debilitated patients.
• Elderly patients are more sensitive to the drug's adverse CNS effects. Assess mental status before initiating therapy.
• Take precautions to prevent hoarding or self-overdosing by patients who are depressed, suicidal, or drug-dependent or who have a history of drug abuse.
• Warn about increased depressant effects of alcohol and against engaging in hazardous activity requiring alertness or physical coordination.
• Supervise walking; raise bed rails, especially for elderly patients.
• May cause less residual sedation ("hangover") the next day than flurazepam or diazepam. Relatively short-acting.
• Onset of action may take as long as 2½ hours.
• If temazepam overdose occurs, give flumazenil (a specific benzodiazepine antagonist). The duration of action of flumazenil is shorter than that of temazepam, so resedation is possible.

buclizine hydrochloride

Bucladin-S**

General

Classification: antiemetic, antivertigo agent (piperazine derivative antihistamine). **Pregnancy risk category:** C.

Mechanism of action

May affect neural pathways originating in the labyrinth to inhibit nausea and vomiting, but the exact mechanism of action is unknown.

Indications and dosage

- Prevention of motion sickness. **Adults:** 50 mg P.O. at least one half hour before beginning travel. If needed, may repeat another 50 mg P.O. after 4 to 6 hours.
- Vertigo. **Adults:** 50 mg P.O., up to 150 mg P.O. daily in severe cases. Maintenance dose is 50 mg b.i.d.

Adverse reactions

CNS: *drowsiness*, headache, dizziness, jitters. **EENT:** blurred vision. **GI:** dry mouth. **GU:** urine retention.

Interactions

Alcohol, CNS depressants: additive CNS depression. Avoid concomitant use.

Nursing diagnoses

- High risk for fluid volume deficit related to motion-sickness-induced nausea and vomiting.
- Altered thought processes related to buclizine-induced drowsiness.
- Knowledge deficit related to buclizine therapy.

Nursing interventions

- *Contraindicated* in patients with hypersensitivity to the drug.
- *Use cautiously* in patients with glaucoma, GU or GI obstruction, and in elderly males with possible prostatic hypertrophy.
- Warn patient against driving and other activities that require alertness until CNS effects of the drug are known.
- Know that buclizine may mask symptoms of ototoxicity, intestinal obstruction, or brain tumor.
- Tablets may be placed in mouth and allowed to dissolve without water. May also be chewed or swallowed whole.

General
Classification: antineoplastic (nonsteroidal antiestrogen). **Pregnancy risk category:** D.

Mechanism of action
Acts as an estrogen antagonist.

Indications and dosage
- Advanced premenopausal and postmenopausal breast cancer. **Women:** 10 mg P.O. b.i.d. to t.i.d.

Adverse reactions
Blood: transient fall in WBC or platelet counts. **GI:** nausea in 10% of patients, vomiting, anorexia. **GU:** vaginal discharge and bleeding. **Metabolic:** hypercalcemia. **Skin:** rash. **Other:** temporary bone or tumor pain, hot flashes in 7% of patients, brief exacerbation of pain from osseous metastasis.

Interactions
None significant.

Nursing diagnoses
- Altered protection related to adverse drug reactions.
- High risk for fluid volume deficit related to adverse drug reactions.
- Knowledge deficit related to tamoxifen therapy.

Nursing interventions
- *Contraindicated* in patients with hypersensitivity to the drug.
- Monitor CBC closely in patients with preexisting leukopenia or thrombocytopenia.
- Acts as an antiestrogen. Best results have been reported in patients with positive estrogen receptors.
- Adverse reactions are usually minor and well tolerated.
- Reassure patient that acute exacerbation of bone pain during tamoxifen therapy usually indicates drug will produce good response. Use analgesic to relieve pain.
- Short-term therapy induces ovulation in premenopausal women. Barrier form of contraception is recommended.
- Monitor serum calcium. Drug may compound hypercalcemia related to bone metastasis during initiation of therapy.
- Also used to treat breast cancer in men and advanced ovarian cancer in women. Has been used to stimulate ovulation in women with oligomenorrhea or amenorrhea who previously used oral contraceptives.

General

Classification: diuretic (loop diuretic). **Pregnancy risk category:** C.

Mechanism of action

Inhibits reabsorption of sodium and chloride at the proximal portion of the ascending loop of Henle.

Indications and dosage

• Edema in congestive heart failure, hepatic or renal disease. **Adults:** 0.5 to 2 mg P.O. once daily; if response inadequate, a second or third dose may be given at 4- to 5-hour intervals. Maximum dosage 10 mg/day. May be administered parenterally when P.O. not feasible. Usual initial dose 0.5 to 1 mg I.V. or I.M.; a second or third dose may be given at 2- to 3-hour intervals. Maximum dosage 10 mg/day. **Children:** 0.02 to 0.1 mg/kg P.O., I.M., or I.V. q 12 hours.

Adverse reactions

CNS: *dizziness,* headache. **CV:** volume depletion and dehydration, orthostatic hypotension, ECG changes. **EENT:** transient deafness. **GI:** nausea. **Metabolic:** *hypokalemia;* hypochloremic alkalosis; *asymptomatic hyperuricemia; fluid and electrolyte imbalances, including dilutional hyponatremia, hypocalcemia, hypomagnesemia; hyperglycemia,* impairment of glucose tolerance. **Skin:** rash. **Other:** muscle pain, tenderness.

Interactions

Aminoglycoside antibiotics: potentiated ototoxicity. **Antihypertensive agents:** increased risk of hypotension. **Probenecid, indomethacin, NSAIDs:** inhibited diuretic response.

Nursing diagnoses

• Fluid volume excess related to the patient's underlying condition as evidenced by edema.
• Altered urinary elimination related to bumetanide therapy (frequency, urgency).
• Knowledge deficit related to bumetanide therapy.

Nursing interventions

• *Contraindicated* in anuria, hepatic coma, or in states of severe electrolyte depletion.
• *Use cautiously* in patients with hepatic cirrhosis and ascites. Supplemental potassium or potassium-sparing diuretics may be used to prevent hypokalemia and metabolic alkalosis in these patients. Use cautiously in patients with depressed renal function. Also use cautiously in patients allergic to sulfonamides, who may show hypersensitivity to bumetanide.
• Use in children is not FDA-approved. Do not use in neonates because it contains benzyl alcohol.
• Potent loop diuretic; can lead to profound water and electrolyte depletion. Monitor blood pressure and pulse rate during rapid diuresis. Use cautiously with other potassium-wasting drugs.
• If oliguria or azotemia develops or increases, doctor may order discontinuation of therapy.
• Monitor serum electrolytes, BUN, and CO_2 frequently.
• Monitor blood glucose levels in patients with diabetes. May treat severe hyperglycemia with oral antidiabetic agents.
• Monitor blood uric acid, especially in patients with a history of gout.
• Watch for signs of hypokalemia. Patients also receiving digitalis glycosides have an increased risk of digitalis toxicity from the potassium-depleting effect of this diuretic.
• Consult with doctor and dietitian to provide high-potassium diet.
• **I.V. use:** Give I.V. doses with 21G or 23G needle over 1 to 2 minutes. For intermittent infusion, give diluted drug through an intermittent infusion device or piggybank into an I.V. line containing a free-flowing compatible solution.
• Advise patients taking bumetanide to stand up slowly to prevent dizziness and to limit alcohol intake and strenuous exercise in hot weather since these exacerbate orthostatic hypotension.
• Bumetanide can be prescribed in patients allergic to furosemide; 1 mg of bumetanide is equal to 40 mg of furosemide (bumetanide may be less ototoxic than furosemide).

General

Classification: nootropic (memory-enhancing) agent (anticholinergic). **Pregnancy risk category:** C.

Mechanism of action

Probably acts by preventing the breakdown of acetylcholine in the CNS, prolonging its actions and enhancing central cholinergic function. Drug also blocks central potassium channels, alters phosphorylation, and blocks presynaptic and postsynaptic cholinergic receptors.

Indications and dosage

• Adjunctive treatment of Alzheimer's disease. **Adults:** initially, 40 to 80 mg P.O. daily in divided doses. If no evidence of hepatotoxicity exists, dosage is increased to 120 mg daily.

Adverse reactions

GI: *diarrhea, increased salivation.* **GU:** *increased urination.* **Other:** ***hepatotoxicity,*** *sweating.*

Interactions

Anticholinergics: decreased effectiveness. Adjust dosage as ordered. **Cholinergic agonists:** enhanced effects. Monitor closely. **Cimetidine:** may interfere with metabolism of tacrine, resulting in increased plasma levels of tacrine. **Theophylline:** decreased hepatic clearance of theophylline. Adjust theophylline dosage as ordered.

Nursing diagnoses

• Diarrhea related to adverse effects of tacrine therapy.
• High risk for injury related to ineffectiveness of tacrine in treating Alzheimer's disease.
• Knowledge deficit related to tacrine therapy.

Nursing interventions

• *Contraindicated* in patients with hypersensitivity to the drug.
• Information is based on current literature and may change with further clinical experience.
• Cholinergic adverse effects are common. Addition of anticholinergic medications, such as glycopyrrolate, may block these adverse effects.

General

Classification: analgesic (narcotic agonist-antagonist, partial opoid agonist). **Pregnancy risk category:** C (D for prolonged use or use of high doses at term). **Controlled substance schedule:** V.

Mechanism of action

Binds with opiate receptors at many sites in the CNS (brain, brain stem, and spinal cord), altering both perception of and emotional response to pain through an unknown mechanism.

Indications and dosage

• Moderate to severe pain. **Adults:** 0.3 mg I.M. or slow I.V. q 6 hours, p.r.n. or around the clock. May administer up to 0.6 mg/dose if necessary.

Adverse reactions

CNS: *dizziness, sedation, headache,* confusion, nervousness, euphoria. **CV:** hypotension. **EENT:** *miosis.* **GI:** *nausea,* vomiting, constipation. **Skin:** pruritus, *sweating.* **Other:** ***respiratory depression,*** hypoventilation.

Interactions

Alcohol, CNS depressants, MAO inhibitors: additive effects. Use together cautiously. **Narcotic analgesics:** avoid concomitant use. Possible decreased analgesic effect.

Nursing diagnoses

• Pain related to patient's underlying condition.
• Ineffective breathing pattern related to buprenorphine-induced respiratory depression.
• Knowledge deficit related to buprenorphine therapy.

Nursing interventions

• *Contraindicated* in patients with hypersensitivity to the drug or other opiate analgesics.
• *Use cautiously* in head injury and increased intracranial pressure; severe respiratory, liver, and kidney impairment; CNS depression; thyroid irregularities; adrenal insufficiency; and prostatic hypertrophy.
• Naloxone will not completely reverse the respiratory depression caused by buprenorphine overdose. Therefore, an overdose may necessitate mechanical ventilation. Larger than customary doses of naloxone (more than 0.4 mg) and doxapram may also be ordered.
• When used postoperatively, encourage turning, coughing, and deep breathing to prevent atelectasis.
• If dependence occurs, withdrawal symptoms may appear up to 14 days after drug is stopped.
• Drug has narcotic antagonist properties. May precipitate abstinence syndrome in narcotic-dependent patients.
• S.C. administration not recommended.
• Buprenorphine 0.3 mg is equal to 10 mg morphine and 75 mg meperidine in analgesic potency. Has longer duration of action than morphine or meperidine.
• Warn the patient to avoid driving and other hazardous activities that require mental alertness until adverse CNS effects of the drug are known.

General

Classification: migraine headache suppressant (serotonin [5-HT] receptor agonist). **Pregnancy risk category:** C.

Mechanism of action

Selectively activates vascular serotonin (5-HT) receptors. Receptor stimulation causes vasoconstriction of these cerebral vessels but has minimal effects on systemic vessels, tissue perfusion, and blood pressure.

Indications and dosage

• Acute migraine attacks (with or without aura). **Adults:** 6 mg S.C. May be repeated after a minimum of 1 hour. Maximum recommended dosage is two 6-mg injections daily.

Adverse reactions

CNS: *dizziness, vertigo,* drowsiness, headache, anxiety, malaise, fatigue, weakness. **CV:** ***atrial fibrillation, ventricular fibrillation, ventricular tachycardia, MI, ECG changes such as ischemic ST-segment elevation*** (rare). **EENT:** discomfort of the throat, nasal cavity or sinus, mouth, jaw, or tongue; visual alterations. **GI:** abdominal discomfort, dysphagia. **Skin:** local reactions, flushing. **Other:** *tingling, warm or hot sensation, burning sensation,* tight feeling in head, cold sensation, pressure or tightness in chest, neck pain, myalgia, muscle cramps, sweating.

Interactions

Ergot and ergot derivatives: prolonged vasospastic effects. Don't use these drugs and sumatriptan within 24 hours of each other.

Nursing diagnoses

• Pain related to patient's underlying condition.
• High risk for injury related to sumatriptan-induced dizziness or vertigo.
• Knowledge deficit related to sumatriptan therapy.

Nursing interventions

• *Contraindicated* in hypertension, hemiplegic or basilar migraine, in patients taking ergotamine, and in patients with ischemic heart disease, such as angina pectoris, Prinzmetal's angina, history of MI, or documented silent ischemia.
• *Use cautiously* in patients who may have unrecognized coronary artery disease (CAD), such as postmenopausal women; men over age 40; or those with risk factors, such as hypertension, hypercholesterolemia, obesity, diabetes, smoking, or a family history of CAD.
• Serious adverse cardiac effects can follow a dose of this drug, but such events are extremely rare. When giving the drug to patients at risk for unrecognized CAD, consider administering the first dose in the doctor's office.
• Onset of pain relief is often rapid (within 10 minutes). Redness or pain at the injection site should subside within 1 hour.
• Although patients may receive a second dose after a minimum of 1 hour, it may not be beneficial.
• Drug is available in a spring-loaded injector system that facilitates self-administration by the patient. Be sure that patient understands how to load the injector, administer the injection, and dispose of the used syringes.
• Be sure patient understands that drug is intended only to treat a migraine attack, not to prevent or reduce the number of attacks.
• Advise female patients not to use this drug if they are pregnant or intend to become pregnant. Advise them to discuss with the doctor the risks and benefits of using the drug during pregnancy.
• Tell patient that drug may be given at any time during a migraine attack, but preferably as soon as symptoms appear.
• Tell patient to stop using the drug and call the doctor immediately if he experiences persistent or severe chest pain; pain or tightness in the throat; wheezing; heart throbbing; swelling of the eyelids, face, or lips; or a skin rash, lumps, or hives.

General

Classification: antidepressant (aminoketone).
Pregnancy risk category: B.

Mechanism of action

Unknown. Bupropion is not a tricyclic antidepressant, does not inhibit MAO, and weakly inhibits norepinephrine, dopamine, and serotonin reuptake.

Indications and dosage

- Treatment of depression. **Adults:** initially, 100 mg P.O. b.i.d. If there is no response after several weeks of therapy, dosage may be increased to 150 mg t.i.d.

Adverse reactions

CNS: *headache,* akathisia, ***seizures,*** *agitation,* anxiety, *confusion,* decreased libido, delusions, euphoria, hostility, impaired sleep quality, insomnia, sedation, sensory disturbance, tremor. **CV:** ***arrhythmias,*** hypertension, hypotension, palpitations, syncope, tachycardia. **GI:** appetite increase, constipation, dyspepsia, nausea, vomiting, dry mouth. **GU:** impotence, menstrual complaints, urinary frequency. **Skin:** pruritus, rash, cutaneous temperature disturbance. **Other:** arthritis, fever and chills, excessive sweating, auditory disturbance, gustatory disturbance, blurred vision.

Interactions

Levodopa, phenothiazines, MAO inhibitors, tricyclic antidepressants; recent and rapid withdrawal of benzodiazepines: increased risk of adverse reactions, including seizures.

Nursing diagnoses

- Ineffective individual coping related to the patient's underlying condition.
- High risk for injury related to bupropion-induced adverse CNS reactions.
- Knowledge deficit related to bupropion therapy.

Nursing interventions

- *Contraindicated* in patients who have taken MAO inhibitors within the previous 14 days and in those with seizure disorders. About 0.4% of patients treated at doses up to 450 mg/day may experience seizures. If dosage is increased to 600 mg/day, the incidence of seizures increases about tenfold. To prevent seizures, do not exceed 450 mg/day and administer in three or four equally divided doses. Also contraindicated in patients with a history of bulimia or anorexia nervosa because of a higher incidence of seizures in these patients.
- Bupropion, like many antidepressants, can cause manic episodes during the depressed phase of bipolar manic depression.
- Clinical trials revealed that 28% of the patients experienced a 5 lb (2.27 kg) or greater weight loss. This drug effect should be considered if weight loss is a major factor in the patient's depressive illness.
- Advise patients to take the drug regularly as scheduled, and to take each day's dosage in three divided doses to minimize the risk of seizures.
- Advise patients to avoid alcohol use, since it may contribute to seizures.
- Advise the patient to avoid hazardous activities that require alertness, including operating heavy machinery or driving a car, until the CNS effects of the drug are known.
- Warn patients not to take any other medications, including OTC medications, without first checking with their doctors.

General

Classification: nonnarcotic analgesic, antipyretic, anti-inflammatory (NSAID). **Pregnancy risk category:** B (D in 3rd trimester).

Mechanism of action

Produces anti-inflammatory, analgesic, and antipyretic effects, possibly through inhibition of prostaglandin synthesis.

Indications and dosage

• Osteoarthritis, rheumatoid arthritis, ankylosing spondylitis. **Adults:** initially, 150 mg P.O. b.i.d.; may increase to 200 mg b.i.d.
• Acute bursitis tendinitis, acute gouty arthritis. **Adults:** 200 mg P.O. b.i.d. for 7 to 14 days. Dose may be reduced as symptoms subside.

Adverse reactions

Blood: prolonged bleeding time, ***aplastic anemia.*** **CNS:** dizziness, headache, nervousness. **EENT:** tinnitus, transient visual disturbances. **GI:** *epigastric distress,* ***peptic ulceration,*** *occult blood loss, nausea.* **Hepatic:** elevated enzymes. **Skin:** rash, pruritus. **Other:** edema.

Interactions

Anticoagulants: increased risk of bleeding. Monitor PT closely. **Aspirin and other salicylates, diflunisal, dimethyl sulfoxide:** decreased metabolism of sulindac to its active metabolite, reducing its effectiveness. Don't use together. **Cyclosporine:** increased nephrotoxicity of cyclosporine. Avoid concomitant use. **Methotrexate:** increased methotrexate toxicity. Avoid concomitant use. **Probenecid:** increased plasma levels of sulindac and its active metabolite. Monitor for toxicity. **Sulfonamides, sulfonylureas, other highly protein-bound drugs:** possible displacement of these drugs from plasma protein-binding sites, leading to increased toxicity. Monitor closely.

Nursing diagnoses

• Pain related to the patient's underlying condition.
• Sensory/perceptual alterations (visual) related to transient adverse effect of sulindac therapy.
• Knowledge deficit related to sulindac therapy.

Nursing interventions

• *Contraindicated* in acute asthmatics whose conditions are precipitated by other NSAIDs or by aspirin and in patients who have active ulcers and GI bleeding.
• *Use cautiously* in patients with a history of ulcers and GI bleeding, renal dysfunction, compromised cardiac function, or hypertension and in those receiving oral anticoagulants or oral antidiabetic agents.
• To reduce adverse GI reactions, give with food, milk, or antacids.
• Serious GI toxicity can occur at any time in patients on long-term NSAID therapy. Teach patient signs and symptoms of GI bleeding, and tell him to report these immediately.
• Patient should notify doctor and have complete eye examination if any visual disturbances occur.
• Periodically monitor hepatic and renal function and CBC in patients receiving long-term therapy.
• Tell patient to notify doctor immediately if easy bruising or prolonged bleeding occurs.
• Drug causes sodium retention but is thought to have less effect on the kidneys than any other NSAID. Patient should report edema and have blood pressure checked monthly.
• Because of its antipyretic and anti-inflammatory actions, sulindac may mask the signs and symptoms of infection.

General

Classification: anxiolytic (azospirodecanedione).
Pregnancy risk category: B.

Mechanism of action

Unknown. However, the drug may inhibit neuronal firing and reduce 5-HT turnover in cortical, amygdaloid, and septohippocampal tissue.

Indications and dosage

• Management of anxiety disorders; short-term relief of anxiety. **Adults:** initially, 5 mg P.O. t.i.d. Dosage may be increased at 3-day intervals. Usual maintenance dosage is 20 to 30 mg daily in divided doses.

Adverse reactions

CNS: *dizziness, drowsiness,* nervousness, insomnia, headache. **GI:** nausea, dry mouth, diarrhea. **Other:** fatigue.

Interactions

Alcohol, other CNS depressants: increased CNS depression. Avoid concomitant use. **MAO inhibitors:** may elevate blood pressure.

Nursing diagnoses

• Anxiety related to the patient's underlying condition.
• High risk for injury related to buspirone-induced CNS reaction.
• Knowledge deficit related to buspirone therapy.

Nursing interventions

• *Contraindicated in* patients with hypersensitivity to the drug.
• *Use cautiously* in patients with hepatic or renal failure.
• Although buspirone is less sedating than other anxiolytics and does not produce any serious functional impairment, CNS effects in an individual patient may be unpredictable. Therefore, warn patients to avoid hazardous activities that require alertness and neuromuscular coordination until CNS effects of the drug are known.
• Unlike the benzodiazepines, buspirone is not an effective anticonvulsant or skeletal muscle relaxant. Its use is limited to the treatment of anxiety.
• Tell patient to take drug with food.
• Before initiating buspirone therapy in patients already being treated with benzodiazepines, warn them against stopping the benzodiazepine abruptly. Abrupt discontinuation may cause a benzodiazepine withdrawal reaction.
• Signs of improvement with buspirone are usually evident within 7 to 10 days; optimal results are achieved after 3 to 4 weeks of therapy.
• This drug has shown no potential for abuse and has not been classified as a controlled substance. However, it is not recommended for use to relieve everyday stress.

General

Classification: antibiotic (sulfonamide). **Pregnancy risk category:** B (D if near term).

Mechanism of action

Inhibits formation of dihydrofolic acid from PABA, decreasing bacterial folic acid synthesis.

Indications and dosage

• Urinary tract and systemic infections. **Adults:** initially, 2 to 4 g P.O., then 1 to 2 g P.O. q.i.d. **Children over 2 months:** initially, 75 mg/kg P.O. daily or 2 g/m² P.O. daily in divided doses q 6 hours, then 150 mg/kg or 4 g/m² P.O. daily in divided doses q 6 hours.

Adverse reactions

Blood: ***agranulocytosis, aplastic anemia,*** megaloblastic anemia, thrombocytopenia, leukopenia, ***hemolytic anemia.*** **CNS:** headache, mental depression, seizures, hallucinations. **GI:** *nausea, vomiting, diarrhea,* abdominal pain, anorexia, stomatitis. **GU:** ***toxic nephrosis with oliguria and anuria,*** crystalluria, hematuria. **Hepatic:** jaundice. **Skin:** ***erythema multiforme (Stevens-Johnson syndrome),*** *generalized skin eruption,* ***epidermal necrolysis, exfoliative dermatitis,*** photosensitivity, urticaria, pruritus. **Other:** ***hypersensitivity,*** *serum sickness, drug fever,* ***anaphylaxis.***

Interactions

Ammonium chloride, ascorbic acid: doses sufficient to acidify urine may cause crystalluria and precipitation of sulfonamide. Don't use together. **Oral anticoagulants:** increased anticoagulant effect. **Oral antidiabetic agents:** increased antidiabetic effect. **Oral contraceptives:** decreased contraceptive effectiveness and increased risk of breakthrough bleeding. **PABA-containing drugs:** inhibit antibacterial action. Don't use together.

Nursing diagnoses

• High risk for injury related to ineffectiveness of sulfisoxazole in eradicating the infection.
• High risk for fluid volume deficit related to adverse GI reactions caused by sulfisoxazole.
• Knowledge deficit related to sulfisoxazole therapy.

Nursing interventions

• *Contraindicated* in porphyria and in infants under 2 months (except in congenital toxoplasmosis).
• *Use cautiously* in impaired hepatic or renal function, severe allergy or bronchial asthma, and G6PD deficiency.
• Obtain specimen for culture and sensitivity tests before first dose. Therapy may begin pending test results.
• Tell patient to drink a full glass of water with each dose and to drink plenty of water throughout the day to prevent crystalluria. Monitor intake and output. Intake should be sufficient to produce output of 1,500 ml daily (between 3,000 and 4,000 ml daily for adults). To aid in prevention of crystalluria, sodium bicarbonate may be administered to alkalinize urine. Monitor urine pH daily.
• Watch for superinfection (fever or other signs of new infection).
• Tell patient to take medication exactly as prescribed, even if he feels better, and to take entire amount prescribed.
• Warn patient to avoid direct sunlight and ultraviolet light to prevent photosensitivity reaction.
• Monitor urine cultures, CBCs, PT, and urinalyses before and during therapy.
• Sulfisoxazole-pyrimethamine combination may be used to treat toxoplasmosis.
• Tell patient to report early signs of blood dyscrasia (sore throat, fever, and pallor) immediately to doctor.
• When given preoperatively, the patient should receive a low-residue diet and a minimal number of enemas and cathartics.

General

Classification: antineoplastic (alkylating agent).
Pregnancy risk category: D.

Mechanism of action

Cross-links strands of cellular DNA and interferes with RNA transcription, causing an imbalance of growth that leads to cell death. Cell cycle-non-specific.

Indications and dosage

• Chronic myelocytic (granulocytic) leukemia. **Adults:** 4 to 8 mg P.O. daily up to maximum 12 mg P.O. daily until WBC count falls to 15,000/mm³. Stop drug until WBC count rises to 50,000/mm³, then resume treatment as before; or 4 to 8 mg P.O. daily until WBC count falls to 10,000 to 20,000/mm³, then reduce daily dosage as needed to maintain WBC count at this level (usually 2 mg daily). **Children:** 0.06 to 0.12 mg/kg or 1.8 to 4.6 mg/m²/day P.O.; adjust dosage to maintain WBC count at 20,000/mm³, but never less than 10,000/mm³.

Adverse reactions

Blood: WBC count falling after about 10 days and continuing to fall for 2 weeks after stopping drug; ***thrombocytopenia, leukopenia, anemia.*** **CNS:** ***seizures.*** **GI:** nausea, vomiting, diarrhea, cheilosis, glossitis. **GU:** amenorrhea, testicular atrophy, impotence. **Metabolic:** Addison-like wasting syndrome, profound hyperuricemia due to increased cell lysis. **Respiratory:** persistent cough, progressive dyspnea with alveolar exudate (may result from drug toxicity). **Skin:** transient hyperpigmentation, rash, urticaria, anhidrosis. **Other:** gynecomastia; alopecia; ***irreversible pulmonary fibrosis, commonly termed "busulfan lung."***

Interactions

None significant.

Nursing diagnoses

• High risk for infection related to the patient's busulfan-induced pancytopenia.
• Altered renal tissue perfusion related to hyperuricemia with resulting uric acid nephropathy.
• Knowledge deficit related to busulfan therapy.

Nursing interventions

• *Contraindicated* in patients with chronic myelogenous leukemia, which is known to be resistant to the drug.
• *Use cautiously* in patients recently given other myelosuppressive drugs or radiation treatment and in those with depressed neutrophil or platelet count. Because high-dose therapy has been associated with seizures, use such therapy cautiously in patients with a history of head trauma or seizures, or in patients receiving other drugs that lower the seizure threshold.
• Warn patient to watch for signs of infection (fever, sore throat, fatigue) and bleeding (easy bruising, nosebleeds, bleeding gums, melena). Take temperature daily.
• Pulmonary fibrosis may occur as late as 4 to 6 months after treatment with busulfan.
• Persistent cough and progressive dyspnea with alveolar exudate may result from drug toxicity, not pneumonia. Instruct patient to report symptoms so dosage adjustments can be made.
• To prevent hyperuricemia with resulting uric acid nephropathy, use with adequate hydration. Monitor serum uric acid.
• Patient response usually begins within 1 to 2 weeks (increased appetite, sense of well-being, decreased total leukocyte count, reduction in size of spleen).
• Anticoagulants and aspirin products should be used cautiously. Watch closely for signs of bleeding. Instruct patient to avoid any OTC product containing aspirin.
• Avoid all I.M. injections when platelet count is below 100,000/mm³.

General
Classification: renal tubular-blocking agent, platelet aggregation inhibitor (uricosuric agent).
Pregnancy risk category: C.

Mechanism of action
Blocks renal tubular reabsorption of uric acid, increasing excretion. Also inhibits platelet aggregation.

Indications and dosage
- Inhibition of platelet aggregation and increased platelet survival time in treatment of thromboembolic disorders, angina, MI, transient cerebral ischemic attacks, peripheral arterial atherosclerosis. **Adults:** 200 mg P.O. q.i.d.
- Maintenance therapy for common gout (reduction, prevention of joint changes and tophi formation). **Adults:** 100 to 200 mg P.O. b.i.d. first week, then 200 to 400 mg P.O. b.i.d. Maximum dosage is 800 mg daily.

Adverse reactions
Blood: ***agranulocytosis, blood dyscrasias (rare).*** **CNS:** dizziness, vertigo, tinnitus. **GI:** *nausea, dyspepsia,* epigastric pain, blood loss, reactivation of peptic ulcers. **Skin:** rash.

Interactions
Oral anticoagulants: increased anticoagulant effect and risk of bleeding. Use together cautiously. **Oral antidiabetic agents:** increased effects. Monitor closely. **Probenecid:** inhibited renal excretion of sulfinpyrazone. Use together cautiously. **Salicylates:** inhibited uricosuric effect of sulfinpyrazone. Don't use together.

Nursing diagnoses
- Pain related to patient's underlying condition.
- High risk for infection related to sulfinpyrazone-induced agranulocytosis.
- Knowledge deficit related to sulfinpyrazone therapy.

Nursing interventions
- *Contraindicated* in hypersensitivity to pyrazole derivatives (including oxyphenbutazone and phenylbutazone); active peptic ulcer; gouty nephropathy; urolithiasis or urinary obstruction; bone marrow suppression; azotemia or hyperuricemia secondary to cancer chemotherapy, radiation therapy or myeloproliferative neoplastic diseases; blood dyscrasias; and during or within 2 weeks after gout attack.
- *Use cautiously* in hepatic or renal impairment.
- Use in treating thromboembolic conditions is investigational and is most often directed at prevention of recurrent MI.
- Recommended for patients unresponsive to probenecid. Suitable for long-term use; neither cumulative effects nor tolerance develops.
- Periodic BUN, CBC, and renal function studies advised during long-term use.
- May increase frequency, severity, and length of acute gout attacks during first 6 to 12 months of therapy. Prophylactic colchicine or another anti-inflammatory agent is given during first 3 to 6 months.
- Therapy may lead to renal colic and formation of uric acid stones. Until acid levels are normal (about 6 mg/dl), monitor intake and output closely.
- Force fluids to maintain minimum daily output of 2 to 3 liters. Alkalinize urine with sodium bicarbonate or other agent ordered by doctor.
- Give with milk, food, or antacids to minimize GI disturbances.
- Patients with gout should restrict foods high in purine: anchovies, liver, sardines, and peas.
- Instruct patient to take drug as ordered to avoid gout attacks. Tell him that blood levels must be monitored and that dosage adjustments may be needed.
- Lifelong therapy may be required in patients with hyperuricemia.
- Warn patient with gout not to take any aspirin-containing medications.

General

Classification: sedative-hypnotic (barbiturate). **Pregnancy risk category:** D. **Controlled substance schedule**: III.

Mechanism of action

Probably interferes with transmission of impulses from the thalamus to the cortex of the brain.

Indications and dosage

- Sedation. **Adults:** 15 to 30 mg P.O. t.i.d. or q.i.d. **Children:** 6 mg/kg P.O. divided t.i.d. Dosage range 7.5 to 30 mg P.O. t.i.d.
- Preoperatively. **Adults:** 50 to 100 mg P.O. 60 to 90 minutes before surgery.
- Insomnia. **Adults:** 50 to 100 mg P.O. h.s.

Adverse reactions

CNS: *drowsiness, lethargy, hangover,* paradoxical excitement in elderly patients. **GI:** nausea, vomiting. **Skin:** rash, urticaria. **Other:** ***Stevens-Johnson syndrome, angioedema,*** exacerbation of porphyria.

Interactions

Alcohol or other CNS depressants, including narcotic analgesics: excessive CNS and respiratory depression. Use together cautiously. **Griseofulvin:** decreased absorption of griseofulvin. **MAO inhibitors:** inhibit the metabolism of barbiturates; may cause prolonged CNS depression. Reduce barbiturate dosage. **Oral anticoagulants, estrogens and oral contraceptives, doxycycline, corticosteroids:** butabarbital may enhance the metabolism of these drugs. Monitor for decreased effect. **Rifampin:** may decrease barbiturate levels. Monitor for decreased effect.

Nursing diagnoses

- Sleep pattern disturbance related to underlying patient problem.
- High risk for trauma related to adverse CNS reactions caused by butabarbital.
- Knowledge deficit related to butabarbital therapy.

Nursing interventions

- *Contraindicated* in uncontrolled severe pain, respiratory disease with dyspnea or obstruction, hypersensitivity to barbiturates, previous addiction to sedatives, or porphyria.
- *Use cautiously* in hepatic or renal impairment.
- Elderly patients are more sensitive to the drug's adverse CNS reactions. Assess mental status before and after initiating therapy.
- Advise caution with activities requiring mental alertness or physical coordination. Supervise walking; raise bed rails, especially for elderly patients.
- Prolonged administration is not recommended: drug loses its efficacy in promoting sleep after 14 days. A drug-free interval of at least 1 week is advised if continued treatment is appropriate.
- Long-term high dosage may cause drug dependence, and patient may experience withdrawal symptoms if drug is suddenly stopped. Withdraw barbiturates gradually.
- Take precautions to prevent hoarding or self-overdosing by patients who are depressed, suicidal, or drug-dependent, or who have a history of drug abuse.
- Watch for signs of barbiturate toxicity: coma, pupillary constriction, cyanosis, clammy skin, and hypotension. Overdose can be fatal.
- Skin eruptions may precede potentially fatal reactions to barbiturate therapy. Discontinue drug when skin reactions occur. In some patients, high fever, stomatitis, headache, or rhinitis may precede skin reactions.
- Morning "hangover" common after hypnotic dose.
- Hypnotic doses suppress REM sleep. Patient may experience nightmares and enhanced dreaming after drug is discontinued.
- Women who use oral contraceptives should consider alternate birth control methods when taking this drug because it may enhance contraceptive hormone metabolism and decrease its effect.

General

Classification: antibiotic (sulfonamide). **Pregnancy risk category:** B (D if near term).

Mechanism of action

Inhibits formation of dihydrofolic acid from PABA, decreasing bacterial folic acid synthesis.

Indications and dosage

- Mild to moderate ulcerative colitis, adjunctive therapy in severe ulcerative colitis. **Adults:** initially, 3 to 4 g P.O. daily in evenly divided doses; usual maintenance dosage is 1.5 to 2 g P.O. daily in divided doses q 6 hours. May need to start with 1 to 2 g initially, with a gradual increase in dosage to minimize adverse effects. **Children over 2 years:** initially, 40 to 60 mg/kg P.O. daily, divided into 3 to 6 doses; then 30 mg/kg daily in 4 doses. May need to start at lower dose if GI intolerance occurs.

Adverse reactions

Blood: ***agranulocytosis, aplastic anemia,*** megaloblastic anemia, thrombocytopenia, leukopenia, ***hemolytic anemia.*** **CNS:** headache, mental depression, ***seizures,*** hallucinations. **GI:** *nausea, vomiting, diarrhea,* abdominal pain, anorexia, stomatitis. **GU:** ***toxic nephrosis with oliguria and anuria,*** crystalluria, hematuria. **Hepatic:** jaundice, hepatotoxicity. **Skin:** ***erythema multiforme (Stevens-Johnson syndrome),*** *generalized skin eruption,* ***epidermal necrolysis, exfoliative dermatitis,*** photosensitivity, urticaria, pruritus. **Other:** ***hypersensitivity,*** *serum sickness, fever,* ***anaphylaxis,*** oligospermia, infertility.

Interactions

Folic acid: absorption may be decreased. **Oral anticoagulants:** increased anticoagulant effect. **Oral antidiabetic agents:** increased antidiabetic effect. **Oral contraceptives:** decreased contraceptive effectiveness and increased risk of breakthrough bleeding.

Nursing diagnoses

- High risk for injury related to ineffectiveness of sulfasalazine in eradicating the infection.
- High risk for fluid volume deficit related to adverse GI reactions.
- Knowledge deficit related to sulfasalazine therapy.

Nursing interventions

- *Contraindicated* in patients with porphyria, intestinal or urinary obstruction, and allergy to salicylates.
- *Use cautiously* and in reduced dosages in impaired hepatic or renal function, severe allergy, bronchial asthma, or G6PD deficiency.
- Obtain specimen for culture and sensitivity tests before first dose. Therapy may begin pending test results.
- Watch for superinfection (fever or other signs of new infection).
- Tell patient to take medication exactly as prescribed, even if he feels better, and to take entire amount prescribed.
- Warn patient to avoid direct sunlight and ultraviolet light to prevent photosensitivity reaction.
- Discolors alkaline urine orange-yellow.
- Most adverse reactions affect GI tract. Minimize symptoms by spacing doses evenly and administering after food intake.

butorphanol tartrate

Stadol, Stadol NS

General

Classification: analgesic, adjunct to anesthesia (opoid partial agonist, narcotic agonist-antagonist). **Pregnancy risk category:** B (D for prolonged use or use of high doses at term).

Mechanism of action

Binds with opiate receptors at many sites in the CNS (brain, brain stem, and spinal cord), altering both perception of and emotional response to pain through an unknown mechanism.

Indications and dosage

- Moderate to severe pain. **Adults:** 1 to 4 mg I.M. q 3 to 4 hours, p.r.n. or around the clock; or 0.5 to 2 mg I.V. q 3 to 4 hours, p.r.n. or around the clock. Alternatively, give 1 mg by nasal spray q 3 to 4 hours (1 spray in one nostril). Repeat in 60 to 90 minutes if pain relief is inadequate.

Adverse reactions

CNS: *sedation, headache, vertigo, floating sensation,* lethargy, confusion, nervousness, unusual dreams, agitation, euphoria, hallucinations, flushing. **CV:** palpitations, fluctuation in blood pressure. **EENT:** diplopia, blurred vision. **GI:** *nausea,* vomiting, dry mouth, constipation. **Skin:** rash, hives, *clamminess, excessive sweating.* **Other:** ***respiratory depression.***

Interactions

Alcohol, CNS depressants: additive effects. Use together cautiously. **Narcotic analgesics:** avoid concomitant use. Possible decreased analgesic effect.

Nursing diagnoses

- Pain related to patient's underlying condition.
- High risk for trauma related to adverse CNS reactions induced by butorphanol.
- Knowledge deficit related to butorphanol therapy.

Nursing interventions

- *Contraindicated* in narcotic addiction; drug has narcotic antagonist properties and may precipitate narcotic abstinence syndrome.
- *Use cautiously* in head injury, increased intracranial pressure, acute MI, ventricular dysfunction, coronary insufficiency, respiratory disease or depression, and renal or hepatic dysfunction.
- Psychological and physical addiction may occur.
- S.C. route not recommended.
- Periodically monitor postoperative vital signs and bladder function. Because drug decreases both rate and depth of respirations, monitoring of arterial oxygen saturation may aid in assessing respiratory depression. However, respiratory depression does not seem to increase with increased dosage.
- Also used as the analgesic component of balanced anesthesia and for relief of postpartum pain.
- Warn the patient to avoid driving and other hazardous activities that require mental alertness until adverse CNS effects of the drug are known.

General

Classification: antibiotic (sulfonamide). **Pregnancy risk category:** B (D if near term).

Mechanism of action

Inhibits formation of dihydrofolic acid from PABA, decreasing bacterial folic acid synthesis.

Indications and dosage

- UTI and systemic infections. **Adults:** initially, 2 g P.O., then 1 g P.O. b.i.d. up to t.i.d. for severe infections. **Children and infants over 2 months:** initially, 50 to 60 mg/kg P.O., then 25 to 30 mg/kg b.i.d. Maximum dosage should not exceed 75 mg/kg daily.
- Lymphogranuloma venereum (genital, inguinal, or anorectal infection). **Adults:** 1 g P.O. daily for at least 3 weeks.

Adverse reactions

Blood: ***agranulocytosis, aplastic anemia,*** megaloblastic anemia, thrombocytopenia, leukopenia, ***hemolytic anemia.*** **CNS:** headache, mental depression, seizures, hallucinations. **GI:** *nausea, vomiting, diarrhea,* abdominal pain, anorexia, stomatitis. **GU:** ***toxic nephrosis with oliguria and anuria,*** crystalluria, hematuria. **Hepatic:** jaundice. **Skin:** ***erythema multiforme (Stevens-Johnson syndrome),*** *generalized skin eruption,* ***epidermal necrolysis, exfoliative dermatitis,*** photosensitivity, urticaria, pruritus. **Other:** ***hypersensitivity,*** *serum sickness, fever,* ***anaphylaxis.***

Interactions

Ammonium chloride, ascorbic acid: doses sufficient to acidify urine may cause precipitation of sulfamethoxazole and crystalluria. Don't use together. **Oral anticoagulants:** increased anticoagulant effect. **Oral antidiabetic agents:** increased antidiabetic effect. **Oral contraceptives:** decreased contraceptive effectiveness and increased risk of breakthrough bleeding. **PABA-containing drugs:** inhibit antibacterial action. Don't use together.

Nursing diagnoses

- High risk for injury related to ineffectiveness of sulfamethoxazole in eradicating the infection.
- High risk for fluid volume deficit related to adverse GI reactions.
- Knowledge deficit related to sulfamethoxazole therapy.

Nursing interventions

- *Contraindicated* in porphyria or in infants under 2 months (except in congenital toxoplasmosis).
- *Use cautiously* and in reduced dosages in impaired hepatic or renal function or severe allergy or bronchial asthma, G6PD deficiency, or blood dyscrasias.
- Tell patient to drink a full glass of water with each dose and to drink plenty of water during the day to prevent crystalluria. Monitor fluid intake and output. Intake should be sufficient to produce output of 1,500 ml daily (between 3,000 and 4,000 ml daily for adults). To aid in prevention of crystalluria, sodium bicarbonate may be administered to alkalinize urine. Monitor urine pH daily.
- Watch for superinfection (fever or other signs of new infection).
- Obtain specimen for culture and sensitivity tests before first dose. Therapy may begin pending test results.
- Tell patient to take medication exactly as prescribed, even if he feels better, and to take entire amount prescribed.
- Warn patient to avoid direct sunlight and ultraviolet light to prevent photosensitivity reaction.
- Monitor urine cultures, CBCs, and urinalyses before and during therapy.
- Sulfamethoxazole is also used as adjunctive treatment for toxoplasmosis.
- Instruct patient to report early signs of blood dyscrasias (sore throat, fever, and pallor) to doctor immediately.

General
Classification: CNS stimulant (methylxanthine).
Pregnancy risk category: B.

Mechanism of action
Inhibits phosphodiesterase, the enzyme that degrades cyclic adenosine monophosphate.

Indications and dosage
- CNS stimulant. **Adults:** 100 to 200 mg anhydrous caffeine P.O.
- Neonatal apnea. **Neonates:** 5 to 10 mg/kg P.O., I.M., or I.V. as a loading dose, then 2.5 to 5 mg P.O., I.M., or I.V. daily, according to patient tolerance and serum caffeine levels (therapeutic range is 5 to 20 mcg/ml).

Adverse reactions
Blood: hyperglycemia. **CNS:** *stimulation, insomnia,* restlessness, nervousness, mild delirium, headache, excitement, agitation, muscle tremors, twitches. **CV:** *tachycardia.* **GI:** nausea, vomiting. **GU:** *diuresis.* **Skin:** hyperesthesia.

Interactions
Theophylline, beta-adrenergic agonists: Excessive CNS stimulation.

Nursing diagnoses
- Sleep pattern disturbance related to stimulant effects of caffeine.
- Altered urinary elimination related to caffeine-induced diuresis.
- Knowledge deficit related to caffeine therapy.

Nursing interventions
- *Contraindicated* in gastric or duodenal ulcer, arrhythmias, or post-myocardial infarction.
- Caffeine-containing beverages should be restricted in patients who experience palpitations.
- Tolerance or psychological dependence may develop.
- Be alert for signs of overdose: GI pain, mild delirium, insomnia, diuresis, dehydration, and fever. Treat with short-acting barbiturates, gastric emesis, or lavage.
- Single dose should not exceed 1 g.
- Caffeine content in cola beverages, 17 to 55 mg/180 ml; tea, 40 to 100 mg/180 ml; instant coffee, 60 to 180 mg/180 ml; brewed coffee, 100 to 150 mg/180 ml; decaffeinated coffee, 1 to 6 mg/180 ml.
- Caffeine does not reverse alcohol intoxication or CNS depressant effects of alcohol. Overvigorous therapy with caffeine may aggravate depression in an already depressed patient.
- Avoid sudden discontinuation of caffeine; may cause headache and irritability.
- Caffeine is included in many OTC analgesic preparations. There's conflicting evidence regarding whether it increases pain relief.
- Treatment of neonatal apnea is an unlabeled indication. Solution may have to be made in pharmacy because most commercially available parenteral caffeine injections contain sodium benzoate, a preservative that may cause kernicterus in neonates.
- Used experimentally to treat certain types of vascular headaches.

General

Classification: antibiotic (sulfonamide). **Pregnancy risk category:** B (D if near term).

Mechanism of action

Inhibits formation of dihydrofolic acid from PABA, decreasing bacterial folic acid synthesis.

Indications and dosage

- UTI. **Adults:** initially, 2 to 4 g P.O., then 500 mg to 1 g P.O. q 6 hours. **Children 2 months and over:** initially, 75 mg/kg or 2 g/m^2 P.O., then 150 mg/kg or 4 g/m^2 P.O. in four to six divided doses daily. Maximum daily dosage is 6 g.
- Rheumatic fever prophylaxis, as an alternative to penicillin. **Children over 30 kg:** 1 g P.O. daily. **Children under 30 kg:** 500 mg P.O. daily.
- Adjunctive treatment in toxoplasmosis. **Adults:** 4 g P.O. in divided doses q 6 hours for 3 to 4 weeks (longer for immunosuppressed patients). Given with pyrimethamine 25 mg P.O. daily. **Children:** 100 mg/kg P.O. in divided doses q 6 hours for 3 to 4 weeks; given with pyrimethamine 2 mg/kg daily for 3 days, then 1 mg/kg daily for 3 to 4 weeks.

Adverse reactions

Blood: ***agranulocytosis, aplastic anemia,*** megaloblastic anemia, thrombocytopenia, leukopenia, ***hemolytic anemia.*** **CNS:** headache, mental depression, seizures, hallucinations. **GI:** *nausea, vomiting, diarrhea,* abdominal pain, anorexia, stomatitis. **GU:** ***toxic nephrosis*** with oliguria and anuria, crystalluria, hematuria. **Hepatic:** jaundice. **Skin:** ***erythema multiforme (Stevens-Johnson syndrome), generalized skin eruption, epidermal necrolysis, exfoliative dermatitis,*** photosensitivity, urticaria, pruritus. **Local:** irritation, extravasation. **Other:** ***hypersensitivity,*** *serum sickness, fever,* ***anaphylaxis.***

Interactions

Ammonium chloride, ascorbic acid: doses sufficient to acidify urine may cause precipitation of sulfadiazine and crystalluria. Don't use together. **Oral anticoagulants:** increased anticoagulant effect. **Oral antidiabetic agents:** increased antidiabetic effect. **Oral contraceptives:** decreased contraceptive effectiveness and increased risk of breakthrough bleeding. **PABA-containing drugs:** inhibit antibacterial action. Don't use together.

Nursing diagnoses

- High risk for injury related to ineffectiveness of sulfadiazine in eradicating the infection.
- High risk for fluid volume deficit related to adverse GI reactions.
- Knowledge deficit related to sulfadiazine therapy.

Nursing interventions

- *Contraindicated* in porphyria or in infants under 2 months (except in congenital toxoplasmosis).
- *Use cautiously* and in reduced dosages in impaired hepatic or renal function, bronchial asthma, history of multiple allergies, G6PD deficiency, or blood dyscrasias.
- Tell patient to drink a full glass of water with each dose and to drink plenty of water throughout the day to prevent crystalluria. Monitor intake and output. Intake should be sufficient to produce output of 1,500 ml daily (between 3,000 and 4,000 ml daily for adults). Sodium bicarbonate may be administered to alkalinize urine (to help prevent crystalluria). Monitor urine pH daily.
- Watch for superinfection.
- Obtain specimen for culture and sensitivity tests before first dose. Therapy may begin pending test results.
- Tell patient to take medication exactly as prescribed and to take entire amount.
- Warn patient to avoid sunlight and ultraviolet light to prevent photosensitivity reaction.
- Monitor for signs of blood dyscrasia and report them immediately.
- Monitor urine cultures, CBCs, and urinalyses before and during therapy.

General
Classification: hypocalcemic (thyroid hormone).
Pregnancy risk category: B.

Mechanism of action
Decreases osteoclastic activity by inhibiting osteocytic osteolysis. Also decreases mineral release and matrix or collagen breakdown in bone.

Indications and dosage
• Paget's disease of bone (osteitis deformans). **Adults:** initially, 100 IU of calcitonin (salmon) daily S.C. or I.M. Maintenance dosage is 50 to 100 IU daily or every other day. Alternatively, give calcitonin (human) 0.5 mg S.C. daily. Some patients may need as much as 1 mg daily. With sufficient improvement, dosage may be reduced to 0.25 mg daily two or three times per week.
• Hypercalcemia. **Adults:** 4 IU/kg of calcitonin (salmon) q 12 hours I.M.
• Postmenopausal osteoporosis. **Women:** 100 IU of calcitonin (salmon) daily I.M. or S.C.

Adverse reactions
CNS: headaches. **GI:** transient nausea with or without vomiting, diarrhea, anorexia. **GU:** transient diuresis. **Metabolic:** hyperglycemia. **Local:** inflammation at injection site, skin rashes. **Other:** *facial flushing;* hypocalcemia; swelling, tingling, and tenderness of hands; unusual taste sensation; ***anaphylaxis.***

Interactions
None significant.

Nursing diagnoses
• High risk for injury related to the patient's underlying bone condition.
• Altered protection related to potential for calcitonin-induced anaphylaxis.
• Knowledge deficit related to calcitonin therapy.

Nursing interventions
• *Contraindicated* in allergy to gelatin diluent used to prepare drug. Not recommended for breast-feeding mothers, or women who are or may become pregnant. Safe use in children not established.
• Calcitonin (human) is indicated in patients who develop resistance to calcitonin (salmon). Calcitonin (human) is associated with risk of diminishing efficacy caused by antibody formation or hypersensitivity reactions.
• Systemic allergic reactions possible since hormone is protein. Skin test is usually done before beginning therapy. Epinephrine should be available.
• Evaluate patients with good initial response to calcitonin who suffer relapse for antibody formation response.
• Transient facial flushing and warmth (lasting about 1 hour) occur in 20% to 30% of all patients within minutes of injection.
• Observe patient for signs of hypocalcemic tetany (muscle twitching, tetanic spasms, and seizures if hypocalcemia is severe).
• Monitor for signs of hypercalcemic relapse: bone pain, renal calculi, polyuria, anorexia, nausea, vomiting, thirst, constipation, lethargy, bradycardia, muscle hypotonicity, pathologic fracture, psychosis, and coma.
• Periodic examinations of urine sediment are advisable. Periodic serum alkaline phosphatase and 24-hour urine hydroxyproline levels should be determined to evaluate drug effect.
• I.M. route is preferred if the volume of the dose exceeds 2 ml.
• Administer at bedtime to minimize nausea and vomiting.
• Treatment usually lasts for at least 6 months; if patient is asymptomatic, drug is discontinued.
• Store calcitonin (human) at room temperature (77° F [25° C]) and calcitonin (salmon) in the refrigerator (36° to 46° F [2° to 8° C]). Use freshly reconstituted solution within 2 hours.
• Patients with postmenopausal osteoporosis may need calcium and vitamin D supplementation.

General

Classification: antibiotic (sulfonamide). **Pregnancy risk category:** C.

Mechanism of action

Prevents uptake of PABA, a metabolite of bacterial folic-acid synthesis.

Indications and dosage

- Inclusion conjunctivitis, corneal ulcers, trachoma, chlamydial infection. **Adults and children:** instill 1 to 2 drops of 10% solution into lower conjunctival sac q 2 to 3 hours during day, less often at night; or 1 to 2 drops of 15% solution into lower conjunctival sac q 1 to 2 hours initially, increasing interval as condition responds; or 1 drop of 30% solution into lower conjunctival sac q 2 hours. Alternatively, instill ½" to 1" of 10% ointment into conjunctival sac q.i.d. and h.s. May use ointment at night along with drops during the day.

Adverse reactions

EENT: slowed corneal wound healing (ointment), *pain on instillation (eyedrop)*, headache or brow pain, photophobia. **Other:** hypersensitivity (including itching or burning), overgrowth of nonsusceptible organisms, ***Stevens-Johnson syndrome***, photosensitivity.

Interactions

Gentamicin (ophthalmic): *in vitro* antagonism. Avoid using together. **Local anesthetics (procaine, tetracaine), para-aminobenzoic acid derivatives:** decreased sulfacetamide action. Wait 30 minutes to 1 hour after instilling anesthetic or para-aminobenzoic acid derivative before instilling sulfacetamide. **Silver preparations:** precipitate formation. Avoid using together.

Nursing diagnoses

- Altered protection related to ocular infection.
- Pain related to burning and stinging induced by instillation of sulfacetamide eyedrops.
- Knowledge deficit related to sulfacetamide therapy.

Nursing interventions

- *Contraindicated* in sulfonamide hypersensitivity. Not recommended for children under 2 months.
- Often used with systemic tetracycline in treating trachoma and inclusion conjunctivitis. Replaced by other antibiotics in treating major ocular infections; still used in minor ocular infections.
- Purulent exudate interferes with sulfacetamide action. Remove as much exudate as possible from lids before instilling sulfacetamide.
- Warn patient that eyedrops burn slightly.
- Tell patient not to share eye medications with family members. If a family member develops the same symptoms, instruct him to contact the doctor.
- Warn patient to avoid sharing washcloths and towels with family members during infection.
- Tell patient to watch for signs of sensitivity, such as itching lids, swelling, or constant burning. Patient who develops such signs should stop drug and notify doctor immediately.
- Teach patient how to instill drug. Advise him to wash hands before and after administering ointment or solution, not to touch tip of dropper to eye or surrounding tissues, and to apply light finger pressure on lacrimal sac for 1 minute after drops are instilled. Stress importance of compliance with recommended therapy. Wait at least 5 minutes before administering other eyedrops.
- Warn patient that solution may stain clothing.
- Store drug in tightly closed, light-resistant container away from heat. Don't use discolored (dark brown) solution.
- Tell patient he may minimize photophobia by wearing sunglasses and avoiding prolonged exposure to sunlight.

calcium polycarbophil

Equalactin◇, FiberCon◇, Mitrolan◇

General

Classification: bulk laxative, antidiarrheal (hydrophilic agent). **Pregnancy risk category:** C.

Mechanism of action

Absorbs water and expands to increase bulk and moisture content of the stool. The increased bulk encourages peristalsis and bowel movement. As an antidiarrheal, absorbs free fecal water, thereby producing formed stools.

Indications and dosage

• Constipation (Equalactin and Mitrolan must be chewed before swallowing). **Adults:** 1 g P.O. q.i.d. as required. Maximum 6 g in 24-hour period. **Children 6 to 12 years:** 500 mg P.O. t.i.d. as required. Maximum 3 g in 24-hour period. **Children 2 to 6 years:** 500 mg P.O. b.i.d. as required. Maximum 1.5 g in 24-hour period.

• Diarrhea associated with irritable bowel syndrome, as well as acute nonspecific diarrhea (Mitrolan must be chewed before swallowing). **Adults:** 1 g P.O. q.i.d. as required. Maximum 6 g in 24-hour period. **Children 6 to 12 years:** 500 mg P.O. t.i.d. as required. Maximum 3 g in 24-hour period. **Children 2 to 6 years:** 500 mg P.O. b.i.d. as required. Maximum 1.5 g in 24-hour period.

Adverse reactions

GI: abdominal fullness and increased flatus, intestinal obstruction. **Other:** laxative dependence in long-term or excessive use.

Interactions

None significant.

Nursing diagnoses

• Constipation related to interruption of normal pattern of elimination characterized by infrequent or absent stools.

• Altered GI tissue perfusion related to drug-induced intestinal obstruction.

• Knowledge deficit related to calcium polycarbophil therapy.

Nursing interventions

• *Contraindicated* in signs of GI obstruction.

• Be alert for rectal bleeding or failure to respond to therapy. May indicate need for surgery.

• Before giving for constipation, determine if patient has adequate fluid intake, exercise, and diet. Tell him that dietary sources of bulk include bran and other cereals, fresh fruit, and vegetables.

• Advise patient to chew the Equalactin or Mitrolan tablets thoroughly and drink a full glass of water with each dose. However, when used as an antidiarrheal, tell patient *not* to drink a glass of water.

• For episodes of severe diarrhea, the dose may be repeated every half hour, but maximum daily dosage should not be exceeded.

General

Classification: anesthetic adjunct to anesthesia (opioid). **Pregnancy risk category:** C (D with prolonged use or high doses at term). **Controlled substance schedule:** II.

Indications and dosage

Binds with opiate receptors at many sites in the CNS (brain, brain stem, and spinal cord), altering both perception of and emotional response to pain through an unknown mechanism.

Indications and dosage

- Adjunct to general anesthetic. **Adults:** 1 to 8 mcg/kg I.V. administered with nitrous oxide or oxygen.
- Primary anesthetic. **Adults:** 8 to 30 mcg/kg I.V. administered with 100% oxygen and a muscle relaxant.

Adverse reactions

CNS: chills. **CV:** *hypotension*, hypertension, bradycardia, tachycardia. **GI:** nausea, vomiting. **Skin:** itching. **Other:** ***chest wall rigidity***, intraoperative muscle movement, ***respiratory depression.***

Interactions

Alcohol, CNS depressants: additive effects. Use together cautiously.

Nursing diagnoses

- Decreased cardiac output related to adverse cardiac effects of therapy.
- Ineffective breathing pattern related to sufentanil-induced respiratory depression or chest wall rigidity.
- Knowledge deficit related to sufentanil therapy.

Nursing interventions

- *Contraindicated* in patients with hypersensitivity to the drug or to other opiate analgesics.
- *Use cautiously* in head injury; pulmonary, hepatic, or renal disease; or decreased respiratory reserve.
- **I.V. use:** Should be administered only by persons specifically trained in the use of I.V. anesthetics.
- When used at doses over 8 mcg/kg, postoperative mechanical ventilation and observation are essential because of prolonged respiratory depression.
- Keep narcotic antagonist (naloxone) and resuscitative equipment available when giving drug.
- Monitor respirations of neonates exposed to the drug during labor.
- Because drug may decrease both rate and depth of respirations, monitoring of arterial oxygen saturation may aid in assessing respiratory depression. Notify doctor if respirations fall below 12 breaths/minute.
- Dose should be reduced in elderly and debilitated patients.
- Monitor postoperative vital signs frequently, including circulatory and respiratory status and urinary function. Drug may cause respiratory depression, hypotension, urine retention, nausea, vomiting, ileus, or altered level of consciousness. Encourage turning, coughing, and deep breathing to prevent atelectasis.
- Has more rapid onset and shorter duration of action than fentanyl.
- High doses can produce muscle rigidity reversible by neuromuscular blockers; however, patient must be artificially ventilated.

calcium salts

Phos-Ex◇, Phos-Lo; Amitone◇, Tums◇; Kalcinate◇; Posture◇

General

Classification: antacid, agent for electrolyte imbalance, cardiotonic (calcium supplement). **Pregnancy risk category:** C.

Mechanism of action

Replaces and maintains calcium.

Indications and dosage

- Hypocalcemia, hypocalcemic tetany, cardiac resuscitation for inotropic effect when epinephrine has failed; magnesium intoxication; hypoparathyroidism. **Adults:** chloride – initially, 500 mg to 1 g I.V. at a maximum rate of 1 ml/minute; gluceptate – 1.2 to 2.4 g I.V. at maximum rate of 2 ml/minute; gluconate – 1 to 2 g I.V. at maximum rate of 5 ml/minute. Additional doses based on serum calcium levels.
- Hypophosphatemia. **Adults:** 1,334 to 2,000 mg P.O. (acetate) t.i.d. with meals.
- Hypocalcemia during exchange transfusions. **Adults and children:** 0.5 ml (gluceptate) I.V. after each 100 ml blood exchanged.
- Calcium supplementation. **Adults:** 1 to 1.5 g (carbonate) P.O. t.i.d., not to exceed 8 g daily.
- Calcium supplementation during total parenteral nutrition. **Adults:** 10 to 15 mEq (chloride) I.V. daily. **Children:** 5 to 20 mEq (chloride) I.V. daily. **Neonates:** 0.5 to 3 mEq/kg (chloride) I.V. daily.

Adverse reactions

CNS: from I.V. use, tingling sensations, sense of oppression or heat waves; with rapid I.V. injection, syncope. **CV:** mild fall in blood pressure; with rapid I.V. injection, vasodilation, bradycardia, ***cardiac arrhythmias, cardiac arrest.*** **GI:** with oral ingestion, irritation, hemorrhage, *constipation;* with I.V. administration, chalky taste; with oral calcium chloride, GI hemorrhage, nausea, vomiting, thirst, abdominal pain. **GU:** hypercalcemia, polyuria, renal calculi. **Skin:** local reaction if given I.M., burning, necrosis, tissue sloughing, cellulitis, soft tissue calcification. **Local:** with S.C. injection, pain and irritation; with I.V., *vein irritation.*

Interactions

Digitalis glycosides: increased digitalis toxicity; administer cautiously (if at all) to digitalized patients. **Oxalic acid, phytic acid, and phosphorus:** may interfere with absorption of calcium.

Nursing diagnoses

- Altered nutrition: Less than body requirements related to insufficient calcium.
- High risk for injury related to calcium-induced hypercalcemia.
- Knowledge deficit related to calcium therapy.

Nursing interventions

- *Contraindicated* in ventricular fibrillation, hypercalcemia, or renal calculi.
- *Use cautiously* in sarcoidosis and renal or cardiac disease and in digitalized patients. Use calcium chloride cautiously in cor pulmonale, respiratory acidosis, and respiratory failure.
- **I.V. use:** Administer slowly through a small needle into a large vein or through an I.V. line containing a free-flowing, compatible solution. Do not use scalp veins in children.
- Calcium chloride should be given I.V. only. When adding to parenteral solutions that contain other additives (especially phosphorus or phosphate), observe for precipitate. Use an in-line filter.
- Monitor ECG when giving calcium I.V. Stop if patient complains of discomfort. Following I.V. injection, patient should lie down for 15 minutes.
- Give I.M. injection in gluteal region in adults; in lateral thigh in infants. I.M. route used only in emergencies when no I.V. route available.
- Warm solutions to body temperature before administration.
- Monitor serum calcium levels frequently.
- If GI upset occurs, give oral calcium products 1 to 1½ hours after meals.
- Crash carts usually contain both gluconate and chloride forms. Make sure doctor specifies form needed.

General
Classification: antiulcer agent (pepsin inhibitor).
Pregnancy risk category: B.

Mechanism of action
Adheres to and protects the ulcer surface by forming a barrier.

Indications and dosage
• Short-term (up to 8 weeks) treatment of duodenal ulcer. **Adults:** 1 g P.O. q.i.d. 1 hour before meals and h.s.
• Maintenance therapy of duodenal ulcer. **Adults:** 1 g P.O. b.i.d.

Adverse reactions
CNS: dizziness, sleepiness. **GI:** *constipation,* nausea, gastric discomfort, diarrhea, bezoar formation.

Interactions
Antacids: may decrease binding of drug to gastroduodenal mucosa, impairing effectiveness. Don't give within 30 minutes of each other. **Ciprofloxacin, norfloxacin, digoxin, cimetidine, ranitidine, phenytoin, tetracycline, theophylline:** decreased absorption. Separate administration times by at least 2 hours.

Nursing diagnoses
• Pain related to the patient's underlying condition.
• Constipation related to adverse GI effects of sucralfate.
• Knowledge deficit related to sucralfate therapy.

Nursing interventions
• No known contraindications.
• Drug is minimally absorbed. Incidence of adverse reactions is low.
• For best results, tell patient to take sucralfate on an empty stomach (1 hour before each meal and at bedtime).
• Pain and ulcer symptoms may subside within first few weeks of therapy. However, for complete healing, be sure patient continues prescribed regimen.
• Monitor for severe, persistent constipation.
• Studies suggest that drug is as effective as cimetidine in healing duodenal ulcers.
• Drug has been used to treat gastric ulcers, but effectiveness of this use is still under investigation.
• Drug contains aluminum but isn't classified as an antacid.
• Urge patient to avoid smoking because this may increase gastric acid secretion and worsen the disease.

General

Classification: antitubercular agent (polypeptide antibiotic). **Pregnancy risk category:** C.

Mechanism of action

Unknown (bacteriostatic).

Indications and dosage

• Adjunctive treatment in pulmonary tuberculosis. **Adults:** 15 mg/kg/day up to 1 g I.M. daily injected deeply into large muscle mass for 60 to 120 days; then 1 g two to three times weekly for 18 to 24 months. Maximum dosage should not exceed 20 mg/kg daily. Must be given in conjunction with another antitubercular drug.

Adverse reactions

Blood: eosinophilia, leukocytosis, leukopenia. **CNS:** headache, ***neuromuscular blockade.*** **EENT:** *ototoxicity* (tinnitus, vertigo, hearing loss). **GU:** *nephrotoxicity* (elevated BUN and nonprotein nitrogen levels, casts, RBC counts, leukocytes; tubular necrosis; proteinuria; decreased creatinine clearance). **Metabolic:** hypokalemia, alkalosis, hepatotoxicity. **Local:** pain, induration, excessive bleeding and sterile abscesses at injection site.

Interactions

None significant.

C

Nursing diagnoses

• High risk for infection related to ineffectiveness of capreomycin to eradicate the infection.
• Sensory/perceptual alterations (auditory) related to capreomycin-induced ototoxicity.
• Knowledge deficit related to capreomycin.

Nursing interventions

• *Contraindicated* in patients receiving other ototoxic or nephrotoxic drugs. Drug is never given I.V. because this use may cause neuromuscular blockade.
• *Use cautiously* in patients with impaired renal function, history of allergies, or hearing impairment.
• Administer deep into large muscle mass to minimize local reactions. Apply ice to injection site p.r.n. for pain.
• Evaluate patient's hearing before and every 1 to 2 weeks during therapy. Notify doctor if patient complains of tinnitus, vertigo, or hearing impairment.
• Monitor renal function (output, specific gravity, urinalysis, BUN level, and serum creatinine level) before and during therapy; notify doctor of decreasing renal function. Dose must be reduced in renal impairment.
• Straw- or dark-colored solution doesn't indicate a loss in potency. Don't administer solutions that contain a precipitate.

General

Classification: skeletal muscle relaxant (depolarizing neuromuscular blocker). **Pregnancy risk category:** C.

Mechanism of action

Prolongs depolarization of the muscle end plate.

Indications and dosage

• Adjunct to anesthesia to induce skeletal muscle relaxation; aid to intubation and mechanical ventilation or orthopedic manipulations; adjunct in induced seizures to lessen muscle contractions. Dosage depends on anesthetic used, individual needs, and response. **Adults:** 25 to 75 mg I.V., then 2.5 mg/minute p.r.n. or 2.5 mg/kg I.M. in deltoid muscle up to maximum of 150 mg I.M.. **Children:** 1 to 2 mg/kg I.M. or I.V. Maximum I.M. dosage is 150 mg.

Adverse reactions

CV: bradycardia, tachycardia, hypertension, hypotension, ***arrhythmias.*** **EENT:** increased intraocular pressure. **Other:** ***prolonged respiratory depression, apnea, malignant hyperthermia,*** muscle fasciculations, *postoperative muscle pain,* myoglobinemia, excessive salivation, allergic or idiosyncratic hypersensitivity reactions.

Interactions

Aminoglycoside antibiotics, cholinesterase inhibitors, general anesthetics, polymyxin antibiotics: potentiated neuromuscular blockade. Use cautiously during surgical and postoperative periods. **Digitalis glycosides:** possible cardiac arrhythmias. Use together cautiously. **Magnesium sulfate (parenterally):** potentiated neuromuscular blockade. Use with caution, preferably with reduced doses. **MAO inhibitors, lithium, cyclophosphamide:** prolonged apnea. Use with caution. **Narcotic analgesics, methotrimeprazine:** potentiated neuromuscular blockade. Use with extreme caution.

Nursing diagnoses

• Ineffective breathing pattern related to adverse drug reaction.
• Knowledge deficit related to succinylcholine therapy.

Nursing interventions

• *Contraindicated* in abnormally low plasma pseudocholinesterase.
• *Use cautiously* in elderly or debilitated patients; patients with personal or family history of malignant hypertension or hyperthermia; hepatic, renal, or pulmonary impairment; and in respiratory depression, severe burns or trauma, electrolyte imbalances, quinidine or digitalis therapy, hyperkalemia, paraplegia, spinal neuraxis injury, degenerative or dystrophic neuromuscular disease, myasthenia gravis, myasthenic syndrome of lung cancer or bronchogenic carcinoma, dehydration, thyroid disorders, collagen diseases, porphyria, fractures, muscle spasms, glaucoma, eye surgery or penetrating eye wounds, pheochromocytoma, and (in large doses) cesarean section.
• Succinylcholine should be used only by personnel experienced in airway management. Resuscitation equipment should be readily available. Don't use reversing agents (neostigmine or edrophonium). They may worsen neuromuscular blockade.
• Continuous I.V. infusion prolongs duration of action. Repeated or continuous infusions of succinylcholine alone may reduce response or prolong muscle relaxation and apnea.
• Monitor baseline electrolyte determinations and vital signs. Sedatives or general anesthetics should be given before neuromuscular blockers.
• Give test dose (10 mg deep I.M. high into deltoid muscle, or I.V.) after patient has been anesthetized. No respiratory depression or transient depression for up to 5 minutes indicates drug may be given. Don't give if patient develops respiratory paralysis sufficient to permit endotracheal intubation. (Recovery occurs in 30 to 60 minutes.)
• Monitor respirations closely until patient is fully recovered from neuromuscular blockade, as evidenced by tests of muscle strength (hand grip, head lift, and ability to cough).

General

Classification: antihypertensive (ACE inhibitor).
Pregnancy risk category: C (D in 2nd and 3rd trimesters).

Mechanism of action

By inhibiting ACE, prevents conversion of angiotensin I to angiotensin II.

Indications and dosage

- Hypertension. **Adults:** initially, 25 mg P.O. b.i.d. or t.i.d. If blood pressure isn't controlled in 1 to 2 weeks, may be increased to 50 mg t.i.d. If not controlled after another 1 to 2 weeks, a diuretic should be added to regimen. If further blood pressure reduction is necessary, dosage may be increased up to 150 mg t.i.d. while continuing the diuretic. Maximum dosage is 450 mg daily. Daily dose may also be administered b.i.d.
- Congestive heart failure. **Adults:** initially, 6.25 to 12.5 mg P.O. t.i.d. May be increased gradually to 50 mg t.i.d. Maximum dosage is 450 mg daily.

Adverse reactions

Blood: ***leukopenia, agranulocytosis, pancytopenia.*** **CNS:** dizziness, fainting. **CV:** *tachycardia, hypotension,* angina pectoris, ***CHF,*** pericarditis. **EENT:** *loss of taste (dysgeusia).* **GI:** anorexia. **GU:** *proteinuria, nephrotic syndrome, membranous glomerulopathy, renal failure* (patients with preexisting renal disease or patients receiving high dosages), urinary frequency. **Metabolic:** hyperkalemia. **Skin:** *urticarial rash, maculopapular rash,* pruritus. **Other:** fever, angioedema of face and extremities, transient increases in liver enzymes, persistent cough.

Interactions

Antacids: decreased captopril effect. Separate administration times. **Digitalis glycosides:** may increase serum digoxin concentration by 15% to 30%. **Insulin, oral hypoglycemic agents:** risk of hypoglycemia when captopril therapy is initiated. Monitor closely. **NSAIDs:** may reduce antihypertensive effect. Monitor blood pressure. **Potassium supplements, potassium-sparing diuretics:** increased risk of hyperkalemia. Avoid these agents unless hypokalemic blood levels are confirmed.

Nursing diagnoses

- High risk for injury related to the patient's underlying condition.
- Altered protection related to captopril-induced blood disorder or renal dysfunction.
- Knowledge deficit related to captopril therapy.

Nursing interventions

- *Contraindicated* during pregnancy because ACE inhibitors can cause fetal and neonatal injury or death. Discontinue ACE inhibitors as soon as pregnancy is detected.
- *Use cautiously* in impaired renal function or serious autoimmune disease (particularly systemic lupus erythematosus) or in patients exposed to other drugs known to affect WBC counts or immune response.
- Proteinuria and nephrotic syndrome may occur. Patients who develop persistent proteinuria or proteinuria exceeding 1 g daily should have their captopril therapy reevaluated.
- Monitor blood pressure and pulse rate frequently.
- Perform WBC and differential counts before starting treatment and regularly thereafter.
- Teach patient about his disease and therapy. Explain the importance of taking this drug as prescribed, even when he's feeling well. Don't discontinue drug suddenly, but call the doctor if unpleasant adverse reactions occur.
- Advise patients to report any sign of infection (sore throat, fever).
- May cause dizziness or fainting, especially during initiation of therapy. Advise patient to avoid sudden postural changes.
- Instruct patient to check with doctor or pharmacist before taking any OTC medications.
- Take 1 hour before meals; food in the GI tract may reduce absorption.

General

Classification: antibiotic (aminoglycoside). **Pregnancy risk category:** D.

Mechanism of action

Inhibits protein synthesis by binding directly to the 30S ribosomal subunit (bactericidal).

Indications and dosage

- Streptococcal endocarditis. **Adults:** 10 mg/kg I.M. (maximum 0.5 g) q 12 hours for 2 weeks with penicillin.
- Primary and adjunctive treatment of tuberculosis. **Adults with normal renal function:** 1 g I.M. daily for 2 to 3 months, then 1 g two or three times a week. Inject deep into upper outer quadrant of buttocks. **Children with normal renal function:** 20 mg/kg daily in divided doses injected deep into large muscle mass. Give concurrently with other antitubercular agents, but *not* with capreomycin, and continue until sputum specimen becomes negative. **Patients with impaired renal function:** first dose is same as for those with normal renal function. Later doses and frequency determined by renal function study results.
- Enterococcal endocarditis. **Adults:** 1 g I.M. q 12 hours for 2 weeks, then 500 mg I.M. q 12 hours for 4 weeks with penicillin.
- Tularemia. **Adults:** 1 to 2 g I.M. daily in divided doses injected deep into upper outer quadrant of buttocks. Continue until patient is afebrile for 5 to 7 days.

Adverse reactions

CNS: ***neuromuscular blockade.*** **EENT:** *ototoxicity (tinnitus, vertigo, hearing loss).* **GU:** some nephrotoxicity. **Local:** pain, irritation, and sterile abscesses at injection site. **Skin:** ***exfoliative dermatitis.*** **Other:** ***hypersensitivity*** (rash, fever, urticaria, and angioneurotic edema), headache, ***transient agranulocytosis.***

Interactions

Cephalothin: increases nephrotoxicity. Use together cautiously. **Dimenhydrinate:** may mask symptoms of streptomycin-induced ototoxicity. Use together cautiously. **General anesthetics, neuromuscular blockers:** may potentiate neuromuscular blockade. **I.V. loop diuretics (such as furosemide):** increase ototoxicity. Use cautiously.

Nursing diagnoses

- High risk for injury related to ineffectiveness of streptomycin in eradicating the infection.
- Sensory/perceptual alterations (auditory) related to streptomycin-induced ototoxicity.
- Knowledge deficit related to streptomycin therapy.

Nursing interventions

- *Contraindicated* in labyrinthine disease.
- *Use cautiously* in renal impairment and in elderly patients.
- Never administer I.V.
- Obtain specimen for culture and sensitivity tests before first dose, except when treating tuberculosis. Therapy may begin pending test results.
- Patient should be well hydrated while taking drug to minimize chemical irritation of renal tubules.
- Evaluate patient's hearing before, during, and 6 months after therapy. Notify doctor if patient complains of hearing loss, roaring noises, or fullness in ears.
- Watch for superinfection (continued fever and other signs of new infections).
- Protect hands when preparing; drug is irritating.
- Endocarditis prophylaxis is recommended for all patients with rheumatic or congenital heart disease or with prosthetic heart valve. These patients should receive prophylactic antibiotics during GI or GU procedures or surgery.
- Draw blood for peak streptomycin level 1 to 2 hours after I.M. injection; for trough levels, draw blood just before next dose. Don't use a heparinized tube because heparin is incompatible with aminoglycosides.

General

Classification: anticonvulsant, analgesic (iminostilbene). **Pregnancy risk category:** C.

Mechanism of action

Stabilizes neuronal membranes and limits seizure activity by decreasing synaptic transmission in the CNS.

Indications and dosage

- Generalized tonic-clonic and complex-partial seizures, mixed seizure patterns. **Adults and children over 12 years:** initially, 200 mg P.O. b.i.d. May increase by 200 mg P.O. daily, in divided doses at 6- to 8-hour intervals. Adjust to minimum effective level when control achieved. **Children under 12 years:** 10 to 20 mg/kg P.O. daily in two to four divided doses.
- Trigeminal neuralgia. **Adults:** initially, 100 mg P.O. b.i.d. with meals. Increase by 100 mg q 12 hours until pain is relieved. Don't exceed 1.2 g daily. Maintenance dose 200 to 400 mg P.O. b.i.d. Attempt to withdraw or reduce dose every 3 months.

Adverse reactions

Blood: ***aplastic anemia, agranulocytosis,*** eosinophilia, leukocytosis, ***thrombocytopenia.*** **CNS:** dizziness, *vertigo, drowsiness,* fatigue, *ataxia,* ***worsening of seizures.*** **CV:** ***CHF,*** hypertension, hypotension, aggravation of coronary artery disease. **EENT:** conjunctivitis, dry mouth and pharynx, blurred vision, diplopia, nystagmus. **GI:** *nausea,* vomiting, abdominal pain, diarrhea, anorexia, *stomatitis,* glossitis. **GU:** urinary frequency, urine retention, impotence, albuminuria, glycosuria, elevated BUN. ***Hepatic:*** abnormal liver function tests, ***hepatitis.*** **Metabolic:** water intoxication. **Skin:** *rash,* urticaria, erythema multiforme, ***Stevens-Johnson syndrome.*** **Other:** diaphoresis, fever, chills, pulmonary hypersensitivity.

Interactions

Lithium: increased CNS toxicity of lithium. Avoid concomitant use. **Phenytoin, primidone, phenobarbital, nicotinic acid:** may decrease carbamazepine levels. Monitor for decreased effect. **Phenytoin, warfarin, doxycycline, theophylline, haloperidol:** carbamazepine may decrease blood levels of these drugs. Monitor for decreased effect. **Propoxyphene, troleandomycin, erythromycin, isoniazid, verapamil:** may increase carbamazepine blood levels. Use cautiously.

Nursing diagnoses

- High risk for injury related to underlying seizure disorder.
- Altered protection related to carbamazepine-induced blood disorders.
- Knowledge deficit related to carbamazepine therapy.

Nursing interventions

- *Contraindicated* in bone marrow suppression or hypersensitivity to carbamazepine or tricyclic antidepressants and in patients who have taken a MAO inhibitor within 14 days of therapy.
- *Use cautiously* in cardiac, renal, or hepatic damage; in increased intraocular pressure; and in children with mixed seizure disorders.
- Institute seizure precautions, when appropriate.
- When administering by nasogastric tube, mix dose with an equal volume of water, 0.9% sodium chloride solution, or D_5W.
- Monitor blood levels and effects closely. Signs of anorexia or subtle appetite changes may indicate excessive blood levels.
- Obtain baseline and periodic urinalyses, BUN levels, liver function, serum iron levels, CBC, and platelet and reticulocyte counts.
- Periodic eye examinations are recommended.
- Never discontinue the drug suddenly.
- Warn patient to avoid activities requiring alertness until CNS effects of drug are known.
- Tell patient to keep tablets in their original container, tightly closed and away from moisture.
- Tell patient to notify doctor immediately if fever, sore throat, mouth ulcers, easy bruising or bleeding, or any other adverse reactions occur.

General

Classification: thrombolytic enzyme (plasminogen activator). **Pregnancy risk category:** C.

Mechanism of action

Plasminogen and streptokinase form a complex that exposes the plasminogen-activating site. Plasminogen is converted to plasmin by cleavage of the peptide bond.

Indications and dosage

• Arteriovenous cannula occlusion. **Adults:** 250,000 IU in 2 ml I.V. solution by I.V. infusion pump into each occluded limb of the cannula over 25 to 35 minutes. Clamp off cannula for 2 hours. Then aspirate contents of cannula, flush with saline solution, and reconnect.

• Venous thrombosis, pulmonary embolism, and arterial thrombosis and embolism. **Adults:** loading dose is 250,000 IU by I.V. infusion over 30 minutes. Sustaining dose is 100,000 IU/hour I.V. infusion for 72 hours for deep vein thrombosis and 100,000 IU/hour over 24 to 72 hours by I.V. infusion pump for pulmonary embolism.

• Lysis of coronary artery thrombi following acute MI. **Adults:** 1.5 million units infused over 60 minutes. Alternatively, a total of 140,000 units administered as a loading dose of 20,000 IU via coronary catheter, followed by a maintenance dose of 2,000 IU/minute for 60 minutes as an infusion.

Adverse reactions

Blood: ***bleeding,*** low hematocrit. **CV:** transient lowering or elevation of blood pressure. **EENT:** periorbital edema. **Skin:** urticaria. **Local:** phlebitis at injection site. **Other:** ***hypersensitivity,*** fever, ***anaphylaxis,*** musculoskeletal pain, minor breathing difficulty, bronchospasms, angioneurotic edema.

Interactions

Anticoagulants: increased risk of bleeding. Monitor closely. **Aspirin, dipyridamole, indomethacin, phenylbutazone, drugs affecting platelet activity:** increased risk of bleeding.

Nursing diagnoses

• Altered cardiopulmonary and peripheral tissue perfusion related to patient's underlying condition.
• Fluid volume deficit related to the adverse effects of streptokinase therapy.
• Knowledge deficit related to drug therapy.

Nursing interventions

• *Contraindicated* in ulcerative wounds, active internal bleeding, and recent CVA; recent trauma with possible internal injuries; visceral or intracranial malignant neoplasms; ulcerative colitis; diverticulitis; severe hypertension; acute or chronic hepatic or renal insufficiency; uncontrolled hypocoagulation; chronic pulmonary disease with cavitation; subacute bacterial endocarditis or rheumatic valvular disease; and recent cerebral embolism, thrombosis, or hemorrhage.
• *Also contraindicated* within 10 days after intra-arterial diagnostic procedure or any surgery, including liver or kidney biopsy, lumbar puncture, thoracentesis, paracentesis, or multiple cutdowns. I.M. injections and other invasive procedures are contraindicated during therapy.
• *Use cautiously* when treating arterial emboli that originate from left side of heart.
• Before initiating therapy, draw blood to determine partial thromboplastin time and PT. Rate of I.V. infusion depends on thrombin time and streptokinase resistance.
• Monitor patient for excessive bleeding. If bleeding is evident, stop therapy. Pretreatment with heparin or drugs affecting platelets increases risk. Have typed and crossmatched packed red cells and whole blood ready to treat possible hemorrhage and aminocaproic acid available to treat bleeding.
• Monitor pulses, color, and sensation of extremities every hour.
• Keep venipuncture sites to a minimum; use pressure dressing on puncture sites for 15 minutes.
• To check for hypersensitivity, give 100 IU intradermally; a wheal and flare response within 20 minutes means patient is probably allergic. Use antihistamines or corticosteroids to treat mild reaction. Stop infusion if severe reaction occurs.

General

Classification: antiparkinson agent (decarboxylase inhibitor and dopamine precursor). **Pregnancy risk category:** C.

Mechanism of action

Counters depletion of dopamine; carbidopa inhibits decarboxylation of levodopa (without affecting levodopa's metabolism within the CNS), making more levodopa available for decarboxylation to dopamine in the brain.

Indications and dosage

• Idiopathic, symptomatic, and postencephalitic parkinsonism. **Adults:** 3 to 6 tablets of 25 mg carbidopa/250 mg levodopa daily in divided doses (not to exceed 8 tablets). Optimum daily dosage is determined by careful individualized titration. Alternatively, 1 tablet (sustained release) P.O. b.i.d. at intervals of not less than 6 hours (up to 8 tablets daily in divided doses of 4 to 8 hours). Allow at least 3 days between dosage adjustments.

Adverse reactions

Blood: ***hemolytic anemia.*** **CNS:** *choreiform, dystonic, dyskinetic movements; involuntary grimacing, head movements, myoclonic body jerks, ataxia,* tremors, muscle twitching; bradykinetic episodes; psychiatric disturbances, memory loss, nervousness, anxiety, disturbing dreams, euphoria, malaise, fatigue; severe depression, ***suicidal tendencies,*** dementia, delirium, hallucinations. **CV:** *orthostatic hypotension,* ***cardiac irregularities,*** flushing, hypertension, phlebitis. **EENT:** blepharospasm, blurred vision, diplopia, mydriasis or miosis, widening of palpebral fissures, activation of latent Horner's syndrome, oculogyric crises, nasal discharge. **GI:** *nausea, vomiting, anorexia,* weight loss (at start), constipation, flatulence, diarrhea, *epigastric pain,* hiccups, sialorrhea, *dry mouth,* bitter taste. **GU:** urinary frequency and incontenence, urine retention, darkened urine, priapism. **Hepatic:** hepatotoxicity. **Other:** dark perspiration, hyperventilation.

Interactions

Antihypertensives: additive hypotensive effects. **Papaverine, phenothiazines and other antipsychotics, phenytoin:** may antagonize antiparkinsonian actions. Use together cautiously. **Sympathomimetics:** increased risk of cardiac arrhythmias.

Nursing diagnoses

• Impaired physical mobility related to underlying parkinsonian syndrome.
• Altered thought processes related to adverse CNS reactions to carbidopa-levodopa.
• Knowledge deficit related to carbidopa-levodopa therapy.

Nursing interventions

• *Contraindicated* in narrow-angle glaucoma, melanoma, or undiagnosed skin lesions.
• *Use cautiously* in cardiovascular, renal, hepatic, and pulmonary disorders; in history of peptic ulcer; psychiatric illness; MI with residual arrhythmias; and endocrine disease.
• Monitor patients taking antihypertensive medication or hypoglycemic agents. Discontinue MAO inhibitors 2 weeks before therapy is begun.
• Observe and monitor vital signs, especially during dosage adjustments.
• Warn patient of possible dizziness and orthostatic hypotension, especially at start of therapy. Have him report any adverse effects.
• Watch for muscle twitching and blepharospasm (twitching of eyelids); they may be an early sign of drug overdosage.
• Long-term therapy requires regular testing for diabetes, acromegaly; and hepatic, renal, and hematopoietic function studies.
• Discontinue levodopa at least 8 hours before starting levodopa-carbidopa.
• Laboratory test interferences include false-positive increases in levels of uric acid, urine ketones, catecholamines, urine glucose, and vanillylmandelic acid, depending on reagent and test method used.

General

Classification: antihypertensive, diuretic (potassium-sparing diuretic). **Pregnancy risk category:** D.

Mechanism of action

Antagonizes aldosterone in the distal tubule, increasing excretion of sodium and water but sparing potassium.

Indications and dosage

• Edema. **Adults:** 25 to 200 mg P.O. daily in divided doses. **Children:** initially, 3.3 mg/kg P.O. daily in divided doses.
• Hypertension. **Adults:** 50 to 100 mg P.O. daily in divided doses.
• Diuretic-induced hypokalemia. **Adults:** 25 to 100 mg P.O. daily when oral potassium supplements are considered inappropriate.
• Detection of primary hyperaldosteronism. **Adults:** 400 mg P.O. daily for 4 days (short test) or 3 to 4 weeks (long test). If hypokalemia and hypertension are corrected, a presumptive diagnosis of primary hyperaldosteronism is made.

Adverse reactions

CNS: headache. **GI:** anorexia, nausea, diarrhea. **Metabolic:** ***hyperkalemia,*** dehydration, hyponatremia, transient elevation in BUN, acidosis. **Skin:** urticaria. **Other:** gynecomastia in men, breast soreness and menstrual disturbances in women.

Interactions

ACE inhibitors, potassium supplements: concomitant use may result in hyperkalemia. Don't use together. **Aspirin:** possible blocked spironolactone effect. Watch for diminished spironolactone response. **Digoxin:** may alter digoxin clearance and increase risk of toxicity. Monitor digoxin levels.

Nursing diagnoses

• Fluid volume excess related to sodium and fluid retention.
• High risk for injury related to spironolactone-induced hyperkalemia.
• Knowledge deficit related to spironolactone therapy.

Nursing interventions

• *Contraindicated* in anuria, acute or progressive renal insufficiency, or hyperkalemia.
• *Use cautiously* in fluid or electrolyte imbalances, impaired renal function, and hepatic disease.
• A mild acidosis may occur during therapy. This may be dangerous in patients with hepatic cirrhosis.
• Monitor serum electrolytes, intake and output, weight, and blood pressure.
• Useful as an adjunct to other diuretic therapy. Less potent diuretic than thiazide and loop types. Diuretic effect delayed 2 to 3 days when used alone.
• Maximum antihypertensive response may be delayed up to 2 weeks.
• Warn patient to avoid excessive ingestion of potassium-rich foods or potassium-containing salt substitutes. Concomitant potassium supplement can lead to serious hyperkalemia.
• Elderly patients are more susceptible to excessive diuresis.
• Protect drug from light.
• Breast cancer reported in some patients taking spironolactone, but cause-and-effect relationship not confirmed. Warn against taking drug indiscriminately.
• Give with meals to enhance absorption.
• Because of its antiandrogenic properties, spironolactone has been prescribed to treat hirsutism. The dose for this indication is 200 mg daily.
• Spironolactone may interfere with some laboratory tests that measure digoxin levels. Inform laboratory that patient is taking spironolactone.

General

Classification: antineoplastic (alkylating agent).
Pregnancy risk category: D.

Mechanism of action

Produces cross-linking of strands of DNA.

Indications and dosage

• Palliative treatment of ovarian carcinoma. **Adults:** 360 mg/m^2 I.V. on day 1 q 4 weeks; doses should not be repeated until platelet count exceeds 100,000/mm^3 and neutrophil count exceeds 2,000/mm^3. Subsequent doses are based on blood counts. Clinical trials have suggested the following dosage adjustments: if platelet count is above 100,000/mm^3 and neutrophil count is above 2,000/mm^3, administer 125% of the recommended starting dose. Reduce dose to 75% if platelet count falls below 50,000/mm^3 or neutrophil count is below 500/mm^3. Adjust dose in severe bone marrow depression (creatinine clearance below 60 ml/min).

Adverse reactions

Blood: ***thrombocytopenia, leukopenia, neutropenia, anemia.*** **CNS:** dizziness, confusion, peripheral neuropathy, ototoxicity, central neurotoxicity. **GI:** constipation, diarrhea, *nausea, vomiting.* **Other:** alopecia, hypersensitivity, hepatotoxicity, *increased BUN, creatinine, AST, or alkaline phosphatase levels.*

Interactions

Bone marrow depressants (including radiotherapy): increased hematologic toxicity. **Nephrotoxic agents:** added nephrotoxicity of carboplatin.

Nursing diagnoses

• Altered nutrition related to nausea, vomiting, and resulting electrolyte imbalances.
• Altered urinary elimination related to nephrotoxic effects of carboplatin.
• Knowledge deficit related to carboplatin therapy.

Nursing interventions

• *Contraindicated* in hypersensitivity to cisplatin, platinum-containing compounds, or mannitol and in severe bone marrow depression or bleeding.
• Exercise extreme caution when preparing or administering carboplatin to avoid mutagenic, teratogenic, and carcinogenic risks.
• Advise women of childbearing age to avoid becoming pregnant or nursing during therapy and to consult with doctor before becoming pregnant.
• Administer carboplatin under the supervision of an oncologist.
• Determine serum electrolytes, creatinine, BUN, CBC, and creatinine clearance levels before the first infusion and before each course.
• Hydration or diuresis before or after treatment is not necessary.
• Transfusions may be necessary during treatment because of cumulative anemia.
• **I.V. use:** Reconstitute with D_5W, 0.9% sodium chloride solution, or sterile water for injection to make a concentration of 10 mg/ml. Drug may be given by continuous or intermittent infusion over at least 15 minutes.
• Avoid needles or I.V. administration sets containing aluminum; drug may precipitate and lose potency.
• Unopened vials should be stored at room temperature. Once reconstituted, drug is stable at room temperature for 8 hours.
• Monitor vital signs during infusion.
• Monitor CBC and platelet count frequently during therapy and, when indicated, until recovery.
• Have epinephrine, corticosteroids, and antihistamines available because anaphylaxis-like reactions may occur within minutes of administration.
• Give antiemetic if patient develops severe emesis.

General

Classification: antibiotic (aminocyclitol). **Pregnancy risk category:** B.

Mechanism of action

Inhibits protein synthesis by binding to the 30S subunit of the ribosome.

Indications and dosage

- Gonorrhea. **Adults:** 2 to 4 g I.M. as single dose injected deeply into the upper outer quadrant of the buttock.

Adverse reactions

CNS: insomnia, dizziness. **GI:** nausea. **GU:** decreased urine output. **Skin:** urticaria. **Local:** pain at injection site. **Other:** fever, chills (may mask or delay symptoms of incubating syphilis).

Interactions

None significant.

Nursing diagnoses

- High risk for injury related to ineffectiveness of spectinomycin in eradicating the infection.
- High risk for fluid volume deficit related to spectinomycin-induced nausea.
- Knowledge deficit related to spectinomycin therapy.

Nursing interventions

- *Contraindicated* in patients with hypersensitivity to the drug.
- *Use cautiously* in patients with strong history of drug allergies.
- Not effective in the treatment of syphilis. Serologic test for syphilis should be done before treatment dose and 3 months after.
- Should be reserved for penicillin-resistant strains of gonorrhea.
- Use 20G needle to administer drug. The 4-g dose (10 ml) should be divided into two 5-ml injections—one in each buttock.
- Shake vial vigorously after reconstitution and before withdrawing dose. Store at room temperature after reconstitution and use within 24 hours.

carboprost tromethamine

Hemabate

General

Classification: oxytocic (prostaglandin). **Pregnancy risk category:** C.

Mechanism of action

Produces strong, prompt contractions of uterine smooth muscle, possibly mediated by calcium and cyclic 3′,5′-adenosine monophosphate.

Indications and dosage

- Abort pregnancy between 13th and 20th weeks of gestation. **Adults:** initially, 250 mcg is administered deep I.M. Subsequent doses of 250 mcg should be administered at intervals of 1½ to 3½ hours, depending on uterine response. Increments in dosage may be increased to 500 mcg if contractility is inadequate after several 250-mcg doses. Total dosage should not exceed 12 mg.
- Postpartum hemorrhage caused by uterine atony that has not responded to conventional management. **Adults:** 250 mcg by deep I.M. injection. May administer repeat doses at 15- to 90-minute intervals. Maximum total dosage is 2 mg.

Adverse reactions

GI: *vomiting, diarrhea,* nausea. **Other:** *fever,* chills.

Interactions

None significant.

Nursing diagnoses

- High risk for fluid volume deficit related to carboprost-induced vomiting and diarrhea.
- High risk for altered body temperature related to possible carboprost-induced fever.
- Knowledge deficit related to carboprost therapy.

Nursing interventions

- *Contraindicated* in pelvic inflammatory disease or active cardiac, pulmonary, renal, or hepatic disease.
- *Use cautiously* in history of asthma; hypertension; cardiovascular, renal, or hepatic disease; anemia; jaundice; diabetes; seizure disorder; and previous uterine surgery.
- Unlike other prostaglandin abortifacients, carboprost is administered by I.M. injection. Injectable form avoids risk of expelling vaginal suppositories, which may occur in the presence of profuse vaginal bleeding.
- I.M. injection of this drug is technically less difficult and poses fewer potential risks than other prostaglandin abortifacients.
- Should be used only in a hospital setting by trained personnel.

General

Classification: antiarrhythmic, antihypertensive, antianginal (nonselective beta-adrenergic blocker).
Pregnancy risk category: B.

Mechanism of action

Depresses sinus heart rate, slows AV conduction, decreases cardiac output, and lowers systolic and diastolic blood pressure.

Indications and dosage

• Documented, life-threatening ventricular arrhythmias. **Adults:** initially, 80 mg P.O. b.i.d. Increase dosage q 2 to 3 days as needed and tolerated; most patients respond to daily dosage of 160 to 320 mg (with selected refractory arrhythmias, up to 640 mg daily).
• Hypertension. **Adults:** initially, 80 mg P.O. b.i.d. Increase dosage at weekly intervals in increments of 80 mg b.i.d. as needed and tolerated. Most patients respond to daily dosage of 160 to 320 mg.
• Angina. **Adults:** initially, 80 mg P.O. b.i.d. Increase dosage at weekly intervals in increments of 80 mg b.i.d. Most patients respond to dosages of 160 mg b.i.d.; maximum daily dosage is 480 mg.

Adverse reactions

CNS: *asthenia, headache, dizziness, weakness, fatigue.* **CV:** *bradycardia,* ***arrhythmias, CHF, AV block.*** **GI:** *nausea.* **Respiratory:** *dyspnea,* ***bronchospasm.***

Interactions

Antiarrhythmics: additive effects. Avoid concomitant use. **Antihypertensives, catecholamine-depleting drugs (such as reserpine and guanethidine):** enhanced hypotensive effects. Monitor closely. **Calcium channel blockers:** enhanced myocardial depression. Avoid concomitant use. **Clonidine:** beta blockers may enhance the rebound effect seen after withdrawal of clonidine. Discontinue sotalol several days before withdrawing clonidine. **General anesthetics:** may cause additional myocardial depression.

Nursing diagnoses

• Pain related to ineffectiveness of sotalol therapy.
• Fluid volume excess related to sotalol-induced CHF.
• Knowledge deficit related to sotalol therapy.

Nursing interventions

• *Contraindicated* in patients with severe sinus node dysfunction, sinus bradycardia, second- or third-degree AV block (unless a functioning pacemaker is present), congenital or acquired QT syndrome, cardiogenic shock, CHF, hypokalemia, hypomagnesemia, bronchial asthma, or allergic rhinitis.
• *Use cautiously* in patients with renal impairment. Because drug is excreted primarily in the urine, dosage adjustments are necessary; for the same reason, such patients take longer to achieve steady-state levels of drug. Dosage adjustments should be scheduled to follow administration of five or six doses. Also use cautiously in patients with diabetes mellitus. Beta-adrenergic blockers may mask signs and symptoms of hypoglycemia.
• Adjust dosage slowly, allowing 2 to 3 days between dosage increases to allow adequate monitoring of QT intervals and for plasma levels of drug to reach steady state.
• Because proarrhythmic events may occur at start of therapy and during dosage adjustments, patient should be hospitalized. Facilities and personnel should be readily available for cardiac rhythm monitoring and interpretation of ECG waveforms.
• Patients receiving I.V. lidocaine have started sotalol therapy without ill effect, but other antiarrhythmic drugs should be withdrawn before sotalol therapy. Delay therapy until two or three half-lives of the withdrawn drug have elapsed. After withdrawal of amiodarone, sotalol shouldn't be administered until the QT interval normalizes.
• Monitor serum electrolytes regularly, especially if patient is receiving diuretics. Electrolyte imbalances (hypokalemia or hypomagnesemia) may enhance prolonged QT interval and increase risk of serious arrhythmias, such as torsades de pointes.

General
Classification: skeletal muscle relaxant (carbamate derivative). **Pregnancy risk category:** C.

Mechanism of action
Precise mechanism unknown; reduces transmission of impulses from the spinal cord to skeletal muscle.

Indications and dosage
- As an adjunct in acute, painful musculoskeletal conditions. **Adults and children over 12 years:** 350 mg P.O. t.i.d. and h.s.

Adverse reactions
CNS: *drowsiness, dizziness,* vertigo, ataxia, tremor, agitation, irritability, headache, depressive reactions, insomnia. **CV:** orthostatic hypotension, tachycardia, facial flushing. **GI:** nausea, vomiting, hiccups, increased bowel activity, epigastric distress. **Skin:** rash, ***erythema multiforme,*** pruritus. **Other:** asthmatic episodes, fever, angioneurotic edema, ***anaphylaxis.***

Interactions
Alcohol, CNS depressants: increased CNS depression. Avoid concomitant use.

Nursing diagnoses
- Pain related to the patient's underlying condition.
- High risk for injury related to drug-induced drowsiness.
- Knowledge deficit related to carisoprodol therapy.

Nursing interventions
- *Contraindicated* in hypersensitivity to related compounds (such as meprobamate, tybamate) or intermittent porphyria. Not recommended for children under 12 years.
- *Use cautiously* in impaired hepatic or renal function.
- Watch for idiosyncratic reactions after first to fourth dose (weakness, ataxia, visual and speech difficulties, fever, skin eruptions, and mental changes) or severe reactions, including bronchospasm, hypotension, and anaphylactic shock. Withhold dose and notify doctor immediately of any unusual reactions.
- Evaluate degree of relief to determine whether dosage can be reduced.
- Warn patient to avoid activities that require alertness until CNS effects of the drug are known. Drowsiness is transient.
- Avoid combining with alcohol or other depressants.
- Advise patient to follow doctor's orders regarding rest and physical therapy.
- Do not stop drug abruptly; mild withdrawal effects, such as insomnia, headache, nausea, and abdominal cramps, may result.

General

Classification: pituitary hormone (polypeptide).
Pregnancy risk category: C.

Mechanism of action

Purified recombinant DNA. Stimulates linear, skeletal muscle, and organ growth.

Indications and dosage

- Long-term treatment of children who have growth failure because of lack of adequate endogenous growth hormone secretion. **Children (prepuberty):** 0.1 mg/kg I.M. or S.C. given three times weekly.

Adverse reactions

Endocrine: hypothyroidism, hyperglycemia.
Other: antibodies to growth hormone.

Interactions

Glucocorticoids: may inhibit growth-promoting action of somatrem. Glucocorticoid dose may need to be adjusted.

Nursing diagnoses

- Self-esteem disturbance related to low growth rate.
- Altered nutrition related to somatrem-induced hyperglyecmia.
- Knowledge deficit related to somatrem therapy.

Nursing interventions

- *Contraindicated* in patients with closed epiphyses, an active underlying intracranial lesion, or known sensitivity to benzyl alcohol.
- *Use cautiously* in patients with hypothyroidism and in those whose growth hormone deficiency results from an intracranial lesion. Patient should be examined frequently for progression or recurrence of the underlying disease.
- Regular checkups with monitoring of height, blood, and radiologic studies are necessary.
- Observe patient for signs of glucose intolerance and hyperglycemia.
- Monitor periodic thyroid function tests for hypothyroidism, which may require treatment with a thyroid hormone.
- This drug replaces pituitary-derived human growth hormone, which was removed from the market in 1985 because of an association with a rare but fatal viral infection (Jakob-Creutzfeldt disease). Reassure your patient and his family that somatrem is *pure* and *safe.*
- To prepare the solution, inject the bacteriostatic water for injection (which is supplied) into the vial containing the drug. Then swirl the vial with a gentle rotary motion until the contents are completely dissolved. *Don't shake* the vial.
- After reconstitution, vial solution should be clear. Don't inject into the patient if the solution is cloudy or contains any particles.
- Store reconstituted vial in refrigerator and use within 7 days. Also be sure to check this product's expiration date.

General

Classification: antihypertensive (beta blocker). **Pregnancy risk category:** C.

Mechanism of action

A nonselective beta-adrenergic blocking agent with intrinsic sympathomimetic activity (ISA). Its antihypertensive effects are probably caused by decreased sympathetic outflow from the brain and decreased cardiac output. Carteolol does not have a consistent effect on renin output.

Indications and dosage

- Hypertension. **Adults:** initially, 2.5 mg P.O. as a single daily dose. Gradually increase dosage as required to 5 mg or 10 mg daily as a single dose. Dosage exceeding 10 mg may decrease response.

Adverse reactions

CNS: lassitude, fatigue, somnolence. **CV:** conduction disturbances. **Other:** *muscle cramps, asthenia.*

Interactions

Calcium channel blockers: increased risk of hypotension, left ventricular failure, and AV conduction disturbances. I.V. calcium antagonists should be used with caution. **General anesthetics:** increased hypotensive effects. Observe carefully for excessive hypotension or bradycardia, or orthostatic hypotension. **Insulin, oral antidiabetic agents:** hypoglycemic response may be altered by beta blockers. Dosage adjustments may be necessary. **Reserpine, catecholamine-depleting drugs:** may have an additive effect when administered with a beta blocker.

Nursing diagnoses

- High risk for injury related to ineffectiveness of carteolol to lower blood pressure.
- Pain related to carteolol-induced muscle cramps.
- Knowledge deficit related to carteolol.

Nursing interventions

- *Contraindicated* in patients with bronchial asthma, severe bradycardia, greater than first-degree heart block, cardiogenic shock, or uncontrolled CHF.
- *Use cautiously* in patients with CHF controlled by digitalis glycosides and diuretics because beta-adrenergic blocking agents do not block the inotropic effects of digitalis derivatives.
- Food may slow the rate, but not the extent, of carteolol absorption. Normally, the patient may take the drug without regard to meals.
- Patients with substantial renal failure should receive the usual dose of carteolol at increased intervals. If creatinine clearance is greater than 60 ml/minute, the drug is given at 24-hour intervals; if creatinine clearance is 20 to 60 ml/minute, the drug is given at 48-hour intervals; if creatinine clearance is less than 20 ml/minute, the drug is given at 72-hour intervals.
- Note that asymptomatic patients with a history of CHF may exhibit signs of cardiac decompensation with beta blocker therapy.
- Patients with unrecognized coronary artery disease may exhibit signs of angina pectoris upon withdrawal of the drug.
- Beta blockade may inhibit glycogenolysis and the signs and symptoms of hypoglycemia (such as tachycardia and blood pressure changes). It may also attenuate insulin release.
- Beta blockers may mask tachycardia associated with hyperthyroidism. In suspected thyrotoxicosis, beta blocker therapy should be withdrawn gradually to avoid thyroid storm.
- The anesthesiologist should be advised that the patient is receiving a beta blocker so that isoproterenol or dobutamine is made readily available for reversal of the cardiac effects of the drug.
- Advise the patient to take the drug exactly as prescribed and not to discontinue the drug suddenly. Emphasize the importance of reporting shortness of breath or difficulty breathing, unusually fast heartbeat, cough, or fatigue with exertion.

General

Classification: nonnarcotic analgesic, antipyretic, anti-inflammatory (salicylate). **Pregnancy risk category:** C.

Mechanism of action

Produces analgesia by an ill-defined effect on the hypothalamus (central action) and by blocking generation of pain impulses (peripheral action). Exerts its anti-inflammatory effect by inhibiting prostaglandin synthesis. Relieves fever by acting on the hypothalamic heat-regulating center to produce peripheral vasodilation, which increases peripheral blood supply and promotes sweating, leading to heat loss and cooling by evaporation.

Indications and dosage

- Minor pain or fever. **Adults:** 325 to 650 mg P.O. q 4 to 6 hours p.r.n., or 500 mg slow I.V. infusion over 4 to 8 hours. Maximum dosage is 1 g daily.
- Arthritis. **Adults:** 3.5 to 5.4 g P.O. daily in divided doses.

Adverse reactions

EENT: *tinnitus, hearing loss.* **GI:** nausea, vomiting, GI distress. **Hepatic:** abnormal liver function studies, hepatitis. **Skin:** *rash.* **Local:** thrombophlebitis (from I.V. use). **Other:** ***hypersensitivity manifested by anaphylaxis or asthma (rare).***

S

Interactions

Alcohol, steroids, other NSAIDs: increased risk of GI distress. Avoid concomitant use. **Ammonium chloride (and other urine acidifiers):** increased blood levels of salicylates. Monitor for salicylate toxicity. **Antacids in large doses (and other urine alkalinizers):** decreased levels of salicylates. Monitor for decreased salicylate effect. **Corticosteroids:** enhance salicylate elimination. Monitor for decreased salicylate effect. **Methotrexate:** increased risk of methotrexate toxicity. Avoid concomitant use. **Oral anticoagulants:** increased risk of bleeding. Avoid using together if possible.

Nursing diagnoses

- Pain related to the patient's underlying condition.
- Altered nutrition: Less than body requirements, related to adverse GI reactions to sodium salicylate therapy.
- Knowledge deficit related to sodium salicylate therapy.

Nursing interventions

- *Contraindicated* in GI ulcer, GI bleeding, or aspirin hypersensitivity.
- *Use cautiously* in hypoprothrombinemia, vitamin K deficiency, bleeding disorders, asthma with nasal polyps (may cause severe bronchospasm), and in CHF and hypertension because of increased sodium load.
- Because of epidemiologic association with Reye's syndrome, the CDC recommends that children or teenagers with chicken pox or influenza-like illness should not be given salicylates.
- Febrile, dehydrated children can develop toxicity rapidly.
- Give with food, milk, antacid, or large glass of water to reduce adverse GI reactions.
- Therapeutic salicylate level in arthritis is 10 to 30 mg/dl. Tinnitus may occur at plasma levels of 30 mg/dl and above, but this is not a reliable indicator of toxicity, especially in very young patients and those over age 60. With chronic therapy, mild toxicity may occur at plasma levels of 20 mg/dl.
- May cause an increase in serum levels of AST, ALT, alkaline phosphatase, and bilirubin.
- Advise patients receiving long-term treatment with large doses to watch for petechiae, bleeding gums, and signs of GI bleeding, and to maintain adequate fluid intake. Obtain hemoglobin and prothrombin tests periodically.
- Unlike aspirin, sodium salicylate does not inhibit platelet aggregation.

General

Classification: stimulant laxative (anthraquinone glycoside mixture). **Pregnancy risk category:** C.

Mechanism of action

Increases peristalsis by direct effect on the smooth muscle of the intestine. Thought either to irritate the musculature or to stimulate the colonic intramural plexus. Also promotes fluid accumulation in the colon and small intestine.

Indications and dosage

• Acute constipation; preparation for bowel or rectal examination. **Adults:** 325 mg tablets P.O. h.s.; or 1 ml fluid extract daily; or 5 ml aromatic fluid extract daily. **Children 2 to 12 years:** ½ adult dose. **Children under 2 years:** ¼ adult dose.

Adverse reactions

GI: *nausea;* vomiting; diarrhea; loss of normal bowel function with excessive use; *abdominal cramps,* especially in severe constipation; malabsorption of nutrients; "cathartic colon" (syndrome resembling ulcerative colitis radiologically and pathologically) after chronic misuse; discoloration of rectal mucosa after long-term use. **Metabolic:** hypokalemia, protein enteropathy, electrolyte imbalance in excessive use. **Other:** laxative dependence in long-term or excessive use.

Interactions

None significant.

Nursing diagnoses

• Constipation related to interruption of normal pattern of elimination.
• Pain related to abdominal cramps induced by cascara sagrada.
• Knowledge deficit related to cascara sagrada therapy.

Nursing interventions

• *Contraindicated* in abdominal pain, nausea, vomiting, or other symptoms of appendicitis or acute surgical abdomen; acute surgical delirium, fecal impaction, intestinal obstruction or perforation. *Use cautiously* when rectal bleeding is present.
• Aromatic cascara fluid extract is less active and less bitter than nonaromatic fluid extract.
• Liquid preparations are more reliable than solid dosage forms.
• Before giving for constipation, determine if patient has adequate fluid intake, exercise, and diet. Tell him that dietary sources of bulk include bran and other cereals, fresh fruit, and vegetables.
• May turn alkaline urine red-pink and acidic urine yellow-brown.
• Monitor serum electrolytes during prolonged use.
• Onset of action is 6 to 12 hours.

General

Classification: potassium-removing resin (cation-exchange resin). **Pregnancy risk category:** C.

Mechanism of action

Exchanges sodium ions for potassium ions in the intestine: 1 g of sodium polystyrene sulfonate is exchanged for 0.5 to 1 mEq of potassium. The resin is then eliminated. Much of the exchange capacity is used for cations other than potassium (calcium and magnesium) and possibly for fats and proteins.

Indications and dosage

• Hyperkalemia. **Adults:** 15 g P.O. daily to q.i.d. in water or sorbitol (3 to 4 ml/g of resin). Alternatively, 30 to 50 g/dl of sorbitol q 6 hours as warm emulsion deep (20 cm) into sigmoid colon. **Children:** 1 g of resin P.O. for each mEq of potassium to be removed.

For nasogastric administration, mix dose with appropriate medium—aqueous suspension or diet appropriate for renal failure; instill in plastic tube.

Adverse reactions

GI: *constipation,* fecal impaction (in elderly patients), anorexia, gastric irritation, nausea, vomiting, *diarrhea (with sorbitol emulsions).* **Other:** ***hypokalemia,*** hypocalcemia, hypomagnesemia, sodium retention.

S

Interactions

Antacids and laxatives (nonabsorbable cation-donating type, including magnesium hydroxide): systemic alkalosis, reduced potassium exchange capability. Don't use together.

Nursing diagnoses

• High risk for injury related to hyperkalemia.
• Altered GI tissue perfusion related to drug-induced fecal impaction.
• Knowledge deficit related to sodium polystyrene sulfonate therapy.

Nursing interventions

• *Use cautiously* in elderly patients, those on digitalis glycoside therapy, and those with severe CHF, severe hypertension, or marked edema.
• Monitor serum potassium level at least once daily. Drug is usually stopped when potassium is reduced to 4 or 5 mEq/liter. Watch for signs of hypokalemia.
• Monitor for symptoms of other electrolyte deficiencies (magnesium, calcium) since drug is nonselective. Monitor serum calcium in patients receiving sodium polystyrene therapy for more than 3 days. Supplementary calcium may be needed.
• Drug contains about 100 mg sodium/g. Watch for sodium overload. About one-third of resin's sodium is retained.
• Premixed forms are available (SPS and others).
• Don't heat resin. Mix resin only with water or sorbitol for P.O. administration and with water and sorbital for rectal use. For oral use, *never* mix with orange juice (high potassium content) to disguise taste. Chill oral suspension for greater palatability. For rectal use, don't use other vehicles (for example, mineral oil) for rectal administration to prevent impactions. Ion exchange requires aqueous medium.
• Consider solid form. Resin cookie and candy recipes are available.
• Watch for constipation in oral or nasogastric administration. Use sorbitol (10 to 20 ml of 70% syrup every 2 hours as needed) to produce one or two watery stools daily.
• Prevent fecal impaction in elderly patients by administering resin rectally. Give cleansing enema before administration. Explain to patient necessity of retaining enema for at least 30 minutes.
• Prepare rectal dose at room temperature. Stir emulsion gently during administration.
• After rectal administration, flush tubing with 50 to 100 ml of nonsodium fluid to ensure delivery of all medication. Flush rectum to remove the resin.
• If hyperkalemia is severe, more drastic modalities should be added—for example, dextrose 50% with regular insulin I.V. push. Do not depend solely on polystyrene resin to lower serum potassium in severe hyperkalemia.

General

Classification: stimulant laxative (glyceride, *Ricinus communis* derivative). **Pregnancy risk category:** X.

Mechanism of action

Increases peristalsis by direct effect on the smooth muscle of the intestine. Thought either to irritate the musculature or to stimulate the colonic intramural plexus. Also promotes fluid accumulation in the colon and small intestine.

Indications and dosage

• Preparation for rectal or bowel examination, or surgery; acute constipation (rarely). **Adults:** 15 to 60 ml P.O. **Children over 2 years:** 5 to 15 ml P.O. **Children under 2 years:** 1.25 to 7.5 ml P.O. **Infants:** up to 4 ml P.O. Increased dose produces no greater effect.

Adverse reactions

GI: *nausea;* vomiting; diarrhea; loss of normal bowel function with excessive use; *abdominal cramps,* especially in severe constipation; malabsorption of nutrients; "cathartic colon" (syndrome resembling ulcerative colitis radiologically and pathologically) in chronic misuse. May cause constipation after catharsis. **GU:** pelvic congestion in menstruating women. **Metabolic:** hypokalemia, protein-losing enteropathy, other electrolyte imbalance in excessive use. **Other:** laxative dependence in long-term or excessive use.

Interactions

None significant.

Nursing diagnoses

• Constipation related to interruption of normal pattern of elimination.
• Pain related to abdominal cramps induced by castor oil.
• Knowledge deficit related to castor oil therapy.

Nursing interventions

• *Contraindicated* in ulcerative bowel lesions; during menstruation; in abdominal pain, nausea, vomiting, or other symptoms of appendicitis or acute surgical abdomen; in anal or rectal fissures, fecal impaction, intestinal obstruction or perforation; and in pregnancy.
• *Use cautiously* in rectal bleeding.
• Failure to respond may indicate acute condition requiring surgery.
• Give with juice or carbonated beverage to mask oily taste. Patient should stir mixture and drink it promptly. Ice held in mouth before taking drug will help prevent tasting it.
• Shake emulsion well. Store below 40° F (4.4° C). Don't freeze.
• Give on empty stomach for best results.
• Produces complete evacuation after 3 hours. Tell patient that after castor oil has emptied bowel he will not have bowel movement for 1 to 2 days.
• Time drug administration so that it doesn't interfere with scheduled activities or sleep.
• Monitor serum electrolytes during prolonged use.
• Generally used before diagnostic testing or therapy requiring thorough evacuation of GI tract.
• Use for short-term treatment. Not recommended for routine use; useful for acute constipation not responsive to milder laxatives.
• Before giving for constipation, determine if patient has adequate fluid intake, exercise, and diet. Tell him that dietary sources of bulk include bran and other cereals, fresh fruit, and vegetables.
• Increased intestinal motility lessens absorption of concomitantly administered P.O. drugs. Reschedule dose.
• Castor oil affects the small intestine. Regular use may cause excessive loss of water and salt.
• Castor oil emulsion is better tolerated but is more expensive.

General

Classification: saline laxative (acid salt). **Pregnancy risk category:** C.

Mechanism of action

Produces an osmotic effect in the small intestine by drawing water into the intestinal lumen.

Indications and dosage

• Constipation. **Adults:** 20 to 30 ml solution mixed with 120 ml cold water P.O.; or 60 to 135 ml P.R. **Children:** 5 to 15 ml mixed with 120 ml cold water P.O.; or 67.5 ml P.R.

Adverse reactions

GI: *abdominal cramping.* **Metabolic:** fluid and electrolyte disturbances (hypernatremia, hyperphosphatemia) if used daily. **Other:** laxative dependence in long-term or excessive use.

Interactions

None significant.

Nursing diagnoses

• Constipation related to interruption of normal pattern of elimination.
• Pain related to abdominal cramping caused by sodium phosphates.
• Knowledge deficit related to sodium phosphates therapy.

Nursing interventions

• *Contraindicated* in abdominal pain, nausea, vomiting, or other symptoms of appendicitis or acute surgical abdomen; intestinal obstruction or perforation; edema; CHF; megacolon; impaired renal function; and in patients on salt-restricted diets.
• *Use cautiously* in patients with large hemorrhoids or anal excoriations.
• Available in oral and rectal forms.
• Before giving for constipation, determine if patient has adequate fluid intake, exercise, and diet. Tell him that dietary sources of bulk include bran and other cereals, fresh fruit, and vegetables.
• Up to 10% of sodium content may be absorbed.
• Enema form elicits response in 5 to 10 minutes.
• Used in preparation for barium enema and sigmoidoscopy, and for treatment of fecal impaction.
• Also prescribed to treat hypercalcemia or as a phosphate replacement.

General

Classification: antibiotic (second-generation cephalosporin). **Pregnancy risk category:** B.

Mechanism of action

Inhibits cell wall synthesis, promoting osmotic instability. Usually bactericidal.

Indications and dosage

• Infections of respiratory or urinary tracts, skin, and soft tissue; and otitis media due to *Haemophilus influenzae* (especially when resistant to ampicillin or amoxicillin), *Streptococcus pneumoniae, S. pyogenes, Escherichia coli, Proteus mirabilis, Klebsiella* species, and staphylococci. **Adults:** 250 to 500 mg P.O. q 8 hours. Total daily dose may also be administered b.i.d (at 12-hour intervals). Total daily dose should not exceed 4 g. **Children:** 20 mg/kg daily P.O. in divided doses q 8 hours. In more serious infections, 40 mg/kg daily are recommended, not to exceed 1 g.

Adverse reactions

Blood: transient leukopenia, lymphocytosis, anemia, eosinophilia. **CNS:** dizziness, headache, somnolence. **GI:** *nausea,* vomiting, *diarrhea,* anorexia, pseudomembranous colitis. **GU:** red and white cells in urine, vaginal moniliasis, vaginitis. **Skin:** *maculopapular rash,* dermatitis. **Other:** ***hypersensitivity,*** fever, cholestatic jaundice.

Interactions

Probenecid: may inhibit excretion and increase blood levels of cefaclor.

Nursing diagnoses

• High risk for injury related to ineffectiveness of cefaclor to eradicate the infection.
• High risk for fluid volume deficit related to adverse GI reactions to cefaclor.
• Knowledge deficit related to cefaclor therapy.

Nursing interventions

• *Contraindicated* in hypersensitivity to other cephalosporins.
• *Use cautiously* in renal impairment and history of sensitivity to penicillin.
• Obtain specimen for culture and sensitivity tests before first dose. Therapy may begin pending test results.
• Tell patient to take medication exactly as prescribed, even after he feels better, and to take entire amount prescribed.
• Call doctor if skin rash develops.
• With large doses or prolonged therapy, monitor for superinfection, especially in high-risk patients.
• Store reconstituted suspension in refrigerator. Stable for 14 days if refrigerated. Shake well before using.
• Drug may be taken with meals.
• Cefaclor is a relatively expensive antibiotic and should be used only when the organism is resistant to other agents.
• Urine glucose determinations may be false-positive with copper sulfate tests only.

General

Classification: systemic and urinary alkalinizer, oral antacid (electrolyte). **Pregnancy risk category:** C.

Mechanism of action

Restores buffering capacity of the body and neutralizes excess acid.

Indications and dosage

- Cardiac arrest. **Adults and children:** 1 mEq/kg I.V. as a 7.5% or 8.4% solution, followed by 0.5 mEq/kg I.V. q 10 minutes depending on ABG levels. Further dosages based on ABG levels. If ABG levels unavailable, use 0.5 mEq/kg I.V. q 10 minutes until spontaneous circulation returns. **Infants up to 2 years:** 4.2% solution by I.V. infusion. Rate not to exceed 8 mEq/kg daily.
- Metabolic acidosis. **Adults and children:** dosage depends on blood carbon dioxide content, pH, and patient's clinical condition. Generally, 2 to 5 mEq/kg I.V. infused over 4- to 8-hour period.
- Systemic or urinary alkalinization. **Adults:** 325 mg to 2 g P.O. q.i.d. **Children:** 12 to 120 mg/kg P.O. daily.
- Antacid. **Adults:** 300 mg to 2 g P.O. chewed and taken with glass of water.

Adverse reactions

GI: gastric distention, belching, flatulence. **GU:** renal calculi or crystals. **Metabolic** (with overdose): ***alkalosis***, hypernatremia, ***hyperkalemia***, hyperosmolarity.

Interactions

I.V. solutions containing calcium: precipitate may form. Don't mix together. Take care to flush I.V. lines adequately.

Nursing diagnoses

- High risk for injury related to acid-base imbalance.
- Altered protection related to sodium bicarbonate overdose.
- Knowledge deficit related to sodium bicarbonate therapy.

Nursing interventions

- *Contraindicated* in hypertension, renal disease, in patients with tendency toward edema, in patients who are losing chlorides by vomiting or from continuous GI suction, in patients receiving diuretics known to produce hypochloremic alkalosis, and in patients on sodium-restricted diets. Not contraindicated in life-threatening emergencies.
- **I.V. use:** May be added to other I.V. fluids. Because sodium bicarbonate inactivates such catecholamines as norepinephrine and dopamine, do not mix with I.V. solutions of these agents.
- To avoid risk of alkalosis, determine blood pH, partial pressure of arterial oxygen, partial pressure of arterial carbon dioxide, and serum electrolytes. Keep doctor informed of serum laboratory results.
- Tell patient not to take with milk. May cause hypercalcemia, alkalosis, and possibly renal calculi.
- Discourage use as an antacid. Offer a nonabsorbable alternative antacid if it is to be used repeatedly.
- May cause enteric-coated drugs to be prematurely released in the stomach.
- Sodium bicarbonate is not routinely recommended for use in cardiac arrest because it may produce paradoxical acidosis from carbon dioxide production. It should not be routinely administered during the early stages of resuscitation unless preexisting acidosis is clearly present. May be used at team leader's discretion after such interventions as defibrillation, cardiac compression, and administration of first-line drugs.
- If sodium bicarbonate is being used to produce alkaline urine, monitor urine pH q 4 to 6 hours (should be > 7.0).

General

Classification: antibiotic (first-generation cephalosporin). **Pregnancy risk category:** B.

Mechanism of action

Inhibits cell wall synthesis, promoting osmotic instability. Usually bactericidal.

Indications and dosage

• Urinary tract infections caused by *Escherichia coli, Proteus mirabilis,* and *Klebsiella* species; infections of skin and soft tissue; and streptococcal pharyngitis. **Adults:** 500 mg to 2 g P.O. per day, depending on the infection being treated. Usually given in once-daily or b.i.d. dosage (because of longer half-life). **Children:** 30 mg/kg P.O. daily in 2 divided doses.

Adverse reactions

Blood: transient neutropenia, eosinophilia, leukopenia, anemia. **CNS:** dizziness, headache, malaise, paresthesias. **GI:** pseudomembranous colitis, *nausea,* anorexia, vomiting, *diarrhea,* glossitis, *dyspepsia,* abdominal cramps, anal pruritus, tenesmus, oral candidiasis (thrush). **GU:** genital pruritus, moniliasis. **Skin:** *maculopapular and erythematous rashes.* **Other:** ***hypersensitivity,*** dyspnea.

Interactions

Probenecid: may inhibit excretion and increase blood levels of cefadroxil.

Nursing diagnoses

• High risk for injury related to ineffectiveness of cefadroxil to eradicate the infection.
• High risk for fluid volume deficit related to adverse GI reactions to cefadroxil.
• Knowledge deficit related to cefadroxil therapy.

Nursing interventions

• *Contraindicated* in patients with hypersensitivity to other cephalosporins.
• *Use cautiously* in history of sensitivity to penicillin.
• Also use cautiously in patients with impaired renal function; dosage adjustments are necessary.
• Obtain specimen for culture and sensitivity tests before first dose. Therapy may begin pending test results.
• If creatinine clearance is below 50 ml/minute, dosage interval should be lengthened so drug doesn't accumulate.
• Tell patient to take medication exactly as prescribed, even after he feels better, and to take entire amount prescribed.
• Call doctor if skin rash develops.
• Since absorption not delayed by presence of food, tell the patient to take with food or milk to lessen GI discomfort.
• Urine glucose determinations may be false-positive with copper sulfate tests only.
• With large doses or prolonged therapy, monitor for superinfection, especially in high-risk patients.

General

Classification: antilipemic, cholesterol-lowering agent (HMG-CoA reductase inhibitor). **Pregnancy risk category:** X.

Mechanism of action

Inhibits the enzyme 3-hydroxy-3-methylglutaryl-coenzyme A (HMG-CoA) reductase, which has rate-limiting action in an early step in the synthetic pathway of cholesterol.

Indications and dosage

- Reduction of low-density lipoprotein (LDL) and total cholesterol levels in patients with primary hypercholesterolemia (types IIa and IIb). **Adults:** initially, 5 to 10 mg daily in the evening. Adjust dosage q 4 weeks based on patient tolerance and response; maximum daily dosage is 40 mg.

Adverse reactions

CNS: headache, asthenia. **GI:** abdominal pain, constipation, diarrhea, dyspepsia, flatulence, nausea. **Other:** upper respiratory infection.

Interactions

Digoxin: simvastatin may elevate digoxin levels. Closely monitor plasma digoxin levels at initiation of therapy. **Drugs that decrease levels or activity of endogenous steroids (such as cimetidine, spironolactone, ketoconazole):** may increase risk of developing endocrine dysfunction. Continue administration of drug, but take complete drug history in patients who develop endocrine dysfunction. **Hepatotoxic drugs, chronic alcohol abuse:** increased risk of hepatotoxicity. Avoid concomitant use. **Immunosuppressive agents (such as cyclosporine), fibric acid derivatives (such as clofibrate or gemfibrozil), high doses of niacin (1 g or more daily), erythromycin:** may increase the risk of rhabdomyolysis. Monitor patient closely if concomitant use cannot be avoided. Limit daily dosage of simvastatin to 10 mg if patient must take cyclosporine. **Warfarin:** anticoagulant effect may be slightly enhanced. Monitor patient's PT at start of therapy and during dosage adjustments.

Nursing diagnoses

- High risk for injury related to ineffectiveness of simvastatin in lowering LDL and total cholesterol levels.
- High risk for injury related to simvastatin-induced rhabdomyolysis.
- Knowledge deficit related to simvastatin therapy.

Nursing interventions

- *Contraindicated* in patients with hypersensitivity to the drug, in patients with active liver disease or conditions that result in unexplained persistent elevations of serum transaminase, in pregnant and breast-feeding women, and in women of childbearing age unless there is no risk of pregnancy.
- Drug may be given with or without food.
- Dosage adjustments should be made about every 4 weeks. If the cholesterol level falls below the target range, dosage may be reduced.
- Perform liver function tests frequently at start of therapy and periodically thereafter. Liver dysfunction my occur. Discontinue drug and monitor patient closely if it occurs.
- Watch for signs of myositis. Myopathy, marked elevations of CK (possibly leading to rhabdomyolysis), and renal failure secondary to myoglobinuria have been reported.
- Temporarily discontinue drug in any patient with an acute condition that suggests a developing myopathy or risk factors that may predispose the patient to renal failure secondary to rhabdomyolysis: severe acute infection; severe endocrine, metabolic, or electrolyte disorders; hypotension; major surgery; or uncontrolled seizures.
- Advise patient to restrict alcohol intake; simvastatin may impair liver function.
- Tell patient to inform doctor of any adverse reactions, particularly muscle aches and pains.
- Teach patient about proper dietary management, weight control, and exercise, and their importance in controlling serum lipids. Cholesterol-lowering diet should be continued during therapy.

General
Classification: antibiotic (second-generation cephalosporin). **Pregnancy risk category:** B.

Mechanism of action
Inhibits cell wall synthesis, promoting osmotic instability. Usually bactericidal.

Indications and dosage
• Serious infections of respiratory and GU tracts, skin and soft-tissue infections, bone and joint infections, septicemia, and peritonitis due to *Escherichia coli* and other coliform bacteria, *S. aureus* (penicillinase- and non-penicillinase-producing), *S. epidermidis,* group A beta-hemolytic streptococci, *Klebsiella, Haemophilus influenzae, Proteus mirabilis,* and *Enterobacter.* **Adults:** 500 mg to 1 g q 4 to 8 hours. In life-threatening infections, up to 2 g q 4 hours may be needed. **Infants and children:** 50 to 100 mg/kg daily in equally divided doses q 4 to 8 hours. May be increased to total daily dose of 150 mg/kg (not to exceed maximum adult dose) for severe infections.

Total daily dosage is same for I.M. or I.V. administration and depends on susceptibility of organism and severity of infection. In patients with impaired renal function, doses or frequency of administration must be modified according to degree of renal impairment, severity of infection, and susceptibility of organism. Should be injected deep I.M. into a large muscle mass, such as gluteus or lateral aspect of thigh.

Adverse reactions
Blood: transient neutropenia, eosinophilia, hemolytic anemia, *hypoprothrombinemia,* bleeding. **CNS:** headache, malaise, paresthesias, dizziness. **GI:** pseudomembranous colitis, nausea, anorexia, vomiting, *diarrhea,* glossitis, dyspepsia, abdominal cramps, tenesmus, anal pruritus, oral candidiasis (thrush). **GU:** genital pruritus and moniliasis. **Skin:** *maculopapular and erythematous rashes, urticaria.* **Local:** *at injection site—pain, induration, sterile abscesses,* temperature elevation, tissue sloughing; *phlebitis and thrombophlebitis with I.V. injection.* **Other:** ***hypersensitivity,*** dyspnea, cholestatic jaundice.

Interactions
Alcohol: may cause a disulfiram-like reaction. Warn patients not to drink alcohol for several days after discontinuing cefamandole. **Oral anticoagulants, aspirin:** increased risk of bleeding. **Probenecid:** may inhibit excretion and increase blood levels of cefamandole.

Nursing diagnoses
• High risk for injury related to ineffectiveness of cefamandole to eradicate the infection.
• High risk for fluid volume deficit related to adverse GI reactions to cefamandole.
• Knowledge deficit related to cefamandole.

Nursing interventions
• *Contraindicated* in patients with hypersensitivity to other cephalosporins.
• *Use cautiously* in impaired renal function and history of sensitivity to penicillin or other cephalosporins.
• Obtain specimen for culture and sensitivity tests before first dose. Therapy may begin pending test results.
• **I.V. use:** Reconstitute 1 g with 10 ml of sterile water for injection, D_5W or 0.9% sodium chloride for injection.
• Don't mix with I.V. infusions containing magnesium or calcium ions; chemically incompatible.
• Reconstituted drug is stable for 24 hours at room temperature or 96 hours under refrigeration.
• If bleeding disorders occur, bleeding can be promptly reversed with administration of vitamin K.
• With large doses or prolonged therapy, monitor for superinfection, especially in high-risk patients.
• Urine glucose determinations may be false-positive with copper sulfate tests only.

General

Classification: antiflatulent (dispersant). **Pregnancy risk category:** C.

Mechanism of action

By its defoaming action, disperses or prevents formation of mucus-surrounded gas pockets in the GI tract.

Indications and dosage

- Flatulence, functional gastric bloating. **Adults and children over 12 years:** 40 to 125 mg after each meal and h.s.

Adverse reactions

GI: expulsion of excessive liberated gas as belching or rectal flatus.

Interactions

None significant.

Nursing diagnoses

- Pain related to excess gas in the digestive tract.
- Knowledge deficit related to simethicone therapy.

Nursing interventions

- Warn patient not to take simethicone indiscriminately.
- Tell patient to chew tablet before swallowing.

General
Classification: antibiotic (first-generation cephalosporin). **Pregnancy risk category:** B.

Mechanism of action
Inhibits cell wall synthesis, promoting osmotic instability. Usually bactericidal.

Indications and dosage
• Serious infections of respiratory, biliary, and GU tracts, skin and soft-tissue infections, bone and joint infections, septicemia, and endocarditis due to *Escherichia coli,* Enterobacteriaceae, gonococci, *Haemophilus influenzae, Klebsiella, Proteus mirabilis, Staphylococcus aureus, Streptococcus pneumoniae,* and group A beta-hemolytic streptococci; and perioperative prophylaxis. **Adults:** 250 mg I.M. or I.V. q 8 hours to 1 g q 6 hours. Maximum 12 g/day in life-threatening situations; 4 g/day in severe renal impairment. **Children over 1 month:** 25 to 100 mg/kg/day I.M. or I.V. in three or four divided doses.

Total daily dosage is same for I.M. or I.V. administration and depends on susceptibility of organism and severity of infection. In patients with renal dysfunction, doses or frequency of administration must be modified according to degree of renal impairment, severity of infection, and susceptibility of organism.

Adverse reactions
Blood: transient neutropenia, leukopenia, eosinophilia, anemia. **CNS:** dizziness, headache, malaise, paresthesia. **GI:** pseudomembranous colitis, nausea, anorexia, vomiting, *diarrhea,* glossitis, dyspepsia, abdominal cramps, anal pruritus, tenesmus, oral candidiasis (thrush). **GU:** genital pruritus and moniliasis, vaginitis. **Skin:** *maculopapular and erythematous rashes, urticaria.* **Local:** *at injection site—pain, induration, sterile abscesses, tissue sloughing; phlebitis and thrombophlebitis with I.V. injection.* **Other:** ***hypersensitivity,*** dyspnea.

Interactions
Probenecid: may inhibit excretion and increase blood levels of cefazolin.

Nursing diagnoses
• High risk for injury related to ineffectiveness of cefazolin to eradicate the infection.
• High risk for fluid volume deficit related to adverse GI reactions to cefazolin.
• Knowledge deficit related to cefazolin therapy.

Nursing interventions
• *Use cautiously* in renal impairment and history of sensitivity to penicillin or other cephalosporins.
• Obtain specimen for culture and sensitivity tests before first dose. Therapy may begin pending test results.
• For I.M. administration, reconstitute with sterile water, bacteriostatic water, or 0.9% sodium chloride solution as follows: 2 ml to 250-mg vial; 2 ml to 500-mg vial; 2.5 ml to 1-g vial. Shake well until dissolved. Resultant concentration: 125 mg/ml, 225 mg/ml, 330 mg/ml, respectively. Inject deep I.M. into a large muscle mass, such as gluteus or lateral aspect of thigh.
• **I.V. use:** Alternate injection sites if I.V. therapy lasts longer than 3 days. Use of small I.V. needles in larger available veins may be preferable.
• For direct injection, further dilute drug with 10 ml of compatible solution; for intermittent infusion, add reconstituted drug to 50 to 100 ml of compatible solution or use premixed solution.
• Reconstituted drug is stable for 24 hours at room temperature or 96 hours under refrigeration.
• Patients receiving cephalosporins may show a false-positive direct Coombs' test; only a few indicate hemolytic anemia.
• With large doses or prolonged therapy, monitor for superinfection.
• Urine glucose determinations may be false-positive only with copper sulfate tests.

General

Classification: antidepressant (serotonin uptake inhibitor). **Pregnancy risk category:** B.

Mechanism of action

Probably acts by blocking the reuptake of serotonin (5-hydroxytryptamine; 5-HT) into presynaptic neurons in the CNS, prolonging the action of 5-HT.

Indications and dosage

- Depression, obsessive-compulsive disorder. **Adults:** 50 mg P.O. daily, either in the morning or evening. Adjust dosage as needed and tolerated, up to 200 mg daily, at intervals of no less than 1 week.

Adverse reactions

CNS: *headache, tremor, dizziness, insomnia, somnolence,* syncope, paresthesia, hypoesthesia, hyperesthesia, twitching, hypertonia, confusion, ataxia, abnormal coordination or gait, nystagmus, vertigo, hyperkinesia, hypokinesia, mania. **CV:** palpitations, chest pain, postural hypotension, hypertension, hypotension, edema, peripheral ischemia, tachycardia. **GI:** *dry mouth, nausea, diarrhea, loose stools, dyspepsia,* vomiting, flatulence, anorexia, abdominal pain, increased appetite, dysphagia. **GU:** male sexual dysfunction. **Skin:** rash, acne, alopecia, pruritus, erythematous or maculopapular rash, dry skin. **Other:** *increased sweating,* cold or clammy skin, flushing, myalgia.

Interactions

Diazepam, tolbutamide: sertraline decreases clearance of these drugs. Monitor patient for increased drug effects. **MAO inhibitors:** may cause serious mental status changes, hyperthermia, autonomic instability, rapid fluctuations of vital signs, delirium, coma, and death. Do not administer sertraline with or within 14 days after discontinuing an MAO inhibitor; also, allow 14 days after discontinuing sertraline before starting an MAO inhibitor. **Warfarin, other highly protein-bound drugs:** interactions may occur, increasing the plasma levels of sertraline or of the other highly bound drug. Small (8%) increases in PT have been seen with concomitant use of warfarin. Monitor closely.

Nursing diagnoses

- High risk for injury related to sertraline-induced dizziness.
- Sleep pattern disturbance related to sertraline-induced insomnia.
- Knowledge deficit related to sertraline therapy.

Nursing interventions

- *Contraindicated* in patients with hypersensitivity to the drug and within 14 days of taking an MAO inhibitor.
- *Use cautiously* in hepatic impairment (drug is extensively metabolized in the liver), seizure disorders, or a history of drug abuse.
- May administer with or without food.
- Because of the risk of suicide in depressed patients, provide close supervision during initiation of drug therapy. Limit the supply of tablets to reduce the risk of overdose.
- Like other antidepressants, the drug can activate mania in patients with major affective disorders.
- Drug may increase serum cholesterol and triglyceride levels and decrease uric acid concentrations. Elevations in serum transaminases (AST, ALT) may occur, usually within the first 9 weeks of therapy; values returned to normal after discontinuing drug.
- Periodically monitor effectiveness during prolonged use. It is unknown if periodic dosage adjustments are necessary to maintain effectiveness.
- Advise patient to use caution when performing hazardous tasks that require alertness, such as driving a car or operating heavy machinery, and to avoid use of alcohol while taking this drug. Drugs that influence the CNS may impair judgment.
- Caution patient to check with the doctor or pharmacist before taking any OTC medications.

General

Classification: antibiotic (third-generation cephalosporin). **Pregnancy risk category:** B.

Mechanism of action

Inhibits cell wall synthesis, promoting osmotic instability. Usually bactericidal.

Indications and dosage

- Uncomplicated urinary tract infections caused by *Escherichia coli* and *Proteus mirabilis;* otitis media caused by *Haemophilus influenzae* (beta-lactam positive and negative strains), *Moraxella (Branhamella) catarrhalis,* and *Streptococcus pyogenes;* pharyngitis and tonsillitis caused by *S. pyogenes;* acute bronchitis and acute exacerbations of chronic bronchitis caused by *S. pneumoniae* and *H. influenzae* (beta-lactamase positive and negative strains). **Adults:** 400 mg/day P.O. as a single 400-mg tablet or 200 mg q 12 hours. **Children:** 8 mg/kg/day suspension P.O. as a single daily dose or 4 mg/kg q 12 hours. Treat children over age 12 and those who weigh more than 50 kg with the recommended adult dose.
- Gonorrhea. **Adults:** 400 mg P.O. as a single dose.

Adverse reactions

Blood: thrombocytopenia, leukopenia, eosinophilia. **CNS:** headaches, dizziness. **GI:** *diarrhea,* loose stools, abdominal pain, nausea, vomiting, dyspepsia, flatulence, pseudomembranous colitis. **GU:** genital pruritus, vaginitis, genital candidiasis. **Skin:** pruritus, rash, urticaria. **Other:** drug fever, ***hypersensitivity reactions.***

Interactions

None significant.

Nursing diagnoses

- High risk for injury related to ineffectiveness of cefixime to eradicate the infection.
- High risk for fluid volume deficit related to adverse GI reactions to cefixime.
- Knowledge deficit related to cefixime therapy.

Nursing interventions

- *Contraindicated* in patients with hypersensitivity to other cephalosporins.
- *Use cautiously* and with reduced dosage in patients with renal dysfunction; reduced dosage is necessary in patients with creatinine clearance below 60 ml/minute.
- Also use cautiously in patients with a history of sensitivity to penicillin.
- Obtain specimen for culture and sensitivity tests before first dose. Therapy may begin pending test results.
- Call doctor if skin rash develops.
- Preparation of oral suspension: add required amount of water to powder in two portions. Shake well after each addition. After mixing, suspension is stable for 14 days. It does not require refrigeration, but keep tightly closed. Shake well before using.
- With large doses or prolonged therapy, monitor for superinfection, especially in high-risk patients.
- Patients receiving cephalosporins may show a false-positive direct Coombs' test; only a few of these tests indicate hemolytic anemia.
- Urine glucose determinations may be false-positive with copper sulfate tests only.

General

Classification: stimulant laxative (anthraquinone derivative). **Pregnancy risk category:** C.

Mechanism of action

Increases peristalsis by direct effect on the smooth muscle of the intestine. Thought either to irritate the musculature or to stimulate the colonic intramural plexus. Also promotes fluid accumulation in the colon and small intestine.

Indications and dosage

• Acute constipation, preparation for bowel or rectal examination. **Adults:** dosage range for Senokot: 1 to 8 tablets P.O.; ½ to 4 teaspoonfuls of granules added to liquid; 1 to 2 suppositories h.s.; 1 to 4 teaspoonfuls syrup h.s. Black-Draught: 2 tablets or ¼ to ½ level teaspoonfuls of granules mixed with water. **Children over 27 kg:** half adult dose of Senokot tablets, granules, or syrup (Black-Draught tablets and granules not recommended for children). **Children 1 month to 1 year:** 1.25 to 2.5 ml Senokot syrup P.O. h.s.

X-Prep Liquid used solely as single dose for preradiographic bowel evacuation. Give 20 g powder dissolved in juice or 75 ml liquid between 2 p.m. and 4 p.m. on day before X-ray procedure. May be given in divided doses for elderly or debilitated patients.

Adverse reactions

GI: *nausea;* vomiting; diarrhea; loss of normal bowel function in excessive use; *abdominal cramps,* especially in severe constipation; malabsorption of nutrients; "cathartic colon" (syndrome resembling ulcerative colitis radiologically) in chronic misuse; may cause constipation after catharsis; yellow, yellow-green cast to feces; diarrhea in nursing infants of mothers receiving senna; darkened pigmentation of rectal mucosa in long-term use, which is usually reversible within 4 to 12 months after stopping drug. **GU:** red-pink discoloration in alkaline urine; yellow-brown color in acidic urine. **Metabolic:** protein-losing enteropathy, electrolyte imbalance, such as hypokalemia, with excessive use. **Other:** laxative dependence in long-term or excessive use.

Interactions

None significant.

Nursing diagnoses

• Constipation related to interruption of normal pattern of elimination.
• Pain related to senna-induced abdominal cramping.
• Knowledge deficit related to senna therapy.

Nursing interventions

• *Contraindicated* in ulcerative bowel lesions; in nausea, vomiting, abdominal pain, or other symptoms of appendicitis or acute surgical abdomen; fecal impaction; or intestinal obstruction or perforation.
• Use for short-term treatment.
• More potent than cascara sagrada. Acts in 6 to 10 hours. X-Prep Liquid produces thorough, strong bowel action beginning in 6 hours.
• Avoid exposing to excessive heat or light.
• Before giving for constipation, determine if patient has adequate fluid intake, exercise, and diet. Tell him that dietary sources of bulk include bran and other cereals, fresh fruit, and vegetables.
• After X-Prep Liquid is taken, diet should be confined to clear liquids.
• Senna is one of the most effective laxatives for counteracting constipation caused by narcotic analgesics.

General

Classification: antibiotic (second-generation cephalosporin). **Pregnancy risk category:** B.

Mechanism of action

Inhibits cell wall synthesis, promoting osmotic instability. Usually bactericidal.

Indications and dosage

• Lower respiratory tract infections caused by *Streptococcus pneumoniae, Staphylococcus aureus* (penicillinase- and non-penicillinase-producing), *Escherichia coli,* and *Haemophilus influenzae* (non-penicillinase-producing); intra-abdominal infections caused by *E. coli* or *Bacteroides fragilis;* skin and skin-structure infections caused by *S. aureus* (penicillinase- and non-penicillinase-producing), *S. epidermidis, Streptococcus pyogenes, S. agalactiae, E. coli, Proteus mirabilis, Klebsiella pneumoniae,* and *B. fragilis.* **Adults:** 2 g I.V. q 6 to 12 hours for 5 to 14 days.
• Urinary tract infections caused by *E. coli.* **Adults:** 2 g I.V. q 12 hours.
• Prophylaxis in patients undergoing vaginal hysterectomy. **Adults:** 2 g I.V. 30 to 90 minutes before surgery as a single dose; or 1 g I.V. 30 to 90 minutes before surgery, repeated in 8 and 16 hours.
• Prophylaxis in patients undergoing abdominal hysterectomy. **Adults:** 1 g I.V. 30 to 90 minutes before surgery, repeated in 8 and 16 hours.
• Prophylaxis in patients undergoing cesarean section. **Adults:** 2 g I.V. as a single dose after clamping cord; or 1 g I.V. after clamping cord, repeated in 8 and 16 hours.
• Prophylaxis in patients undergoing colorectal surgery. **Adults:** 2 g I.V. as a single dose 30 to 90 minutes before surgery. Some clinicians follow with additional 2-g doses in 8 and 16 hours.
• Prophylaxis in patients undergoing cholecystectomy (high risk). **Adults:** 1 g I.V. 30 to 90 minutes before surgery, repeated in 8 and 16 hours.

Adverse reactions

CNS: headache. **CV:** ***shock,*** hypotension. **EENT:** epistaxis, altered color perception. **GI:** nausea, vomiting, *diarrhea,* epigastric pain, pseudomembranous colitis. **GU:** vaginitis. **Respiratory:** pleural effusion, dyspnea, respiratory distress. **Skin:** rash, pruritus, generalized erythema. **Local:** *pain at injection site,* phlebitis. **Other:** fever, bacterial or fungal superinfection, ***hypersensitivity.***

Interactions

Alcohol: disulfiram-like reaction. Avoid alcohol within 24 hours of administration. **Aminoglycosides:** increased risk of nephrotoxicity.

Nursing diagnoses

• High risk for injury related to ineffectiveness of cefmetazole to eradicate the infection.
• High risk for fluid volume deficit related to adverse GI reactions to cefmetazole.

Nursing interventions

• *Contraindicated* in history of hypersensitivity to other cephalosporins.
• *Use cautiously* in history of sensitivity to penicillin.
• Obtain specimen for culture and sensitivity before first dose. Therapy may begin pending test results.
• Monitor patient for bacterial and fungal superinfections (prolonged use).
• Monitor prothrombin time and administer vitamin K, as ordered, if bleeding disorders occur.
• May cause false-positive results for urine glucose with copper sulfate tests only.
• **I.V. use:** Reconstitute with bacteriostatic water for injection, sterile water for injection, or 0.9% sodium chloride for injection. May be further diluted by adding 0.9% sodium chloride injection, D_5W, or lactated Ringer's injection. Reconstituted or diluted solutions are stable for 24 hours at room temperature or 1 week if refrigerated.

General

Classification: antiparkinsonian agent (MAO inhibitor). **Pregnancy risk category:** C.

Mechanism of action

Probably acts by selectively inhibiting MAO type B (found mostly in the brain). At higher-than-recommended doses, it is a nonselective inhibitor of MAO, including MAO type A (found in the GI tract). It also may directly increase dopaminergic activity by decreasing the reuptake of dopamine into nerve cells. Its pharmacologically active metabolites (amphetamine and methamphetamine) may contribute to this effect.

Indications and dosage

• Adjunct to carbidopa-levodopa in the management of the symptoms associated with Parkinson's disease. **Adults:** 10 mg P.O. daily, taken as 5 mg at breakfast and 5 mg at lunch. After 2 or 3 days of therapy, begin gradual decrease of carbidopa-levodopa dosage.

Adverse reactions

CNS: *dizziness,* increased tremor, chorea, loss of balance, restlessness, blepharospasm, increased bradykinesia, facial grimace, stiff neck, dyskinesia, involuntary movements, increased apraxia, behavioral changes, tiredness, headache. **CV:** orthostatic hypotension, hypertension, hypotension, ***arrhythmias,*** palpitations, new or increased anginal pain, tachycardia, peripheral edema, syncope. **GI:** *nausea,* vomiting, constipation, weight loss, anorexia or poor appetite, dysphagia, diarrhea, heartburn, dry mouth, taste alteration. **GU:** slow urination, transient nocturia, prostatic hyperplasia, urinary hesitancy, urinary frequency, urine retention, sexual dysfunction. **Skin:** rash, alopecia, sweating. **Other:** malaise.

Interactions

Adrenergic agents: possible increased pressor response, particularly in patients who have taken an overdose of selegiline.

Nursing diagnoses

• Impaired physical mobility related to underlying parkinsonian syndrome.
• High risk for injury related to adverse CNS reactions to drug therapy.
• Knowledge deficit related to selegiline therapy.

Nursing interventions

• *Contraindicated* in patients with hypersensitivity to the drug.
• Warn patients to move about cautiously at the start of therapy because they may experience dizziness and risk falling.
• Some patients experience increased adverse reactions associated with levodopa (including muscle twitches) and require reduction of carbidopa-levodopa dosage (commonly by 10% to 30%.)
• Because the drug is an MAO inhibitor, patients should be told about the possibility of an interaction with tyramine-containing foods. They should immediately report any signs or symptoms of hypertension, including severe headache. However, there is no evidence that this interaction occurs at recommended dosage because, at 10 mg daily, the drug inhibits only MAO type B. No dietary restrictions appear necessary if the patient does not exceed the recommended dose.
• Advise patient not to take more than 10 mg daily, because there is no evidence that a greater amount improves efficacy and it may increase adverse reactions.

General

Classification: antibiotic (second-generation cephalosporin). **Pregnancy risk category:** B.

Mechanism of action

Inhibits cell wall synthesis, promoting osmotic instability. Usually bactericidal.

Indications and dosage

• Serious infections of the lower respiratory and urinary tract; skin and skin structure infections; septicemia; bone and joint infections; and perioperative prophylaxis. Susceptible microorganisms include *Streptococcus pneumoniae, Klebsiella pneumoniae, Escherichia coli, Haemophilus influenzae, Proteus mirabilis, Staphylococcus aureus, S. epidermidis,* and *Streptococcus pyogenes.* **Adults:** usual dosage is 1 g I.V. or I.M. q 24 hours. In life-threatening infections, 2 g q 24 hours.

Total daily dosage is same for I.M. or I.V. administration and depends on susceptibility of organism and severity of infection. In patients with renal dysfunction, doses or frequency of administration must be modified according to degree of renal impairment, severity of infection, and susceptibility of organism.

Adverse reactions

Blood: transient neutropenia, leukopenia, eosinophilia, anemia. **CNS:** dizziness, headache, malaise, paresthesia. **GI:** pseudomembranous colitis, nausea, anorexia, vomiting, diarrhea, glossitis, dyspepsia, abdominal cramps, anal pruritus, tenesmus, oral candidiasis (thrush). **GU:** genital pruritus and moniliasis, vaginitis. **Skin:** *maculopapular and erythematous rashes, urticaria.* **Local:** *at injection site—pain, induration, sterile abscesses, tissue sloughing; phlebitis and thrombophlebitis with I.V. injection.* **Other:** ***hypersensitivity,*** dyspnea.

Interactions

Probenecid: may inhibit excretion and increase blood levels of cefonicid.

Nursing diagnoses

• High risk for injury related to ineffectiveness of cefonicid to eradicate the infection.
• High risk for fluid volume deficit related to adverse GI reactions to cefonicid.
• Knowledge deficit related to cefonicid therapy.

Nursing interventions

• *Contraindicated* in patients with hypersensitivity to other cephalosporins.
• *Use cautiously* in impaired renal function and history of sensitivity to penicillin.
• Obtain specimen for culture and sensitivity tests before first dose. Therapy may begin pending test results.
• When given I.M., inject deep I.M. into a large muscle mass, such as gluteus or lateral aspect of thigh.
• When administering 2-g I.M. doses once daily, divide the dose equally and inject deeply in two large muscle sites.
• **I.V. use:** Reconstitute 500-mg vial with 2 ml of sterile water for injection (yields a concentration of 220 mg/ml) and 1-g vial with 2.5 ml of sterile water for injection (yields a concentration of 325 mg/ml). Shake well. Reconstitute piggyback vials with 50 to 100 ml of sterile water for injection, bacteriostatic water for injection, or 0.9% sodium chloride.
• With large doses or prolonged therapy, monitor for superinfection, especially in high-risk patients.
• Has been promoted as a cost-effective agent for surgical prophylaxis.

General
Classification: sedative-hypnotic, anticonvulsant (barbiturate). **Pregnancy risk category:** D. **Controlled substance schedule:** II.

Mechanism of action
Interferes with transmission of impulses from the thalamus to the cortex of the brain.

Indications and dosage
- Preoperative sedation. **Adults:** 200 to 300 mg P.O. 1 to 2 hours before surgery. **Children:** 50 to 100 mg P.O. or 4 to 5 mg/kg P.R. 1 to 2 hours before surgery.
- Insomnia. **Adults:** 100 to 200 mg P.O. or I.M. **Children:** 3 to 5 mg/kg I.M., not to exceed 100 mg, with no more than 5 ml injected in any one site; or 4 to 5 mg/kg P.R.
- Acute tetanus seizure. **Adults and children:** 5.5 mg/kg I.M. or slow I.V., repeated q 3 to 4 hours if needed; I.V. injection rate not to exceed 50 mg/15 seconds.
- Acute psychotic agitation. **Adults:** 50 mg/minute I.V. up to 250 mg; give additional doses cautiously after 5 minutes if desired response is not obtained. Not to exceed 500 mg total.
- Status epilepticus. **Adults and children:** 250 to 350 mg I.M. or I.V.

Adverse reactions
CNS: *drowsiness, lethargy, hangover,* paradoxical excitement in elderly patients. **GI:** nausea, vomiting. **Skin:** rash, urticaria. **Other:** ***Stevens-Johnson syndrome, angioedema,*** exacerbation of porphyria.

Interactions
Alcohol or other CNS depressants, including narcotic analgesics: excessive CNS and respiratory depression. Use together cautiously. **Griseofulvin:** decreased absorption of griseofulvin. **MAO inhibitors:** inhibit metabolism of secobarbital; may cause prolonged CNS depression. Reduce secobarbital dosage. **Oral anticoagulants, estrogens and oral contraceptives, doxycycline, corticosteroids:** secobarbital may enhance the metabolism of these drugs. Monitor for decreased effect. **Rifampin:** may decrease secobarbital levels. Monitor for decreased effect.

Nursing diagnoses
- Sleep pattern disturbance related to patient's underlying problem.
- High risk for trauma related to adverse CNS reactions to drug therapy.
- Knowledge deficit related to secobarbital therapy.

Nursing interventions
- *Contraindicated* in uncontrolled severe pain, respiratory disease with dyspnea or obstruction, hypersensitivity to barbiturates, previous addiction to sedatives, or porphyria.
- *Use cautiously* in hepatic or renal impairment and in pregnant women with toxemia or history of bleeding.
- Assess elderly patients' mental status before giving drug (more sensitive to adverse CNS effects).
- Take appropriate seizure precautions if secobarbital is used to manage seizures.
- **I.V. use:** reserve for emergency treatment; give under close supervision. Administer slowly at a rate not exceeding 50 mg/15 seconds.
- I.V. administration may cause severe respiratory depression, laryngospasm, or hypotension. Have emergency resuscitation equipment available.
- Give I.M. injection deeply. Superficial injection may cause pain, sterile abscess, and sloughing.
- Supervise walking and raise bed rails.
- May cause drug dependence and severe withdrawal symptoms. Withdraw gradually.
- Prevent hoarding or self-overdosing by patients who are depressed, suicidal, or drug-dependent or who have a history of drug abuse.
- Watch for signs of barbiturate toxicity: coma, pupillary constriction, cyanosis, clammy skin, and hypotension. Overdose can be fatal.
- Morning "hangover" is common after hypnotic dose, which also suppresses REM sleep.
- Skin eruptions may precede potentially fatal reactions to barbiturate therapy; discontinue drug when they occur.

General

Classification: antibiotic (third-generation cephalosporin). **Pregnancy risk category:** B.

Mechanism of action

Inhibits cell wall synthesis, promoting osmotic instability. Usually bactericidal.

Indications and dosage

• Serious infections of the respiratory tract; intra-abdominal, gynecologic, and skin infections; bacteremia, septicemia. Susceptible microorganisms include *Streptococcus pneumoniae* and *S. pyogenes; Staphylococcus aureus* (penicillinase and non-penicillinase-producing) and *S. epidermidis;* enterococcus; *Escherichia coli; Klebsiella; Haemophilus influenzae; Enterobacter; Citrobacter; Proteus;* some *Pseudomonas,* including *Pseudomonas aeruginosa;* and *Bacteroides fragilis.* **Adults:** usual dosage is 1 to 2 g q 12 hours I.M. or I.V. In severe infections, or infections caused by less sensitive organisms, the total daily dosage or frequency may be increased up to 16 g/day in certain situations.

No dosage adjustment is usually necessary in patients with renal impairment. However, doses of 4 g/day should be given very cautiously in patients with hepatic disease. Should be injected deep I.M. into a large muscle mass, such as gluteus or lateral aspect of the thigh.

Adverse reactions

Blood: transient neutropenia, eosinophilia, hemolytic anemia, hypoprothrombinemia, bleeding. **CNS:** headache, malaise, paresthesias, dizziness. **GI:** pseudomembranous colitis, nausea, anorexia, vomiting, *diarrhea,* glossitis, dyspepsia, abdominal cramps, tenesmus, anal pruritus, oral candidiasis (thrush). **Hepatic:** mildly elevated liver enzymes. **GU:** genital pruritus and moniliasis. **Skin:** *maculopapular and erythematous rashes, urticaria.* **Local:** *at injection site—pain, induration, sterile abscesses, temperature elevation, tissue sloughing; phlebitis and thrombophlebitis with I.V. injection.* **Other:** ***hypersensitivity,*** dyspnea.

Interactions

Alcohol: may cause a disulfiram-like reaction. Warn patients not to drink alcohol for several days after discontinuing cefoperazone. **Oral anticoagulants, aspirin:** increased risk of bleeding. **Probenecid:** may inhibit excretion and increase blood levels of cefoperazone.

Nursing diagnoses

• High risk for injury related to ineffectiveness of cefoperazone to eradicate the infection.
• High risk for fluid volume deficit related to adverse GI reactions to cefoperazone.
• Knowledge deficit related to cefoperazone therapy.

Nursing interventions

• *Contraindicated* in patients with hypersensitivity to other cephalosporins.
• *Use cautiously* in renal impairment and history of sensitivity to penicillin.
• Obtain specimen for culture and sensitivity tests before first dose. Therapy may begin pending test results.
• **I.V. use:** Infuse by intermittent infusion over 15 to 30 minutes into tubing containing a compatible solution.
• Cefoperazone has greater activity than first-generation cephalosporins against gram-negative organisms, but less activity against gram-positive organisms.
• Because of high degree of biliary excretion, may cause more diarrhea than other cephalosporins.
• If bleeding disorders occur, bleeding can be promptly reversed with administration of vitamin K. Monitor prothrombin time regularly.
• With large doses or prolonged therapy, monitor for superinfection, especially in high-risk patients.
• Urine glucose determinations may be false-positive with copper sulfate tests only.

General

Classification: antimuscarinic, antiemetic/antivertigo agent, antiparkinsonian agent (anticholinergic). **Pregnancy risk category:** C.

Mechanism of action

Inhibits muscarinic actions of acetylcholine on autonomic effectors innervated by postganglionic cholinergic neurons. Affects neural pathways originating in the labyrinth to inhibit nausea and vomiting.

Indications and dosage

- Postencephalitic parkinsonism and other spastic states. **Adults:** 0.5 to 1 mg (hydrobromide) P.O. t.i.d. or q.i.d.; or 0.3 to 0.6 mg S.C., I.M., or I.V. (with suitable dilution) t.i.d. or q.i.d. **Children:** 0.006 mg/kg or 0.2 mg/m^2 (hydrobromide) P.O. or S.C. t.i.d. or q.i.d.
- Preoperatively to reduce secretions and block cardiac vagal reflexes. **Adults:** 0.4 to 0.6 mg (hydrobromide) S.C. 30 to 60 minutes before induction of anesthesia.
- Prevention of nausea and vomiting associated with motion sickness. **Adults:** apply one Transderm-Scōp patch, which delivers 0.5 mg scopolamine daily over 72 hours, to the skin behind the ear 3 to 12 hours before antiemetic effect is required, or apply one Transderm-V patch, which delivers 1 mg scopolamine daily over 72 hours, behind the ear 12 hours before antiemetic effect is required. Not recommended for children.

Adverse reactions

Adverse reactions may be caused by pending atropine-like toxicity and are dose-related. **CNS:** disorientation, restlessness, irritability, dizziness, drowsiness, headache. **CV:** palpitations, tachycardia, paradoxical bradycardia. **EENT:** dilated pupils, blurred vision, photophobia, increased intraocular pressure, difficulty swallowing. **GI:** *constipation, dry mouth, nausea, vomiting, epigastric distress.* **GU:** urinary hesitancy, urine retention. **Skin:** rash, flushing, dryness. **Other:** bronchial plugging, fever, depressed respirations.

Interactions

Alcohol, CNS depressants: increased CNS depression. **Centrally acting anticholinergics (TCAs, phenothiazines):** increased CNS adverse reactions. **Digoxin:** increased digoxin levels.

Nursing diagnoses

- Altered thought processes related to scopolamine-induced confusion.
- Constipation related to adverse reaction to scopolamine hydrobromide.
- Knowledge deficit related to scopolamine therapy.

Nursing interventions

- *Contraindicated* in narrow-angle glaucoma, obstructive uropathy, GI obstruction, asthma, chronic pulmonary disease, myasthenia gravis, paralytic ileus, intestinal atony, unstable CV status in acute hemorrhage, or toxic megacolon.
- *Use cautiously* in patients with autonomic neuropathy, hyperthyroidism, coronary artery disease, cardiac arrhythmias, CHF, hypertension, hiatal hernia associated with reflux esophagitis, hepatic or renal disease, or ulcerative colitis; in patients over age 40; in children under age 6; and in hot or humid environments.
- Some patients become temporarily excited or disoriented. Raise side rails as a precaution.
- Drug may produce amnesia, drowsiness, and euphoria, which are desirable effects when it is used as an adjunct to anesthesia. Reorient patient.
- Warn patient to avoid activities requiring alertness until CNS effects of the drug are known.
- Tolerance may develop with long-term use.
- Advise patient to report urinary reactions.
- **I.V. use:** Dilute with sterile water for injection and inject at ordered rate through patent I.V. line.
- Wash and dry hands before applying the transdermal patch on dry skin. After removal, discard patch, and wash application site and hands thoroughly. If patch is displaced, apply a new one on a fresh site.

General

Classification: antibiotic (third-generation cephalosporin). **Pregnancy risk category:** B.

Mechanism of action

Inhibits cell wall synthesis, promoting osmotic instability. Usually bactericidal.

Indications and dosage

- Serious infections of the lower respiratory and urinary tracts, CNS infections, gynecologic infections, bacteremia, septicemia, skin infections, and perioperative prophylaxis. Among susceptible microorganisms are streptococci, including *Streptococcus pneumoniae* and *S. pyogenes; Staphylococcus aureus* (penicillinase- and non-penicillinase-producing) and *S. epidermidis; Escherichia coli; Klebsiella; Haemophilus influenzae; Enterobacter; Proteus;* and *Peptostreptococcus.* **Adults:** usual dose is 1 g I.V. or I.M. q 6 to 8 hours. Up to 12 g daily can be administered in life-threatening infections. **Children 1 month to 12 years:** 50 to 180 mg/kg/day I.M. or I.V. in 4 to 6 divided doses. **Neonates 1 to 4 weeks:** 50 mg/kg I.V. q 8 hours. **Neonates to 1 week:** 50 mg/kg I.V. q 12 hours.

Total daily dosage is same for I.M. or I.V. administration and depends on susceptibility of organism and severity of infection. In patients with renal dysfunction, doses or frequency of administration must be modified according to degree of renal impairment, severity of infection, and susceptibility of organism.

Adverse reactions

Blood: transient neutropenia, eosinophilia, hemolytic anemia. **CNS:** headache, malaise, paresthesias, dizziness. **GI:** pseudomembranous colitis, nausea, anorexia, vomiting, *diarrhea,* glossitis, dyspepsia, abdominal cramps, tenesmus, anal pruritus, oral candidiasis (thrush). **GU:** genital pruritus and moniliasis. **Skin:** *maculopapular and erythematous rashes, urticaria.* **Local:** *at injection site—pain, induration, sterile abscesses, temperature elevation, tissue sloughing; phlebitis and thrombophlebitis with I.V. injection.* **Other:** ***hypersensitivity,*** dyspnea, elevated temperature.

Interactions

Probenecid: may inhibit excretion and increase blood levels of cefotaxime. Use together cautiously.

Nursing diagnoses

- High risk for injury related to ineffectiveness of cefotaxime to eradicate the infection.
- High risk for fluid volume deficit related to adverse GI reactions to cefotaxime.
- Knowledge deficit related to cefotaxime therapy.

Nursing interventions

- *Contraindicated* in patients with hypersensitivity to other cephalosporins.
- *Use cautiously* in impaired renal function and in history of sensitivity to penicillin.
- Obtain specimen for culture and sensitivity tests before first dose. Therapy may begin pending test results.
- **I.V. use:** Reconstitute infusion vials with 50 to 100 ml of D_5W or 0.9% sodium chloride. Interrupt flow of primary I.V. solution during infusion.
- Inject deep I.M. into a large muscle mass, such as gluteus or lateral aspect of thigh.
- With large doses or prolonged therapy, monitor for superinfection, especially in high-risk patients.
- Cefotaxime has increased antibacterial activity against gram-negative microorganisms and has an active metabolite.
- Some doctors may prescribe cefotaxime in clinical situations in which they formerly prescribed aminoglycosides. However, this drug is usually not effective against infections caused by *Pseudomonas* organisms.
- Urine glucose determinations may be false-positive with copper sulfate tests.

General

Classification: colony stimulating factor (biological response modifier). **Pregnancy risk category:** C.

Mechanism of action

A glycoprotein containing 127 amino acids manufactured by recombinant DNA technology. It differs from the natural human granulocyte-macrophage colony stimulating factor by substitution of leucine for arginine at position 23. Sargramostim binds to specific receptors on cell surfaces of target cells.

Indications and dosage

- Acceleration of hematopoietic reconstitution after autologous bone marrow transplantation in patients with malignant lymphoma or acute lymphoblastic leukemia or during autologous bone marrow transplantation in patients with Hodgkin's disease. **Adults:** 250 mcg/m² daily for 21 consecutive days, given as a 2-hour I.V. infusion beginning 2 to 4 hours after the transplant.

Adverse reactions

CNS: malaise, CNS disorder. **CV:** *blood dyscrasias,* hemorrhage. **GI:** nausea, vomiting, diarrhea, anorexia, hemorrhage, GI disorder, stomatitis, liver damage. **GU:** urinary tract disorder, abnormal kidney function. **Respiratory:** dyspnea, lung disorder. **Skin:** alopecia, transient rash. **Other:** fever, mucous membrane disorder, asthenia, edema, peripheral edema, ***sepsis.***

Interactions

Lithium, corticosteroids: may potentiate myeloproliferative effects of sargramostim. Use together cautiously.

Nursing diagnoses

- High risk for infection related to the patient's underlying condition.
- Knowledge deficit related to sargramostim therapy.

Nursing interventions

- *Contraindicated* in patients with excessive leukemic myeloid blasts in bone marrow or peripheral blood and in those with hypersensitivity to the drug or to yeast-derived products.
- *Use cautiously* in patients with preexisting cardiac disease, hypoxia, preexisting fluid retention, pulmonary infiltrates, CHF, or impaired renal or hepatic function.
- Don't administer within 24 hours of last dose of chemotherapy or within 12 hours of last dose of radiation therapy. These cytotoxic therapies make the drug ineffective.
- Reduce dose by half or temporarily discontinue if severe adverse reactions occur. Resume therapy when reactions abate.
- Drug's effect may be limited in patients who have received extensive radiation therapy for treatment of primary disease in the abdomen or chest or who have been exposed to multiple agents (alkylating, anthracycline antibiotics, antimetabolites) before autologous bone marrow transplantation.
- Stimulation of marrow precursors may result in rapid rise of WBC count; biweekly monitoring of CBC with differential, including examination for presence of blast cells, is recommended. If blast cells appear or increase to 10% or more of the WBC count or if progression of the underlying disease occurs, discontinue therapy. If the absolute neutrophil count is above 20,000 cells/mm³ or if platelet counts are above 50,000 cells/mm³, discontiue therapy or reduce dose by half. Blood counts return to normal or baseline levels within 3 to 7 days after stopping treatment.
- Sargramostim can act as a growth factor for any tumor type, particularly myeloid malignancies.
- **I.V. use:** Reconstitute according to pharmacy directions. Don't reenter or reuse the single-dose vial. Direct stream of sterile water against side of vial and *gently swirl* contents to minimize foaming. Avoid excessive or vigorous agitation or shaking. Administer reconstituted or diluted solution within 6 hours. Discard any unused portion. Don't add other medications to infusion solution.

General

Classification: antibiotic (second-generation cephalosporin). **Pregnancy risk category:** B.

Mechanism of action

Inhibits cell wall synthesis, promoting osmotic instability. Usually bactericidal.

Indications and dosage

• Serious infections of the urinary and lower respiratory tracts, and gynecologic, skin and skin structure, intra-abdominal, and bone and joint infections, and perioperative prophylaxis. Among susceptible microorganisms are streptococci, *Staphylococcus aureus* (penicillinase- and non-penicillinase-producing) and *S. epidermidis, Escherichia coli, Klebsiella, Enterobacter, Proteus, Haemophilus influenzae, Neisseria gonorrhoeae,* and *Bacteroides,* including *B. fragilis.* **Adults:** 1 to 2 g I.V. or I.M. q 12 hours for 5 to 10 days. Up to 6 g daily in life-threatening infections.

Total daily dosage is same for I.M. or I.V. administration and depends on susceptibility of organism and severity of infection. In patients with renal dysfunction, doses or frequency of administration must be modified according to degree of renal impairment, severity of infection, and susceptibility of organism.

Adverse reactions

Blood: transient neutropenia, eosinophilia, hemolytic anemia, hypoprothrombinemia, bleeding. **CNS:** headache, malaise, paresthesias, dizziness. **GI:** pseudomembranous colitis, nausea, anorexia, vomiting, *diarrhea,* glossitis, dyspepsia, abdominal cramps, tenesmus, anal pruritus. **GU:** genital pruritus and moniliasis. **Skin:** *maculopapular and erythematous rashes, urticaria.* **Local:** *at injection site — pain, induration, sterile abscesses, tissue sloughing; phlebitis and thrombophlebitis with I.V. injection.* **Other:** ***hypersensitivity,*** dyspnea, elevated temperature.

Interactions

Alcohol: may cause a disulfiram-like reaction. Warn patients not to drink alcohol for several days after discontinuing cefotetan. **Oral anticoagulants, aspirin:** increased risk of bleeding. **Probenecid:** may inhibit excretion and increase blood levels of cefotetan.

Nursing diagnoses

• High risk for injury related to ineffectiveness of cefotetan to eradicate the infection.
• High risk for fluid volume deficit related to adverse GI reactions to cefotetan.
• Knowledge deficit related to cefotetan therapy.

Nursing interventions

• *Contraindicated* in patients with hypersensitivity to other cephalosporins.
• *Use cautiously* in renal impairment and in history of sensitivity to penicillin.
• Obtain specimen for culture and sensitivity tests before first dose. Therapy may begin pending test results.
• **I.V. use:** Reconstitute with sterile water for injection. Then, may be mixed with 50 to 100 ml of D_5W or 0.9% sodium chloride solution. Interrupt flow of primary I.V. solution during cefotetan infusion.
• I.M. injection may be reconstituted with sterile water or bacteriostatic water for injection, 0.9% sodium chloride solution, 0.5% or 1% lidocaine hydrochloride. Shake to dissolve and let stand until clear. Inject deep I.M. into a large muscle mass, such as gluteus or lateral aspect of thigh.
• Reconstituted drug is stable for 24 hours at room temperature or 96 hours when refrigerated.
• Bleeding has not been reported with this drug.
• With large doses or prolonged therapy, monitor for superinfection, especially in high-risk patients.
• Cefotetan is particularly useful in intra-abdominal and gynecologic infections (highly active against *B. fragilis*).

General

Classification: nonnarcotic analgesic, antipyretic, anti-inflammatory (salicylate). **Pregnancy risk category:** C.

Mechanism of action

Produces analgesia by an ill-defined effect on the hypothalamus (central action) and by blocking generation of pain impulses (peripheral action). The peripheral action may involve inhibition of prostaglandin synthesis. Exerts its anti-inflammatory effect by inhibiting prostaglandin synthesis; may also inhibit the synthesis or action of other mediators of the inflammatory response.

Indications and dosage

• Arthritis. **Adults:** 3 g P.O. daily, divided b.i.d. or t.i.d. Usual maintenance dose is 2 to 4 g daily.

Adverse reactions

EENT: *tinnitus and hearing loss.* **GI:** nausea, vomiting, GI distress, occult bleeding (rare). **Hepatic:** abnormal liver function studies, hepatitis. **Skin:** *rash,* bruising. **Other:** *hypersensitivity manifested by anaphylaxis and asthma.*

Interactions

Alcohol, corticosteroids, NSAIDs: increased risk of GI bleeding. Avoid concomitant use. **Ammonium chloride (and other urine acidifiers):** increased blood levels of salicylates. Monitor for salicylate toxicity. **Antacids in high doses (and other urine alkalinizers):** decreased levels of salicylates. Monitor for decreased salicylate effect. **Corticosteroids:** compete for binding sites. Monitor for decreased salicylate effect. **Methotrexate:** increased risk of methotrexate toxicity. Avoid concomitant use. **Oral anticoagulants:** possible increased risk of bleeding. Avoid using together if possible.

Nursing diagnoses

• Pain related to the patient's underlying condition.
• High risk for fluid volume deficit related to adverse GI reactions to long-term, high-dose salsalate therapy.
• Knowledge deficit related to salsalate therapy.

Nursing interventions

• *Contraindicated* in salsalate hypersensitivity.
• *Use cautiously* in GI bleeding, aspirin hypersensitivity, renal insufficiency, hypoprothrombinemia, vitamin K deficiency, and bleeding disorders.
• Because of epidemiologic association with Reye's syndrome, CDC recommends that children or teenagers with chicken pox or influenza-like illness should not be given salicylates.
• Give with food, milk, antacid, or large glass of water to reduce possible GI adverse reactions.
• Therapeutic blood salicylate level in arthritis is 10 to 30 mg/dl. Tinnitus may occur at plasma levels of 30 mg/dl and above, but this is not a reliable indicator of toxicity, especially in very young patients and those over age 60. With long-term therapy, mild toxicity may occur at plasma levels of 20 mg/dl.
• May cause an increase in serum levels of AST, ALT, alkaline phosphatase, and bilirubin.
• Advise patients receiving long-term treatment with large doses to watch for petechiae, bleeding gums, and signs of GI bleeding, and to maintain adequate fluid intake. Obtain hemoglobin and prothrombin tests periodically.

General
Classification: antibiotic (second-generation cephalosporin). **Pregnancy risk category:** B.

Mechanism of action
Inhibits cell wall synthesis, promoting osmotic instability. Usually bactericidal.

Indications and dosage
- Serious infections of respiratory and GU tracts, skin and soft-tissue infections, bone and joint infections, bloodstream and intra-abdominal infections, and perioperative prophylaxis. Among susceptible organisms are *Escherichia coli* and other coliform bacteria, *Staphylococcus aureus* (penicillinase- and non-penicillinase-producing) and *S. epidermidis*, streptococci, *Klebsiella*, *Haemophilus influenzae*, and *Bacteroides*, including *B. fragilis*. **Adults:** 1 to 2 g q 6 to 8 hours for uncomplicated forms of infection. Up to 12 g daily in life-threatening infections. **Children:** 80 to 160 mg/kg daily given in 4 to 6 equally divided doses.

Total daily dosage is same for I.M. or I.V. administration and depends on susceptibility of organism and severity of infection. In patients with renal dysfunction, doses or frequency of administration must be modified according to degree of renal impairment, severity of infection, and susceptibility of organism.

Adverse reactions
Blood: transient neutropenia, eosinophilia, ***hemolytic anemia.*** **CNS:** headache, malaise, paresthesias, dizziness. **GI:** pseudomembranous colitis, nausea, anorexia, vomiting, *diarrhea,* glossitis, dyspepsia, abdominal cramps, tenesmus, anal pruritus, oral candidiasis (thrush). **GU:** genital pruritus and moniliasis. **Skin:** *maculopapular and erythematous rashes, urticaria.* **Local:** *at injection site—pain, induration, sterile abscesses, tissue sloughing; phlebitis and thrombophlebitis with I.V. injection.* **Other:** ***hypersensitivity,*** dyspnea, elevated temperature.

Interactions
Probenecid: may inhibit excretion and increase blood levels of cefoxitin.

Nursing diagnoses
- High risk for injury related to ineffectiveness of cefoxitin to eradicate the infection.
- High risk for fluid volume deficit related to adverse GI reactions to cefoxitin.
- Knowledge deficit related to cefoxitin therapy.

Nursing interventions
- *Contraindicated* in patients with hypersensitivity to other cephalosporins.
- *Use cautiously* in renal impairment and in history of sensitivity to penicillin.
- Obtain specimen for culture and sensitivity tests before first dose. Therapy may begin pending test results.
- A very useful cephalosporin when anaerobic or mixed aerobic-anaerobic infection is suspected, especially *B. fragilis.*
- Associated with development of thrombophlebitis. Assess I.V. site frequently.
- **I.V. use:** Reconstitute 1 g with at least 10 ml of sterile water for injection, and 2 g with 10 to 20 ml. Solutions of D_5W and 0.9% sodium chloride for injection can also be used. Interrupt flow of primary I.V. solution during infusion.
- I.M. injection can be reconstituted with 0.5% or 1% lidocaine hydrochloride (without epinephrine) to minimize pain. Inject deep I.M. into a large muscle mass, such as gluteus or lateral aspect of thigh.
- Reconstituted drug is stable for 24 hours at room temperature or 1 week under refrigeration.
- With large doses or prolonged therapy, monitor for superinfection, especially in high-risk patients.
- Urine glucose determinations may be false-positive with copper sulfate tests (Clinitest).

General

Classification: antiviral (vaccine). **Pregnancy risk category:** X.

Mechanism of action

Promotes immunity to rubella by inducing production of antibodies.

Indications and dosage

- Measles immunization. **Adults and children over 1 year:** 1 vial (1,000 units) S.C.

Adverse reactions

Local: pain, erythema, induration, lymphadenopathy. **Systemic:** *joint pain,* fever, rash, thrombocytopenic purpura, urticaria, arthritis, arthralgia, polyneuritis, ***anaphylaxis.***

Interactions

Immune serum globulin, whole blood, plasma: antibodies in serum may interfere with immune response. Don't use vaccine within 3 months of transfusion. Immune serum globulin may be given 2 weeks before vaccine. **Tuberculin skin test:** may temporarily decrease response to test. Defer skin testing.

Nursing diagnoses

- Altered protection related to lack of immunity to rubella virus.
- Pain (joint) related to vaccine-induced adverse reaction.
- Knowledge deficit related to rubella virus vaccine therapy.

Nursing interventions

- *Contraindicated* in immunosuppression; cancer; blood dyscrasias; corticosteroid or radiation therapy; gamma globulin disorders; active, untreated tuberculosis; or fever.
- *Use cautiously* in patients with hypersensitivity to neomycin, chickens, ducks, eggs, or feathers. Defer in acute illness and after administration of human immune serum globulin, blood, or plasma.
- Stress importance of avoiding pregnancy for 3 months after immunization. If necessary, provide contraceptive information.
- Store in refrigerator and protect from light. Solution may be used if red, pink, or yellow (but must be clear).
- Use only diluent supplied. Discard 8 hours after reconstituting.
- Obtain history of allergies, especially to ducks and rabbits, and reaction to immunization.
- Inject into outer aspect of upper arm. Don't inject I.V.
- Keep epinephrine 1:1,000 available.
- Allow an interval of at least 3 weeks between bacille Calmette-Guérin and rubella vaccines.

General
Classification: antibiotic (second-generation cephalosporin). **Pregnancy risk category:** B.

Mechanism of action
Inhibits cell wall synthesis, promoting osmotic instability. Usually bactericidal.

Indications and dosage
- Acute, community-acquired pneumonia caused by non-beta-lactamase-producing strains of *Haemophilus influenzae* or *Streptococcus pneumoniae.* **Adults:** 200 mg P.O. q 12 hours for 14 days.
- Uncomplicated gonorrhea in men and women; rectal gonococcal infections in women. **Adults:** 200 mg P.O. as a single dose. Follow with doxycycline 100 mg P.O. b.i.d. for 7 days.
- Uncomplicated skin and skin structure infections caused by *Staphylococcus aureus* or *Streptococcus pyogenes.* **Adults:** 400 mg P.O. q 12 hours for 7 to 14 days.
- Acute otitis media caused by *S. pneumoniae, H. influenzae,* or *Moraxella (Branhamella) catarrhalis.* **Children 6 months and over:** 5 mg/kg (not to exceed 200 mg) P.O. q 12 hours for 10 days.
- Pharyngitis or tonsillitis caused by *S. pyogenes.* **Adults:** 100 mg P.O. q 12 hours for 10 days. **Children 6 months and over:** 5 mg/kg (not to exceed 100 mg) P.O. q 12 hours for 10 days.

- Uncomplicated urinary tract infections caused by *Escherichia coli, Klebsiella pneumoniae, Proteus mirabilis,* or *Staphylococcus saprophyticus.* **Adults:** 100 mg P.O. q 12 hours for 7 days.

Adverse reactions
CNS: headache. **GI:** *diarrhea,* nausea, vomiting, abdominal pain. **GU:** vaginal fungal infections. **Skin:** rash. **Other:** ***anaphylaxis.***

Interactions
Antacids, H_2 antagonists: decreased absorption of cefpodoxime. Avoid concomitant use. **Probenecid:** decreased excretion of cefpodoxime. Monitor for toxicity.

Nursing diagnoses
- High risk for injury related to ineffectiveness of cefpodoxime to eradicate the infection.
- High risk for fluid volume deficit related to adverse GI reactions to cefpodoxime.
- Knowledge deficit related to cefpodoxime therapy.

Nursing interventions
- *Contraindicated* in patients with hypersensitivity to the drug or other cephalosporins. Safety and efficacy in children under 6 months have not been established.
- *Use cautiously* in patients with a history of penicillin hypersensitivity because of the risk of cross-sensitivity and in patients receiving nephrotoxic drugs because other cephalosporins have been shown to have nephrotoxic potential. Because drug is excreted in human breast milk, also use cautiously in breast-feeding women.
- Dosage frequency should be altered in patients with severe renal impairment. When creatinine clearance is below 30 ml/minute, dosage interval should be increased to q 24 hours. Patients receiving dialysis should get the drug three times weekly, after dialysis.
- Studies have shown that drug's pharmacokinetics aren't altered in patients with hepatic impairment, including those with ascites.
- Absorption of drug is enhanced when it's taken with food.
- Store suspension in the refrigerator (36° to 46° F [2° to 8° C]). Shake well before using. Discard unused portion after 14 days.

General
Classification: antiviral (vaccine). **Pregnancy risk category:** X.

Mechanism of action
Promotes immunity to rubella and mumps by inducing production of antibodies.

Indications and dosage
• Measles and mumps immunization. **Adults and children over 1 year:** 1 vial (1,000 units) S.C.

Adverse reactions
Local: pain, erythema, induration, lymphadenopathy. **Systemic:** fever, rash, thrombocytopenic purpura, urticaria, arthritis, arthralgia, polyneuritis, ***anaphylaxis.***

Interactions
Immune serum globulin, whole blood, plasma: antibodies in serum may interfere with immune response. Don't give vaccine within 3 months of transfusion. **Tuberculin skin test:** vaccine may temporarily decrease response to test. Defer skin testing.

Nursing diagnoses
• Altered protection related to lack of immunity to rubella and mumps virus.

• Ineffective breathing pattern related to vaccine-induced anaphylaxis.
• Knowledge deficit related to rubella and mumps virus vaccine therapy.

Nursing interventions
• *Contraindicated* in immunosuppression; cancer; blood dyscrasias; corticosteroid or radiation therapy; gamma globulin disorders; active, untreated tuberculosis; fever; or pregnancy.
• *Use cautiously* in patients with hypersensitivity to neomycin, chickens, ducks, eggs, or feathers. Defer in acute illness and after administration of immune serum globulin, blood, or plasma.
• Stress importance of avoiding pregnancy for 3 months after immunization. If necessary, provide contraceptive information.
• Store in refrigerator and protect from light. Solution may be used if red, pink, or yellow (but must be clear).
• Use only diluent supplied. Discard 8 hours after reconstituting.
• Obtain history of allergies, especially to ducks, rabbits, and antibiotics, and reaction to immunization.
• Inject into outer aspect of upper arm. Don't inject I.V.
• Keep epinephrine 1:1,000 available.
• Allow an interval of at least 3 weeks between bacille Calmette-Guérin and rubella vaccines.

General

Classification: antibiotic (second-generation cephalosporin). **Pregnancy risk category:** B.

Mechanism of action

Interferes with bacterial cell wall synthesis during cell replication, leading to osmotic instability and cell lysis. Bactericidal.

Indications and dosage

• Pharyngitis or tonsillitis caused by *Streptococcus pyogenes*. **Adults:** 500 mg P.O. daily for at least 10 days.
• Otitis media caused by *S. pneumoniae, Haemophilus influenzae,* and *Moraxella (Branhamella) catarrhalis*. **Infants and children 6 months to 12 years:** 15 mg/kg powder in 50 or 100 ml sterile water or D_5W P.O. q 12 hours for 10 days.
• Secondary bacterial infections of acute bronchitis and acute bacterial exacerbation of chronic bronchitis caused by *S. pneumoniae, H. influenzae,* and *M. catarrhalis*. **Adults:** 500 mg P.O. q 12 hours for 10 days.
• Uncomplicated skin and skin structure infections caused by *Staphylococcus aureus* and *Streptococcus pyogenes*. **Adults:** 250 mg P.O. b.i.d., or 500 mg P.O. daily to b.i.d.

Adverse reactions

Blood: decreased leukocyte count, eosinophilia. **CNS:** dizziness, hyperactivity, headache, nervousness, insomnia. **GI:** *diarrhea, nausea,* vomiting, abdominal pain. **GU:** elevated BUN level, elevated serum creatinine level, genital pruritus, vaginitis. **Hepatic:** elevated liver enzymes, cholestatic jaundice (rare). **Skin:** rash, urticaria, diaper rash. **Other:** superinfection, hypersensitivity, ***anaphylaxis.***

Interactions

None reported.

Nursing diagnoses

• High risk for injury related to ineffectiveness of cefprozil to eradicate the infection.
• High risk for fluid volume deficit related to adverse GI reactions to cefprozil.
• Knowledge deficit related to cefprozil therapy.

Nursing interventions

• *Contraindicated* in patients with hypersensitivity to the drug or any other cephalosporin.
• *Use cautiously* in patients with a history of hypersensitivity to penicillin because up to 10% of these patients will exhibit cross-sensitivity to a cephalosporin or a hypersensitivity reaction. Also use cautiously in patients with impaired hepatic or renal function.
• Oral powder for suspensions features a bubblegum flavor to improve palatability and compliance in children. Reconstituted suspension should be stored in the refrigerator, and unused drug should be discarded after 14 days.
• Drug is removed by hemodialysis; administer after treatment is completed.
• Obtain appropriate specimen for culture and sensitivity tests before first dose. Therapy may begin pending test results.
• May cause overgrowth of nonsusceptible bacteria or fungi. Monitor for signs and symptoms of superinfection.
• Tell patient to shake suspension well before measuring dose.

ritodrine hydrochloride

Yutopar

General

Classification: tocolytic (beta-receptor agonist).
Pregnancy risk category: B.

Mechanism of action

Stimulates the beta$_2$-adrenergic receptors in uterine smooth muscle, inhibiting contractility.

Indications and dosage

• Management of preterm labor. **Women:** dilute 150 mg (3 ampules) in 500 ml of fluid, yielding a final concentration of 0.3 mg/ml. Usual initial dose is 0.1 mg/minute I.V., to be gradually increased according to results by 0.05 mg/minute q 10 minutes until desired result obtained. Effective dosage usually ranges from 0.15 to 0.35 mg/minute.

Note: I.V. infusion should be continued for 12 to 24 hours after contractions have stopped. Oral maintenance: 1 tablet (10 mg) may be given approximately 30 minutes before termination of I.V. therapy. Usual dosage for first 24 hours of maintenance is 10 mg P.O. q 2 hours. Thereafter, usual dosage is 10 to 20 mg P.O. q 4 to 6 hours. Total daily dosage should not exceed 120 mg.

Adverse reactions

I.V.: **CNS:** nervousness, anxiety, headache. **CV:** *dose-related alterations in blood pressure, palpitations,* ***pulmonary edema,*** *tachycardia,* ECG changes. **GI:** nausea, vomiting. **Metabolic:** *hyperglycemia,* hypokalemia. **Other:** erythema.
Oral: **CNS:** tremors, nervousness. **CV:** palpitations. **GI:** nausea, vomiting. **Skin:** rash.

Interactions

Beta-adrenergic blockers: may inhibit ritodrine's action. Avoid concurrent administration. **Corticosteroids:** may produce pulmonary edema in mother. When these drugs are used concomitantly, monitor closely. **Inhalational anesthetics:** potentiated adverse cardiac effects, arrhythmias, hypotension. **Sympathomimetics:** additive effects. Use together cautiously.

Nursing diagnoses

• Anxiety related to the patient's underlying condition.
• Decreased cardiac output related to adverse reaction to drug.
• Knowledge deficit related to ritodrine hydrochloride therapy.

Nursing interventions

• *Contraindicated* before 20th week of pregnancy and in the following conditions: antepartum hemorrhage, eclampsia, intrauterine fetal death, chorioamnionitis, maternal cardiac disease, pulmonary hypertension, maternal hyperthyroidism, or uncontrolled maternal diabetes mellitus.
• **I.V. use:** Because cardiovascular responses are common and more pronounced during I.V. administration, cardiovascular effects—including maternal pulse rate and blood pressure, and fetal heart rate—should be closely monitored. Maternal tachycardia of over 140 beats/minute or persistent respiratory rate of over 20 breaths/minute may be a sign of impending pulmonary edema.
• Monitor amount of fluids administered I.V., to prevent circulatory overload.
• Don't use ritodrine I.V. if solution is discolored or contains a precipitate.
• Monitor blood glucose concentrations during ritodrine infusions, especially in diabetic mothers.
• Discontinue drug if pulmonary edema develops.
• Drug's effectiveness in preterm labor is currently being reviewed by the FDA.

General

Classification: antibiotic (third-generation cephalosporin). **Pregnancy risk category:** B.

Mechanism of action

Inhibits cell wall synthesis, promoting osmotic instability. Usually bactericidal.

Indications and dosage

- Serious infections of the lower respiratory and urinary tracts, gynecologic infections, bacteremia, septicemia, intra-abdominal infections, CNS infections, and skin infections. Susceptible microorganisms include streptococci, including *Streptococcus pneumoniae* and *S. pyogenes; Staphylococcus aureus* (penicillinase- and non-penicillinase-producing); *Escherichia coli; Klebsiella; Proteus; Enterobacter; Haemophilus influenzae; Pseudomonas;* and some strains of *Bacteroides.* **Adults:** 1 g I.V. or I.M. q 8 to 12 hours; up to 6 g daily in life-threatening infections. **Children 1 month to 12 years:** 30 to 50 mg/kg I.V. q 8 hours. **Neonates to 4 weeks:** 30 mg/kg I.V. q 12 hours.

Total daily dosage is same for I.M. or I.V. administration and depends on susceptibility of organism and severity of infection. In patients with renal dysfunction, doses or frequency of administration must be modified according to degree of renal impairment, severity of infection, and susceptibility of organism.

Adverse reactions

Blood: eosinophilia; thrombocytosis, leukopenia. **CNS:** headache, dizziness. **GI:** pseudomembranous colitis, nausea, vomiting, diarrhea, dysgeusia, abdominal cramps. **GU:** genital pruritus and moniliasis. **Hepatic:** transient elevation in liver enzymes. **Skin:** *maculopapular and erythematous rashes, urticaria.* **Local:** *at injection site—pain, induration, sterile abscesses, tissue sloughing; phlebitis and thrombophlebitis with I.V. injection.* **Other:** ***hypersensitivity,*** dyspnea, elevated temperature.

Interactions

Sodium bicarbonate-containing solutions: make ceftazidime unstable. Don't mix together.

Nursing diagnoses

- High risk for injury related to ineffectiveness of ceftazidime to eradicate the infection.
- High risk for fluid volume deficit related to adverse GI reactions to ceftazidime.
- Knowledge deficit related to ceftazidime therapy.

Nursing interventions

- *Contraindicated* in patients with hypersensitivity to other cephalosporins.
- *Use cautiously* in history of sensitivity to penicillin.
- Obtain specimen for culture and sensitivity tests before first dose. Therapy may begin pending test results.
- **I.V. use:** Vials of ceftazidime are supplied under reduced pressure. When the antibiotic is dissolved, carbon dioxide is released and a positive pressure develops. Each brand of ceftazidime includes specific instructions for reconstitution. Read and follow these instructions carefully.
- When given I.M., inject deep into a large muscle mass, such as gluteus or lateral aspect of thigh.
- This third-generation cephalosporin has excellent activity against infections caused by *Pseudomonas aeruginosa.* May be prescribed for these infections, especially when aminoglycosides are potentially too dangerous.
- With large doses or prolonged therapy, monitor for superinfection, especially in high-risk patients.

General

Classification: antitubercular (rifamycin B derivative. **Pregnancy risk category:** C.

Mechanism of action

Inhibits DNA-dependent RNA polymerase, thus impairing RNA synthesis (bactericidal).

Indications and dosage

• Primary treatment in pulmonary tuberculosis. **Adults:** 600 mg P.O. or I.V. daily in single dose 1 hour before or 2 hours after meals. **Children over 5 years:** 10 to 20 mg/kg P.O. or I.V. daily in single dose 1 hour before or 2 hours after meals. Maximum dosage is 600 mg daily. Concomitant administration of other effective antitubercular drugs is recommended.

• Meningococcal carriers. **Adults:** 600 mg P.O. or I.V. b.i.d. for 2 days. **Children 1 month to 12 years:** 10 mg/kg P.O. or I.V. b.i.d. for 2 days, not to exceed 600 mg/dose. **Infants under 1 month:** 5 mg/kg P.O. or I.V. b.i.d. for 2 days.

• Prophylaxis of *Haemophilus influenzae* type b. **Adults and children:** 20 mg/kg P.O. daily for 4 days. Do not exceed 600 mg/day.

Adverse reactions

Blood: eosinophilia, thrombocytopenia, transient leukopenia, ***hemolytic anemia.*** **CNS:** headache, fatigue, *drowsiness,* ataxia, dizziness, mental confusion, generalized numbness. **GI:** epigastric distress, anorexia, nausea, vomiting, abdominal pain, diarrhea, flatulence, sore mouth and tongue. **Metabolic:** hyperuricemia. **Hepatic:** ***serious hepatotoxicity,*** *transient abnormalities in liver function tests.* Skin: pruritus, urticaria, rash. **Other:** flulike syndrome, discoloration of body fluids.

Interactions

Alcohol: may increase risk of hepatotoxicity. **Para-aminosalicylate sodium, ketoconazole:** may interfere with absorption of rifampin. Give these drugs 8 to 12 hours apart. **Probenecid:** may increase rifampin levels. Use cautiously.

Nursing diagnoses

• High risk for injury related to dosage regimen inadequate to eradicate the infection.
• Noncompliance related to prolonged therapy.
• Knowledge deficit related to rifampin therapy.

Nursing interventions

• *Contraindicated* in clinically active hepatitis.
• *Use cautiously* in hepatic disease or in patients receiving other hepatotoxic drugs.
• Monitor hepatic function, hematopoietic studies, and serum uric acid.
• Watch closely for signs of hepatic impairment (loss of appetite, fatigue, malaise, jaundice, dark urine, liver tenderness). Notify doctor if these occur.
• Warn patient about drowsiness and the possibility of red-orange discoloration of urine, feces, saliva, sweat, sputum, and tears. Soft contact lenses may be permanently stained.
• Rifampin may cause hemorrhaging in neonates of rifampin-treated mothers.
• Advise patient to avoid alcoholic beverages while taking this drug; they may increase risk of hepatotoxicity.
• Give 1 hour before or 2 hours after meals for optimal absorption; however, if GI irritation occurs, patient may take rifampin with meals.
• Increases enzyme activity of liver; may require increased doses of warfarin, corticosteroids, oral contraceptives, and oral antidiabetics. See each drug entry for specific drug interactions.
• **I.V. use:** Reconstitute vial with 10 ml sterile water for injection to make a solution containing 60 mg/ml. Add to 100 ml D_5W and infuse over 30 minutes, or add to 500 ml D_5W and infuse over 3 hours. When dextrose is contraindicated, drug may be diluted with 0.9% sodium chloride solution. Do not use other I.V. solutions.

General

Classification: antibiotic (third-generation cephalosporin). **Pregnancy risk category:** B.

Mechanism of action

Inhibits cell wall synthesis, promoting osmotic instability. Usually bactericidal.

Indications and dosage

• Serious infections of the lower respiratory and urinary tracts, gynecologic infections, bacteremia, septicemia, meningitis, intra-abdominal infections, bone and joint infections, and skin infections. Among susceptible microorganisms are streptococci, including *Streptococcus pneumoniae* and *S. pyogenes; Staphylococcus aureus* (penicillinase- and non-penicillinase-producing) *and S. epidermidis; Escherichia coli; Klebsiella; Haemophilus influenzae; Enterobacter; Proteus;* some *Pseudomonas;* and *Peptostreptococcus.* **Adults:** usual dosage is 1 to 2 g I.V. or I.M. q 8 to 12 hours. In life-threatening infections, up to 2 g q 4 hours.

Total daily dosage is same for I.M. or I.V. administration and depends on susceptibility of organism and severity of infection. In patients with renal dysfunction, doses or frequency of administration must be modified according to degree of renal impairment, severity of infection, and susceptibility of organism.

Adverse reactions

Blood: transient neutropenia, eosinophilia, hemolytic anemia. **CNS:** headache, malaise, paresthesias, dizziness. **GI:** pseudomembranous colitis, nausea, anorexia, vomiting, *diarrhea,* glossitis, dyspepsia, abdominal cramps, tenesmus, anal pruritus. **GU:** genital pruritus and moniliasis. **Skin:** *maculopapular and erythematous rashes, urticaria.* **Local:** *at injection site—pain, induration, sterile abscesses, tissue sloughing; phlebitis and thrombophlebitis with I.V. injection.* **Other:** ***hypersensitivity,*** dyspnea, elevated temperature.

Interactions

Probenecid: may inhibit excretion and increase blood levels of ceftizoxime.

Nursing diagnoses

• High risk for injury related to ineffectiveness of ceftizoxime to eradicate the infection.
• High risk for fluid volume deficit related to adverse GI reactions to ceftizoxime.
• Knowledge deficit related to ceftizoxime therapy.

Nursing interventions

• *Contraindicated* in patients with hypersensitivity to other cephalosporins.
• *Use cautiously* in renal impairment and in history of sensitivity to penicillin.
• Obtain specimen for culture and sensitivity tests before first dose. Therapy may begin pending test results.
• With large doses or prolonged therapy, monitor for superinfection, especially in high-risk patients.
• When given I.M., inject deep into a large muscle mass, such as gluteus or lateral aspect of thigh.
• Larger doses (2 g) administered I.M. should be divided into two doses and administered at separate sites in a large muscle.
• No significant degree of bleeding or disulfiram-type reaction has been reported with the use of ceftizoxime.
• **I.V. use:** To reconstitute powder, add 10 ml of sterile water to 1-g vial and 20 ml to 2-g vial. Reconstitute piggyback vials with 50 to 100 ml of 0.9% sodium chloride or D_5W. Shake vial well.

General

Classification: antiviral (synthetic nucleoside).
Pregnancy risk category: X.

Mechanism of action

Inhibits viral activity by an unknown mechanism. Thought to inhibit RNA and DNA synthesis by depleting intracellular nucleotide pools.

Indications and dosage

• Hospitalized infants and young children infected by RSV. **Infants and young children:** solution in concentration of 20 mg/ml delivered via the Viratek Small Particle Aerosol Generator (SPAG-2). Treatment is carried out for 12 to 18 hours/day for at least 3, and no more than 7, days.

Adverse reactions

Blood: anemia, reticulocytosis. **EENT:** conjunctivitis. **Respiratory:** worsening of respiratory state. **Other:** rash or erythema of eyelids.

Interactions

None significant.

Nursing diagnoses

• High risk for injury related to ineffectiveness of ribavirin in eradicating the infection.
• Impaired gas exchange related to adverse respiratory reactions to ribavirin therapy.
• Knowledge deficit related to ribavirin therapy.

Nursing interventions

• *Contraindicated* in women who are or may become pregnant during treatment with drug.
• Ribavirin aerosol is indicated only for severe lower respiratory tract infection due to RSV. Although treatment may be started while awaiting diagnostic test results, existence of RSV infection must be documented eventually.
• Most infants and children with RSV infection don't require treatment because the disease is often mild and self-limiting. Infants with underlying conditions, such as prematurity or cardiopulmonary disease, get RSV in its severest form and benefit most from treatment with ribavirin aerosol.
• This treatment must be accompanied by, and does not replace, supportive respiratory and fluid management.
• Ribavirin aerosol *must* be administered by the SPAG-2. Don't use any other aerosol generating device.
• Ribavirin may precipitate in ventilator apparatus, which may result in equipment malfunction with serious consequences. The use of ribavirin in ventilator-dependent patients is not recommended.
• The water used to reconstitute this drug must not contain any antimicrobial agent. Use sterile USP water for injection, *not* bacteriostatic water.
• Discard solutions placed in the SPAG-2 unit at least every 24 hours before adding newly reconstituted solution.
• Store reconstituted solutions at room temperature for 24 hours.

ceftriaxone sodium

Rocephin

General

Classification: antibiotic (third-generation cephalosporin). **Pregnancy risk category:** B.

Mechanism of action

Inhibits cell wall synthesis, promoting osmotic instability. Usually bactericidal.

Indications and dosage

• Serious infections of the CNS (meningitis), lower respiratory and urinary tracts, gynecologic infections, bone and joint infections, bacteremia, septicemia, intra-abdominal infections, preoperative prophylaxis, and skin infections and Lyme disease. Susceptible microorganisms are streptococci, including *Streptococcus pneumoniae* and *S. pyogenes; Staphylococcus aureus* (penicillinase- and non-penicillinase-producing) and *S. epidermidis; Escherichia coli; Klebsiella; Haemophilus influenzae; Neisseria meningitidis; N. gonorrhoeae; Enterobacter; Proteus; Pseudomonas; Peptostreptococcus;* and *Serratia marcescens.* **Adults:** 1 to 2 g I.M. or I.V. daily or in equally divided doses b.i.d.; not to exceed 4 g daily. **Children:** 50 to 75 mg/kg, given in divided doses q 12 hours.

• Meningitis. **Adults and children:** 100 mg/kg given in divided doses q 12 hours. May give loading dose of 75 mg/kg.

Total daily dose is same for I.M. or I.V. administration and depends on susceptibility of organism and severity of infection.

Adverse reactions

Blood: eosinophilia; thrombocytosis, leukopenia. **CNS:** headache, dizziness. **GI:** pseudomembranous enterocolitis, nausea, vomiting, diarrhea, dysgeusia, abdominal cramps. **GU:** genital pruritus and moniliasis. **Hepatic:** transient elevation in liver enzymes. **Skin:** *maculopapular and erythematous rashes, urticaria.* **Local:** *at injection site—pain, induration, sterile abscesses, tissue sloughing; phlebitis and thrombophlebitis with I.V. injection.* **Other:** ***hypersensitivity,*** dyspnea, elevated temperature.

Interactions

Probenicid: high doses (1 or 2 g/day) may enhance hepatic clearance of ceftriaxone and shorten half-life. Avoid concomitant use.

Nursing diagnoses

• High risk for injury related to ineffectiveness of ceftriaxone to eradicate the infection.
• High risk for fluid volume deficit related to adverse GI reactions to ceftriaxone.
• Knowledge deficit related to ceftriaxone therapy.

Nursing interventions

• *Contraindicated* in patients with hypersensitivity to other cephalosporins.
• *Use cautiously* in history of sensitivity to penicillin.
• Obtain specimen for culture and sensitivity tests before first dose. Therapy may begin pending test results.
• **I.V. use:** Reconstitute with sterile water for injection, 0.9% sodium chloride injection, dextrose 5% or 10% injection, or a combination of sodium chloride and dextrose injection or other compatible solutions. Reconstitute by adding 2.4 ml diluent to the 250-mg vial, 4.8 ml to the 500-mg vial, 9.6 ml to the 1-g vial, and 19.2 ml to the 2-g vial. All reconstituted solutions yield a concentration that averages 100 mg/ml. Dilute further for intermittent infusion. I.V. dilutions are stable for 24 hours at room temperature.
• When given I.M., inject deep into a large muscle mass, such as gluteus or lateral aspect of thigh.
• Long half-life allows once-daily dose regimen.
• Dosage adjustment generally not needed in patients with renal insufficiency.
• Commonly used for outpatient treatment of serious infections, such as osteomyelitis.
• With large doses or prolonged therapy, monitor for superinfection, especially in high-risk patients.

General

Classification: anti-$Rh_0(D)$-positive prophylaxis agent (immune serum). **Pregnancy risk category:** C.

Mechanism of action

Suppresses the active antibody response and formation of anti-$Rh_0(D)$ in $Rh_0(D)$-negative, D^u-negative patients exposed to Rh-positive blood.

Indications and dosage

- Rh exposure. **Women:** give after abortion, miscarriage, ectopic pregnancy, or delivery. Transfusion unit or blood bank determines fetal packed RBC volume entering woman's blood, then gives one vial I.M. if fetal packed RBC volume is less than 15 ml. More than one vial I.M. may be required if fetomaternal hemorrhage is large. Must be given within 72 hours of delivery or miscarriage.
- Transfusion accidents. **Adults and children:** consult blood bank or transfusion unit at once. Must be given within 72 hours.
- Prevention of Rh antibody formation after abortion or miscarriage. **Women:** consult transfusion unit or blood bank. One microdose vial will suppress immune reaction to 2.5 ml $Rh_0(D)$-positive RBCs. Ideally should be given within 3 hours, but may be given up to 72 hours after abortion or miscarriage.

Adverse reactions

Local: discomfort at injection site. **Other:** slight fever, ***anaphylaxis.***

Interactions

Live virus vaccines: possible interference with response. Defer vaccination for 3 months after administration of $Rh_0(D)$ immune globulin.

Nursing diagnoses

- Altered protection related to the presence of active Rh antibodies.
- Pain related to local discomfort at injection site.
- Knowledge deficit related to $Rh_0(D)$ immune globulin.

Nursing interventions

- *Contraindicated* in $Rh_0(D)$-positive or D^u-positive patients and those previously immunized to $Rh_0(D)$ blood factor.
- Immediately after delivery, send a sample of infant's cord blood to laboratory for typing and cross matching. Confirm if mother is $Rh_0(D)$-negative and D^u-negative. Infant must be $Rh_0(D)$-positive or D^u-positive.
- Obtain history of allergies and reaction to immunization.
- MICRhoGAM is recommended for every woman undergoing abortion or miscarriage up to 12 weeks' gestation unless she is $Rh_0(D)$-positive or D^u-positive, has Rh antibodies, or the father or fetus is Rh-negative.
- Store at 36° to 46° F (2° to 8° C).
- Immune serum provides passive immunity to the woman exposed to Rh_0-positive fetal blood during pregnancy. Prevents formation of maternal antibodies (active immunity), which would endanger future Rh_0-positive pregnancies.
- Explain to the patient how drug protects future Rh_0-positive infants.

General

Classification: antibiotic (second-generation cephalosporin). **Pregnancy risk category:** B.

Mechanism of action

Inhibits cell wall synthesis, promoting osmotic instability. Usually bactericidal.

Indications and dosage

• Injectable form – serious infections of the lower respiratory and urinary tracts; skin and skin structure infections; bone and joint infections, septicemia, meningitis, gonorrhea, and perioperative prophylaxis; oral form – otitis media, pharyngitis, tonsillitis, infections of the urinary and lower respiratory tracts, and skin and skin structure infections. Among susceptible organisms are *Streptococcus pneumoniae* and *S. pyogenes, Haemophilus influenzae, Klebsiella, Staphylococcus aureus, Escherichia coli, Enterobacter,* and *Neisseria gonorrhoeae.* **Adults:** 750 mg to 1.5 g (sodium) I.M. or I.V. q 8 hours, usually for 5 to 10 days; for life-threatening infections and infections caused by less susceptible organisms, 1.5 g I.M. or I.V. q 6 hours; for bacterial meningitis, up to 3 g I.V. q 6 hours. Alternatively, give 250 mg (axetil) P.O. q 12 hours; for severe infections or less susceptible organisms, dosage may be increased to 500 mg P.O. q 12 hours. **Children and infants over 3 months:** 50 to 100 mg/kg/day (sodium) I.M. or I.V. Higher doses are administered when treating meningitis. Alternatively, give 125 mg (axetil) P.O. q 12 hours.

• Uncomplicated urinary tract infections. **Adults:** 125 to 250 mg P.O. q 12 hours.

• Otitis media. **Children under 2 years:** 125 mg P.O. q 12 hours. **Children 2 years and over:** 250 mg P.O. q 12 hours.

Total daily dosage is same for I.M. or I.V. administration and depends on susceptibility of organism and severity of infection. In patients with renal dysfunction, doses or frequency of administration must be modified according to degree of impairment, severity of infection, and susceptibility of organism.

Adverse reactions

Blood: transient neutropenia, eosinophilia, ***hemolytic anemia,*** decrease in hemoglobin and hematocrit. **CNS:** headache, malaise, paresthesia, dizziness. **GI:** pseudomembranous colitis, nausea, anorexia, vomiting, *diarrhea,* glossitis, dyspepsia, abdominal cramps, tenesmus, anal pruritus. **GU:** genital pruritus and moniliasis. **Skin:** *maculopapular and erythematous rashes, urticaria.* **Local:** *at injection site – pain, induration, sterile abscesses, temperature elevation, tissue sloughing; phlebitis and thrombophlebitis with I.V. injection.* **Other:** ***hypersensitivity,*** dyspnea.

Interactions

Probenecid: may inhibit excretion and increase blood levels of cefuroxime.

Nursing diagnoses

• High risk for injury related to ineffectiveness of cefuroxime to eradicate the infection.
• High risk for fluid volume deficit related to adverse GI reactions to cefuroxime.
• Knowledge deficit related to cefuroxime.

Nursing interventions

• *Contraindicated* in hypersensitivity to other cephalosporins.
• *Use cautiously* in patients with renal impairment and in those with history of sensitivity to penicillin.
• Inject deep I.M. into a large muscle mass, such as gluteus or lateral aspect of thigh.
• Cefuroxime axetil is available only as tablets, which can be crushed if needed. Absorption is enhanced by food.
• Obtain specimen for culture and sensitivity tests before first dose. Begin therapy pending test results.
• Monitor patient for signs of superinfection.

General

Classification: antihypertensive (rauwolfia alkaloid, peripherally acting antiadrenergic agent).
Pregnancy risk category: C.

Mechanism of action

Acts peripherally, inhibiting norepinephrine release and depleting norepinephrine stores in adrenergic nerve endings.

Indications and dosage

- Mild to moderate essential hypertension. **Adults:** 0.1 to 0.25 mg P.O. daily. **Children:** 5 to 20 mcg/kg P.O. daily.

Adverse reactions

CNS: mental confusion, *depression, drowsiness, nervousness, paradoxical anxiety, nightmares,* extrapyramidal symptoms, sedation. **CV:** *orthostatic hypotension, bradycardia, syncope.* **EENT:** *nasal stuffiness,* glaucoma. **GI:** *dry mouth, hyperacidity, nausea, vomiting,* GI bleeding. **Skin:** pruritus, rash. **Other:** *impotence, weight gain.*

Interactions

MAO inhibitors: may cause excitability and hypertension. Use together cautiously.

Nursing diagnoses

- Altered tissue perfusion (renal, cerebral, cardiopulmonary, peripheral) related to the patient's underlying condition.
- High risk for injury related to adverse CV reactions to reserpine.
- Knowledge deficit related to reserpine therapy.

Nursing interventions

- *Contraindicated* in depression.
- *Use cautiously* in severe cardiac or cerebrovascular disease, history of seizures, peptic ulcer, ulcerative colitis, gallstones, or mental depressive disorders; in patients undergoing surgery; and in those taking other antihypertensive drugs.
- Monitor patient's blood pressure and pulse rate frequently.
- Teach patient about his disease and therapy. Explain the importance of taking this drug as prescribed, even when he's feeling well. Tell outpatient not to discontinue this drug suddenly, but to call doctor if unpleasant adverse reactions occur.
- Instruct patient to check with doctor or pharmacist before taking OTC medications.
- Warn patient that this drug can cause drowsiness. Tell him to avoid hazardous activities that require alertness and coordination until CNS effects of the drug are known.
- Warn female patient to notify doctor if she becomes pregnant.
- Watch patient closely for signs of mental depression. Warn him to notify doctor promptly if he experiences nightmares.
- Inform patient that orthostatic hypotension can be minimized by rising slowly and avoiding sudden position changes. Dry mouth can be relieved with sugarless chewing gum, sour hard candy, or ice chips. Tell patient to contact doctor if relief is needed for nasal stuffiness.
- Give this drug with meals.
- Patient should weigh himself daily and notify doctor of any weight gain.
- Effects of this drug may last for 10 days after it's discontinued.
- Advise patient to have periodic eye examinations.

General

Classification: antibiotic (first-generation cephalosporin). **Pregnancy risk category:** B.

Mechanism of action

Inhibits cell wall synthesis, promoting osmotic instability. Usually bactericidal.

Indications and dosage

• Infections of respiratory and GU tracts, skin and soft-tissue infections, bone and joint infections, and otitis media due to *Escherichia coli* and other coliform bacteria, group A beta-hemolytic streptococci, *Haemophilus influenzae, Klebsiella, Proteus mirabilis, Streptococcus pneumoniae,* and staphylococci. **Adults:** 250 mg to 1 g P.O. q 6 hours. **Children:** 6 to 12 mg/kg P.O. q 6 hours. Maximum 25 mg/kg q 6 hours.

Adverse reactions

Blood: transient neutropenia, eosinophilia, anemia. **CNS:** dizziness, headache, malaise, paresthesia. **GI:** pseudomembranous colitis, *nausea, anorexia,* vomiting, *diarrhea,* glossitis, dyspepsia, abdominal cramps, anal pruritus, tenesmus, oral candidiasis (thrush). **GU:** genital pruritus and moniliasis, vaginitis. **Skin:** *maculopapular and erythematous rashes, urticaria.* **Other:** ***hypersensitivity,*** dyspnea.

Interactions

Probenecid: may increase blood levels of cephalexin.

Nursing diagnoses

• High risk for injury related to ineffectiveness of cephalexin to eradicate the infection.
• High risk for fluid volume deficit related to adverse GI reactions to cephalexin.
• Knowledge deficit related to cephalexin therapy.

Nursing interventions

• *Use cautiously* in renal impairment and in history of sensitivity to penicillin.
• Obtain specimen for culture and sensitivity tests before first dose. Therapy may begin pending test results.
• Tell patient to take medication exactly as prescribed, even after he feels better. Group A beta-hemolytic streptococcal infections should be treated for a minimum of 10 days.
• Tell patient to take with food or milk to lessen GI discomfort.
• Call doctor if skin rash develops.
• Preparation of oral suspension: add required amount of water to powder in two portions. Shake well after each addition. After mixing, store in refrigerator. Stable for 14 days without significant loss of potency. Keep tightly closed and shake well before using.
• With large doses or prolonged therapy, monitor for superinfection, especially in high-risk patients.
• Patients receiving cephalosporins may show a false-positive direct Coombs' test; only a few of these indicate hemolytic anemia.
• Urine glucose determinations may be false-positive with copper sulfate tests (Clinitest).

General

Classification: antihypertensive (adrenergic neuron blocking agent). **Pregnancy risk category:** D.

Mechanism of action

Acts peripherally, inhibiting norepinephrine release and depleting norepinephrine stores in adrenergic nerve endings.

Indications and dosage

• Mild to moderate hypertension. **Adults:** initially and for 1 to 3 weeks thereafter, 200 to 400 mg P.O. daily as a single dose or in two divided doses.

Maintenance dosage is 50 to 300 mg daily. No dosing recommendations for children.

Adverse reactions

CNS: confusion, *depression, drowsiness, nervousness, paradoxical anxiety,* nightmares, sedation, headache, extrapyramidal symptoms. **CV:** orthostatic hypotension, bradycardia, syncope. **EENT:** *nasal stuffiness,* glaucoma. **GI:** *dry mouth, hypersecretion of gastric acid, nausea, vomiting,* GI bleeding. **Skin:** pruritus, rash. **Other:** impotence, weight gain.

Interactions

Digitalis glycosides: possible digitalis glycoside-induced arrhythmias. Use together cautiously.

MAO inhibitors: possible excitability and hypertension. Use together cautiously.

Nursing diagnoses

• Altered tissue perfusion (renal, cerebral, cardiopulmonary, peripheral) related to the patient's underlying condition.
• High risk for injury related to the drug's adverse CNS effects.
• Knowledge deficit related to rauwolfia therapy.

Nursing interventions

• *Contraindicated* in depression.
• *Use cautiously* in patients with severe cardiac or cerebrovascular disease, impaired renal function, peptic ulcer, ulcerative colitis, gallstones; in those undergoing surgery; in elderly or debilitated patients; and in those taking other antihypertensives or TCAs.
• Monitor the patient's blood pressure and pulse rate frequently.
• Teach the patient about his disease and therapy. Explain the importance of taking this drug as prescribed, even when he's feeling well. Tell the outpatient not to discontinue this drug suddenly, but to call the doctor if unpleasant reactions occur.
• Instruct the patient to check with the doctor or pharmacist before taking OTC medications.
• Warn that this drug can cause drowsiness. Patient should not drive or perform other activities that require alertness and coordination until CNS effects are known.
• Watch the patient closely for signs of depression. Warn him to notify the doctor promptly if he has nightmares.
• Inform the patient that orthostatic hypotension can be minimized by rising slowly and avoiding sudden position changes.
• Tell him that dry mouth can be relieved with sugarless chewing gum, sour hard candy, or ice chips.
• Advise him to contact the doctor if relief is needed for nasal stuffiness.
• Give this drug with meals.
• Instruct the patient to weigh himself daily and to notify the doctor of any weight gain.
• Effects of this drug may last for 10 days after it's discontinued.
• Advise the patient to have periodic eye examinations.

General

Classification: antibiotic (first-generation cephalosporin). **Pregnancy risk category:** B.

Mechanism of action

Inhibits cell wall synthesis, promoting osmotic instability. Usually bactericidal.

Indications and dosage

• Serious infections of respiratory, GU, or GI tract; skin and soft-tissue infections (including peritonitis); bone and joint infections; septicemia; endocarditis; and perioperative prophylaxis. Susceptible organisms include *Escherichia coli* and other coliform bacteria, Enterobacteriaceae, enterococci, gonococci, group A beta-hemolytic streptococci, *Haemophilus influenzae, Klebsiella, Proteus mirabilis, Salmonella, Staphylococcus aureus, Shigella, Streptococcus pneumoniae* and *S. viridans*, and staphylococci. **Adults:** 500 mg to 1 g I.M. or I.V. (or intraperitoneally) q 4 to 6 hours; in life-threatening infections, up to 2 g q 4 hours. **Children:** 100 mg/kg/day I.V. in divided doses q 4 or 6 hours. Adjust dose in accordance with age, weight, and severity of infection.

Dosage schedule is determined by degree of renal impairment, severity of infection, and susceptibility of causative organism. I.V. route is preferable in severe or life-threatening infections.

Adverse reactions

Blood: transient neutropenia, eosinophilia, ***hemolytic anemia.*** **CNS:** headache, malaise, paresthesia, dizziness. **GI:** pseudomembranous colitis, nausea, anorexia, vomiting, *diarrhea,* glossitis, dyspepsia, abdominal cramps, tenesmus, anal pruritus, oral candidiasis (thrush). **GU:** nephrotoxicity, genital pruritus and moniliasis. **Skin:** *maculopapular and erythematous rashes, urticaria.* **Local:** *at injection site—pain, induration, sterile abscesses, tissue sloughing; phlebitis and thrombophlebitis with I.V. injection.* **Other:** ***hypersensitivity,*** dyspnea, fever.

Interactions

Aminoglycosides: increased nephrotoxicity. Monitor kidney function tests carefully. **Probenecid:** may increase blood levels of cephalosporins. Use together cautiously.

Nursing diagnoses

• High risk for injury related to ineffectiveness of cephalothin in eradicating the infection.
• High risk for fluid volume deficit related to adverse GI reactions to cephalothin.
• Knowledge deficit related to cephalothin therapy.

Nursing interventions

• *Use cautiously* in renal impairment and in history of sensitivity to penicillin.
• Obtain specimen for culture and sensitivity tests before first dose. Therapy may begin pending test results.
• For I.M. administration, reconstitute each gram of drug with 4 ml of sterile water for injection, providing 500 mg in each 2.2 ml. If not completely dissolved, add an additional 0.2 to 0.4 ml diluent, and warm contents slightly. Inject deep I.M. into a large muscle mass, such as gluteus or lateral aspect of thigh. Extremely painful when given I.M.
• **I.V. use:** When given I.V., check for vein irritation and phlebitis. Alternate injection sites if therapy lasts longer than 3 days.
• For I.V. administration, dilute contents of 4-g vial with at least 20 ml of sterile water for injection, D_5W, or 0.9% sodium chloride injection and add to an I.V. solution. Choose solution and fluid volume according to patient's fluid and electrolyte status.
• With large doses or prolonged therapy, monitor for superinfection.
• Patients receiving drug may show a false-positive direct Coombs' test; only a few indicate hemolytic anemia.
• Urine glucose determinations may be false-positive with copper sulfate tests.

General

Classification: antiulcer agent (H_2-receptor antagonist). **Pregnancy risk category:** B.

Mechanism of action

Competitively inhibits the action of H_2 at receptor sites of the parietal cells, decreasing gastric acid secretion.

Indications and dosage

- Duodenal and gastric ulcer (short-term treatment); pathological hypersecretory conditions, such as Zollinger-Ellison syndrome. **Adults:** 150 mg P.O. b.i.d. or 300 mg daily h.s. Dosages up to 6 g daily may be prescribed in patients with Zollinger-Ellison syndrome. When administered parenterally, give 50 mg I.V. or I.M. q 6 to 8 hours. When giving I.V. push, dilute to a total volume of 20 ml and inject over a period of 5 minutes. No dilution necessary when administering I.M. If giving by intermittent infusion, dilute 50 mg ranitidine in 100 ml of D_5W and infuse over 15 to 20 minutes. If giving by continuous infusion, dilute 150 mg of ranitidine in 250 mg of a compatible solution. Administer at 6.25 mg/hour using an infusion pump.
- Maintenance therapy of duodenal ulcer. **Adults:** 150 mg P.O. h.s.
- Gastroesophageal reflux disease. **Adults:** 150 mg P.O. b.i.d.
- Erosive esophagitis. **Adults:** 150 mg P.O. q.i.d.

Adverse reactions

Blood: ***neutropenia, thrombocytopenia.*** **CNS:** headache, malaise, dizziness, confusion. **CV:** bradycardia. **GI:** nausea, constipation. **Hepatic:** elevated liver enzymes, jaundice. **Skin:** rash. **Local:** burning and itching at injection site.

Interactions

Antacids: possible interference with absorption of ranitidine (conflicting data). Stagger doses if possible. **Diazepam:** decreased absorption when administered with ranitidine. **Glipizide:** possibly increased hypoglycemic effect. Dosage adjustment of glipizide may be necessary. **Procainamide:** possible decreased renal clearance (conflicting data). **Warfarin:** possible interference with warfarin clearance (conflicting data).

Nursing diagnoses

- Pain related to the patient's underlying condition.
- Constipation related to adverse GI reactions to ranitidine.
- Knowledge deficit related to ranitidine therapy.

Nursing interventions

- *Use cautiously* in hepatic dysfunction. Dosage should be adjusted in patients with impaired renal function.
- Drug can be taken without regard to meals. Absorption isn't affected by food.
- Remind the patient that if he's taking ranitidine once daily, he should take it at bedtime for best results.
- Urge the patient to avoid smoking, as this may increase gastric acid secretion and worsen disease.
- I.V. use: When administering premixed I.V. infusion, give by slow I.V. drip (over 15 to 20 minutes). Do not add other drugs to the solution. If the patient is receiving a primary I.V. solution, discontinue this solution during the infusion.
- To prepare I.V. injection, dilute 50 mg (2 ml) in 100 ml of compatible solution and infuse over 15 to 20 minutes. Compatible solutions include 0.9% sodium chloride injection, 5% or 10% dextrose injection, 5% sodium bicarbonate injection, or lactated Ringer's injection.
- Drug is incompatible with aluminum. Avoid using aluminum-based needles or other equipment when mixing or administering drug.

cephapirin sodium

Cefadyl

General

Classification: antibiotic (first-generation cephalosporin). **Pregnancy risk category:** B.

Mechanism of action

Inhibits cell wall synthesis, promoting osmotic instability. Usually bactericidal.

Indications and dosage

• Serious infections of respiratory, GU, or GI tract; skin and soft-tissue infections; bone and joint infections (including osteomyelitis); septicemia; and endocarditis due to *Streptococcus pneumoniae, Escherichia coli,* group A beta-hemolytic streptococci, *Haemophilus influenzae, Klebsiella, Proteus mirabilis, Staphylococcus aureus,* and *Streptococcus viridans.* **Adults:** 40 to 80 mg/kg/day I.V. or I.M. in divided doses q 4 to 6 hours. **Children over 3 months:** 10 to 20 mg/kg I.V. or I.M. q 6 hours; dose depends on age, weight, and severity of infection.

Depending on causative organism and severity of infection, patients with reduced renal function may be treated adequately with a lower dose (7.5 to 15 mg/kg q 12 hours). Patients with severely reduced renal function and who are to be dialyzed should receive same dose just before dialysis and q 12 hours thereafter.

Adverse reactions

Blood: transient neutropenia, eosinophilia, anemia. **CNS:** dizziness, headache, malaise, paresthesia. **GI:** pseudomembranous colitis, nausea, anorexia, vomiting, *diarrhea,* glossitis, dyspepsia, abdominal cramps, tenesmus, anal pruritus, oral candidiasis (thrush). **GU:** genital pruritus and moniliasis, vaginitis. **Skin:** *maculopapular and erythematous rashes, urticaria.* **Local:** *at injection site—pain, induration, sterile abscesses, tissue sloughing; phlebitis and thrombophlebitis with I.V. injection.* **Other:** ***hypersensitivity,*** dyspnea.

Interactions

Probenecid: may increase blood levels of cephalosporins.

Nursing diagnoses

• High risk for injury related to ineffectiveness of cephapirin to eradicate the infection.
• High risk for fluid volume deficit related to adverse GI reactions to cephapirin.
• Knowledge deficit related to cephapirin therapy.

Nursing interventions

• *Use cautiously* in renal impairment and history of sensitivity to penicillin.
• Obtain specimen for culture and sensitivity tests before first dose. Therapy may begin pending test results.
• For I.M. administration, reconstitute 1-g vial with 2 ml sterile water for injection or bacteriostatic water for injection so that 1.2 ml contains 500 mg of cephapirin. I.M. injection is painful. Inject deep I.M. into a large muscle mass, such as gluteus or lateral aspect of thigh.
• **I.V. use:** When given I.V., check frequently for vein irritation and phlebitis. Alternate injection sites if I.V. therapy lasts longer than 3 days.
• Prepare I.V. infusion using dextrose injection, sodium chloride injection, or bacteriostatic water for injection as diluent: 20 ml yields 1 g/10 ml; 50 ml yields 1 g/25 ml; 100 ml yields 1 g/50 ml.
• I.V. infusion with Y-tubing: during infusion of cephapirin solution, stop other solution. Check volume of cephapirin solution carefully so that calculated dose is infused. When Y-tubing is used, dilute 4-g vial with 40 ml of diluent.
• Reconstituted drug is stable for 10 days under refrigeration and for 24 hours at room temperature.
• With large doses or prolonged therapy, monitor for superinfection.
• Patients receiving cephalosporins may show a false-positive direct Coombs' test; only a few indicate hemolytic anemia.
• Urine glucose determinations may be false-positive with copper sulfate tests.

General

Classification: antihypertensive (ACE inhibitor).
Pregnancy risk category: D.

Mechanism of action

Prevents conversion of angiotensin I to angiotensin II, thereby reducing aldosterone secretion, decreasing sodium and water retention and blood pressure.

Indications and dosage

• Essential hypertension (alone or with diuretics). **Adults:** initially, 2.5 mg P.O. once daily. Increase dosage as needed based on response. Maintenance of 2.5 to 20 mg daily in single or divided doses.

Adverse reactions

CNS: headache, dizziness, fatigue, asthenia, malaise, light-headedness, anxiety, amnesia, ***seizures,*** depression, insomnia, neuralgia, neuropathy, paresthesia, somnolence, tremor, vertigo. **CV:** orthostatic hypotension, syncope, angina, ***arrhythmia,*** chest pain, palpitations, ***MI.*** **EENT:** epistaxis. **GI:** nausea, vomiting, abdominal pain, anorexia, constipation, diarrhea, dry mouth, dyspepsia, dysphagia, gastroenteritis, increased salivation, taste disturbance. **GU:** impotence. **Respiratory:** dry, persistent, tickling, nonproductive cough; dyspnea. **Skin:** hypersensitivity, rash, dermatitis, pruritus, photosensitivity, purpura. **Other:** ***angioedema,*** arthralgia, arthritis, edema, increased sweating, myalgia, weight gain.

Interactions

Diuretics: excessive hypotension, especially at start of therapy. Discontinue diuretic at least 3 days earlier, increase sodium intake, or reduce the starting dose of ramipril. **Insulin, oral antidiabetic agents:** risk of hypoglycemia, especially when starting ramipril. Monitor closely. **Lithium:** increased serum lithium levels. Use together cautiously and monitor lithium levels. **Potassium-sparing diuretics, potassium supplements, sodium substitutes containing potassium:** increased risk of hyperkalemia because ramipril attenuates potassium loss. Avoid use or monitor plasma potassium closely.

Nursing diagnoses

• Altered tissue perfusion (renal, cerebral, cardiopulmonary, peripheral) related to the patient's underlying condition.
• High risk for injury related to adverse reactions to ramipril.
• Knowledge deficit related to ramipril therapy.

Nursing interventions

• *Contraindicated* in patients with history of angioedema and during pregnancy. ACE inhibitors can cause fetal morbidity and mortality; their use during second and third trimesters has been associated with oligohydramnios, neonatal hypotension, renal failure, skull hypoplasia, and death.
• *Use cautiously* in renal insufficiency or diabetes mellitus, in patients receiving potassium supplements or potassium-sparing diuretics, and in those using potassium-containing sodium substitutes because these patients have a higher risk for hyperkalemia.
• Patients with renal insufficiency should start at 1.25 mg P.O. daily. Titrate gradually according to response. Maximum daily dosage is 5 mg.
• In patients with severe CHF or hypertension with renal artery stenosis, renal function may worsen at start of therapy. Closely assess renal function in such patients during first few weeks of therapy.
• Regularly check serum creatinine and BUN.
• Monitor WBC count in renal impairment or collagen vascular disease because of possible agranulocytosis and bone marrow depression after ACE inhibitor therapy.
• Tell patient to continue taking the drug even if he feels better and to check with the doctor or pharmacist before taking OTC drugs.
• Tell patient not to change position suddenly to avoid orthostatic hypotension.
• Advise him to report light-headedness, signs of infection, difficulty breathing, edema or swelling, or any unusual bruising or bleeding.
• Tell the patient to avoid sodium substitutes containing potassium unless recommended by doctor.

General

Classification: antibiotic (first-generation cephalosporin). **Pregnancy risk category:** B.

Mechanism of action

Inhibits cell wall synthesis, promoting osmotic instability. Usually bactericidal.

Indications and dosage

• Serious infections of respiratory, GU, or GI tract; skin and soft-tissue infections; bone and joint infections; septicemia; endocarditis; otitis media; and perioperative prophylaxis. Among susceptible organisms are *Escherichia coli* and other coliform bacteria, group A beta-hemolytic streptococci, *Haemophilus influenzae, Klebsiella, Proteus mirabilis, Staphylococcus aureus, Streptococcus pneumoniae* and *S. viridans*, and staphylococci. **Adults:** 500 mg to 1 g I.M. or I.V. b.i.d. to q.i.d., not to exceed 8 g daily. Or 250 to 500 mg P.O. q 6 hours. Severe or chronic infections may require larger and/or more frequent doses (up to 1 g P.O. q 6 hours). **Children over 1 year:** 6 to 12 mg/kg P.O. q 6 hours, or 12 to 25 mg/kg I.M. or I.V. q 6 hours.

• Otitis media. 19 to 25 mg/kg P.O. q 6 hours. Do not exceed 4 g daily.

Larger doses (up to 1 g q.i.d.) may be given for severe or chronic infections (regardless of age and weight). Parenteral therapy may be followed by oral.

Adverse reactions

Blood: transient neutropenia, eosinophilia. **CNS:** dizziness, headache, malaise, paresthesia. **GI:** pseudomembranous colitis, *nausea, anorexia,* vomiting, heartburn, glossitis, dyspepsia, abdominal cramping, *diarrhea,* tenesmus, anal pruritus, oral candidiasis (thrush). **GU:** genital pruritus and moniliasis, vaginitis. **Skin:** *maculopapular and erythematous rashes, urticaria.* **Local:** *at injection site—pain, induration, sterile abscesses, tissue sloughing; phlebitis and thrombophlebitis with I.V. injection.* **Other:** ***hypersensitivity,*** dyspnea.

Interactions

Probenecid: may increase blood levels of cephalosporins.

Nursing diagnoses

• High risk for injury related to ineffectiveness of cephradine to eradicate the infection.

• High risk for fluid volume deficit related to adverse GI reactions to cephradine.

• Knowledge deficit related to cephradine therapy.

Nursing interventions

• *Contraindicated* in patients with hypersensitivity to other cephalosporins.

• *Use cautiously* in renal impairment and history of sensitivity to penicillin.

• Obtain specimen for culture and sensitivity tests. Therapy may begin pending test results.

• Oral form may be taken with food or milk to lessen GI discomfort.

• For I.M. administration, reconstitute with sterile water or with bacteriostatic water for injection as follows: 1.2 ml to 250-mg vial; 2 ml to 500-mg vial; 4 ml to 1-g vial. Use solution within 2 hours if kept at room temperature and within 24 hours if refrigerated.

• When given I.M., inject deep into a large muscle mass, such as gluteus or lateral aspect of thigh.

• **I.V. use:** When given I.V., check frequently for vein irritation and phlebitis. Alternate injection sites if I.V. therapy lasts longer than 3 days. Follow product directions carefully when reconstituting drug.

• With large doses or prolonged therapy, monitor for superinfection.

• Patients receiving cephalosporins may show a false-positive direct Coombs' test; only a few tests indicate hemolytic anemia.

• Urine glucose determinations may be false-positive with copper sulfate tests.

General
Classification: antimalarial (cinchona alkaloid).
Pregnancy risk category: X.

Mechanism of action
Mechanism of antiprotozoal action is unknown, but the drug is often referred to as a generalized protoplasmic poison. As a muscle relaxant, quinine appears to have a direct effect on muscle fibers that decreases their response to repetitive stimulation.

Indications and dosage
- Malaria due to *Plasmodium falciparum* (chloroquine-resistant). **Adults:** 650 mg P.O. q 8 hours for 10 days, with 25 mg pyrimethamine q 12 hours for 3 days, and with 500 mg sulfadiazine q.i.d. for 5 days.
- Nocturnal leg cramps. **Adults:** 260 to 300 mg P.O. h.s. or after the evening meal.

Adverse reactions
Blood: hemolytic anemia, thrombocytopenia, ***agranulocytosis***, hypoprothrombinemia. **CNS:** severe headache, apprehension, excitement, confusion, delirium, syncope, hypothermia, seizures (with toxic doses). **CV:** hypotension, ***CV collapse*** with overdose or rapid I.V. administration. **EENT:** altered color perception, photophobia, blurred vision, night blindness, amblyopia, scotoma, diplopia, mydriasis, optic atrophy, tinnitus, impaired hearing. **GI:** epigastric distress, diarrhea, nausea, vomiting. **GU:** renal tubular damage, anuria. **Skin:** rashes, pruritus. **Local:** thrombosis at infusion site. **Other:** asthma, flushing.

Interactions
Antacids containing aluminum: decreased absorption of quinine. Separate administration times by at least 2 hours. **Cimetidine:** decreased hepatic metabolism of quinine. Monitor for toxicity. **Digoxin:** possible increased serum digoxin levels. Monitor for toxicity. **Mefloquine:** risk of seizures, ECG changes, and cardiac arrest. Don't use together. **Neuromuscular blockers:** prolonged muscle paralysis. Monitor for respiratory distress or excessive weakness. **Oral anticoagulants:** enhanced anticoagulant effect. Monitor for bleeding. **Sodium bicarbonate:** elevated quinine levels because of decreasing quinine excretion. Use together cautiously.

Nursing diagnoses
- High risk for injury related to the ineffectiveness of quinine in eradicating the infection.
- Altered protection related to quinine-induced hematologic abnormalities.
- Knowledge deficit related to quinine therapy.

Nursing interventions
- *Contraindicated* in patients with G6PD deficiency.
- *Use cautiously* in patients with CV conditions.
- Discontinue drug if any signs of idiosyncrasy or toxicity occur.
- Quinine is no longer used for acute attacks of malaria due to *Plasmodium vivax* or for suppression of malaria due to organism resistance.
- Administer drug after meals to minimize GI distress. Do not crush tablets, as the drug is irritating to gastric mucosa.

chloral hydrate

Aquachloral Supprettes, Novochlorhydrate†

General

Classification: sedative-hypnotic (general CNS depressant). **Pregnancy risk category:** C. **Controlled substance schedule:** IV.

Mechanism of action

Unknown. Sedative effects may be caused by its primary metabolite, trichloroethanol.

Indications and dosage

- Sedation. **Adults:** 250 mg P.O. or P.R. t.i.d. after meals. **Children:** 8.3 mg/kg or 250 mg/m^2 P.O. or P.R. t.i.d. Maximum dosage is 500 mg t.i.d.
- Insomnia. **Adults:** 500 mg to 1 g P.O. or P.R. 15 to 30 minutes before bedtime. **Children:** 50 mg/kg or 1.5 g/m^2 P.O. or P.R. 15 to 30 minutes before bedtime. Maximum single dose is 1 g.
- Premedication for EEG. **Children:** 20 to 25 mg/kg P.O. or P.R. Maximum single dose is 1 g.
- Management of alcohol withdrawal symptoms. **Adults:** 500 mg to 1 g P.O. or P.R. q 6 hours, not to exceed 2 g daily.

Adverse reactions

Blood: eosinophilia. **CNS:** *hangover, drowsiness,* nightmares, dizziness, ataxia, paradoxical excitement. **GI:** *nausea,* vomiting, diarrhea, flatulence. **Skin:** hypersensitivity reactions.

Interactions

Alcohol or other CNS depressants, including narcotic analgesics: excessive CNS depression or vasodilation reaction. Use together cautiously. **Furosemide I.V.:** sweating, flushes, variable blood pressure, and uneasiness. Use together cautiously or use a different hypnotic drug. **Oral anticoagulants:** increased risk of bleeding. Monitor patient closely.

Nursing diagnoses

- Sleep pattern disturbance related to underlying patient problem.
- High risk for trauma related to adverse CNS reactions caused by chloral hydrate.
- Knowledge deficit related to chloral hydrate therapy.

Nursing interventions

- *Contraindicated* in marked hepatic or renal impairment and hypersensitivity to chloral hydrate or trichloroacetic acid. Oral administration contraindicated in gastric disorders.
- *Use cautiously* in severe cardiac disease, mental depression, and suicidal tendencies.
- Prolonged administration is not recommended. Drug loses efficacy in promoting sleep after 14 days of continued use. Long-term use may cause drug dependence, and patient may experience withdrawal symptoms if drug is suddenly discontinued.
- Dilute or administer with liquid to minimize unpleasant taste and stomach irritation. Administer after meals.
- Note two strengths of oral liquid form. Double check dose, especially when administering to children. Fatal overdoses have occurred.
- Take precautions to prevent hoarding or self-overdosing by patients who are depressed, suicidal, or drug-dependent or who have a history of drug abuse.
- Advise caution with activities requiring mental alertness or physical coordination. Supervise walking; raise bed rails, especially for elderly patients.
- Large dosage may raise BUN levels.
- May interfere with fluorometric tests for urine catecholamines and Reddy-Jenkins-Thorn test for urine 17-hydroxycorticosteroids. Do not administer drug for 48 hours before fluorometric test. May also cause false-positive tests for urine glucose when using copper sulfate tests. Use glucose enzymatic tests instead.
- Aqueous solutions are incompatible with alkaline substances.
- Store in dark container; store suppositories in refrigerator.

General

Classification: ventricular, supraventricular antiarrhythmic (cinchona alkaloid). **Pregnancy risk category:** C.

Mechanism of action

Class Ia antiarrhythmic that depresses phase 0; prolongs action potential and stabilizes membranes.

Indications and dosage

• Atrial flutter or fibrillation. **Adults:** 200 mg quinidine sulfate or equivalent P.O. q 2 to 3 hours for 5 to 8 doses with subsequent daily increases until rhythm restored or toxicity develops. Give after digitalization to avoid increasing AV conduction. Maximum dosage 3 to 4 g daily.
• Paroxysmal supraventricular tachycardia. **Adults:** 400 to 600 mg I.M. gluconate q 2 to 3 hours until toxic reactions develop or arrhythmia subsides.
• Premature atrial and ventricular contractions; junctional rhythm; paroxysmal atrial tachycardia; maintenance after cardioversion of atrial fibrillation or flutter. **Adults:** test dose is 50 to 200 mg P.O., then monitor vital signs before therapy. Quinidine sulfate or equivalent base 200 to 400 mg P.O. q 4 to 6 hours; or initially, quinidine gluconate 600 mg I.M., then up to 400 mg q 2 hours, p.r.n.; or quinidine gluconate 800 mg added to 40 ml D_5W, infused at 16 mg (1 ml)/minute. **Children:** test dose is 2 mg/kg; 3 to 6 mg/kg q 2 to 3 hours for 5 doses P.O. daily.
• Severe *Plasmodium falciparum* malaria. **Adults:** 10 mg/kg I.V. (gluconate) diluted in 250 ml 0.9% sodium chloride injection and infused over 1 to 2 hours; then maintenance infusion of 0.02 mg/kg/minute for 72 hours or until parasitemia is reduced to less than 1%.

Adverse reactions

Blood: ***hemolytic anemia, thrombocytopenia, agranulocytosis.*** **CNS:** *vertigo, headache, light-headedness,* confusion, restlessness, cold sweat, pallor, fainting, dementia. **CV:** ***premature ventricular contractions; severe hypotension;*** *SA and AV block;* ***ventricular fibrillation,*** *tachycardia;* ***aggravated CHF;*** *ECG changes.* **EENT:** *tinnitus,* excessive salivation, blurred vision. **GI:** *diarrhea, nausea, vomiting,* anorexia, abdominal pain. **Hepatic:** hepatotoxicity. **Skin:** rash, hemorrhage of buccal mucosa, pruritus. **Other:** angioedema, asthma attack, respiratory arrest, *fever, cinchonism.*

Interactions

Acetazolamide, antacids, sodium bicarbonate: possible increased quinidine levels. **Amiodarone, cimetidine:** increased quinidine levels. **Barbiturates, phenytoin, rifampin:** possible antagonized quinidine activity. **Digoxin:** increased digoxin levels after initiating quinidine. **Nifedipine:** possible reduced quinidine levels. **Other antiarrhythmics, such as lidocaine and propranolol:** increased toxicity. **Verapamil:** possible hypotension. **Warfarin:** increased anticoagulant effect.

Nursing diagnoses

• Decreased cardiac output related to ineffectiveness of quinidine therapy.
• Altered protection related to quinidine-induced proarrhythmias.
• Knowledge deficit related to quinidine.

Nursing interventions

• *Contraindicated* in digitalis toxicity with grossly impaired AV conduction and in complete AV block with AV nodal or idioventricular pacemaker.
• *Use cautiously* in myasthenia gravis.
• Check apical pulse rate and blood pressure before therapy. If extremes noted, tell doctor.
• Check liver function for first 4 to 8 weeks.
• When changing route of administration, alter dosage to compensate for variations in quinidine base content.
• GI reactions, especially diarrhea, signal toxicity. Notify doctor. Serum levels over 8 mcg/ml are toxic.
• Have patient notify doctor if rash, fever, unusual bleeding, bruising, tinnitus, or vision changes.
• Give anticoagulant before restoring rhythm to prevent thromboembolism.
• Store away from heat and direct light; never use discolored quinidine.

General
Classification: antineoplastic (alkylating agent). **Pregnancy risk category:** D.

Mechanism of action
Cross-links strands of cellular DNA and interferes with RNA transcription, causing an imbalance of growth that leads to cell death. Cell cycle-nonspecific.

Indications and dosage
• Chronic lymphocytic leukemia, diffuse lymphocytic lymphoma, nodular lymphocytic lymphoma, Hodgkin's disease, ovarian carcinoma, mycosis fungoides, polycythemia vera, nephrotic syndrome, testicular carcinoma. **Adults:** 0.1 to 0.2 mg/kg P.O. daily for 3 to 6 weeks, then adjust for maintenance (usually 4 to 10 mg daily). **Children:** 0.1 to 0.2 mg/kg P.O. daily or 4.5 mg/m^2 daily as a single dose or in divided doses.

Adverse reactions
Blood: ***leukopenia,*** delayed up to 3 weeks, lasting up to 10 days after last dose; ***thrombocytopenia; anemia;*** myelosuppression (usually moderate, gradual, and rapidly reversible). **CNS:** seizures (with overdose). **GI:** *nausea, vomiting, stomatitis.* **GU:** *azoospermia, infertility.* **Metabolic:** hyperuricemia, hepatotoxicity (rare). **Respiratory:** interstitial pneumonitis or ***pulmonary fibrosis*** (rare). **Skin:** ***exfoliative dermatitis,*** rash. **Other:** allergic febrile reaction.

Interactions
Anticoagulants, aspirin: increased risk of bleeding. Watch for signs of bleeding.

Nursing diagnoses
• Infection related to chlorambucil-induced neutropenia.
• Impaired skin integrity related to resultant exfoliative dermatitis.
• Knowledge deficit related to chlorambucil therapy.

Nursing interventions
• *Contraindicated* in patients with hypersensitivity or resistance to previous therapy. Patients hypersensitive to melphalan may also be hypersensitive to chlorambucil. Dosage adjustment is recommended in hematologic impairment.
• *Use cautiously* in patients with a history of seizures or head trauma or with use of epileptogenic drugs.
• Place patient on neutropenia precautions if WBC falls below 2,000/mm^3 or granulocytes fall below 1,000/mm^3.
• Severe neutropenia reversible up to cumulative dosage of 6.5 mg/kg in a single course.
• Warn patient to watch for signs of infection (fever, sore throat, fatigue) and bleeding (easy bruising, nosebleeds, bleeding gums, melena). Take temperature daily.
• Monitor CBC.
• To prevent hyperuricemia with resulting uric acid nephropathy, allopurinol may be used with adequate hydration. Monitor serum uric acid.
• Avoid all I.M. injections when platelets are below 100,000/mm^3.
• Instruct patient to avoid OTC products containing aspirin.
• Therapeutic effects are often accompanied by toxicity.

quinethazone Hydromox

General
Classification: diuretic (quinazoline derivative). **Pregnancy risk category:** D.

Mechanism of action
Although not a thiazide diuretic, quinethazone acts in a similar fashion. It increases urine excretion of sodium and water by inhibiting sodium reabsorption in the cortical diluting site of the nephron.

Indications and dosage
• Edema or hypertension. **Adults:** 50 to 100 mg P.O. daily or 50 mg P.O. b.i.d. Occasionally, up to 150 to 200 mg P.O. daily may be needed.

Adverse reactions
Blood: ***aplastic anemia, agranulocytosis,*** leukopenia, thrombocytopenia. **CV:** volume depletion and dehydration, orthostatic hypotension. **GI:** anorexia, nausea, pancreatitis. **Hepatic:** hepatic encephalopathy. **Metabolic:** hypokalemia, asymptomatic hyperuricemia, hyperglycemia and impairment of glucose tolerance, fluid and electrolyte imbalances including dilutional hyponatremia and hypochloremia, metabolic alkalosis, hypercalcemia, gout. **Skin:** dermatitis, photosensitivity, rash. **Other:** hypersensitivity reactions, such as pneumonitis and vasculitis.

Interactions
Cholestyramine, colestipol: intestinal absorption of thiazides decreased. Keep doses as separate as possible. **Diazoxide:** increased antihypertensive, hyperglycemic, and hyperuricemic effects. Use together cautiously. **Digitalis glycosides:** increased risk of toxicity because of quinethazone's potassium-depleting effect. Use a potassium-sparing diuretic instead.

Nursing diagnoses
• Fluid volume excess related to the patient's underlying condition.
• Altered urinary elimination related to quinethazone therapy.
• Knowledge deficit related to quinethazone therapy.

Nursing interventions
• *Contraindicated* in anuria or hypersensitivity to quinethazones, thiazides, or other sulfonamide-derived drugs.
• *Use cautiously* in severe renal disease, impaired hepatic function, and allergies.
• Monitor the patient's intake and output, weight, blood pressure, and serum electrolytes.
• Consult with the doctor and dietitian to provide a high-potassium diet. Foods rich in potassium include citrus fruits, tomatoes, bananas, dates, and apricots.
• Watch for signs of hypokalemia, such as muscle weakness and cramps.
• Monitor serum creatinine and BUN levels regularly.
• Check insulin requirements in patients with diabetes. May treat severe hyperglycemia with oral antidiabetic agents.
• Monitor serum uric acid levels, especially in patients with a history of gout.
• In hypertension, therapeutic response may be delayed several days.
• Give drug in the morning to prevent nocturia.
• Elderly patients are especially susceptible to excessive diuresis.
• Stop drug before parathyroid function tests are performed.
• Advise patient to avoid sudden posture changes and rise slowly to avoid orthostatic hypotension.
• Also advise him to use a sunscreen.

General

Classification: antibiotic (dichloracetic acid derivative). **Pregnancy risk category:** C.

Mechanism of action

Inhibits bacterial protein synthesis by binding to the 50S subunit of the ribosome (bacteriostatic).

Indications and dosage

• *Haemophilus influenzae* meningitis, acute *Salmonella typhi* infection, and meningitis, bacteremia, or other severe infections caused by sensitive *Salmonella* species, *Rickettsia*, lymphogranuloma, psittacosis, or various sensitive gram-negative organisms. **Adults and children:** 50 to 100 mg/kg P.O. (base, palmitate) or I.V. (sodium succinate) daily, divided q 6 hours, up to 100 mg/kg daily. **Premature infants and neonates 2 weeks or younger:** 25 mg/kg P.O. (base, palmitate) or I.V. (sodium succinate) once daily. I.V. route must be used to treat meningitis.

Adverse reactions

Blood: ***aplastic anemia,*** hypoplastic anemia, *granulocytopenia,* thrombocytopenia. **CNS:** headache, mild depression, confusion, delirium, peripheral neuropathy with prolonged therapy. **EENT:** optic neuritis (in patients with cystic fibrosis), glossitis, decreased visual acuity. **GI:** nausea, vomiting, stomatitis, diarrhea, enterocolitis. **Other:** infections from nonsusceptible organisms, hypersensitivity reaction (fever, rash, urticaria, ***anaphylaxis***), jaundice, ***gray syndrome in neonates (abdominal distention, gray cyanosis, vasomotor collapse, respiratory distress, death within a few hours of onset of symptoms).***

Interactions

Acetaminophen: elevates chloramphenicol levels. Monitor for chloramphenicol toxicity. **Chlorpropamide, dicumarol, phenobarbital, phenytoin, tolbutamide:** blood levels of these agents may be increased by chloramphenicol. Monitor for toxicity. **Iron supplements, vitamin B_{12}, folic acid:** chloramphenicol may delay the response to these drugs in patients with anemia. Monitor closely.

Nursing diagnoses

• High risk for injury related to ineffectiveness of chloramphenicol to eradicate the infection.
• Altered protection related to chloramphenicol-induced aplastic anemia.
• Knowledge deficit related to chloramphenicol therapy.

Nursing interventions

• *Use cautiously* in patients with impaired hepatic or renal function, acute intermittent porphyria, and G6PD deficiency and with other drugs causing bone marrow depression or blood disorders.
• Use drug only when clearly indicated for severe infection.
• Obtain specimen for culture and sensitivity tests before first dose. Therapy may begin pending test results.
• Monitor CBC, platelets, serum iron, and reticulocytes before and every 2 days during therapy. Stop drug immediately if anemia, reticulocytopenia, leukopenia, or thrombocytopenia develops.
• Instruct patient to report adverse reactions to the doctor, especially nausea, vomiting, diarrhea, fever, confusion, sore throat, or mouth sores.
• Tell patient to take all of the medication, exactly as directed, even after he feels better.
• **I.V. use:** Give I.V. slowly over at least 1 minute. Check injection site daily for phlebitis and irritation.
• Reconstitute 1-g vial of powder for injection with 10 ml sterile water for injection. Concentration will be 100 mg/ml. Stable for 30 days at room temperature, but refrigeration recommended. Don't use cloudy solutions.
• Monitor for superinfection.

General
Classification: estrogen replacement (estrogen).
Pregnancy risk category: X.

Mechanism of action
Increases the synthesis of DNA, RNA, and protein in responsive tissues. Also reduces release of follicle-stimulating hormone and luteinizing hormone from the pituitary.

Indications and dosage
• Moderate to severe vasomotor symptoms associated with menopause, and for atrophic vaginitis, kraurosis vulvae, female hypogonadism, female castration, and primary ovarian failure. **Women:** 100 mcg P.O. once daily for 7 days, followed by 100 mcg weekly as maintenance dosage beginning 2 weeks after start of treatment. Dosage may be increased to 200 mcg weekly.

Adverse reactions
CNS: headache, dizziness, chorea, migraine, depression, libido changes. **CV:** thrombophlebitis; ***thromboembolism;*** hypertension; edema; ***increased risk of stroke, pulmonary embolism, and myocardial infarction.*** **EENT:** worsening of myopia or astigmatism, intolerance to contact lenses. **GI:** *nausea,* vomiting, abdominal cramps, bloating, diarrhea, constipation, anorexia, increased appetite, excessive thirst, weight changes. **GU:** breakthrough bleeding, altered menstrual flow, dysmenorrhea, amenorrhea, cervical erosion or abnormal secretions, enlargement of uterine fibromas, vaginal candidiasis. **Hepatic:** cholestatic jaundice. **Metabolic:** hyperglycemia, hypercalcemia, folic acid deficiency. **Skin:** melasma, urticaria, acne, seborrhea, oily skin, hirsutism or loss of hair. **Other:** leg cramps, purpura, breast changes (tenderness, enlargement, secretion).

Interactions
Bromocriptine: possible amenorrhea, interfering with the effects of bromocriptine. Avoid concomitant use. **Carbamazepine, phenobarbital, rifampin:** decreased effectiveness of quinestrol. Monitor closely. **Corticosteroids:** possible enhanced effects. Monitor closely. **Cyclosporine:** increased risk of toxicity. Use together with caution and frequently monitor cyclosporine levels. **Dantrolene, other hepatotoxic medications:** increased risk of hepatotoxicity. Monitor closely. **Oral anticoagulants:** dosage adjustments may be necessary. Monitor PT. **Tamoxifen:** possible impaired effectiveness of tamoxifen. Avoid concomitant use.

Nursing diagnoses
• Sexual dysfunction related to hormonal imbalance.
• Altered tissue perfusion (cerebral, peripheral, cardiopulmonary) related to possible drug-induced thromboembolism.
• Knowledge deficit related to quinestrol therapy.

Nursing interventions
• *Contraindicated* in thrombophlebitis or thromboembolic disorders, cancer of breast or reproductive organs, undiagnosed abnormal genital bleeding, and pregnancy.
• *Use cautiously* in hypertension, mental depression, migraine, seizures, diabetes mellitus, amenorrhea, hepatic or renal dysfunction, or family history (mother, grandmother, sister) of breast or genital tract cancer.
• Patients should have a thorough physical examination before therapy; those receiving long-term therapy should have repeat examinations yearly.
• Diabetic patients should report elevated blood glucose levels so antidiabetic dosage can be adjusted.
• Try to discontinue drug at 3- to 6-month intervals.
• Similar in effectiveness to conjugated estrogens. Biggest advantage is that quinestrol can be taken once a week.
• Explain to patients that, although menstrual-like bleeding or spotting may occur, fertility has not been restored.

General

Classification: sedative-hypnotic (benzodiazepine). **Pregnancy risk category:** D. **Controlled substance schedule:** IV.

Mechanism of action

Depresses the CNS at limbic and subcortical levels of the brain.

Indications and dosage

• Mild to moderate anxiety and tension. **Adults:** 5 to 10 mg P.O. t.i.d. or q.i.d. **Children over 6 years:** 5 mg P.O. b.i.d. to q.i.d. Maximum dosage is 10 mg b.i.d. to t.i.d.
• Severe anxiety and tension. **Adults:** 20 to 25 mg P.O. t.i.d. or q.i.d.
• Withdrawal symptoms of acute alcoholism. **Adults:** 50 to 100 mg P.O., I.M., or I.V., up to 300 mg daily.
• Preoperative apprehension and anxiety. **Adults:** 5 to 10 mg P.O. t.i.d. or q.i.d. on day preceding surgery; or 50 to 100 mg I.M. 1 hour before surgery.

Note: Parenteral form not recommended in children under 12 years.

Adverse reactions

CNS: *drowsiness, lethargy, hangover,* fainting. **CV:** transient hypotension. **GI:** nausea, vomiting, abdominal discomfort. **Local:** *thrombophlebitis, swelling, pain at injection site.*

Interactions

Alcohol, other CNS depressants: increased CNS depression. Avoid concomitant use. **Cigarette smoking:** increased clearance of benzodiazepines. Monitor for lack of effect. **Cimetidine:** increased sedation. Monitor carefully. **Digoxin:** increased serum digoxin levels and risk of toxicity. Monitor closely.

Nursing diagnoses

• Anxiety related to the patient's underlying condition.
• High risk for injury related to chlordiazepoxide-induced CNS reactions.
• Knowledge deficit related to chlordiazepoxide therapy.

Nursing interventions

• *Contraindicated* in acute narrow-angle glaucoma, psychoses, or anxiety-free psychiatric disorders.
• *Use cautiously* in mental depression, psychiatric disturbances, blood dyscrasias, porphyria, and hepatic or renal disease or in those taking anticoagulants.
• Reduce dosage in elderly or debilitated patients.
• Possibility of abuse and addiction. Don't withdraw drug abruptly; withdrawal symptoms may occur.
• Warn patient to avoid activities requiring alertness until CNS effects of the drug are known.
• Recommended for I.M. use only, but may be given I.V.
• Injectable form (as hydrochloride) comes as two ampules – diluent and powdered drug. Read directions carefully. Don't mix injectable form with any other parenteral drug. For I.M. use, add 2 ml of diluent to powder and agitate gently until clear. Use immediately.
• **I.V. use:** Use 5 ml of saline injection or sterile water for injection as diluent; don't give packaged diluent I.V. Give slowly over 1 minute.
• Make sure that emergency airway management equipment and personnel are available when giving drug I.V. Monitor respirations every 5 to 15 minutes and before each repeated I.V. dose.
• If overdose occurs, give flumazenil (a specific benzodiazepine antagonist). The duration of action of chlordiazepoxide is longer than that of flumazenil, so resedation is possible.
• Caution patient against giving medication to others.
• May cause false-positive reaction in the Gravindex pregnancy test and interfere with certain tests for urine 17-ketosteroids.
• Perform periodic hepatic, renal, and hematopoietic function studies in patients on repeated or prolonged therapy.

quinacrine hydrochloride

Atabrine

General

Classification: anthelmintic, antiprotozoal, antimalarial (acridine derivative). **Pregnancy risk category:** C.

Mechanism of action

Inhibits DNA metabolism in susceptible parasites.

Indications and dosage

• Giardiasis. **Adults:** 300 mg P.O. in 3 divided doses for 5 to 7 days. **Children:** 7 mg/kg/day P.O. given in 3 divided doses after meals for 5 days. Maximum 300 mg/day. Dosage may be repeated in 2 weeks.
• Tapeworms (beef, pork, and fish). **Adults and children over 14 years:** 4 doses of 200 mg P.O. given 10 minutes apart (800 mg total). **Children 11 to 14 years:** 600 mg P.O. total dosage, administered in 3 or 4 divided doses, 10 minutes apart. **Children 5 to 10 years:** 400 mg P.O. total dosage, administered in 3 or 4 divided doses, 10 minutes apart.

Adverse reactions

CNS: *headache, dizziness, nervousness, vertigo, mood shifts, nightmares,* ***seizures.*** **GI:** *diarrhea, anorexia, nausea, abdominal cramps,* vomiting. **GU:** yellow urine. **Skin:** pleomorphic skin eruptions, yellow discoloration.

Interactions

Primaquine: enhanced toxicity of primaquine. Don't use together.

Nursing diagnoses

• Altered health maintenance related to the ineffectiveness of quinacrine in eradicating the infection.
• High risk for fluid volume deficit related to quinacrine-induced adverse GI reactions.
• Knowledge deficit related to quinacrine therapy.

Nursing interventions

• *Use with extreme caution* in patients with porphyria or psoriasis because quinacrine may exacerbate these conditions.
• *Use cautiously* in patients with hepatic, renal, or cardiac disease, alcoholism, psychosis, and G6PD deficiency. Also use cautiously in those over 60 years or under 1 year.
• Give the drug after meals with a large glass of water, tea, or fruit juice to reduce GI irritation. Bitter taste may be disguised by jam or honey.
• Give a saline cathartic 1 to 2 hours after drug is given to expel the worm.
• Collect all of stool after treatment. Look for the scolex (attachment organ), which will be stained yellow.
• Warn the patient about temporary yellow color of skin and urine.
• Keep the patient on a bland, nonfat, semisolid diet for 24 hours. Then have him fast after the evening meal before treatment.

General

Classification: antimalarial, amebicide, (4-aminoquinoline). **Pregnancy risk category:** C.

Mechanism of action

May bind to and alter the properties of DNA in susceptible parasites.

Indications and dosage

Doses are expressed as chloroquine base: 1 mg of chloroquine base is equal to 1.67 mg chloroquine phosphate or 1.25 mg chloroquine hydrochloride.

- Treatment of acute attacks of malaria caused by *Plasmodium vivax, P. malariae, P. ovale,* and susceptible strains of *P. falciparum.* **Adults:** initially, 600 mg (base) P.O., then 300 mg at 6, 24, and 48 hours. Or 160 to 200 mg (base) I.M. initially; repeat in 6 hours if needed. Switch to oral therapy as soon as possible. **Children:** initially, 10 mg (base)/kg P.O., then 5 mg (base)/kg at 6, 24, and 48 hours (not to exceed adult dose). Or 5 mg (base)/kg I.M. initially; repeat in 6 hours if needed. Switch to oral therapy as soon as possible.
- Malaria suppressive treatment. **Adults and children:** 5 mg (base)/kg P.O. (not to exceed 300 mg) weekly on same day of the week (begin 2 weeks before entering endemic area and continue for 8 weeks after leaving). If treatment begins after exposure, double the initial dose (600 mg for adults, 10 mg/kg for children) in two divided doses 6 hours apart.
- Extraintestinal amebiasis. **Adults:** 1 g (600 mg base) chloroquine phosphate P.O. daily for 2 days; then 500 mg (300 mg base) daily for at least 2 to 3 weeks. Treatment is usually combined with an effective intestinal amebicide. **Children:** 16.7 mg/kg chloroquine phosphate (10 mg/kg base) P.O. once daily for 2 to 3 weeks. Maximum dosage is 500 mg phosphate (300 mg base) daily.
- Rheumatoid arthritis and lupus erythematosus. **Adults:** 250 mg chloroquine phosphate daily with evening meal.

Adverse reactions

Blood: ***agranulocytosis, aplastic anemia,*** hemolytic anemia, thrombocytopenia. **CNS:** mild and transient headache, neuromyopathy, psychic stimulation, fatigue, irritability, nightmares, seizures, dizziness. **CV:** hypotension, ECG changes. **EENT:** *visual disturbances* (often severe), ototoxicity. **GI:** anorexia, abdominal cramps, diarrhea, nausea, vomiting, stomatitis. **Skin:** pruritus, skin eruptions, skin and mucosal pigmentary changes.

Interactions

Cimetidine: decreased hepatic metabolism of chloroquine. Monitor for toxicity. **Magnesium and aluminum salts, kaolin:** decreased GI absorption. Separate administration times.

Nursing diagnoses

- High risk for injury related to ineffective drug dosage.
- Sensory/perceptual alterations (visual or auditory) related to adverse reactions to chloroquine.
- Knowledge deficit related to chloroquine therapy.

Nursing interventions

- *Contraindicated* in retinal or visual field changes or porphyria.
- *Use with extreme caution* in presence of severe GI, neurologic, or blood disorders.
- *Use cautiously* in hepatic disease, alcoholism G6PD deficiency, and psoriasis.
- Periodically perform CBCs and liver function studies in prolonged therapy.
- Overdosage quickly leads to toxic symptoms: headache, drowsiness, visual disturbances, CV collapse, and seizures, followed by respiratory and cardiac arrest. Monitor carefully.
- Baseline and periodic ophthalmologic and audiometric examinations needed. Tell patient to report any symptoms of visual disturbances or ototoxicity.

General

Classification: anxiolytic, sedative-hypnotic (benzodiazepine). **Pregnancy risk category:** X. **Controlled substance schedule:** IV.

Mechanism of action

Acts on the limbic system and thalamus of the CNS by binding to specific benzodiazepine receptors.

Indications and dosage

- Insomnia. **Adults:** 15 mg P.O. h.s. Some patients may respond to lower doses. Decrease dosage in elderly patients to 7.5 mg P.O. h.s. after 2 days of therapy.

Adverse reactions

CNS: *fatigue, dizziness, daytime drowsiness, headache.*

Interactions

Alcohol or other CNS depressants, including antihistamines, opiate analgesics, and other benzodiazepines: increased CNS depression.

Nursing diagnoses

- Sleep pattern disturbance related to the patient's underlying problem.
- High risk for trauma related to adverse CNS reactions to quazepam.
- Knowledge deficit related to quazepam therapy.

Nursing interventions

- *Contraindicated* in patients allergic to benzodiazepines, in pregnant patients, and in patients with suspected or established sleep apnea.
- *Use cautiously* in patients with hepatic, renal, or respiratory disease and in elderly patients.
- Warn the patient about the possible additive depressant effects that can occur with alcohol consumption. Additive effects can occur if alcohol is consumed on the day after the use of quazepam.
- Patients who receive prolonged therapy with benzodiazepines may experience withdrawal symptoms if the drug is suddenly stopped (possibly after 6 weeks of continuous therapy).
- Check the patient's CBC before and periodically during long-term therapy. Observe for signs of hematologic toxicity, such as easy bruising or bleeding, or signs of infection.
- Take precautions to prevent hoarding or self-overdosing by patients who are depressed, suicidal, or known drug abusers.
- Supervise walking and use bed rails, especially for elderly patients.
- Warn the patient to avoid driving and other hazardous activities that require alertness until the CNS effects of the drug are known.
- Caution the patient not to increase the drug dosage but to inform the doctor if he feels that the drug is no longer effective.
- If quazepam overdose occurs, administer flumazenil (a specific benzodiazepine antagonist). Know that the duration of action of flumazenil is shorter than that of quazepam; as a consequence, the patient may become resedated.

General

Classification: diuretic, antihypertensive (thiazide). **Pregnancy risk category:** D.

Mechanism of action

Increases urine excretion of sodium and water by inhibiting sodium reabsorption.

Indications and dosage

• Edema, hypertension. **Adults:** 500 mg to 2 g P.O. or I.V. daily or in two divided doses.
• Diuresis. **Children over 6 months:** 20 mg/kg P.O. or I.V. daily in divided doses. **Children under 6 months:** may require 30 mg/kg P.O. or I.V. daily in two divided doses.

Adverse reactions

Blood: ***aplastic anemia, agranulocytosis,*** leukopenia, thrombocytopenia. **CV:** volume depletion and dehydration, orthostatic hypotension. **GI:** anorexia, nausea, pancreatitis. **Hepatic:** hepatic encephalopathy. **Metabolic:** hypokalemia, asymptomatic hyperuricemia, hyperglycemia and glucose tolerance impairment, fluid and electrolyte imbalances including dilutional hyponatremia and hypochloremia, metabolic alkalosis, hypercalcemia, gout. **Skin:** dermatitis, photosensitivity, rash. **Other:** hypersensitivity reactions, such as pneumonitis and vasculitis.

Interactions

Cholestyramine, colestipol: intestinal absorption of thiazides decreased. Separate doses. **Diazoxide:** increased antihypertensive, hyperglycemic, and hyperuricemic effects. Use together cautiously. **NSAIDs:** decreased diuretic effectiveness. Avoid concomitant use.

Nursing diagnoses

• Fluid volume excess related to the patient's underlying condition as evidenced by edema.
• Altered urinary elimination related to chlorothiazide therapy.
• Knowledge deficit related to chlorothiazide therapy.

Nursing interventions

• *Contraindicated* in anuria, hypersensitivity to other thiazides or other sulfonamide-derived drugs, impaired hepatic function, or progressive hepatic disease.
• *Use cautiously* in severe renal disease.
• Monitor intake and output, weight, blood pressure, and serum electrolytes.
• Consult with doctor and dietitian to provide high-potassium diet. Watch for signs of hypokalemia.
• Patients on digitalis glycosides have an increased risk of digitalis toxicity from the potassium-depleting effect of the diuretic. Drug may be used with potassium-sparing diuretic to prevent potassium loss.
• Foods rich in potassium include citrus fruits, tomatoes, bananas, dates, and apricots.
• Monitor blood glucose levels. Check insulin requirements in patients with diabetes. May treat severe hyperglycemia with oral antidiabetic agents.
• Monitor serum creatinine and BUN regularly. Not as effective if levels are more than twice normal.
• Monitor blood uric acid, especially in patients with a history of gout, and serum calcium. Watch for progressive renal impairment.
• **I.V. use:** For I.V. use only—not I.M. or S.C. Reconstitute 500 mg with 18 ml of sterile water for injection. May store reconstituted solutions at room temperature up to 24 hours. Compatible with I.V. dextrose or sodium chloride solutions. Inject reconstituted drug directly into vein, through an I.V. line containing a free-flowing compatible solution, or through an intermittent infusion device. Avoid I.V. infiltration; may be painful.
• Give in a.m. to prevent nocturia. Administer oral form with food (may enhance absorption).
• Elderly patients are prone to excessive diuresis.
• Stop drug before performing parathyroid function tests.
• Advise patient to avoid sudden posture changes and rise slowly to prevent orthostatic hypotension.
• Advise patient to use a sunscreen.

General

Classification: antimalarial (folic acid antagonist with sulfonamide). **Pregnancy risk category:** C.

Mechanism of action

Inhibits the enzyme dihydrofolate reductase, thereby impeding reduction of dihydrofolic acid to tetrahydrofolic acid. Sulfadoxine competitively inhibits PABA.

Indications and dosage

- Acute attacks of malaria. **Adults:** 2 to 3 tablets as a single dose, either alone or in sequence with quinine or primaquine. **Children 9 to 14 years:** 2 tablets. **Children 4 to 8 years:** 1 tablet. **Children under 4 years:** ½ tablet.
- Malaria prophylaxis. **Adults:** 1 tablet weekly, or 2 tablets q 2 weeks. **Children 9 to 14 years:** ¾ tablet weekly, or 1½ tablets q 2 weeks. **Children 4 to 8 years:** ½ tablet weekly, or 1 tablet q 2 weeks. **Children under 4 years:** ¼ tablet weekly, or ½ tablet q 2 weeks.

Adverse reactions

Blood: ***agranulocytosis, aplastic anemia,*** megaloblastic anemia, bone marrow suppression, leukopenia, thrombocytopenia, pancytopenia. **CNS:** stimulation and seizures (acute toxicity). **GI:** anorexia, vomiting, diarrhea, atrophic glossitis. **Skin:** rashes, ***erythema multiforme (Stevens-Johnson syndrome), toxic epidermal necrolysis.***

Interactions

Folic acid, PABA: decreased antitoxoplasmic effects. May require dosage adjustment. **Sulfonamides, co-trimoxazole, methotrexate:** increased adverse effects. Use together cautiously.

Nursing diagnoses

- High risk for injury related to the ineffectiveness of drug to eradicate the infection.
- High risk for impaired skin integrity related to adverse skin reactions to drug.
- Knowledge deficit related to therapy with pyrimethamine with sulfadoxine.

Nursing interventions

- Fansidar is *contraindicated* in porphyria because it contains sulfadoxine, a sulfonamide. *Use cautiously* in impaired hepatic or renal function, severe allergy or bronchial asthma, or G6PD deficiency.
- *Use cautiously* in seizure disorders after treatment with chloroquine.
- Dosages for toxoplasmosis approach toxic levels. Twice-weekly blood counts, including platelets, are needed. If folic or folinic acid deficiency develop, lower dosage or stop drug while the patient receives parenteral folinic acid until blood counts normalize.
- First dose of prophylactic Fansidar should be taken 1 to 2 days before travel to an endemic area.

General

Classification: estrogen replacement, antineoplastic (estrogen). **Pregnancy risk category:** X.

Mechanism of action

Increases the synthesis of DNA, RNA, and protein in responsive tissues. Also reduces release of follicle-stimulating hormone and luteinizing hormone from the pituitary.

Indications and dosage

- Prostatic cancer. **Men:** 12 to 25 mg P.O. daily.
- Atrophic vaginitis. **Women:** 12 to 25 mg P.O. daily for 30 to 60 days.
- Female hypogonadism. **Women:** 12 to 25 mg P.O. for 21 days, followed by 1 dose of progesterone 100 mg I.M. or 5 days of oral progestogen (such as medroxyprogesterone) given concurrently with last 5 days of chlorotrianisene.
- Menopausal symptoms. **Women:** 12 to 25 mg P.O. daily for 30 days or cyclic (3 weeks on, 1 week off).
- Vulvar squamous hyperplasia. **Women:** 12 to 25 mg P.O. daily.

Adverse reactions

CNS: headache, dizziness, chorea, migraine, depression, libido changes. **CV:** thrombophlebitis; ***thromboembolism;*** hypertension; edema; ***increased risk of stroke, pulmonary embolism, and MI.*** **EENT:** worsening of myopia or astigmatism, intolerance to contact lenses. **GI:** *nausea,* vomiting, abdominal cramps, bloating, diarrhea, constipation, anorexia, increased appetite, excessive thirst, weight changes, pancreatitis. **GU:** in women—breakthrough bleeding, altered menstrual flow, dysmenorrhea, amenorrhea, cervical erosion or abnormal secretions, enlargement of uterine fibromas, vaginal candidiasis. In men—*gynecomastia, testicular atrophy, impotence.* **Hepatic:** cholestatic jaundice. **Metabolic:** hyperglycemia, hypercalcemia, folic acid deficiency. **Skin:** melasma, urticaria, acne, seborrhea, oily skin, hirsutism or loss of hair. **Other:** leg cramps, purpura, breast changes.

Interactions

Bromocriptine: may cause amenorrhea, interfering with the effects of bromocriptine. Avoid concomitant use. **Carbamazepine, phenobarbital, rifampin:** decreased effectiveness of estrogen therapy. Monitor closely. **Corticosteroids:** possible enhanced effects. Monitor closely. **Cyclosporine:** increased risk of toxicity. Use together with caution and frequently monitor cyclosporine levels. **Dantrolene, other hepatotoxic medications:** increased risk of hepatotoxicity. Monitor closely. **Oral anticoagulants:** dosage adjustments may be necessary. Monitor PT. **Tamoxifen:** estrogens may interfere with the effectiveness of tamoxifen. Avoid concomitant use.

Nursing diagnoses

- Sexual dysfunction related to the patient's hormonal deficiency.
- Altered tissue perfusion (cerebral, peripheral, cardiopulmonary) related to potential for chlorotrianisene to cause thromboembolism.
- Knowledge deficit related to chlorotrianisene therapy.

Nursing interventions

- *Contraindicated* in thrombophlebitis or thromboembolic disorders; cancer of breast, reproductive organs, or genitals; undiagnosed abnormal genital bleeding; and pregnancy.
- *Use cautiously* in hypertension, asthma, mental depression, bone diseases, blood dyscrasias, gallbladder disease, migraine, seizure disorders, diabetes mellitus, amenorrhea, heart failure, hepatic or renal dysfunction, uterine fibroids, hypercalcemia from metastatic breast disease, and family history (mother, grandmother, sister) of breast or genital tract cancer.
- With long-term therapy, schedule regular physical examinations. Monitor blood pressure, hepatic function, serum lipid levels, and weight.
- Warn patient to immediately report any adverse reactions or suspected pregnancy.

General

Classification: muscle stimulant (cholinesterase inhibitor). **Pregnancy risk category:** C.

Mechanism of action

Inhibits the destruction of acetylcholine released from the parasympathetic and somatic efferent nerves. Acetylcholine accumulates, promoting increased stimulation of the receptor.

Indications and dosage

• Antidote for nondepolarizing neuromuscular blockers. **Adults:** 10 to 20 mg I.V. preceded by atropine sulfate 0.6 to 1.2 mg I.V.

• Myasthenia gravis. **Adults:** 60 to 120 mg P.O. q 3 or 4 hours. Usual dosage is 600 mg daily but higher dosage may be needed (up to 1,500 mg daily). Give ⅓ of oral dose I.M. or I.V. Dosage must be adjusted for each patient, depending on response and tolerance of adverse reactions. Alternatively, may give 180 to 540 mg timed-release tablets (1 to 3 tablets) P.O. b.i.d., with at least 6 hours between doses.

Adverse reactions

CNS: headache (with high doses), weakness, sweating, ***seizures.*** **CV:** bradycardia, hypotension. **EENT:** miosis. **GI:** abdominal cramps, nausea, vomiting, diarrhea, excessive salivation. **Skin:** rash. **Local:** thrombophlebitis. **Other:** ***bronchospasm, bronchoconstriction,*** increased bronchial secretions, muscle cramps, muscle fasciculations.

Interactions

Aminoglycosides, anesthetics: possible decreased response to pyridostigmine. Use together cautiously. **Atropine, anticholinergics, procainamide, quinidine:** possible reversal of cholinergic effects. Observe for lack of drug effect.

Nursing diagnoses

• Altered health maintenance related to the patient's underlying condition.

• Ineffective breathing pattern related to adverse reactions.

• Knowledge deficit related to pyridostigmine therapy.

Nursing interventions

• *Contraindicated* in mechanical obstruction of intestine or urinary tract, bradycardia, or hypotension. *Use with extreme caution* in bronchial asthma.

• *Use cautiously* in seizure disorder, recent coronary occlusion, vagotonia, hyperthyroidism, cardiac arrhythmias, and peptic ulcer. Avoid large doses in decreased GI motility.

• Stop all other cholinergics before giving this drug.

• **I.V. use:** Administer I.V. injection slowly, no faster than 1 mg/minute. If I.V. administration is too rapid, bradycardia and seizures may result. Monitor vital signs frequently, and check respirations carefully. Position patient to ease breathing. Have atropine injection readily available and be prepared to give as ordered; provide respiratory support as needed.

• If weakness is severe, the doctor will determine if it's caused by drug toxicity or exacerbation of myasthenia gravis. Test dose of edrophonium I.V. will aggravate drug-induced weakness but will temporarily relieve weakness caused by disease.

• When used for myasthenia gravis, stress the importance of taking the drug exactly as ordered, on time, in evenly spaced doses.

• Used orally to treat senility associated with Alzheimer's disease.

• Don't crush the timed-release (Timespan or SR) tablets.

• Available as a syrup for patients who have difficulty swallowing. Syrup is sweet; give over ice chips if patient can't tolerate flavor.

• Store tablets in a tightly capped bottle, away from moisture.

chlorphenesin carbamate

Maolate**

General

Classification: skeletal muscle relaxant (carbamate derivative). **Pregnancy risk category:** C.

Mechanism of action

Reduces transmission of impulses from the spinal cord to skeletal muscle.

Indications and dosage

- As an adjunct in short-term, acute, painful musculoskeletal conditions. **Adults:** initial dose is 800 mg P.O. t.i.d. Maintenance dose is 400 mg P.O. q.i.d. for maximum of 8 weeks.
- Trigeminal neuralgia. **Adults:** 400 mg P.O. t.i.d. Usually given upon awakening, at noon, and h.s.

Adverse reactions

Blood: thrombocytopenia, leukopenia, ***agranulocytosis.*** **CNS:** *drowsiness, dizziness,* confusion, headache, weakness. Dose-related adverse reactions include paradoxical stimulation, agitation, insomnia, nervousness, headache. **GI:** *nausea, GI distress.* **Other:** ***anaphylaxis.***

Interactions

Alcohol, CNS depressants: increased CNS depression. Avoid concomitant use.

Nursing diagnoses

- Pain related to the patient's underlying condition.
- High risk for injury related to drug-induced drowsiness.
- Knowledge deficit related to chlorphenesin therapy.

Nursing interventions

- *Use cautiously* in hepatic disease or impaired renal function and in patients with hypersensitivity to aspirin.
- Take with meals or milk to prevent GI distress.
- Amount of relief determines if dosage (and drowsiness) can be reduced.
- Watch for sensitivity reactions, such as fever, skin eruptions, and respiratory distress. Withhold dose and notify doctor of unusual reactions.
- Monitor CBC and platelet studies in patients on long-term therapy. Watch for unusual bleeding and infections that may indicate blood dyscrasias.
- Tell patient to avoid activities that require mental alertness until adverse CNS effects of the drug are known.

pyrazinamide

PMS Pyrazinamide†, Tebrazid†

General

Classification: antitubercular (synethetic pyrazine analogue of nicotinamide). **Pregnancy risk category:** C.

Mechanism of action

Unknown (bacteriostatic).

Indications and dosage

• Adjunctive treatment of tuberculosis (when primary and secondary antitubercular drugs cannot be used or have failed). **Adults:** 20 to 35 mg/kg P.O. daily, divided in three to four doses. Maximum dosage is 3 g daily.

Adverse reactions

Blood: sideroblastic anemia, possible bleeding tendency because of thrombocytopenia. **GI:** anorexia, nausea, vomiting, diarrhea. **GU:** dysuria. **Hepatic:** hepatitis. **Metabolic:** interference with control in diabetes mellitus, *hyperuricemia.* **Other:** malaise, fever, arthralgia.

Interactions

None significant.

Nursing diagnoses

• High risk for injury related to the ineffectiveness of pyrazinamide to eradicate the infection.
• Altered health maintenance related to pyrazinamide-induced gout.
• Knowledge deficit related to pyrazinamide therapy.

Nursing interventions

• *Contraindicated* in patients with severe hepatic disease.
• *Use cautiously* in patients with diabetes mellitus or gout.
• Nearly 100% of the drug is excreted in urine; as a consequence, reduce the dosage in patients with renal impairment.
• Perform liver function studies and examination for jaundice, liver tenderness, or enlargement before and frequently during therapy.
• Watch closely for signs of gout and of hepatic impairment (loss of appetite, fatigue, malaise, jaundice, dark urine, and liver tenderness). Notify doctor at once.
• Question doses that exceed 35 mg/kg because they may cause liver damage.
• Monitor the patient's hematopoietic studies and serum uric acid level.
• When used with surgical management of tuberculosis, start pyrazinamide 1 to 2 weeks before surgery and continue for 4 to 6 weeks postoperatively.

General

Classification: antihistamine (histamine$_1$-receptor antagonist). **Pregnancy risk category:** B.

Mechanism of action

Competes with histamine for H_1-receptor sites on effector cells. Prevents but does not reverse histamine-mediated responses.

Indications and dosage

• Rhinitis, allergy symptoms. **Adults:** 4 mg P.O. q 4 to 6 hours, not to exceed 24 mg/day; or (timed-release) 8 mg P.O. q 12 hours; or 5 to 40 mg I.M., I.V., or S.C. daily. Give I.V. injection over 1 minute. **Children 6 to 12 years:** 2 mg P.O. q 4 to 6 hours, not to exceed 12 mg/day. Alternatively, may give 8 mg (timed-release) h.s. **Children 2 to 6 years:** 1 mg P.O. q 4 to 6 hours.

Note: Children under 12 years should use only as directed by a doctor.

Adverse reactions

CNS: *stimulation,* sedation, *drowsiness* (especially in elderly patients), excitability (in children). **CV:** hypotension, palpitations. **GI:** epigastric distress, *dry mouth.* **GU:** urine retention. **Skin:** rash, urticaria. **Other:** thick bronchial secretions. **After parenteral administration:** local stinging, burning sensation, pallor, weak pulse, transient hypotension.

Interactions

CNS depressants: increased sedation. Use together cautiously. **MAO inhibitors:** increased anticholinergic effects. Don't use together.

Nursing diagnoses

• Ineffective airway clearance related to the patient's underlying condition.
• High risk for injury related to chlorpheniramine-induced adverse CNS reactions.
• Knowledge deficit related to chlorpheniramine therapy.

Nursing interventions

• *Contraindicated* in acute asthmatic attacks.
• *Use cautiously* in elderly patients and in increased intraocular pressure, hyperthyroidism, CV or renal disease, hypertension, bronchial asthma, urine retention, prostatic hypertrophy, bladder-neck obstruction, and stenosing peptic ulcers.
• Warn patient against drinking alcoholic beverages and using other CNS depressants during therapy and against driving or other activities that require alertness until CNS response to drug is determined.
• Coffee or tea may reduce drowsiness. Sugarless gum or sour hard candy or ice chips may relieve dry mouth.
• If tolerance develops, another antihistamine may be substituted.
• Warn patient to stop taking drug 4 days before allergy skin tests to preserve accuracy of tests.
• **I.V. use:** Only injectable forms without preservatives can be given I.V. Give slowly.
• If symptoms occur during or after parenteral dose, discontinue drug. Notify doctor.
• Because of the potential risk to the infant, antihistamines are not recommended for use by women who are breast-feeding because small amounts of drug are excreted in breast milk.

pyrantel pamoate

Antiminth, Combantrin†

General

Classification: anthelmintic (pyrimidine derivative). **Pregnancy risk category:** C.

Mechanism of action

Blocks neuromuscular action, paralyzing the worm and causing its expulsion by normal peristalsis.

Indications and dosage

• Roundworm and pinworm. **Adults and children over 2 years:** single dosage of 11 mg/kg P.O. Maximum dosage 1 g. For pinworm, dosage should be repeated in 2 weeks.

Adverse reactions

CNS: headache, dizziness, drowsiness, insomnia. **GI:** anorexia, nausea, vomiting, gastralgia, cramps, diarrhea, tenesmus. **Hepatic:** transient elevation of AST (SGOT). **Skin:** rashes. **Other:** fever, weakness.

Interactions

Piperazine salts: possible antagonism; don't give together.

Nursing diagnoses

• Altered health maintenance related to ineffectiveness of pyrantel.
• Knowledge deficit related to pyrantel therapy.

Nursing interventions

• *Use cautiously* in severe malnutrition or anemia or in hepatic dysfunction. Treat for anemia, dehydration, or malnutrition before giving drug.
• No dietary restrictions, laxatives, or enemas are necessary.
• May be taken with food, milk, or fruit juices. Shake suspension well.
• Treat all family members.
• Teach patient about the need for good personal hygiene, especially good handwashing technique. To avoid reinfection, teach him to wash perianal area daily, to change undergarments and bedclothes daily, and to wash hands and clean fingernails before meals and after bowel movements. Advise patient to refrain from preparing food during infestation.
• Protect drug from light. Store below 86° F (30° C).

chlorpromazine hydrochloride

Chlorpromanyl†, Novo-Chlorpromazine†, Thorazine

General

Classification: antipsychotic, antiemetic (phenothiazine). **Pregnancy risk category:** C.

Mechanism of action

Blocks postsynaptic dopamine receptors in the brain and inhibits the chemoreceptor trigger zone.

Indications and dosage

- Intractable hiccups. **Adults:** 25 to 50 mg P.O. or I.M. t.i.d. or q.i.d.
- Mild alcohol withdrawal, acute intermittent porphyria, tetanus. **Adults:** 25 to 50 mg I.M. t.i.d. or q.i.d.
- Psychosis. **Adults:** initially, 30 to 75 mg P.O. daily in two to four divided doses, increased by 20 to 50 mg twice weekly until symptoms are controlled; some patients may require up to 800 mg daily. Or give 25 to 50 mg I.M. q 1 to 4 hours p.r.n. Switch to oral therapy as soon as possible. **Children:** 0.25 mg/kg P.O. q 4 to 6 hours; or 0.25 mg/kg I.M. q 6 to 8 hours; or 0.5 mg/kg P.R. q 6 to 8 hours. Maximum I.M. dose – 40 mg in children under 5 years; 75 mg in children 5 to 12 years.
- Nausea and vomiting. **Adults:** 10 to 25 mg P.O. or I.M. q 4 to 6 hours, p.r.n.; or 50 to 100 mg P.R. q 6 to 8 hours, p.r.n. **Children:** 0.25 mg/kg P.O. q 4 to 6 hours; or 0.25 mg/kg I.M. q 6 to 8 hours; or 0.5 mg/kg P.R. q 6 to 8 hours.

C

Adverse reactions

Blood: transient leukopenia, ***agranulocytosis.*** **CNS:** *extrapyramidal reactions, sedation, tardive dyskinesia,* pseudoparkinsonism, EEG changes, dizziness. **CV:** *orthostatic hypotension,* tachycardia, ECG changes. **EENT:** ocular changes, *blurred vision.* **GI:** dry mouth, constipation. **GU:** *urine retention, dark urine, menstrual irregularities, gynecomastia, inhibited ejaculation.* **Hepatic:** cholestatic jaundice, abnormal liver function tests. **Metabolic:** hyperprolactinemia. **Skin:** *photosensitivity,* allergic reactions. **Local:** *pain on I.M. injection,* sterile abscess. **Other:** weight gain; increased appetite; rarely, ***neuroleptic malignant syndrome.*** **After abrupt withdrawal of long-term therapy:** gastritis, nausea, vomiting, dizziness, tremor, sweating, tachycardia, headache, insomnia.

Interactions

Alcohol, other CNS depressants: increased CNS depression. Avoid concomitant use. **Antacids:** inhibit absorption of oral phenothiazines. Separate doses of each by 2 hours. **Anticholinergics (including antidepressant and antiparkinsonian agents):** increased anticholinergic activity, aggravated parkinsonian symptoms. Use with caution. **Antihypertensives:** decreased a antihypertensive effect. **Barbiturates, lithium:** may decrease phenothiazine effect. Observe patient. **Oral anticoagulants:** decreased anticoagulant effect. **Propranolol:** increased levels of both drugs.

Nursing diagnoses

- Altered health maintenance related to patient's underlying condition.
- Impaired physical mobility related to extrapyramidal effects of adverse drug reactions.
- Knowledge deficit related to chlorpromazine therapy.

Nursing interventions

- *Contraindicated* in CNS depression, bone marrow suppresion, subcortical damage, Reye's syndrome, and coma and with use of spinal or edidural anesthetics or adrenergic blockers.
- *Use cautiously* in hepatic or CV disease, arteriosclerosis, exposure to extreme heat or cold, respiratory disorders, hypocalcemia, seizure disorders, suspected brain tumor or GI obstruction, glaucoma, and prostatic hypertrophy; in elderly or debilitated patients; and in ill or dehydrated children. Use parenteral form cautiously in asthma and hypersensitivity to sulfites.
- Hold dose and notify doctor if patient develops jaundice, symptoms of blood dyscrasias, or persistent extrapyramidal reactions.
- Periodically evaluate bilirubin level, CBC, liver function tests, and ocular examination.

General
Classification: bulk laxative (adsorbant). **Pregnancy risk category:** C.

Mechanism of action
Absorbs water and expands to increase bulk and moisture content of the stool. The increased bulk encourages peristalsis and bowel movement.

Indications and dosage
• Constipation; bowel management. **Adults:** 1 to 2 rounded teaspoonfuls P.O. in full glass of liquid daily, b.i.d. or t.i.d., followed by second glass of liquid; or 1 packet P.O. dissolved in water daily, b.i.d. or t.i.d. **Children over 6 years:** 1 level teaspoonful P.O. in half a glass of liquid h.s.

Adverse reactions
GI: nausea, vomiting, diarrhea, all after excessive use; esophageal, gastric, small intestinal, or colonic strictures when drug taken in dry form; abdominal cramps, especially in severe constipation.

Interactions
None significant.

Nursing diagnoses
• Constipation related to interruption of the normal pattern of elimination characterized by infrequent or absent stools.
• Pain related to psyllium-induced abdominal cramping.
• Knowledge deficit related to psyllium therapy.

Nursing interventions
• *Contraindicated* in abdominal pain, nausea, vomiting, or other signs and symptoms of appendicitis and in intestinal obstruction or ulceration, disabling adhesion, or difficulty swallowing.
• In diabetic patients, use brand of psyllium that does not contain sugar. Check label.
• Mix with at least 8 oz (240 ml) of cold, pleasant-tasting liquid such as orange juice to mask grittiness, and stir only a few seconds. Patient should drink the mixture immediately or it will congeal. Follow with an additional glass of liquid.
• Before giving for constipation, determine if the patient has adequate fluid intake, exercise, and diet. Tell him that dietary sources of bulk include bran and other cereals, fresh fruit, and vegetables.
• May reduce appetite if taken before meals.
• Laxative effect usually seen in 12 to 24 hours, but may be delayed for 3 days.
• Psyllium isn't absorbed systemically; nontoxic. Especially useful in postpartum constipation, debilitated patients, chronic laxative abuse, irritable bowel syndrome, and diverticular disease and in combination with other laxatives to empty colon before barium enema examinations.

chlorpropamide

Apo-Chlorpropamide†, Diabinese, Glucamide, Novo-propamide†

General

Classification: antidiabetic, antidiuretic (sulfonylurea). **Pregnancy risk category:** D.

Mechanism of action

Stimulates insulin release from the pancreatic beta cells and reduces glucose output by the liver. An extrapancreatic effect increases peripheral sensitivity to insulin. Also exerts an antidiuretic effect in patients with pituitary-deficient diabetes insipidus.

Indications and dosage

- Adjunct to diet in type II (non-insulin-dependent) diabetes to lower blood glucose. **Adults:** 250 mg P.O. daily with breakfast or in divided doses if GI upset occurs. First dosage increase may be made after 5 to 7 days because of extended duration of action, then dosage may be increased q 3 to 5 days by 50 to 125 mg, if needed, up to 750 mg daily. **Adults over 65 years:** initially, 100 to 125 mg P.O. daily, increased as needed and tolerated.
- Change from insulin to oral therapy. **Adults:** if insulin dosage is less than 40 units daily, stop insulin and start oral therapy as above. If insulin dosage is 40 units or more daily, start oral therapy as above with insulin reduced 50%. Base further reductions on patient response.

Adverse reactions

GI: nausea, heartburn, vomiting. **GU:** tea-colored urine. **Metabolic:** ***prolonged hypoglycemia, dilutional hyponatremia.*** **Skin:** rash, pruritus, facial flushing. **Other:** ***hypersensitivity reactions.***

Interactions

Anabolic steroids, chloramphenicol, clofibrate, guanethidine, MAO inhibitors, phenylbutazone, salicylates, sulfonamides: increased hypoglycemic activity. Monitor blood glucose level. **Beta blockers, clonidine:** prolonged hypoglycemic effect and masked symptoms of hypoglycemia. Use together cautiously. **Corticosteroids, glucagon, rifampin, thiazide diuretics:** decreased hypoglycemic response. Monitor blood glucose level. **Hydantoins:** increased blood levels of hydantoins. Monitor blood levels. **Oral anticoagulants:** increased hypoglycemic activity or enhanced anticoagulant effect. Monitor blood glucose and prothrombin time.

Nursing diagnoses

- Altered nutrition: More than body requirements, related to the patient's inability to release insulin to maintain normal blood glucose levels.
- High risk for injury related to chlorpropamide-induced hypoglycemia.
- Knowledge deficit related to chlorpropamide therapy.

Nursing interventions

- *Contraindicated* in pregnancy and breast-feeding and in treatment of type I (insulin-dependent) diabetes, diabetes mellitus adequately controlled by diet, and type II (non-insulin-dependent) diabetes complicated by fever, ketosis, acidosis, diabetic coma, major surgery, severe trauma, Raynaud's disease, gangrene, renal or hepatic impairment, or thyroid or other endocrine dysfunction.
- *Use cautiously* in patients with sulfonamide hypersensitivity.
- Instruct patient about nature of the disease; importance of following therapeutic regimen; adhering to diet, weight reduction, exercise, and personal hygiene programs; precautions to avoid infection; how and when to perform self-monitoring of blood glucose level; and recognition of and intervention for hypoglycemia and hyperglycemia.
- Hospitalization during transition from insulin therapy to an oral antidiabetic may be needed; monitor blood glucose levels t.i.d. before meals.
- Report signs of renal insufficiency, such as dysuria, anuria, and hematuria, to doctor.
- Advise patient to check with doctor before changing drug dosage or taking any other medications, including OTC drugs.
- Advise patient to carry a medical identification bracelet identifying him as a diabetic patient.

pseudoephedrine

Cenafed◇, Children's Sudafed Liquid◇, Pediacare Infant's Oral Decongestant Drops◇, Sinufed◇, Sudafed◇; Afrinol Repetabs

General

Classification: decongestant (adrenergic). **Pregnancy risk category:** C.

Mechanism of action

Stimulates alpha-adrenergic receptors in the respiratory tract, producing vasoconstriction.

Indications and dosage

- Nasal and eustachian tube decongestant. **Adults:** 60 mg P.O. (hydrochloride) q 4 hours. Maximum dosage is 240 mg daily. **Children 6 to 12 years:** 30 mg P.O. (hydrochloride) q 4 to 6 hours. Maximum dosage is 120 mg daily. **Children 2 to 6 years:** 15 mg P.O. (hydrochloride) q 4 hours. Maximum dosage is 60 mg/day.
- Extended-release tablets (hydrochloride, sulfate). **Adults and children over 12 years:** 120 mg P.O. q 12 hours. This form is contraindicated for children under 12 years.
- Relief of nasal congestion. **Adults:** 120 mg P.O. (hydrochloride) q 12 hours.

Adverse reactions

CNS: transient stimulation, tremor, dizziness, headache, insomnia, *nervousness*. **CV:** arrhythmias, *palpitations*, tachycardia. **GI:** dry mouth, anorexia, nausea, vomiting. **GU:** difficulty in urinating. **Skin:** pallor.

Interactions

Antihypertensives: possible attenuated hypotensive effect. **MAO inhibitors:** possible hypertensive crisis. Don't use together.

Nursing diagnoses

- Ineffective airway clearance related to the patient's underlying condition.
- Altered oral mucous membrane related to adverse drug reaction.
- Knowledge deficit related to pseudoephedrine therapy.

Nursing interventions

- *Contraindicated* in severe hypertension or severe coronary artery disease; in patients receiving MAO inhibitors; and in breast-feeding women.
- *Use cautiously* in hypertension, cardiac disease, diabetes, glaucoma, hyperthyroidism, and prostatic hypertrophy.
- Elderly patients are more sensitive to the drug's effects.
- Tell the patient to stop the drug if he becomes unusually restless and to notify the doctor promptly.
- Warn against using OTC products containing other sympathomimetics.
- Tell the patient not to take the drug within 2 hours of bedtime because it can cause insomnia.
- Tell patient to relieve dry mouth with sugarless gum or hard candy.
- Don't crush or break extended-release dosage forms.

General
Classification: antipsychotic (thiothexene). **Pregnancy risk category:** C.

Mechanism of action
Blocks postsynaptic dopamine receptors in the brain.

Indications and dosage
- Psychotic disorders. **Adults:** initially, 10 mg P.O. t.i.d. or q.i.d., increased as needed to maximum of 600 mg daily. **Children over 6 years:** 10 to 25 mg P.O. t.i.d. or q.i.d.
- Agitation of severe neurosis, depression, schizophrenia. **Adults:** 25 to 50 mg P.O. or I.M. t.i.d. or q.i.d., increased as needed up to maximum of 600 mg daily.

Adverse reactions
Blood: transient leukopenia, ***agranulocytosis.*** **CNS:** extrapyramidal reactions, tardive dyskinesia, *sedation,* pseudoparkinsonism, EEG changes, dizziness. **CV:** *orthostatic hypotension,* tachycardia, ECG changes. **EENT:** ocular changes, *blurred vision.* **GI:** dry mouth, constipation. **GU:** *urine retention,* dark urine, menstrual irregularities, gynecomastia, inhibited ejaculation. **Hepatic:** cholestatic jaundice, abnormal liver function tests. **Metabolic:** hyperprolactinemia. **Skin:** *photosensitivity,* allergic reactions. **Local:** pain on I.M. injection, sterile abscess. **Other:** weight gain; increased appetite; rarely, ***neuroleptic malignant syndrome.*** **After abrupt withdrawal of long-term therapy:** gastritis, nausea, vomiting, dizziness, tremor, sweating, tachycardia, headache, insomnia.

Interactions
Alcohol, other CNS depressants: increased CNS depression. Avoid concomitant use. **Anticholinergics:** potentiated central anticholinergic effects. Use together cautiously. **Centrally acting antihypertensives:** decreased antihypertensive effect.

Nursing diagnoses
- Impaired thought processes related to the patient's underlying condition.
- Urinary retention related to adverse drug reaction.
- Knowledge deficit related to chlorprothixene therapy.

Nursing interventions
- *Contraindicated* in coma, CNS depression, bone marrow suppression, circulatory collapse, CHF, cardiac decompensation, coronary artery or cerebrovascular disorders, and subcortical damage and with use of spinal or epidural anesthetic or adrenergic blockers.
- *Use cautiously* in elderly or debilitated patients; in hepatic or renal disease, arteriosclerosis or CV disease, exposure to extreme heat or cold, respiratory disorders, hypocalcemia, seizure disorders, suspected brain tumor or GI obstruction, glaucoma, or prostatic hypertrophy; and in acutely ill or dehydrated children.
- Watch for signs of neuroleptic malignant syndrome.
- Hold dose and notify doctor if patient develops symptoms of blood dyscrasias, jaundice, or persistent extrapyramidal reactions.
- Periodically evaluate bilirubin levels, CBC, liver function tests, and ocular examinations.
- Warn against activities requiring alertness until CNS effects of the drug are known. Advise patient to use sunscreen.
- Obtain baseline measures of blood pressure before therapy and monitor regularly. Watch for orthostatic hypotension. Keep patient in a supine position for 1 hour afterward and advise him to change positions slowly.
- Give deep I.M. only in upper outer quadrant of buttocks or midlateral thigh. Massage injection site afterward to prevent sterile abscess.
- Dilute liquid concentrate with fruit juice, milk, or semisolid food just before administration.
- Keep drug off skin and clothes.
- A 100-mg dose of chlorprothixene is the therapeutic equivalent of 100 mg of chlorpromazine.

General

Classification: antidepressant (tricyclic). **Pregnancy risk category:** C.

Mechanism of action

Increases the amount of norepinephrine or serotonin, or both, in the CNS by blocking their reuptake by the presynaptic neurons. This allows these neurotransmitters to accumulate.

Indications and dosage

- Depression. **Adults:** 15 to 40 mg P.O. daily in divided doses, increasing gradually to maximum of 60 mg daily.

Adverse reactions

CNS: excitation, ***seizures,*** tremor, weakness, confusion, headache, nervousness, EEG changes, extrapyramidal reactions. **CV:** *tachycardia, ECG changes, orthostatic hypotension, hypertension.* **EENT:** *blurred vision,* tinnitus, mydriasis. **GI:** *dry mouth, constipation,* nausea, vomiting, anorexia, paralytic ileus. **GU:** *urine retention.* **Skin:** rash, urticaria, photosensitivity. **Other:** *sweating,* allergy. **After abrupt withdrawal of long-term therapy:** nausea, headache, malaise (does not indicate addiction).

Interactions

Barbiturates: decreased TCA blood levels. Monitor for decreased antidepressant effect. **Cimetidine:** possible increased protriptyline levels. Monitor for increased adverse reactions. **Epinephrine, norepinephrine:** increased hypertensive effect. Use with caution. **MAO inhibitors:** possible severe excitation, hyperpyrexia, seizures, and death, usually with high dose. Use together cautiously. **Methylphenidate:** increased TCA blood levels. Monitor for enhanced antidepressant effect.

Nursing diagnoses

- Ineffective individual coping related to the patient's underlying condition.
- Constipation related to adverse GI reactions to protriptyline.
- Knowledge deficit related to protriptyline.

Nursing interventions

- *Contraindicated* during acute recovery phase of MI, in prostatic hypertrophy, and in seizure disorders.
- *Use cautiously* in elderly patients and in CV disease, urine retention, increased intraocular tension, thyroid disease, or blood dyscrasias; in patients at risk for suicide; and in those receiving electroshock therapy, thyroid drugs, or elective surgery.
- Protriptyline has anticholinergic effects. Dry mouth may be relieved with sugarless hard candy or gum, or saliva substitutes if necessary.
- Check for urine retention and constipation. Increase fluids to lessen constipation. Suggest stool softener or high-fiber diet, if needed.
- Protriptyline has low potential for producing orthostatic hypotension and is the least sedating of the TCAs. It may even have amphetamine-like effects. Avoid late-day dosing to prevent insomnia.
- Reduce dosage in elderly or debilitated patients and adolescents.
- Do not withdraw drug abruptly.
- Watch for increased psychotic signs, anxiety, agitation, or CV reactions; dosage should be reduced if they occur. Record mood changes. Watch for suicidal tendencies. To lessen suicide risk, allow minimum supply of tablets.
- Expect a delay of 2 weeks or more before noticeable effect; 4 weeks or more before full effect.
- Warn patient not to use other drugs without first consulting the doctor. Avoid combining with alcohol or other depressants.
- Used investigationally to treat obstructive sleep apnea.
- Because hypertensive episodes have occurred during surgery in patients receiving TCAs, these drugs should be discontinued several days before surgery.
- Some patients may experience photosensitivity reactions.

chlorthalidone

Apo-Chlorthalidone†, Hygroton, Novo-Thalidone†, Thalitone, Uridon†

General

Classification: diuretic, antihypertensive (thiazide-like diuretic). **Pregnancy risk category:** D.

Mechanism of action

Although not a thiazide, chlorthalidone acts in a similar fashion. It increases urine excretion of sodium and water by inhibiting sodium reabsorption in the cortical diluting site of the nephron.

Indications and dosage

• Edema, hypertension. **Adults:** 25 to 100 mg P.O. daily, or 100 mg 3 times weekly or on alternate days. **Children:** 2 mg/kg P.O. 3 times weekly.

Adverse reactions

Blood: ***aplastic anemia, agranulocytosis,*** leukopenia, thrombocytopenia. **CV:** volume depletion and dehydration, orthostatic hypotension. **GI:** anorexia, nausea, pancreatitis. **GU:** impotence. **Hepatic:** hepatic encephalopathy. **Metabolic:** hypokalemia, asymptomatic hyperuricemia, hyperglycemia and impairment of glucose tolerance, fluid and electrolyte imbalances including dilutional hyponatremia and hypochloremia, metabolic alkalosis, hypercalcemia, gout. **Skin:** dermatitis, photosensitivity, rash. **Other:** hypersensitivity reactions, such as pneumonitis and vasculitis.

Interactions

Cholestyramine, colestipol: intestinal absorption of thiazides decreased. Keep doses as separate as possible. **Diazoxide:** increased antihypertensive, hyperglycemic, and hyperuricemic effects. Use together cautiously. **NSAIDs:** decreased diuretic effectiveness. Avoid concomitant use.

Nursing diagnoses

• Fluid volume excess related to the patient's underlying condition as evidenced by edema.
• Altered urinary elimination related to chlorthalidone therapy.
• Knowledge deficit related to chlorthalidone therapy.

Nursing interventions

• *Contraindicated* in anuria or in hypersensitivity to thiazides or other sulfonamide-derived drugs.
• *Use cautiously* in severe renal disease, progressive hepatic disease, and impaired hepatic function.
• Monitor intake and output, weight, blood pressure, and serum electrolytes.
• Consult with doctor and dietitian to provide high-potassium diet. Watch for signs of hypokalemia (for example, muscle weakness and cramps). Patients on digitalis glycosides have an increased risk of digitalis toxicity from the potassium-depleting effect of this diuretic. Drug may be used with potassium-sparing diuretic to prevent potassium loss.
• Foods rich in potassium include citrus fruits, tomatoes, bananas, dates, and apricots.
• Monitor serum creatinine and BUN levels regularly. Drug isn't as effective if these are more than twice normal.
• Monitor blood uric acid, especially in patients with a history of gout.
• Monitor blood glucose levels. Check insulin requirements in patients with diabetes. May treat severe hyperglycemia with oral antidiabetic agents.
• In hypertension, therapeutic response may be delayed several days.
• Give in a.m. to prevent nocturia.
• Elderly patients are especially susceptible to excessive diuresis.
• Discontinue chlorthalidone before parathyroid function tests.
• Advise patient to avoid sudden postural changes and rise slowly to prevent orthostatic hypotension.
• Advise patient to use a sunscreen.
• Notice that Uridon tablets (available in Canada only) should not be confused with the urinary anti-infective Uridon Modified (available in the United States).

General

Classification: antihyperthyroid agent (thyroid hormone antagonist). **Pregnancy risk category:** D.

Mechanism of action

Inhibits oxidation of iodine in the thyroid gland, blocking iodine's ability to combine with tyrosine to form thyroxine. May also prevent the coupling of monoiodotyrosine and diiodotyrosine to form thyroxine and triiodothyronine.

Indications and dosage

- Hyperthyroidism. **Adults:** 100 mg P.O. t.i.d.; up to 300 mg q 8 hours have been used in severe cases. Continue until patient is euthyroid, then start maintenance dosage of 100 mg daily to t.i.d. **Children over 10 years:** 100 mg P.O. t.i.d. Continue until patient is euthyroid, then start maintenance dosage of 25 mg t.i.d. to 100 mg b.i.d. **Children 6 to 10 years:** 50 to 150 mg P.O. divided doses q 8 hours.
- Preparation for thyroidectomy. **Adults and children:** same doses as for hyperthyroidism, then iodine may be added 10 days before surgery.
- Thyrotoxic crisis. **Adults and children:** same doses as for hyperthyroidism, with concomitant iodine therapy and propranolol.

Adverse reactions

Blood: ***agranulocytosis,*** leukopenia, thrombocytopenia (appear to be dose-related). **CNS:** headache, drowsiness, vertigo. **EENT:** visual disturbances. **GI:** diarrhea, *nausea, vomiting* (may be dose-related). **Hepatic:** jaundice, ***hepatotoxicity.*** **Skin:** rash, urticaria, skin discoloration, pruritus. **Other:** arthralgia, myalgia, salivary gland enlargement, loss of taste, drug fever, lymphadenopathy, vasculitis.

Interactions

None significant.

Nursing diagnoses

- Activity intolerance related to inceased metabolic rate.
- High risk for fluid volume deficit related to propylthiouracil-induced GI reaction.
- Knowledge deficit related to propylthiouracil therapy.

Nursing interventions

- *Use cautiously* in pregnancy. Less drug may be required as pregnancy progresses. Monitor thyroid function studies closely; thyroid may be added to regimen. Drugs may be stopped during last few weeks of pregnancy.
- Also use cautiously in breast-feeding women. Although drug appears in small amounts in breast milk, it appears safe for use by breast-feeding mothers if the infant's thyroid function is monitored at weekly or biweekly intervals.
- Watch for signs of hypothyroidism (depression; cold intolerance; hard, nonpitting edema). Dosage may need to be adjusted.
- Monitor CBC periodically to detect impending leukopenia, thrombocytopenia, and agranulocytosis.
- Warn patient to report immediately: fever, sore throat, or mouth sores (possible signs of developing agranulocytosis). Agranulocytosis can develop too rapidly to be detected by periodic blood cell counts.
- Tell patient to also report skin eruptions (sign of hypersensitivity) immediately.
- Stop drug if severe rash or enlarged cervical lymph nodes develop.
- Tell patient to ask doctor about using iodized salt and eating shellfish during treatment.
- Warn patient against OTC cough medicines; many contain iodine.
- Give drug with meals to reduce adverse GI reactions.
- Store drug in light-resistant container.

General
Classification: skeletal muscle relaxant (benzoxazole derivative). **Pregnancy risk category:** C.

Mechanism of action
Precise mechanism unknown; reduces transmission of impulses from the spinal cord to skeletal muscle.

Indications and dosage
- As an adjunct in acute, painful musculoskeletal conditions. **Adults:** 250 to 750 mg P.O. t.i.d. or q.i.d. **Children:** 20 mg/kg P.O. daily in divided doses t.i.d. or q.i.d.

Adverse reactions
Blood: anemia, granulocytopenia. **CNS:** *drowsiness, dizziness, light-headedness,* malaise, headache, overstimulation. **GI:** anorexia, nausea, vomiting, heartburn, abdominal distress, constipation, diarrhea. **GU:** urine discoloration (orange or purple-red). **Hepatic:** hepatic dysfunction. **Skin:** urticaria, redness, itching, petechiae, bruising.

Interactions
Alcohol and CNS depressants: increased CNS depression. Avoid concomitant use.

Nursing diagnoses
- Pain related to the patient's underlying condition.
- High risk for injury related to chlorzoxazone-induced drowsiness.
- Knowledge deficit related to chlorzoxazone therapy.

Nursing interventions
- *Contraindicated* in impaired hepatic function.
- *Use cautiously* in history of drug allergies.
- Amount of relief determines if dosage (and drowsiness) can be reduced.
- Watch for signs of hepatic dysfunction. Withhold dose and notify doctor.
- Warn patient to avoid activities that require alertness until CNS effects of the drug are known.
- Avoid combining with alcohol or other depressants.
- Tell patient that the drug may discolor urine orange or purple-red.
- Advise patient to follow doctor's orders regarding physical activity.
- Give with meals or milk to prevent GI distress.

General

Classification: antihypertensive, antianginal, antiarrhythmic; adjunctive therapy for migraine or MI (beta-adrenergic blocker). **Pregnancy risk category:** C.

Mechanism of action

Reduces cardiac oxygen demand by blocking catecholamine-induced increases in heart rate, blood pressure, and force of myocardial contraction. Depresses renin secretion. Prevents vasodilation of cerebral arteries.

Indications and dosage

• Angina pectoris. **Adults:** 10 to 20 mg P.O. t.i.d. or q.i.d. Or one 80-mg sustained-release capsule daily. Dosage may be increased at 7- to 10-day intervals. The average optimum dosage is 160 mg daily.

• Reduction of mortality after MI. **Adults:** 180 to 240 mg P.O. daily in divided doses. Usually given t.i.d. to q.i.d.

• Supraventricular, ventricular, and atrial arrhythmias; tachyarrhythmias caused by excessive catecholamine action during anesthesia, hyperthyroidism, and pheochromocytoma. **Adults:** 1 to 3 mg by slow I.V. push, not to exceed 1 mg/minute. After 3 mg have been given, another dose may be given in 2 minutes; subsequent doses, no sooner than q 4 hours. Drug may be given by direct injection or diluted in 50 ml D_5W or 0.9% sodium chloride solution and infused slowly. Usual maintenance dose is 10 to 80 mg P.O. t.i.d. to q.i.d.

• Hypertension. **Adults:** initially, 80 mg P.O. daily in two to four divided doses or sustained-release form once daily. Increase at 3- to 7-day intervals to maximum daily dosage of 640 mg. Usual maintenance dosage is 160 to 480 mg daily.

• Prevention of frequent, severe, uncontrollable, or disabling migraine or vascular headache. **Adults:** initially, 80 mg P.O. daily in divided doses or 1 sustained-release capsule daily. Usual maintenance dosage is 160 to 240 mg daily, divided t.i.d. or q.i.d.

Adverse reactions

CNS: *fatigue, lethargy,* hallucinations, vivid dreams.
CV: *bradycardia, hypotension,* ***CHF,*** peripheral vascular disease. **GI:** nausea, vomiting, diarrhea. **Metabolic:** hypoglycemia. **Skin:** rash. **Other:** *increased airway resistance, fever, arthralgia.*

Interactions

Aminophylline: antagonized beta-blocking effects. **Cimetidine:** inhibited propranolol metabolism. **Digitalis glycosides, verapamil:** excessive bradycardia and increased myocardial depression. **Epinephrine:** severe vasoconstriction. **Insulin, oral antidiabetic agents:** altered requirements for these in previously stable diabetics. **Isoproterenol, glucagon:** antagonized propranolol effect.

Nursing diagnoses

• Pain related to ineffectiveness of propranolol.
• Fluid volume excess related to drug-induced CHF.
• Knowledge deficit related to propranolol therapy.

Nursing interventions

• *Contraindicated* in diabetes mellitus, asthma, allergic rhinitis, sinus bradycardia, heart block greater than first degree, cardiogenic shock, and right ventricular failure from pulmonary hypertension.
• *Use cautiously* in CHF or respiratory disease.
• If you detect extremes in apical pulse rates, withhold drug and call the doctor immediately.
• Monitor blood pressure, ECG, heart rate and rhythm frequently, especially with I.V. use.
• After prolonged atrial fibrillation, restoring normal rhythm may cause thromboembolism. Anticoagulants often advised before restoring normal rhythm.
• Tell patient to take drug as prescribed, even when he's feeling well; abrupt cessation of drug can exacerbate angina and MI.
• Masks common signs of shock and hypoglycemia.
• Food may increase absorption. Give with meals.
• For overdose, may give I.V. isoproterenol or atropine; refractory cases may require pacemaker.

General

Classification: antilipemic, bile acid sequestrant (anion exchange resin). **Pregnancy risk category:** C.

Mechanism of action

Combines with bile acid to form an insoluble compound that is excreted. The liver must synthesize new bile acid from cholesterol; this leads to reduced low-density-lipoprotein cholesterol levels.

Indications and dosage

• Primary hyperlipidemia, pruritus, and diarrhea due to excess bile acid; as adjunctive therapy for reduction of elevated serum cholesterol in patients with primary hypercholesterolemia; to reduce risk of atherosclerotic coronary artery disease and MI. **Adults:** 4 g before meals and h.s., not to exceed 32 g daily. Each scoop or packet of Questran contains 4 g cholestyramine. Also available as Cholybar, a chewable candy bar (raspberry or caramel flavored) containing 4 g cholestyramine. **Children:** 240 mg/kg daily P.O. in three divided doses with beverage or food. Safe dosage not established for children under 6 years.

Adverse reactions

GI: *constipation,* fecal impaction, hemorrhoids, *abdominal discomfort,* flatulence, *nausea,* vomiting, steatorrhea. **Skin:** *rashes;* irritation of skin, tongue, and perianal area. **Other:** *vitamin A, D, and K deficiency from decreased absorption;* hyperchloremic acidosis (long-term or high dosage).

Interactions

Acetaminophen, coumarin anticoagulants, beta-adrenergic blockers, corticosteroids, digitalis glycosides, fat-soluble vitamins (A, D, E, and K), iron preparations, thiazide diuretics, thyroid hormone: absorption may be substantially decreased by cholestyramine. Separate administration times by at least 2 hours.

Nursing diagnoses

• High risk for injury related to ineffectiveness of cholestyramine to lower blood lipid and cholesterol levels.
• Constipation related to adverse drug reactions.
• Knowledge deficit related to cholestyramine.

Nursing interventions

• *Contraindicated* in hypersensitivity to bile acid sequestering resins and in complete biliary obstruction.
• *Use cautiously* in patients predisposed to constipation and in patients with conditions that may be aggravated by constipation, such as severe, symptomatic coronary artery disease. Long-term use may be associated with deficiency of vitamins A, D, E, and K and folic acid.
• Inform patients who are taking this drug to reduce the risks of atherosclerotic heart disease and to be aware of other cardiac disease risk factors. Recommend weight control and stop-smoking programs.
• Monitor serum cholesterol and triglyceride levels regularly. Teach the patient about proper dietary management (restricting total fat and cholesterol intake), weight control, and exercise and their importance in controlling elevated serum lipids.
• To mix powder, sprinkle powder on surface of beverage or wet food. Let stand a few minutes, then stir.
• Mixing with carbonated beverages may result in excess foaming. Use large glass and mix slowly.
• Administer all other medications at least 1 hour before or 4 to 6 hours after cholestyramine to avoid blocking their absorption.
• Monitor bowel habits. If constipation develops, decrease dosage, add a stool softener, or discontinue drug. Encourage high-fiber diet and fluids.
• Monitor serum levels of digitalis glycosides in patients receiving both medications concurrently.
• Watch for signs of folic acid and vitamin A, D, E, and K deficiency.
• May bind to many drugs and cause decreased absorption. Check drug interactions of individual drugs.

General
Classification: analgesic (opioid). **Pregnancy risk category:** C (D for prolonged use). **Controlled substance schedule:** IV.

Mechanism of action
Binds with opiate receptors at many sites in the CNS (brain, brain stem, and spinal cord), altering both the perception of pain and the emotional response to it through an unknown mechanism.

Indications and dosage
- Mild to moderate pain. **Adults:** 65 mg (hydrochloride) P.O. q 4 hours p.r.n.; or 100 mg (napsylate) q 4 hours p.r.n.

Adverse reactions
CNS: *dizziness,* headache, sedation, euphoria, paradoxical excitement, insomnia. **GI:** nausea, vomiting, constipation. **Other:** ***respiratory depression,*** psychological and physical dependence.

Interactions
Alcohol, CNS depressants: additive effects. Use together cautiously.

Nursing diagnoses
- Pain related to the patient's underlying condition.
- High risk for trauma related to possible sedation or dizziness from adverse CNS reaction to propoxyphene.
- Knowledge deficit related to propoxyphene therapy.

Nursing interventions
- *Contraindicated* in patients with hypersensitivity to opiate analgesics.
- *Use cautiously* in patients with hepatic or renal disease, emotional instability, or a history of drug abuse.
- Respiratory depression, hypotension, profound sedation, and coma may result if used in excessive doses or with other CNS depressants. Studies have shown that propoxyphene-containing products alone or in combination with other drugs are a major cause of drug-related overdose and death. Warn patient not to exceed recommended dosage.
- Not to be prescribed for maintenance purposes in narcotic addiction.
- Warn ambulatory patient to avoid hazardous activities that require alertness or coordination until CNS effects of the drug are known.
- Do not use caffeine or amphetamines to treat overdose; may cause fatal seizures. Use narcotic antagonist instead.
- 65 mg propoxyphene hydrochloride equals 100 mg propoxyphene napsylate.
- Can be considered a mild narcotic analgesic, but pain relief is equivalent to aspirin. Tolerance and physical dependence have been observed. Used with aspirin or acetaminophen to maximize analgesia.
- To minimize GI upset, advise patient to take drug with food or milk.
- Advise patient to limit alcohol intake when taking this drug.

General

Classification: nonnarcotic analgesic, antipyretic, anti-inflammatory (salicylate). **Pregnancy risk category:** C.

Mechanism of action

Produces analgesia by an ill-defined central effect; produces a peripheral anti-inflammatory effect by inhibiting prostaglandin synthesis. Relieves fever by acting on the hypothalamic heat-regulating center.

Indications and dosage

- Arthritis, mild. **Adults:** 1 to 2 teaspoonfuls or tablets P.O. b.i.d. Total daily dosage can also be given at one time (usually h.s.).
- Rheumatoid arthritis and osteoarthritis. **Adults:** initially, 3 g P.O. daily either as a single dose h.s. or b.i.d. Dosage is adjusted according to patient response, ranging from 1 to 4.5 g daily.
- Juvenile rheumatoid arthritis. **Children** (12 to 37 kg): 50 mg/kg/day P.O. in divided doses. **Children** (more than 37 kg): 2,250 mg P.O. in divided doses.
- Mild to moderate pain and fever. **Adults:** 2 to 3 g P.O. daily divided b.i.d. **Children** (12 to 37 kg): 50 mg/kg/day P.O. in divided doses.

Adverse reactions

EENT: tinnitus and hearing loss. **GI:** GI distress. **Skin:** rash. **Other:** ***hypersensitivity manifested by anaphylaxis (rare).***

Interactions

Alcohol, steroids, and other NSAIDs: enhanced risk of adverse GI effects. **Ammonium chloride (and other urine acidifiers):** increased blood levels of salicylates. Monitor for salicylate toxicity. **Antacids in high doses (and other urine alkalinizers):** decreased levels of salicylates. Monitor for decreased salicylate effect. **Corticosteroids:** enhance salicylate elimination. Monitor for decreased salicylate effect. **Methotrexate:** increased risk of methotrexate toxicity. Avoid concomitant use. **Oral anticoagulants:** increased risk of bleeding. Use together cautiously.

Nursing diagnoses

- Pain related to the patient's underlying condition.
- Sensory/perceptual alterations (auditory) related to adverse drug reactions.
- Knowledge deficit related to salicylate therapy.

Nursing interventions

- *Use cautiously* in chronic renal failure, peptic ulcer disease, and gastritis and in patients with a known allergy to salicylates.
- Each 500-mg tablet or teaspoonful is equal in salicylate content to 650 mg aspirin; each 750-mg tablet, 975 mg aspirin; each 1,000-mg tablet, 1,300 mg aspirin.
- The CDC recommends that children or teenagers with chicken pox or influenza-like illness should not be given salicylates (associated with Reye's syndrome).
- Causes less GI distress than aspirin. Give choline magnesium trisalicylate before meals and antacids, if needed, 2 hours after meals.
- Salicylate salts don't affect platelet function. Therefore, don't substitute these agents for aspirin during antithrombotic therapy.
- Tell patient to take tablets with food or a full glass of water. Solution may be mixed with fruit juice, but not antacids.
- Toxicity can develop rapidly in febrile, dehydrated children.
- Therapeutic blood salicylate level in arthritis is 10 to 30 mg/100 ml. Tinnitus may occur at plasma levels of 30 mg/100 ml and above. However, mild toxicity may occur at plasma levels of 20 mg/100 ml (especially in those who are young or over age 60).
- Periodically monitor hemoglobin and PT in patients receiving long-term treatment with large doses.

General

Classification: antimuscarinic, GI antispasmodic (anticholinergic). **Pregnancy risk category:** C.

Mechanism of action

Competitively blocks acetylcholine, which decreases GI motility and inhibits gastric acid secretion.

Indications and dosage

- Adjunctive treatment of peptic ulcer, irritable bowel syndrome, and other GI disorders; to reduce duodenal motility during diagnostic radiologic procedures. **Adults:** 15 mg P.O. t.i.d. before meals, and 30 mg h.s. up to 60 mg q.i.d. For elderly patients, 7.5 mg P.O. t.i.d. before meals.

Adverse reactions

CNS: headache, insomnia, drowsiness, dizziness, *confusion or excitement in elderly patients,* nervousness, weakness. **CV:** palpitations, tachycardia. **EENT:** *blurred vision,* mydriasis, increased ocular tension, cycloplegia, photophobia. **GI:** *dry mouth,* dysphagia, constipation, heartburn, loss of taste, nausea, vomiting, paralytic ileus. **GU:** *urinary hesitancy, urine retention,* impotence. **Skin:** urticaria, decreased sweating or possible anhidrosis, other dermal manifestations. **Other:** fever, allergic reactions.

P

Overdosage may cause curare-like symptoms.

Interactions

Amantadine, antihistamines, antiparkinsonian agents, disopyramide, glutethimide, meperidine, phenothiazines, procainamide, quinidine: additive adverse effects. Avoid concomitant use. **Ketoconazole:** possible interference with ketoconazole absorption. Avoid concomitant use. **Methotrimeprazine:** possible enhanced risk of extrapyramidal reactions. Avoid concomitant use.

Nursing diagnoses

- Pain related to the patient's underlying condition.
- High risk for injury related to drug-induced adverse reaction.
- Knowledge deficit related to propantheline therapy.

Nursing interventions

- *Contraindicated* in narrow-angle glaucoma, obstructive uropathy, obstructive disease of GI tract, severe ulcerative colitis, myasthenia gravis, hypersensitivity to anticholinergics, paralytic ileus, intestinal atony, unstable CV status in acute hemorrhage, or toxic megacolon.
- *Use cautiously* in autonomic neuropathy, hyperthyroidism, coronary artery disease, cardiac arrhythmias, CHF, hypertension, hiatal hernia associated with reflux esophagitis, hepatic or renal disease, and ulcerative colitis or in patients over 40 years because of the increased incidence of glaucoma. Also use cautiously in hot or humid environments. Drug-induced heatstroke can develop.
- Give 30 minutes to 1 hour before meals and at bedtime. Bedtime dose can be larger and should be given at least 2 hours after the last meal of the day.
- Monitor patient's vital signs and urine output carefully.
- Instruct patient to avoid driving and other hazardous activities if he is drowsy or dizzy or has blurred vision; to drink plenty of fluids to help prevent constipation; and to report any rash or skin eruption.
- Gum or sugarless hard candy may relieve dry mouth.

General

Classification: antiulcer agent (histamine$_2$-receptor antagonist). **Pregnancy risk category:** B.

Mechanism of action

Inhibits histamine (H_2) action at receptor sites of parietal cells, reducing gastric acid secretion.

Indications and dosage

- Duodenal ulcer (short-term treatment). **Adults and children over 16 years:** 800 mg P.O. h.s., 400 mg b.i.d., or 300 mg q.i.d. (with meals and h.s.). Continue therapy for 4 to 6 weeks unless endoscopy shows healing. Maintenance: 400 mg h.s. Parenteral: 300 mg I.M. or I.V. q 6 hours. Maximum dosage is 2,400 mg daily. Alternatively, give by continuous infusion: 900 mg/day (37.5 mg/hour) diluted in 100 to 1,000 ml of compatible solution.
- Duodenal ulcer prophylaxis. **Adults and children over 16 years:** 400 mg P.O. h.s.
- Active benign gastric ulcer. **Adults:** 300 mg P.O. q.i.d. with meals and h.s. for up to 8 weeks.
- Pathologic hypersecretory conditions (such as Zollinger-Ellison syndrome). **Adults and children over 16 years:** 300 mg P.O. q.i.d. with meals and h.s.; adjust to individual needs. Maximum daily dosage is 2,400 mg. Parenteral: 300 mg I.V. q 6 hours. Maximum dosage is 2,400 mg daily.
- Gastroesophageal reflux disease. **Adults:** 800 mg P.O. b.i.d. or 400 mg q.i.d. before meals and h.s.
- Prevention of upper GI bleeding in critically ill patients. **Adults:** 50 mg/hour by continuous infusion for up to 7 days; 25 mg/hour, if creatinine clearance below 30 ml/minute/1.73 m^2.

Adverse reactions

Blood: ***agranulocytosis, neutropenia, thrombocytopenia, aplastic anemia.*** **CNS:** confusion, dizziness, headaches, peripheral neuropathy. **CV:** bradycardia. **GI:** *mild diarrhea.* **GU:** transient elevations in serum creatinine. **Skin:** acnelike rash, urticaria. **Other:** hypersensitivity, muscle pain, mild gynecomastia after use longer than 1 month.

Interactions

Antacids: impaired cimetidine absorption. Separate cimetidine and antacids by at least 1 hour. **Warfarin, phenytoin, lidocaine, propranolol, some benzodiazepines, theophylline:** possible inhibited hepatic microsomal enzyme metabolism.

Nursing diagnoses

- Pain related to the patient's condition.
- Diarrhea related to cimetidine use.
- Knowledge deficit related to cimetidine therapy.

Nursing interventions

- I.M. administration may be painful.
- Hemodialysis reduces blood levels of cimetidine. Schedule dose at end of hemodialysis treatment.
- Taking with meals ensures consistent therapeutic effect. If patient is taking drug once daily, he should take it at bedtime for best results.
- Urge patient not to smoke, because this may increase gastric acid secretion and worsen disease.
- **I.V. use:** Don't infuse I.V. too rapidly. May cause bradycardia or circulatory overload. Some experts recommend infusion over at least 30 minutes to lower risk of adverse cardiac effects. Use an infusion pump for volume of 250 ml/24 hours or less.
- Compatible I.V. solutions: 0.9% sodium chloride, dextrose 5% and 10% in water, lactated Ringer's, 5% sodium bicarbonate injection.
- Investigational use: before anesthesia for prophylaxis of aspiration pneumonitis; treatment of hyperparathyroidism, herpes zoster, chronic hives; adjunctive treatment of acetaminophen overdose.

General

Classification: antiarrhythmic (sodium channel antagonist). **Pregnancy risk category:** C.

Mechanism of action

A class Ic antiarrhythmic that stabilizes cardiac cell membranes, probably by decreasing sodium influx. It also has weak beta-adrenergic blocking properties.

Indications and dosage

• Suppression of life-threatening ventricular arrhythmias, such as sustained ventricular tachycardia. **Adults:** initially, 150 mg P.O. q 8 hours. Dosage may be increased to 225 mg q 8 hours after 3 or 4 days; if necessary, increase dosage to 300 mg q 8 hours. Maximum daily dosage 900 mg.

Adverse reactions

CNS: anxiety, ataxia, dizziness, drowsiness, fatigue, headache, insomnia, syncope, tremor, weakness. **CV:** angina, atrial fibrillation, bradycardia, bundle branch block, ***CHF,*** chest pain, edema, first-degree AV block, hypotension, increased QRS duration, intraventricular conduction delay, palpitations, ***proarrhythmic events (ventricular tachycardia, premature ventricular contractions).*** **EENT:** blurred vision. **GI:** abdominal pain or cramps, constipation, diarrhea, dyspepsia, flatulence, nausea, vomiting, dry mouth, anorexia, unusual taste. **Respiratory:** dyspnea. **Skin:** rash. **Other:** diaphoresis, joint pain.

Interactions

Antiarrhythmics: increased potential for CHF. **Cimetidine:** decreased metabolism of propafenone. **Digitalis glycosides, oral anticoagulants:** possible increased serum levels of these agents, resulting in toxicity. **Local anesthetics:** increased risk of CNS toxicity. **Propranolol, metoprolol:** slowed metabolism of these agents. Dosage adjustments may be necessary. **Quinidine:** slowed metabolism of propafenone. Avoid concomitant use.

Nursing diagnoses

• Decreased cardiac output related to the ineffectiveness of propafenone therapy.
• Altered protection related to propafenone-induced proarrhythmias.
• Knowledge deficit related to propafenone therapy.

Nursing interventions

• *Contraindicated* in severe or uncontrolled CHF; cardiogenic shock; SA, AV, or intraventricular disorders of impulse conduction; sinus node dysfunction in the absence of a pacemaker; severe bradycardia (50 beats/minute or less); marked hypotension; bronchospastic disorders; severe obstructive pulmonary disease; severe electrolyte imbalance; severe hepatic failure; and hypersensitivity to the drug.
• *Use cautiously* in patients with CHF because propafenone can exert a negative inotropic effect on the heart, in patients receiving other cardiac depressant drugs, and in those with hepatic or renal failure.
• Because plasma levels do not increase linearly with dose, dosage should be increased stepwise at 3- to 4-day intervals.
• Some patients metabolize propafenone rapidly, and early studies indicate that the drug may have a plasma half-life of 5 to 6 hours in fast metabolizers and 17 hours or more in slow metabolizers.
• Continuously monitor cardiac status during initiation of therapy and during dosage adjustments. If PR interval or QRS duration increase by more than 25%, a reduction in dosage may be necessary.
• Administer drug with food to minimize adverse GI reactions.
• During use with digoxin, frequently monitor ECG and serum digoxin levels because propafenone increases serum digoxin levels by 35% to 85%.

General

Classification: urinary tract antiseptic (quinolone). **Pregnancy risk category:** B.

Mechanism of action

Inhibits microbial DNA synthesis.

Indications and dosage

• Treatment of initial and recurrent urinary tract infections caused by susceptible strains of *Escherichia coli, Klebsiella, Enterobacter, Proteus mirabilis, P. vulgaris, Morganella morganii, Serratia,* and *Citrobacter.* **Adults and children over 12 years:** 1 g P.O. daily, in two to four divided doses for 7 to 14 days.

Not recommended for children under 12 years.

Adverse reactions

CNS: *dizziness, headache,* drowsiness, insomnia, seizures. **EENT:** photosensitivity, tinnitus. **GI:** *nausea, vomiting, abdominal pain,* diarrhea. **Skin:** rash, urticaria, pruritus, photosensitivity.

Interactions

Probenecid: may decrease urine levels of cinoxacin by inhibiting renal tubular secretion. Monitor for increased toxicity and reduced antibacterial effectiveness.

Nursing diagnoses

• High risk for injury related to ineffectiveness of cinoxacin to eradicate the infection.
• High risk for fluid volume deficit related to adverse GI reactions caused by cinoxacin.
• Knowledge deficit related to cinoxacin therapy.

Nursing interventions

• *Contraindicated* in patients with hypersensitivity to nalidixic acid.
• *Use cautiously* in patients with impaired renal and hepatic function.
• Not effective against *Pseudomonas,* enterococci, or staphylococci.
• Obtain clean-catch urine specimen for culture and sensitivity before therapy and repeat p.r.n. Therapy may begin pending test results.
• Remind the patient to continue taking this drug, even when he feels better, and to take the entire amount prescribed.
• High urine levels permit twice-daily dosing.
• Report adverse CNS reactions to doctor immediately. They indicate serious toxicity and usually dictate the cessation of drug therapy.
• Because the drug can cause dizziness or drowsiness, warn the patient to avoid driving and other hazardous activities that require alertness until the drug's CNS effects are known.
• Advise the patient to take cinoxacin with meals to help decrease adverse GI reactions.
• Monitor hydration status if adverse GI reactions occur.
• Warn the patient about photosensitizing effects of the drug, and advise him to avoid bright sunlight and to use sunblock.

promethazine hydrochloride

Anergan, Histantil†, Phenameth, Phenazine, Phencen-50, Phenergan*, Prometh-25, Prometh-50, V-Gan-25, V-Gan-50

General

Classification: antiemetic, antivertigo agent, antihistamine (H_1-receptor antagonist); preoperative, postoperative, or obstetric sedative and adjunct to analgesics (phenothiazine derivative).
Pregnancy risk category: C.

Mechanism of action

Competes with histamine for H_1-receptor sites on effector cells. Prevents but does not reverse histamine-mediated responses.

Indications and dosage

- Motion sickness. **Adults:** 25 mg P.O. b.i.d. **Children:** 1 mg/kg P.O., I.M., or P.R. b.i.d.
- Nausea. **Adults:** 12.5 to 25 mg P.O., I.M., or P.R. q 4 to 6 hours, p.r.n. **Children:** 1 mg/kg I.M. or P.R. q 4 to 6 hours, p.r.n.
- Rhinitis, allergy symptoms. **Adults:** 12.5 mg P.O. q.i.d.; or 25 mg P.O. h.s. **Children:** 6.25 to 12.5 mg P.O. t.i.d. or 25 mg P.O. or P.R. h.s.
- Sedation. **Adults:** 25 to 50 mg P.O. or I.M. h.s. or p.r.n. **Children:** 12.5 to 25 mg P.O., I.M., or P.R. h.s.
- Routine preoperative or postoperative sedation or as an adjunct to analgesics. **Adults:** 25 to 50 mg I.M., I.V., or P.O. **Children:** 12.5 to 25 mg I.M., I.V., or P.O.

Adverse reactions

Blood: leukopenia, ***agranulocytosis.*** **CNS:** (especially in elderly patients) *sedation,* confusion, restlessness, tremor, *drowsiness.* **CV:** hypotension. **EENT:** transient myopia, nasal congestion. **GI:** anorexia, nausea, vomiting, constipation, *dry mouth.* **GU:** urine retention. **Other:** photosensitivity.

Interactions

Alcohol, CNS depressants: increased sedation. **Anticholinergics, TCAs, phenothiazines:** increased effects. **MAO inhibitors:** increased anticholinergic effects. **Levodopa:** possible decreased antiparkinsonian action. **Lithium:** possible reduced absorption or enhanced elimination of lithium.

Nursing diagnoses

- Altered nutrition: Less than body requirements, related to nausea and motion sickness.
- High risk for infection related to promethazine-induced agranulocytosis.
- Knowledge deficit related to drug therapy.

Nursing interventions

- *Contraindicated* in increased intraocular pressure, intestinal obstruction, prostatic hypertrophy, bladder-neck obstruction, seizures, bone marrow depression, coma, CNS depression, stenosing peptic ulcers, and in neonates and acutely ill or dehydrated children.
- *Use cautiously* in pulmonary, hepatic, or CV disease; asthma; elderly or debilitated patients; and patients with a history of seizures.
- Warn patient against drinking alcohol during therapy and against driving or other activities that require alertness until CNS response to drug is determined.
- Reduce GI distress by giving with food or milk.
- Coffee or tea may reduce drowsiness. Sugarless gum or hard candy or ice chips may relieve dry mouth.
- Pronounced sedative effect limits use in many ambulatory patients.
- When treating motion sickness, tell patient to take first dose 30 to 60 minutes before travel. On succeeding days of travel, he should take dose upon arising and with evening meal.
- Inject deep I.M. into large muscle mass. Don't administer S.C. Rotate injection sites.
- **I.V. use:** May be given I.V., but not at a concentration greater than 25 mg/ml, nor at a rate exceeding 25 mg/minute. Shield I.V. infusion from direct light.
- Warn patient about possible photosensitivity and precautions to avoid it.
- Antihistamines are not recommended for use by women who are breast-feeding because small amounts of drug are excreted in breast milk.

General

Classification: broad-spectrum antibiotic (quinolone). **Pregnancy risk category:** C.

Mechanism of action

Exact mechanism unknown, but bactericidal effects may result from drug's ability to inhibit bacterial DNA gyrase and to prevent DNA replication in susceptible bacteria.

Indications and dosage

- Mild to moderate urinary tract infections. **Adults:** 250 mg P.O. or 200 mg I.V. q 12 hours.
- Severe or complicated urinary tract infections; mild to moderate bone and joint infections; mild to moderate respiratory tract infections; mild to moderate skin and skin structure infections; infectious diarrhea. **Adults:** 500 mg P.O. or 400 mg I.V. q 12 hours.
- Severe or complicated bone or joint, respiratory, skin, or skin structure infections. **Adults:** 750 mg P.O. q 12 hours.

Adverse reactions

Blood: eosinophilia. **CNS:** headache, restlessness, tremor, light-headedness, confusion, hallucinations, *seizures*. **EENT:** photosensitivity. **GI:** *nausea, diarrhea,* vomiting, abdominal discomfort, oral candidiasis. **GU:** crystalluria. **Local:** (with I.V. administration) thrombophlebitis, burning, pruritus, paresthesia, erythema, swelling. **Skin:** rash.

Interactions

Antacids containing magnesium hydroxide or aluminum hydroxide, sucralfate, iron supplements: decreased ciprofloxacin absorption. Separate administration by at least 2 hours. **Probenecid:** may elevate serum level of ciprofloxacin. **Theophylline:** increased plasma theophylline levels and prolonged theophylline half-life. Monitor theophylline levels and observe for adverse effects.

Nursing diagnoses

- High risk for injury related to ineffectiveness of ciprofloxacin to eradicate the infection.
- High risk for fluid volume deficit related to adverse GI reactions to ciprofloxacin.
- Knowledge deficit related to ciprofloxacin therapy.

Nursing interventions

- *Contraindicated* in patients sensitive to quinolones, in pregnant or breast-feeding women, and in children under 18 years. Quinolone antibiotics cause arthropathy in young laboratory animals.
- *Use with extreme caution* with theophylline. Serious (even fatal) reactions have occurred in patients receiving I.V. theophylline and ciprofloxacin. If a patient must receive theophylline or aminophylline with ciprofloxacin, closely monitor serum theophylline levels and adjust dosage accordingly.
- *Use cautiously* in CNS disorders, such as severe cerebral arteriosclerosis or seizure disorders, and in seizure-prone patients. May stimulate CNS.
- Obtain specimen for culture and sensitivity tests before first dose. Therapy may begin pending results.
- Give oral doses 2 hours after a meal. Food doesn't affect absorption but may delay peak serum levels.
- **I.V. use:** Dilute I.V. vials before use. Infuse slowly (over 60 minutes) into a large vein.
- Dosage adjustments are needed in renal dysfunction.
- Prolonged use may result in overgrowth of organisms that are resistant to ciprofloxacin.
- Advise patient that hypersensitivity may occur even after first dose. If the patient develops a skin rash or any allergic-type reaction, he should stop taking drug immediately and notify his doctor.
- Tell patient to avoid caffeine while taking the drug because of possible cumulative caffeine effects.
- Drug is excreted in breast milk. Patient should discontinue breast-feeding during treatment or should be treated with another drug.
- Warn patient to avoid hazardous tasks that require alertness, such as driving, until drug's CNS effects are known.
- Advise patient to drink plenty of fluids to reduce the risk of crystalluria.

General
Classification: antipsychotic, antiemetic (phenothiazine). **Pregnancy risk category:** C.

Mechanism of action
Blocks postsynaptic dopamine receptors in brain.

Indications and dosage
• Psychosis. **Adults:** 10 to 200 mg P.O. or I.M. q 4 to 6 hours, up to 1 g daily. I.V. maximum of 25 mg/ml for acutely agitated patients. Initial dose is 50 to 150 mg; repeat within 10 minutes if needed. **Children over 12 years:** 10 to 25 mg P.O. or I.M. q 4 to 6 hours.

Adverse reactions
Blood: transient leukopenia, ***agranulocytosis.*** **CNS:** *extrapyramidal reactions, tardive dyskinesia, sedation,* pseudoparkinsonism, dizziness. **CV:** *orthostatic hypotension,* tachycardia. **EENT:** ocular changes, *blurred vision.* **GI:** *dry mouth, constipation.* **GU:** *urine retention,* dark urine, menstrual irregularities, gynecomastia, inhibited ejaculation. **Hepatic:** jaundice. **Skin:** *mild photosensitivity,* allergic reactions. **Local:** pain at I.M. site, sterile abscess. **Other:** weight gain; increased appetite; rarely, ***neuroleptic malignant syndrome.*** **After abrupt withdrawal of long-term therapy:** gastritis, nausea, vomiting, dizziness, tremor, sweating, tachycardia, headache, insomnia.

Interactions
Alcohol, other CNS depressants: increased CNS depression. **Antacids:** inhibited absorption of oral phenothiazines. **Anticholinergics (including antidepressants and antiparkinsonian agents):** increased anticholinergic activity, aggravated parkinsonian symptoms. **Barbiturates, lithium:** possible decreased phenothiazine effect. **Centrally acting antihypertensives:** reduced antihypertensive effect. **Oral anticoagulants:** reduced effectiveness. **Propranolol:** increased serum levels of propranolol and promazine.

Nursing diagnoses
• Impaired thought processes related to the patient's underlying condition.
• Urinary retention related to adverse reaction.
• Knowledge deficit related to promazine therapy.

Nursing interventions
• *Contraindicated* in coma, CNS depression, bone marrow suppression, and subcortical damage.
• *Use cautiously* in elderly or debilitated patients and in hepatic or CV disease, extreme heat or cold, respiratory disorders, seizures, suspected brain tumor or intestinal obstruction, glaucoma, prostatic hypertrophy, and acutely ill or dehydrated children.
• Tardive dyskinesia may occur after prolonged use, sometimes months or years later; may stop spontaneously or last for life despite drug cessation.
• Give I.V. diphenhydramine for acute dystonic reaction.
• Hold dose and notify doctor if patient develops jaundice, blood dyscrasias, persistent extrapyramidal reactions, or such reactions in pregnancy or childhood.
• Monitor therapy by weekly bilirubin tests during first month; periodic CBC and liver function; and ophthalmic tests (long-term use).
• Have patient report urine retention or constipation.
• Warn against activities requiring alertness or coordination until CNS effects known. Drowsiness and dizziness usually subside after few weeks.
• Monitor blood pressure with patient lying and standing before therapy, and routinely during it.
• Watch for orthostatic hypotension, especially with parenteral use. Keep patient supine for 1 hour afterward. Advise changing positions slowly.
• Give deep I.M. in upper outer quadrant of buttocks.
• Protect drug from light. Slight yellowing doesn't affect potency.
• Don't stop drug abruptly unless severe reactions occur.
• Sugarless gum or hard candy may relieve dry mouth.

General

Classification: antiemetic, GI stimulant (serotonin-receptor agonist). **Pregnancy risk category:** C.

Mechanism of action

Stimulates serotonin-4 (5-HT_4) receptors and enhances the release of acetylcholine. Increases lower esophageal sphincter pressure and increases gastric emptying.

Indications and dosage

• Nocturnal heartburn caused by gastroesophageal reflux disease. **Adults:** 10 mg P.O. q.i.d. at least 15 minutes before meals and h.s., to a maximum of 20 mg P.O. q.i.d.

Adverse reactions

CNS: headache. **EENT:** rhinitis. **GI:** diarrhea, abdominal pain, constipation, dyspepsia.

Interactions

Alcohol, benzodiazepines: increased sedative effect. Avoid concurrent use. **Anticholinergics:** decreased effectiveness. Avoid concurrent use. **Cimetidine:** increased cisapride absorption. **Digoxin:** may alter absorption of digoxin. Monitor serum levels closely. **Oral anticoagulants:** increased risk of bleeding. Monitor PT closely.

Nursing diagnoses

• Pain related to patient's condition.
• Knowledge deficit related to cisapride therapy.

Nursing interventions

• *Contraindicated* in patients hypersensitive to the drug for whom and in those for whom increased GI motility may be harmful, such as patients with GI hemorrhage, mechanical obstruction, or perforation.
• *Use cautiously* in breast-feeding women.
• Cisapride accelerates gastric emptying time. This may affect the absorption of other orally administered drugs; check with doctor or pharmacist.

General
Classification: contraceptive (progestin). **Pregnancy risk category:** X.

Mechanism of action
Suppresses ovulation, possibly by inhibiting pituitary gonadotropin secretion. Also forms a thick cervical mucus.

Indications and dosage
- Amenorrhea. **Women:** 5 to 10 mg I.M. daily for 6 to 8 days.
- Dysfunctional uterine bleeding. **Women:** 5 to 10 mg I.M. daily for six doses.
- Premenstrual syndrome (PMS). **Women:** 200 to 400 mg as a suppository administered either rectally or vaginally.

Adverse reactions
CNS: dizziness, migraine headache, lethargy, depression. **CV:** hypertension, thrombophlebitis, ***pulmonary embolism,*** edema. **GI:** nausea, vomiting, abdominal cramps. **GU:** breakthrough bleeding, dysmenorrhea, amenorrhea, cervical erosion, abnormal secretions, uterine fibromas, vaginal candidiasis. **Hepatic:** cholestatic jaundice. **Local:** pain at injection site. **Metabolic:** hyperglycemia. **Skin:** melasma, rash. **Other:** breast tenderness, enlargement, or secretion; decreased libido.

Interactions
Barbiturates, carbamazepine, rifampin: decreased progestin effects. Monitor for diminished therapeutic response. **Bromocriptine:** possible amenorrhea, interfering with bromocriptine effects. Avoid concomitant use.

Nursing diagnoses
- High risk for fluid volume deficit related to excessive abnormal uterine bleeding.
- Fluid volume excess related to progesterone-induced edema.
- Knowledge deficit related to progesterone therapy.

Nursing interventions
- *Contraindicated* in thromboembolic disorders, breast cancer, undiagnosed abnormal vaginal bleeding, severe hepatic disease, or missed abortion.
- *Use cautiously* in diabetes mellitus, seizure disorder, migraine, cardiac or renal disease, asthma, and mental illness.
- FDA regulations require that, before receiving first dose, patients read package insert explaining possible progestin adverse reactions. Provide verbal explanation also.
- Instruct the patient to report any unusual symptoms immediately and to stop the drug and call the doctor if visual disturbances or migraine occur.
- Give oil solutions (peanut oil or sesame oil) deep I.M. Check sites frequently for irritation. Rotate injection sites.
- Preliminary estrogen treatment is usually needed in menstrual disorders.
- Teach the patient how to perform a monthly breast self-examination.
- Progesterone suppositories are not commercially available and must be made by the pharmacist.
- Progesterone has been used during the first trimester of pregnancy to treat habitual abortion or pending spontaneous abortion.

General

Classification: antineoplastic agent (alkylating agent). **Pregnancy risk category:** D.

Mechanism of action

Cross-links strands of cellular DNA and interferes with RNA transcription, causing growth imbalance leading to cell death. Cell cycle-nonspecific.

Indications and dosage

• Adjunctive therapy in metastatic testicular cancer. **Adults:** 20 mg/m² I.V. daily for 5 days. Repeat q 3 weeks for 3 cycles or longer.
• Adjunctive therapy in metastatic ovarian cancer. **Adults:** 100 mg/m² I.V. Repeat q 4 weeks; or 50 mg/m² q 3 weeks with doxorubicin therapy.
• Advanced bladder cancer. **Adults:** 50 to 70 mg/m² I.V. once q 3 to 4 weeks. Patients receiving other antineoplastics or radiation therapy should receive 50 mg/m² q 4 weeks.

Adverse reactions

Blood: *mild myelosuppression (25% to 30%),* ***leukopenia, thrombocytopenia, hypomagnesemia, hypocalcemia, anemia;*** nadirs in circulating platelets and leukocytes (days 18 to 23; recovery by day 39). **CNS:** peripheral neuritis, loss of taste, ***seizures.*** **EENT:** *tinnitus, hearing loss.* **GI:** *nausea, vomiting;* diarrhea; metallic taste. **GU:** *more prolonged and severe renal toxicity with repeated courses of therapy.* **Other:** ***anaphylactic reaction.***

Note: Prehydration and mannitol diuresis may reduce renal toxicity and ototoxicity significantly.

Interactions

Aminoglycosides: additive nephrotoxicity. Monitor renal function studies carefully. **Bumetanide, ethacrynic acid, furosemide:** additive ototoxicity. **Phenytoin:** decreased serum phenytoin levels.

Nursing diagnoses

• High risk for fluid volume deficit and renal impairment related to physiologic renal needs.
• Sensory/perceptual alterations (auditory) related to ototoxicity manifested by tinnitus and hearing loss.
• Knowledge deficit related to cisplatin therapy.

Nursing interventions

• *Contraindicated* in patients with hypersensitivity to carboplatin and in severe renal disease, hearing impairment, or myelosuppression.
• Maintain urine output of 100 ml/hour for 4 consecutive hours before and 24 hours after therapy.
• **I.V. use:** Manufacturer recommends that drug be given I.V. in 2 liters 0.9% sodium chloride solution with 37.5 g mannitol over 6 to 8 hours.
• Don't use needles or I.V. sets containing aluminum because it will displace the platinum, causing loss of potency and formation of a black precipitate.
• Mannitol may be given as 12.5-g I.V. bolus before cisplatin infusion. Follow, if ordered, by mannitol infusion of up to 10 g/hour p.r.n. to maintain output during and 24 hours after cisplatin infusion. To prevent deficiencies, add 10 to 20 mEq/liter potassium chloride to I.V. fluids before and after cisplatin therapy.
• I.V. sodium thiosulfate may minimize toxicity.
• Don't repeat dosage unless platelets > 100,000/mm³, WBC > 4,000/mm³, creatinine < 1.5 mg/dl, or BUN < 25 mg/dl. Avoid I.M. injections when platelets < 100,000/mm³.
• Monitor CBC, electrolytes (especially potassium and magnesium), platelets, and renal function studies before initial and subsequent dosages.
• Tell patient to report tinnitus immediately to prevent permanent hearing loss. Do audiometry prior to initial dosage and subsequent courses.
• Delayed-onset vomiting (3 to 5 days after treatment) has been reported. Nausea and vomiting may be severe and last up to 24 hours. Give antiemetics as ordered. Continue I.V. hydration until patient can tolerate adequate oral intake.
• Ondansetron or high-dose metoclopramide effectively treats and prevents nausea and vomiting. Some clinicians combine metoclopramide with dexamethasone and antihistamines.
• Preparation of parenteral form is associated with carcinogenic, mutagenic, and teratogenic risks. Follow institutional policy to reduce risks.

General

Classification: antiparkinsonian agent (anticholinergic). **Pregnancy risk category:** C.

Mechanism of action

Blocks central cholinergic receptors, helping to balance cholinergic activity in the basal ganglia.

Indications and dosage

- Parkinsonism, muscle rigidity. **Adults:** initially, 2 to 2.5 mg P.O. t.i.d., after meals. Increase dosage gradually p.r.n. Usual dosage range is 20 to 30 mg/day, but some patients may require up to 60 mg daily.

Drug is also used to relieve extrapyramidal dysfunction that accompanies treatment with phenothiazines and rauwolfia derivatives. In addition, it controls excessive salivation from neuroleptic medications.

Adverse reactions

CNS: light-headedness, giddiness. **EENT:** blurred vision, mydriasis. **GI:** *constipation, dry mouth,* nausea, vomiting, epigastric distress. **Skin:** rash. **Other:** muscle weakness.

Interactions

None significant.

Nursing diagnoses

- Impaired physical immobility related to underlying parkinsonism.
- Altered oral mucous membrane related to dry mouth induced by procyclidine.
- Knowledge deficit related to procyclidine therapy.

Nursing interventions

- *Contraindicated* in patients with narrow-angle glaucoma because procyclidine-induced cyclopegia and mydriasis may increase intraocular pressure.
- *Use cautiously* in patients with tachycardia, hypotension, urine retention, and prostatic hypertrophy because procyclidine may aggravate these conditions.
- Watch closely for confusion, disorientation, agitation, hallucinations, and psychotic symptoms, especially in elderly patients. Call the doctor promptly if these occur.
- Monitor the drug's effectiveness by regularly checking the patient's body movements for signs of improvement.
- Make certain that the patient receives gonioscopic evaluation and close monitoring of intraocular pressure, especially if he's over age 40.
- In severe parkinsonism, tremor may increase as spasticity is relieved.
- Give procyclidine after meals to minimize GI distress.
- Warn the patient to avoid activities that require alertness until the CNS effects of the drug are known.
- Regularly check the patient's oral mucous membranes for dryness.
- Relieve dry mouth with cool drinks, ice chips, sugarless gum, or hard candy.

General

Classification: antibiotic (macrolide). **Pregnancy risk category:** C.

Mechanism of action

A derivative of erythromycin; binds to the 50S subunit of bacterial ribosomes, blocking protein synthesis. Bacteriostatic or bactericidal, depending on concentration.

Indications and dosage

- Pharyngitis or tonsillitis caused by *Streptococcus pyogenes.* **Adults:** 250 mg P.O. q 12 hours for 10 days.
- Acute maxillary sinusitis caused by *S. pneumoniae.* **Adults:** 500 mg P.O. q 12 hours for 14 days.
- Acute exacerbations of chronic bronchitis caused by *Moraxella (Branhamella) catarrhalis* or *S. pneumoniae;* pneumonia caused by *S. pneumoniae* or *Mycoplasma pneumoniae.* **Adults:** 250 mg P.O. q 12 hours for 7 to 14 days.
- Acute exacerbations of chronic bronchitis caused by *Haemophilus influenzae.* **Adults:** 500 mg P.O. q 12 hours for 7 to 14 days.
- Uncomplicated skin and skin structure infections caused by *Staphylococcus aureus* or *Streptococcus pyogenes.* **Adults:** 250 mg P.O. q 12 hours for 7 to 14 days.

Adverse reactions

CNS: headache. **GI:** *diarrhea, nausea, abnormal taste,* dyspepsia, abdominal pain or discomfort.

Interactions

Carbamazepine: possible increase in serum levels of carbamazepine. Monitor blood levels. **Theophylline:** possible increase in plasma theophylline levels. Monitor theophylline levels carefully. **Warfarin:** possible increase in PT. Monitor PT carefully.

Nursing diagnoses

- High risk for injury related to ineffectiveness of clarithromycin to eradicate the infection.
- High risk for fluid volume deficit related to clarithromycin-induced adverse GI reactions.
- Knowledge deficit related to clarithromycin therapy.

Nursing interventions

- *Contraindicated* in patients with hypersensitivity to erythromycin or other macrolide antibiotics.
- *Use cautiously* in patients with hepatic or renal impairment.
- Obtain specimen for culture and sensitivity tests before first dose. Therapy may begin pending test results.
- Drug may be taken without regard to meals.
- May cause overgrowth of nonsusceptible bacteria or fungi. Monitor for signs and symptoms of superinfection.
- Tell patient to take all of the medication prescribed, even after he feels better.

General
Classification: antipsychotic, antiemetic, anxiolytic (phenothiazine). **Pregnancy risk category:** C.

Mechanism of action
Acts on the chemoreceptor trigger zone to inhibit nausea and vomiting; in larger doses, partially depresses the vomiting center as well.

Indications and dosage
• Preoperative nausea control. **Adults:** 5 to 10 mg I.M. 1 to 2 hours before induction, repeat once in 30 minutes, if needed; or 5 to 10 mg I.V. 15 to 30 minutes before induction (repeat once if needed); or 20 mg/liter D_5W and 0.9% sodium chloride solution by infusion, added to infusion 15 to 30 minutes before induction. Maximum parenteral dosage: 40 mg daily.
• Severe nausea, vomiting. **Adults:** 5 to 10 mg P.O. (maleate, edisylate) t.i.d. or q.i.d.; or 15 mg sustained-release form (maleate) on arising; or 10 mg sustained-release form q 12 hours; or 25 mg P.R. b.i.d.; or 5 to 10 mg I.M. injected deeply into upper outer quadrant of gluteal region. Repeat q 3 to 4 hours p.r.n. Maximum I.M. dosage: 40 mg daily. **Children 18 to 39 kg:** 2.5 mg P.O. or P.R. t.i.d.; or 5 mg P.O. or P.R. b.i.d. Maximum 15 mg daily; or 0.132 mg/kg deep I.M. **Children 14 to 17 kg:** 2.5 mg P.O. or P.R. b.i.d. or t.i.d. Maximum 10 mg daily; or 0.132 mg/kg deep I.M.. **Children 9 to 13 kg:** 2.5 mg P.O. or P.R. daily or b.i.d. Maximum 7.5 mg daily; or 0.132 mg/kg deep I.M.
• Management of psychotic disorders. **Adults:** 5 to 10 mg, P.O. t.i.d. or q.i.d. **Children 2 to 12 years:** 2.5 mg P.O. or P.R. b.i.d. or t.i.d. Increase slowly to maximum (if needed). **Children 6 to 10 years:** maximum 25 mg P.O. daily.
• Management of severe psychoses. **Adults:** 10 to 20 mg I.M. May repeat in 1 to 4 hours. Rarely, patients may receive 10 to 20 mg q 4 to 6 hours. Use oral therapy after symptoms controlled. **Children:** 0.13 mg/kg I.M.
• Excessive anxiety. **Adults:** 5 to 10 mg deep I.M. q 3 to 4 hours, not to exceed 40 mg daily; or 5 to 10 mg P.O. t.i.d. or q.i.d.; or 15 mg (sustained-release) once daily or 10 mg q 12 hours.

Adverse reactions
Blood: *transient leukopenia,* ***agranulocytosis.*** **CNS:** *extrapyramidal reactions,* pseudoparkinsonism, sedation, dizziness. **CV:** *orthostatic hypotension,* tachycardia. **EENT:** *ocular changes, blurred vision.* **GI:** *dry mouth, constipation.* **GU:** *urine retention,* dark urine, menstrual irregularities, gynecomastia, inhibited ejaculation. **Hepatic:** *cholestatic jaundice.* **Skin:** *mild photosensitivity,* allergic reactions, ***exfoliative dermatitis.*** **Other:** weight gain, increased appetite.

Interactions
Antacids: inhibited oral phenothiazine absorption. **Anticholinergics, including antiparkinsonian agents:** increased anticholinergic activity and aggravated parkinsonian symptoms. **Barbiturates:** possible decreased phenothiazine effect.

Nursing diagnoses
• High risk for fluid volume deficit related to nausea and vomiting.
• Altered thought processes related to prochlorperazine-induced CNS depression.
• Knowledge deficit related to prochlorperazine.

Nursing interventions
• *Contraindicated* in CNS depression, phenothiazine hypersensitivity, bone marrow suppression, or subcortical damage; during pediatric surgery, use of spinal or epidural anesthetic or adrenergic blockers, alcohol use, and coma or depression.
• *Use cautiously* in hepatic or CV disease, extreme heat or cold, respiratory disease, seizures, glaucoma, suspected brain tumor or intestinal obstruction, and prostatic hypertrophy; in acutely ill or dehydrated children; and in elderly or debilitated patients.
• Use only when vomiting can't be controlled by other measures or when only a few doses are required.
• **I.V. use:** Infuse slowly, never as a bolus injection.
• Watch for orthostatic hypotension.

General

Classification: antihistamine (ethanolamine-derivative antihistamine). **Pregnancy risk category:** C.

Mechanism of action

Competes with histamine for H_1-receptor sites on effector cells. Prevents but does not reverse histamine-mediated responses.

Indications and dosage

• Rhinitis, allergy symptoms. **Adults and children 12 years and over:** 1.34 mg P.O. q 12 hours. *Note:* Children under 12 years should use only as directed by a doctor.

Adverse reactions

Blood: hemolytic anemia, thrombocytopenia, ***agranulocytosis.*** **CNS:** (especially in elderly patients) *sedation, drowsiness.* **CV:** hypotension, palpitations, tachycardia. **GI:** epigastric distress, anorexia, nausea, vomiting, constipation, *dry mouth.* **GU:** urine retention. **Skin:** rash, urticaria. **Other:** thick bronchial secretions.

Interactions

CNS depressants: increased sedation. Use together cautiously. **MAO inhibitors:** increased anticholinergic effects. Don't use together.

Nursing diagnoses

• Ineffective airway clearance related to allergy symptoms.
• Hyperthermia related to potential clemastine-induced agranulocytosis.
• Knowledge deficit related to clemastine therapy.

Nursing interventions

• *Contraindicated* in acute asthmatic attacks.
• *Use cautiously* in elderly patients and in patients with increased intraocular pressure, hyperthyroidism, CV or renal disease, hypertension, bronchial asthma, urine retention, prostatic hypertrophy, bladder-neck obstruction, and stenosing peptic ulcers.
• Avoid use in breast-feeding women because small amounts of drug are excreted in breast milk.
• Warn patient against drinking alcoholic beverages during therapy and against driving or other activities that require alertness until CNS response to drug is determined.
• Tell patient that coffee or tea may reduce drowsiness and that sugarless gum, sour hard candy, or ice chips may relieve dry mouth.
• If tolerance develops, another antihistamine may be substituted.
• Warn patient to stop taking drug 4 days before allergy skin tests to preserve accuracy of tests.
• Monitor blood counts during long-term therapy; observe for signs of blood dyscrasias.

General

Classification: antiarrhythmic (procaine derivative). **Pregnancy risk category:** C.

Mechanism of action

A class Ia antiarrhythmic that depresses phase 0. It prolongs the action potential.

Indications and dosage

• Premature ventricular contractions, ventricular tachycardia, atrial arrhythmias unresponsive to quinidine, paroxysmal atrial tachycardia. **Adults:** 100 mg q 5 minutes slow I.V. push, no faster than 25 to 50 mg/minute until arrhythmias disappear, adverse reactions develop, or 1 g has been given. (Usual effective dose is 500 to 600 mg.) When arrhythmias disappear, give continuous infusion of 2 to 6 mg/minute. If arrhythmias recur, repeat bolus as above and increase infusion rate; 0.5 to 1 g I.M. q 4 to 8 hours until oral therapy begins.

• Loading dose for atrial fibrillation or paroxysmal atrial tachycardia. **Adults:** 1 to 1.25 g P.O. If arrhythmias persist after 1 hour, give additional 750 mg. If no change occurs, give 500 mg to 1 g q 2 hours until arrhythmias disappear or adverse reactions occur.

• Loading dose for ventricular tachycardia. **Adults:** 1 g P.O. Maintenance dosage is 50 mg/kg daily q 3 hours; average is 250 to 500 mg q 3 hours.

Note: Sustained-release tablet may be used for maintenance in ventricular tachycardia, atrial fibrillation, and paroxysmal atrial tachycardia. Dosage is 500 mg to 1 g q 6 hours.

Adverse reactions

Blood: thrombocytopenia, ***neutropenia, agranulocytosis,*** hemolytic anemia. **CNS:** hallucinations, confusion, ***seizures,*** depression. **CV:** ***severe hypotension,*** *bradycardia,* AV block, ***ventricular fibrillation (after parenteral use).*** **GI:** *nausea, vomiting, anorexia, diarrhea, bitter taste.* **Skin:** *maculopapular rash.* **Other:** *fever,* lupus-like syndrome, myalgia.

Interactions

Amiodarone: increased procainamide levels and possible drug toxicity. **Anticholinergics:** additive anticholinergic effects. **Anticholinesterase agents:** anticholinesterase dosage may need to be increased. **Cimetidine:** possible increased procainamide levels. **Neuromuscular blockers:** increased skeletal muscle relaxation.

Nursing diagnoses

• Decreased cardiac output related to the drug's ineffectiveness or its CV reactions.
• Altered protection related to procainamide-induced blood disorders.
• Knowledge deficit related to procainamide.

Nursing interventions

• *Contraindicated* in complete, second-, or third-degree heart block unassisted by electrical pacemaker or in myasthenia gravis.
• *Use cautiously* in CHF, other conduction disturbances, and hepatic or renal insufficiency.
• **I.V. use:** Patients receiving infusions must be attended at all times. Use an infusion pump.
• Monitor serum electrolytes, especially potassium. Hypokalemia predisposes patient to arrhythmias.
• Monitor blood pressure and ECG continuously during I.V. administration. Watch for prolonged QT and QRS intervals, heart block, or increased arrhythmias. If these occur, withhold drug, obtain rhythm strip, and notify doctor immediately.
• Keep patients supine for I.V. administration if hypotension occurs.
• Monitor CBC frequently during first 3 months.
• Decrease dose in hepatic and renal dysfunction, and give over 6 hours.
• Positive antinuclear antibody titer is common in about 60% of patients who don't have signs of lupus-like syndrome. Response seems related to prolonged use, not dosage.
• After prolonged atrial fibrillation, restoration of normal rhythm may result in thromboembolism. Anticoagulation usually advised before restoration of normal sinus rhythm.
• Emphasize taking drug exactly as prescribed.

General

Classification: antimuscarinic, GI antispasmodic (anticholinergic). **Pregnancy risk category:** C.

Mechanism of action

Competitively blocks acetylcholine, which decreases GI motility and inhibits gastric acid secretion.

Indications and dosage

• Adjunctive therapy for peptic ulcers. *Dosage should be individualized according to severity of symptoms and occurrence of adverse reactions.* **Elderly or debilitated patients:** 2.5 to 5 mg P.O. t.i.d. or q.i.d. before meals and h.s.

Adverse reactions

CNS: headache, insomnia, drowsiness, dizziness, *confusion or excitement in elderly patients,* nervousness, weakness. **CV:** *palpitations,* tachycardia. **EENT:** *blurred vision,* mydriasis, increased ocular tension, cycloplegia, photophobia. **GI:** *dry mouth,* dysphagia, heartburn, loss of taste, nausea, vomiting, *paralytic ileus, constipation.* **GU:** *urinary hesitancy, urine retention,* impotence. **Skin:** urticaria, decreased sweating or possible anhidrosis, other dermal manifestations. **Other:** fever, allergic reactions. Overdosage may cause curare-like symptoms.

C

Interactions

Amantadine, antihistamines, antiparkinsonian agents, disopyramide, glutethimide, meperidine, phenothiazines, procainamide, quinidine: additive adverse effects. Avoid concomitant use. **Ketoconazole:** possible interference with ketoconazole absorption. Avoid concomitant use. **Methotrimeprazine:** possible enhanced risk of extrapyramidal reactions. Avoid concomitant use.

Nursing diagnoses

• Altered health maintenance related to the patient's underlying condition.
• Constipation related to adverse drug reactions.
• Knowledge deficit related to clidinium therapy.

Nursing interventions

• *Contraindicated* in narrow-angle glaucoma, obstructive uropathy, obstructive disease of the GI tract, severe ulcerative colitis, myasthenia gravis, hypersensitivity to anticholinergics, paralytic ileus, intestinal atony, unstable CV status in acute hemorrhage, or toxic megacolon.
• *Use cautiously* in autonomic neuropathy, hyperthyroidism, coronary artery disease, cardiac arrhythmias, CHF, hypertension, hiatal hernia associated with reflux esophagitis, hepatic or renal disease, and ulcerative colitis or in patients over 40 years because of increased incidence of glaucoma. Also use cautiously in hot or humid environments; drug-induced heatstroke may develop.
• Give 30 minutes to 1 hour before meals and at bedtime. Bedtime dose can be larger and should be given at least 2 hours after last meal of day.
• Monitor patient's vital signs and urine output carefully.
• Instruct patient to avoid driving and other hazardous activities if he is drowsy or dizzy or has blurred vision; to drink plenty of fluids to help prevent constipation; and to report any rash or skin eruption.
• Sugarless gum or hard candy may relieve dry mouth.
• Dysphagia may cause aspiration.
• No conclusive evidence exists that clidinium aids in healing peptic ulcers, decreases their recurrence, or prevents their complications.

General

Classification: cholesterol-lowering agent (bisphenol derivative). **Pregnancy risk category:** B.

Mechanism of action

Inhibits cholesterol transport from the intestine, prevents oxidation of low-density lipoprotein, and may also decrease cholesterol synthesis. Appears to be more effective in patients with mild cholesterol elevations than in those with severe hypercholesterolemia.

Indications and dosage

- Primary hypercholesterolemia. **Adults:** 500 mg P.O. b.i.d. with morning and evening meals. Do not exceed 1 g/day.

  Drug is not recommended for children.

Adverse reactions

CV: prolonged QT interval, arrhythmias. **GI:** *diarrhea, flatulence, abdominal pain, nausea, vomiting.* **Other:** *hyperhidrosis,* fetid sweat, ***angioneurotic edema.***

Interactions

Clofibrate: additive effects. **Tricyclic antidepressants, class Ia antiarrhythmics, phenothiazines, beta blockers, digitalis glycosides, calcium channel blocking agents:** increased risk of arrhythmias.

Nursing diagnoses

- High risk for injury related to elevated serum lipid and cholesterol levels.
- Diarrhea related to an adverse reaction brought on by probucol.
- Knowledge deficit related to probucol therapy.

Nursing interventions

- *Contraindicated* in patients with arrhythmias. Discontinue the drug in any patient whose ECG shows a prolonged QT interval. Monitor the patient's ECG periodically.
- Recognize that the drug's effect is enhanced when taken with food.
- Teach the patient about proper dietary management, weight control, and exercise. Explain the importance of following these measures to help control serum lipid levels.
- Monitor the patient's intake and output if vomiting and diarrhea occur. Provide fluids.
- If a female patient wishes to become pregnant, tell her that withdrawal of the drug and effective contraception is recommended for 6 months because of the persistence of the drug in the body.

General

Classification: antibiotic (lincomycin derivative).
Pregnancy risk category: B.

Mechanism of action

Inhibits bacterial protein synthesis by binding to the 50S subunit of the ribosome.

Indications and dosage

- Moderate to severe infections caused by sensitive staphylococci, streptococci, pneumococci, *Bacteroides, Fusobacterium, Clostridium perfringens,* and other sensitive aerobic and anaerobic organisms.

Adults: 150 to 450 mg P.O. (palmitate hydrochloride, hydrochloride) q 6 hours; or 300 mg I.M. or I.V. (phosphate) q 6, 8, or 12 hours. Up to 2,700 mg I.M. or I.V. daily, divided q 6, 8, or 12 hours.
Children over 1 month: 8 to 20 mg/kg P.O. (palmitate) daily, divided q 6 to 8 hours; or 15 to 40 mg/kg I.M. or I.V. daily, divided q 6 hours.

Adverse reactions

Blood: transient leukopenia, eosinophilia, thrombocytopenia. **GI:** *nausea,* vomiting, abdominal pain, *diarrhea,* pseudomembranous colitis, esophagitis, flatulence, anorexia, *bloody or tarry stools, dysphagia.* **Hepatic:** elevated AST, alkaline phosphatase, bilirubin. **Skin:** maculopapular rash, urticaria. **Local:** *pain,* induration, *sterile abscess with I.M. injection;* thrombophlebitis, erythema, and pain after I.V. administration. **Other:** unpleasant or bitter taste, ***anaphylaxis.***

Interactions

Erythromycin: antagonist that may block access of clindamycin to its site of action. Don't use together.
Kaolin: decreased absorption of oral clindamycin. Separate administration times. **Neuromuscular blockers:** potentiated neuromuscular blockade. Monitor closely.

Nursing diagnoses

- High risk for injury related to ineffectiveness of clindamycin to eradicate the infection.
- High risk for fluid volume deficit related to clindamycin-induced adverse GI reactions.
- Knowledge deficit related to clindamycin therapy.

Nursing interventions

- *Contraindicated* in patients with hypersensitivity to lincomycin antibiotics and in patients with history of GI disease, especially colitis.
- *Use cautiously* in neonates and patients with renal or hepatic disease, asthma, or significant allergies.
- Monitor renal, hepatic, and hematopoietic functions during prolonged therapy.
- Obtain specimen for culture and sensitivity tests before first dose. Therapy may begin pending test results.
- Don't use in meningitis. Drug does not penetrate blood-brain barrier.
- Don't refrigerate reconstituted oral solution because it will thicken. Drug remains stable for 2 weeks at room temperature.
- Clindamycin has been associated with the development of pseudomembranous colitis caused by overgrowth of *Clostridium difficile.* Diarrhea is an early symptom; if patient develops diarrhea, tell him that additional antibiotic therapy may be necessary.
- Advise patient taking the capsule form to take with a full glass of water to prevent dysphagia.
- Give deep I.M. Rotate sites. Warn that I.M. injection may be painful. Doses greater than 600 mg per injection are not recommended.
- **I.V. use:** Check site daily for phlebitis and irritation. For I.V. infusion, dilute each 300 mg in 50 ml solution; give no faster than 30 mg/minute (over 10 to 60 minutes). Never give undiluted as a bolus.
- Watch for superinfection (fever or other signs of new infection).
- I.M. injection may cause CK level to rise because of muscle irritation.

General

Classification: uricosuric agent (sulfonamide derivative). **Pregnancy risk category:** B.

Mechanism of action

Blocks renal tubular reabsorption of uric acid, increasing excretion.

Indications and dosage

• Adjunct to penicillin or cephalosporin therapy. **Adults and children over 50 kg:** 500 mg P.O. q.i.d. **Children 2 to 14 years or under 50 kg:** initially, 25 mg/kg P.O., then 40 mg/kg divided q.i.d.

• Single-dose treatment of gonorrhea. **Adults:** 3.5 g ampicillin P.O. with 1 g probenecid P.O. given together; or 1 g probenecid P.O. 30 minutes before dose of 4.8 million units of aqueous penicillin G procaine I.M., injected at two different sites.

• Treatment of hyperuricemia of gout, gouty arthritis. **Adults:** 250 mg P.O. b.i.d. for first week, then 500 mg b.i.d., to maximum of 2 g daily. Maintenance dosage is 500 mg daily for 6 months.

Adverse reactions

Blood: ***hemolytic anemia.*** **CNS:** *headache,* dizziness. **CV:** hypotension. **GI:** anorexia, nausea, vomiting, *gastric distress.* **GU:** urinary frequency, renal colic. **Skin:** dermatitis, pruritus, alopecia. **Other:** flushing, sore gums, fever.

Interactions

Indomethacin: decreased indomethacin excretion. Lower indomethacin dosages may be required. **Methotrexate:** decreased methotrexate excretion. Lower methotrexate dosage may be required. **Oral antidiabetic agents:** enhanced hypoglycemic effect. Monitor blood glucose levels closely. **Salicylates:** inhibited uricosuric effect of probenecid, causing urate retention. Do not use together.

Nursing diagnoses

• Pain related to patient's underlying condition.
• Altered tissue perfusion (cardiopulmonary, renal, GI, cerebral, peripheral) related to probenecid-induced hemolytic anemia.
• Knowledge deficit related to probenecid therapy.

Nursing interventions

• *Contraindicated* in blood dyscrasias, acute gout attack, penicillin therapy in renal impairment, gouty nephropathy, urinary tract stones or obstruction, and azotemia or hyperuricemia from cancer chemotherapy, radiation, or myeloproliferative diseases.
• *Use cautiously* in peptic ulcer and renal impairment.
• Usually preferred over sulfinpyrazone because probenecid produces fewer and less severe GI and hematologic reactions.
• Contains no analgesic or anti-inflammatory agents and is of no value during acute gout attacks. Don't initiate therapy until acute attack subsides.
• Suitable for long-term use.
• Not effective with chronic renal insufficiency.
• Periodically monitor BUN and renal function during long-term therapy.
• May increase frequency, severity, and length of acute gout attacks during first 6 to 12 months of therapy. Prophylactic anti-inflammatory agent is given during first 3 to 6 months.
• Tell patient to avoid alcohol (it increases urate level) and all aspirin compounds (these may precipitate gout).
• Warn patient with gout to restrict foods high in purine.
• Instruct patient and his family that drug must be taken regularly to prevent gout attacks. Tell him to visit doctor regularly so uric acid can be monitored and dosage can be adjusted if necessary. Lifelong therapy may be required in patients with hyperuricemia.
• Force fluids to maintain minimum daily output of 2 to 3 liters. Alkalinize urine with sodium bicarbonate or potassium citrate as ordered. These measures prevent hematuria, renal colic, urate stone development, and costovertebral pain.
• Give with milk, food, or antacids to minimize GI distress.

General

Classification: antilipemic (fibric acid derivative).
Pregnancy risk category: C.

Mechanism of action

Seems to inhibit biosynthesis of cholesterol at an early stage, but the exact mechanism is unknown.

Indications and dosage

- Hyperlipidemia and xanthoma tuberosum; type III hyperlipidemia that doesn't respond adequately to diet; treatment of patients with extremely high serum triglyceride levels (type IV or V hyperlipidemia). **Adults:** 2 g P.O. daily in two or four divided doses. Some patients may respond to lower doses as evaluated by serum lipid monitoring.

Adverse reactions

Blood: leukopenia. **CNS:** fatigue, weakness. **CV:** ***arrhythmias.*** **GI:** *nausea, diarrhea, vomiting,* stomatitis, *dyspepsia,* flatulence. **GU:** impotence and decreased libido, acute renal failure. **Hepatic:** gallstones, *transient and reversible elevations of liver function tests.* **Skin:** rashes, urticaria, pruritus, dry skin and hair. **Other:** myalgia and arthralgia, resembling a flulike syndrome; *weight gain; polyphagia;* fever; decreased libido.

Interactions

Furosemide, sulfonylureas: clofibrate may potentiate the effect of these agents. Monitor patient closely. **Lovastatin, simvastatin, pravastatin:** risk of myositis, rhabdomyolysis, and renal failure. Avoid concomitant use. **Oral anticoagulants:** clofibrate may potentiate the effects of warfarin or dicumarol. Decrease anticoagulant dosage. **Oral contraceptives, rifampin:** may antagonize clofibrate's lipid-lowering effect. Monitor serum lipids. **Probenecid:** increased clofibrate effect. Monitor for toxicity.

Nursing diagnoses

- High risk for injury related to the ineffectiveness of clofibrate in reducing blood lipid and cholesterol levels.
- Diarrhea related to adverse drug reaction.
- Knowledge deficit related to clofibrate therapy.

Nursing interventions

- *Contraindicated* in severe renal or hepatic disease.
- Should not be used in children.
- Warn patient to report flulike symptoms to doctor immediately.
- Monitor renal and hepatic function, blood counts, and serum electrolyte and blood glucose levels. If liver function tests show steady rise, clofibrate should be discontinued.
- Drug should not be used indiscriminately. May pose an increased risk of gallstones, heart disease, and cancer.
- Used to treat patients with high serum triglyceride levels (type IV or V hyperlipidemia). These patients typically have serum triglyceride levels over 2,000 mg/dl.
- Monitor serum cholesterol and triglycerides regularly during clofibrate therapy.
- Teach patient about proper dietary management (restricting total fat and cholesterol intake), weight control, and exercise. Explain their importance in lowering serum lipids.
- If significant reduction in serum lipids isn't achieved within 3 months, drug should be discontinued.
- Clofibrate has been used investigationally to treat diabetes insipidus at doses of 1.5 to 2 g daily.

General
Classification: anticonvulsant (barbiturate).
Pregnancy risk category: D.

Mechanism of action
Unknown, but some activity may be caused by phenobarbital, which is an active metabolite.

Indications and dosage
• Generalized tonic-clonic seizures, complex-partial seizures. **Adults and children over 8 years:** 250 mg P.O. daily. Increase by 250 mg weekly, up to a maximum of 2 g daily, divided q.i.d. **Children under 8 years:** 125 mg P.O. daily. Increase by 125 mg weekly, up to a maximum of 1 g daily, divided q.i.d.

Adverse reactions
Blood: leukopenia, eosinophilia. **CNS:** *drowsiness, ataxia,* emotional disturbances, vertigo, hyperirritability, fatigue. **EENT:** diplopia, nystagmus, edema of the eyelids. **GI:** anorexia, *nausea, vomiting.* **GU:** impotence, polyuria. **Skin:** morbilliform rash, alopecia. **Other:** edema, thirst.

Interactions
Carbamazepine: increased primidone levels. Observe for toxicity. **Phenytoin:** stimulates conversion of primidone to phenobarbital. Observe for increased phenobarbital effect.

Nursing diagnoses
• High risk for injury related to the patient's underlying seizure disorder.
• Sensory/perceptual alterations (visual) related to primidone-induced diplopia.
• Knowledge deficit related to primidone therapy.

Nursing interventions
• *Contraindicated* in patients with phenobarbital hypersensitivity or porphyria.
• Don't withdraw the drug suddenly. Call the doctor if adverse reactions develop.
• If adverse CNS or visual disturbances occur, institute safety precautions, such as assisting the patient with ambulation and keeping the bed's side rails raised.
• Warn the patient to avoid hazardous activities that require alertness and good psychomotor coordination until the CNS effects of the drug are known. Full therapeutic response may take 2 weeks or more.
• Therapeutic blood level of primidone is 5 to 12 mcg/ml. Therapeutic blood level of phenobarbital is 15 to 40 mcg/ml.
• Inform the patient that a CBC and routine blood chemistry studies should be performed every 6 months during therapy.
• Primidone is partially converted to phenobarbital; consequently, use the drug cautiously with phenobarbital.
• Shake the liquid suspension well.

General

Classification: anticonvulsant (benzodiazepine). **Pregnancy risk category:** C. **Controlled substance schedule:** IV.

Mechanism of action

Appears to act on the limbic system, thalamus, and hypothalamus to produce anticonvulsant effects.

Indications and dosage

- Lennox-Gastaut syndrome and atypical absence seizures; akinetic and myoclonic seizures. **Adults:** initial dosage shouldn't exceed 1.5 mg P.O. daily in three divided doses. May be increased by 0.5 to 1 mg q 3 days until seizures are controlled. If given in unequal doses, the largest dose should be given h.s. Maximum recommended daily dosage is 20 mg. **Children up to 10 years or 30 kg:** 0.01 to 0.03 mg/kg P.O. daily (not to exceed 0.05 mg/kg daily), divided q 8 hours. Increase dosage by 0.25 to 0.5 mg q third day to a maximum maintenance dosage of 0.1 to 0.2 mg/kg daily.

Adverse reactions

Blood: leukopenia, thrombocytopenia, eosinophilia. **CNS:** *drowsiness, ataxia, behavioral disturbances (especially in children),* slurred speech, tremor, confusion. **EENT:** *increased salivation,* diplopia, nystagmus, abnormal eye movements. **GI:** constipation, gastritis, change in appetite, nausea, abnormal thirst, sore gums. **GU:** dysuria, enuresis, nocturia, urine retention. **Skin:** rash. **Other:** ***respiratory depression.***

Interactions

Alcohol, CNS depressants: increased CNS depression. Monitor closely.

Nursing diagnoses

- High risk for injury related to patient's underlying seizure disorder.
- Activity intolerance related to clonazepam-induced sedation.
- Knowledge deficit related to clonazepam therapy.

Nursing interventions

- *Contraindicated* in hepatic disease; chlordiazepoxide, diazepam, or other benzodiazepine sensitivity; or acute narrow-angle glaucoma.
- *Use cautiously* in patients with mixed seizure types because drug may precipitate generalized tonic-clonic seizures and in those with chronic respiratory disease, impaired renal function, and open-angle glaucoma.
- Therapeutic blood level is 20 to 80 ng/ml.
- Elderly patients are more sensitive to the drug's CNS effects.
- Warn patient to avoid activities that require alertness and good psychomotor coordination until CNS effects of the drug are known.
- Never withdraw drug suddenly. Call doctor at once if adverse reactions develop.
- Obtain periodic CBC and liver function tests.
- Monitor patient for oversedation.
- Withdrawal symptoms similar to those of barbiturates.
- Clonazepam may interfere with children's attentiveness in school. Instruct parents to monitor child's school performance.

General

Classification: anti-inflammatory, immunosuppressant (glucocorticoid). **Pregnancy risk category:** B.

Mechanism of action

Decreases inflammation, mainly by stabilizing leukocyte lysosomal membranes. Also suppresses the immune response, stimulates bone marrow, and influences protein, fat, and carbohydrate metabolism.

Indications and dosage

- Severe inflammation or immunosuppression. **Adults:** 2.5 to 15 mg P.O. b.i.d., t.i.d., or q.i.d. Maintenance dosage given once daily or every other day. Dosage must be individualized. **Children:** 0.14 to 2 mg/kg P.O. daily divided q.i.d.
- Acute exacerbations of multiple sclerosis. **Adults:** 200 mg P.O. daily for 1 week, then 80 mg every other day for 1 month.

Adverse reactions

Most reactions are dose- or duration-dependent. **CNS:** depression, *euphoria, insomnia,* psychotic behavior, pseudotumor cerebri. **CV:** ***CHF,*** hypertension, edema. **EENT:** cataracts, glaucoma. **GI:** *peptic ulcer,* GI irritation, increased appetite. **Metabolic:** hypokalemia, hyperglycemia and carbohydrate intolerance. **Skin:** delayed wound healing, acne, skin eruptions. **Other:** weakness, osteoporosis, pancreatitis, hirsutism, susceptibility to infections. Acute adrenal insufficiency may occur with increased stress (infection, surgery, or trauma) or abrupt withdrawal after long-term therapy. **Withdrawal symptoms:** rebound inflammation, fatigue, weakness, arthralgia, fever, dizziness, lethargy, depression, fainting, orthostatic hypotension, dyspnea, anorexia, hypoglycemia. ***Sudden withdrawal may be fatal.***

Interactions

Barbiturates, phenytoin, rifampin: decreased corticosteroid effect. **NSAIDs, indomethacin, aspirin:** increased risk of GI distress and bleeding. **Oral anticoagulants:** altered dosage requirements. **Potassium-depleting drugs:** enhanced potassium-wasting effects of prednisone. **Skin-test antigens:** decreased response. **Vaccines and toxoids:** decreased antibody response and increased risk of neurologic complications.

Nursing diagnoses

- Impaired tissue integrity related to the patient's underlying condition.
- High risk for injury related to adverse reactions to prednisone.
- Knowledge deficit related to prednisone therapy.

Nursing interventions

- *Contraindicated* in systemic fungal infections.
- *Use cautiously* in GI ulceration or renal disease, hypertension, osteoporosis, varicella, vaccinia, exanthema, diabetes mellitus, Cushing's syndrome, thromboembolic disorders, seizures, myasthenia gravis, metastatic cancer, CHF, tuberculosis, ocular herpes simplex, emotional instability, psychosis.
- Have patient on long-term therapy exercise or undergo physical therapy. Give vitamin D or calcium supplements as ordered.
- Gradually reduce drug dosage after long-term therapy, always titrating to lowest effective dose.
- Monitor blood pressure, sleep pattern, serum potassium. Weigh patient daily; report sudden gain.
- May mask or exacerbate infections, including latent amebiasis. Tell patient to report slow healing.
- Give a daily dose in the morning for better results and less toxicity.
- Teach patient signs of early adrenal insufficiency.
- Recommend periodic ophthalmic examinations for patients receiving long-term therapy.
- Unless contraindicated, give low-sodium diet high in potassium and protein. Supplement potassium.
- Unless contraindicated, give with food when possible to reduce GI irritation.
- May be used for alternate-day therapy.
- Warn patients on long-term therapy about cushingoid symptoms.

General

Classification: antihypertensive (antiadrenergic agent). **Pregnancy risk category:** C.

Mechanism of action

Inhibits the central vasomotor centers, thereby decreasing sympathetic outflow.

Indications and dosage

- Essential, renal, and malignant hypertension. **Adults:** initially, 0.1 mg P.O. b.i.d. Then increase by 0.1 to 0.2 mg daily on a weekly basis. Usual dosage range is 0.2 to 0.8 mg daily in divided doses; infrequently, dosages as high as 2.4 mg daily may be ordered. No dosage recommendations for children. Alternatively, apply transdermal patch to a hairless area of intact skin on the upper arm or torso, once q 7 days.
- Prophylactic treatment of migraine; treatment of menopausal flushing. **Adults:** 0.025 mg P.O. b.i.d. If remission doesn't occur within 2 weeks, increase dosage to 0.05 mg b.i.d.
- Suppression of abstinence symptoms during narcotics withdrawal. **Adults:** 0.1 mg P.O. t.i.d.

Adverse reactions

CNS: *drowsiness,* dizziness, fatigue, sedation, nervousness, headache, vivid dreams. **CV:** orthostatic hypotension, bradycardia, ***severe rebound hypertension.*** **GI:** *dry mouth, constipation.* **GU:** urine retention, impotence. **Metabolic:** transient glucose intolerance (after large doses). **Skin:** *pruritus, dermatitis* (from transdermal patch).

Interactions

CNS depressants: enhanced CNS depression. Use together cautiously. **Propranolol and other beta blockers:** paradoxical hypertensive response. Monitor carefully. **Tricyclic antidepressants and MAO inhibitors:** possible decreased antihypertensive effect. Use together cautiously.

Nursing diagnoses

- High risk for injury related to the ineffectiveness of clonidine in lowering blood pressure.
- Altered protection related to severe rebound hypertension caused by abrupt cessation of clonidine.
- Knowledge deficit related to clonidine therapy.

Nursing interventions

- *Use cautiously* in severe coronary insufficiency, diabetes, MI, cerebrovascular disease, chronic renal failure or depression or with other antihypertensives.
- Monitor blood pressure and pulse rate frequently. Dosage is usually adjusted to patient's blood pressure and tolerance.
- Don't stop clonidine therapy for surgery.
- Reduce dosage gradually over 2 to 4 days. If stopped abruptly, may cause severe hypertension.
- In patients receiving both clonidine and a beta blocker, the beta blocker should be gradually withdrawn before clonidine to minimize adverse reactions.
- Tell patient not to stop drug suddenly if unpleasant reactions occur; this can cause severe rebound hypertension. He should call doctor instead. Warn that drug can cause drowsiness, but tolerance will develop.
- Instruct the patient to check with the doctor or pharmacist before taking OTC medications.
- Observe for tolerance to the drug's therapeutic effects that may require an increased dosage.
- Rising slowly and avoiding sudden position chances can minimize orthostatic hypotension.
- Recommend periodic eye examinations.
- Last dose should be taken just before retiring.
- Transdermal patch available in three strengths: TTS-1 contains 2.5 mg of clonidine and releases 0.1 mg/24 hours; TTS-2 contains 5 mg of clonidine and releases 0.2 mg/24 hours; TTS-3 contains 7.5 mg of clonidine and releases 0.3 mg/24 hours.
- Patch usually adheres despite showering and other routine daily activities. Instruct the patient to place the patch at a different site each week.
- Antihypertensive effects of transdermal clonidine may take 2 to 3 days to occur. Oral antihypertensive therapy may have to be continued in the interim.
- Remove patch before defibrillation to prevent arcing.

General

Classification: anti-inflammatory, immunosuppressant (glucocorticoid). **Pregnancy risk category:** B.

Mechanism of action

Decreases inflammation, mainly by stabilizing leukocyte lysosomal membranes. Also suppresses the immune response, stimulates bone marrow, and influences protein, fat, and carbohydrate metabolism.

Indications and dosage

• Severe inflammation, immunosuppression. **Adults:** 2.5 to 15 mg P.O. b.i.d., t.i.d., or q.i.d.; 2 to 30 mg I.M. (acetate, phosphate), or I.V. (phosphate) q 12 hours; or 2 to 30 mg (phosphate) into joints, lesions, and soft tissue; or 4 to 40 mg (tebutate) into joints and lesions; or 0.25 to 1 ml (acetate-phosphate suspension) into joints weekly, p.r.n.

Adverse reactions

Most reactions are dose- or duration-dependent. **CNS:** depression, *euphoria, insomnia,* psychotic behavior, pseudotumor cerebri. **CV:** ***CHF,*** hypertension, edema. **EENT:** cataracts, glaucoma. **GI:** *peptic ulcer,* GI irritation, increased appetite. **Metabolic:** hypokalemia, hyperglycemia, carbohydrate intolerance. **Skin:** delayed wound healing, acne, skin eruptions. **Other:** weakness, osteoporosis, pancreatitis, hirsutism, susceptibility to infections. Acute adrenal insufficiency may occur with increased stress (infection, surgery, trauma) or abrupt withdrawal after long-term use. **Withdrawal symptoms:** rebound inflammation, fatigue, weakness, arthralgia, fever, dizziness, lethargy, depression, fainting, orthostatic hypotension, dyspnea, anorexia, hypoglycemia. ***Sudden withdrawal may be fatal.***

Interactions

Barbiturates, phenytoin, rifampin: decreased corticosteroid effect. **NSAIDs, indomethacin, aspirin:** increased risk of GI distress and bleeding. **Oral anticoagulants:** altered dosage requirements. **Potassium-depleting drugs:** enhanced potassium-wasting effects of prednisolone. **Skin-test antigens:** reduced response. **Vaccines and toxoids:** decreased antibody response and increased risk of neurologic complications.

Nursing diagnoses

• Impaired tissue integrity related to the patient's underlying condition.
• High risk for injury related to adverse reactions.
• Knowledge deficit related to prednisolone therapy.

Nursing interventions

• *Contraindicated* in systemic fungal infections.
• *Use cautiously* in GI ulcers, renal disease, hypertension, osteoporosis, varicella, vaccinia, exanthema, diabetes mellitus, Cushing's syndrome, thromboembolic disorders, seizures, myasthenia gravis, metastatic cancer, CHF, tuberculosis, ocular herpes simplex, emotional instability, and psychosis.
• Tell patient on long-term therapy to exercise or have physical therapy. Supplement vitamin D or calcium.
• Slowly lower dosage after long-term use, always titrating to lowest effective dose.
• May be used for alternate-day therapy.
• Monitor weight, blood pressure, serum electrolytes.
• May mask or exacerbate infections.
• Teach patient signs of early adrenal insufficiency.
• **I.V. use:** Use only prednisolone sodium phosphate; never give acetate form I.V.
• Give I.M. injection deep into gluteal muscle. Rotate injection sites to prevent muscle atrophy. Avoid S.C. injection, as atrophy and sterile abscesses may occur.
• Unless contraindicated, give low-sodium diet high in potassium and protein. Supplement potassium as needed.
• Warn patient on long-term therapy about cushingoid effects.

General

Classification: anxiolytic, anticonvulsant, sedative-hypnotic (benzodiazepine). **Pregnancy risk category:** C. **Controlled substance schedule:** IV.

Mechanism of action

Depresses the CNS at limbic and subcortical levels of the brain. As an anticonvulsant, suppresses the spread of seizure activity produced by epileptogenic foci in the cortex, thalamus, and limbic structures.

Indications and dosage

• Acute alcohol withdrawal. **Adults:** day 1 – 30 mg P.O. initially, followed by 30 to 60 mg in divided doses; day 2 – 45 to 90 mg P.O. in divided doses; day 3 – 22.5 to 45 mg P.O. in divided doses; day 4 – 15 to 30 mg P.O. in divided doses; gradually reduce daily dosage to 7.5 to 15 mg.
• Anxiety. **Adults:** 15 to 60 mg P.O. daily.
• Adjunctive treatment of seizure disorder. **Adults and children over 12 years:** Maximum recommended initial dosage is 7.5 mg P.O. t.i.d. Dosage increases should be no greater than 7.5 mg/week. Maximum daily dosage should not exceed 90 mg daily. **Children between 9 and 12 years:** Maximum recommended initial dosage is 7.5 mg P.O. b.i.d. Dosage increases should be no greater than 7.5 mg/week. Maximum daily dosage should not exceed 60 mg/day.

Adverse reactions

CNS: *drowsiness, lethargy, hangover,* fainting. **CV:** transient hypotension. **GI:** nausea, vomiting, abdominal discomfort.

Interactions

Alcohol, other CNS depressants: increased CNS depression. Avoid concomitant use. **Cigarette smoking:** increased clearance of benzodiazepines. Monitor for lack of effect. **Cimetidine:** increased sedation. Monitor carefully. **Digoxin:** possible increased serum levels of digoxin, increasing risk of toxicity. Monitor closely.

Nursing diagnoses

• Anxiety related to the patient's underlying condition.
• High risk for injury related to clorazepate-induced adverse reactions.
• Knowledge deficit related to clorazepate therapy.

Nursing interventions

• *Contraindicated* in acute narrow-angle glaucoma, depressive neuroses, and psychotic reactions and in children under 9 years.
• *Use cautiously* when hepatic or renal damage is present.
• Dosage should be reduced in elderly or debilitated patients.
• Possibility of abuse and addiction exists. Do not withdraw drug abruptly after prolonged use; withdrawal symptoms may occur.
• Warn patient to avoid activities requiring alertness and good psychomotor coordination until CNS effects of the drug are known.
• Warn patient not to combine drug with alcohol or other depressants.
• Suggest sugarless chewing gum or hard candy to relieve dry mouth.
• Caution patient against giving medication to others.
• Drug should not be prescribed regularly for everyday stress.
• Periodic hepatic, renal, and hematopoietic function studies should be performed in patients receiving repeated or prolonged therapy.
• If clorazepate overdose occurs, flumazenil (a specific benzodiazepine antagonist) may be useful. Know that the duration of action of clorazepate is longer than that of flumazenil, and resedation is possible.

General

Classification: antihypertensive (alpha-adrenergic blocking agent). **Pregnancy risk category:** C.

Mechanism of action

Relaxes both arteriolar and venous smooth muscle probably by blocking postsynaptic alpha receptors.

Indications and dosage

- Mild to moderate hypertension; used alone or with a diuretic or other antihypertensive drugs; also used to decrease afterload in severe chronic CHF. **Adults:** P.O. test dose is 1 mg given before bedtime to prevent "first-dose syncope." Initial dose is 1 mg t.i.d. Increase dosage slowly. Maximum daily dosage is 20 mg. Maintenance dosage is 3 to 20 mg daily in three divided doses. A few patients have required dosages larger than this (up to 40 mg daily). If other antihypertensive drugs or diuretics are added to this drug, decrease prazosin dosage to 1 to 2 mg t.i.d. and retitrate.

Adverse reactions

CNS: *dizziness,* headache, drowsiness, weakness, *"first-dose syncope,"* depression. **CV:** orthostatic hypotension, *palpitations.* **EENT:** blurred vision. **GI:** dry mouth, vomiting, diarrhea, abdominal cramps, constipation, *nausea.* **GU:** priapism, impotence.

Interactions

Propranolol and other beta blockers: syncope with loss of consciousness may occur more frequently. Advise the patient to sit or lie down if he feels dizzy.

Nursing diagnoses

- Altered tissue perfusion (renal, cerebral, cardiopulmonary, peripheral) related to the patient's underlying condition.
- High risk for injury related to adverse CNS reactions to prazosin.
- Knowledge deficit related to prazosin therapy.

Nursing interventions

- *Use cautiously* in patients receiving other antihypertensives.
- Monitor the patient's blood pressure and pulse rate frequently.
- If the initial dose is greater than 1 mg, the patient may develop severe syncope with loss of consciousness (first-dose syncope). Increase dosage slowly. Instruct him to sit or lie down if he experiences dizziness.
- Elderly patients may be more sensitive to hypotensive effects.
- Teach the patient about his disease and therapy. Explain the importance of taking this drug as prescribed, even when he's feeling well. Tell the outpatient not to discontinue this drug suddenly, but to call the doctor if adverse reactions occur.
- Instruct the patient to check with his doctor or pharmacist before taking any OTC medications.
- Inform the patient that orthostatic hypotension can be minimized by rising slowly and avoiding sudden position changes.
- Explain that dry mouth can be relieved with sugarless chewing gum, sour hard candy, or ice chips.
- Compliance may be improved by giving this drug once a day. Check with doctor.
- Drug has been used to treat Raynaud's disease.

cloxacillin sodium

Apo-Cloxit†, Cloxapen, Novocloxin†, Orbenin†, Tegopen

General

Classification: antibiotic (penicillinase-resistant penicillin). **Pregnancy risk category:** B.

Mechanism of action

Bactericidal against microorganisms by inhibiting cell wall synthesis during active multiplication. Bacteria resist penicillins by producing penicillinases—enzymes that convert penicillins to inactive penicilloic acid. Cloxacillin resists these enzymes.

Indications and dosage

- Systemic infections caused by penicillinase-producing staphylococci. **Adults:** 2 to 4 g P.O. daily, divided into doses given q 6 hours. **Children:** 50 to 100 mg/kg P.O. daily, divided into doses given q 6 hours.

Adverse reactions

Blood: eosinophilia. **GI:** *nausea*, vomiting, *epigastric distress, diarrhea.* **Skin:** *rash.* **Other:** *hypersensitivity (rash, urticaria, chills, fever, sneezing, wheezing,* ***anaphylaxis****)*, intrahepatic cholestasis, overgrowth of nonsusceptible organisms.

Interactions

Probenecid: increases blood levels of cloxacillin and other penicillins. Probenecid may be used for this purpose.

Nursing diagnoses

- High risk for injury related to ineffectiveness of cloxacillin to eradicate the infection.
- High risk for fluid volume deficit related to cloxacillin-induced adverse GI reactions.
- Knowledge deficit related to cloxacillin therapy.

Nursing interventions

- *Use cautiously* in patients with other drug allergies, especially to cephalosporins (possible cross-allergenicity).
- Obtain specimen for culture and sensitivity tests before first dose. Therapy may begin pending test results.
- Before giving cloxacillin, ask the patient if he's had any allergic reactions to penicillin. However, a negative history of penicillin allergy is no guarantee against a future allergic reaction.
- Tell the patient to take medication exactly as prescribed, even if he feels better. Entire quantity prescribed should be taken.
- Instruct the patient to call the doctor if rash, fever, or chills develop. A rash is the most common allergic reaction.
- Drug may cause GI disturbances. Food may interfere with absorption, so give 1 to 2 hours before meals or 2 to 3 hours after them.
- Advise the patient to take each dose with a full glass of water, not fruit juice or carbonated beverage, because acid will inactivate the drug.
- With large doses and prolonged therapy, bacterial and fungal superinfections may occur, especially in elderly, debilitated, or immunosuppressed patients. Close observation is essential.
- Warn the patient never to use leftover cloxacillin for a new illness or to share it with family and friends.
- Give cloxacillin at least 1 hour before bacteriostatic antibiotics.

General

Classification: anxiolytic (benzodiazepine). **Pregnancy risk category:** C. **Controlled substance schedule:** IV.

Mechanism of action

Depresses the CNS at the limbic and subcortical levels of the brain.

Indications and dosage

- Anxiety. **Adults:** 20 to 60 mg P.O. daily in divided doses, or 20 mg h.s.

Adverse reactions

CNS: *drowsiness, lethargy, hangover,* dizziness, ataxia, fainting. **CV:** transient hypotension. **GI:** dry mouth, nausea, vomiting, abdominal discomfort. **Skin:** rash.

Interactions

Alcohol, other CNS depressants: increased CNS depression. Avoid concomitant use. **Cigarette smoking:** increased clearance of benzodiazepines. Monitor for lack of effect. **Cimetidine:** increased sedation. Monitor carefully. **Digoxin:** possible increased serum levels of digoxin, increasing risk of toxicity. Monitor closely.

Nursing diagnoses

- Anxiety related to the patient's underlying condition.
- High risk for injury related to adverse CNS reactions to prazepam.
- Knowledge deficit related to prazepam therapy.

Nursing interventions

- *Contraindicated* in patients with acute narrow-angle glaucoma, psychoses, or anxiety-free psychiatric disorders.
- *Use cautiously* in patients with renal or hepatic impairment.
- Dosage should be reduced in elderly or debilitated patients.
- Possibility of prazapem abuse and addiction exists. Don't stop drug abruptly because withdrawal symptoms may occur.
- Warn the patient to avoid activities that require alertness and coordination until the CNS effects of the drug are known.
- Prazepam should not be prescribed for everyday stress.
- Periodically monitor hepatic, renal, and hematopoietic function studies in patients receiving repeated or prolonged therapy.
- If prazepam overdose occurs, administer flumazenil (a specific benzodiazepine antagonist). Keep in mind that the duration of action of prazepam is longer than that of flumazenil, and resedation is possible.

General

Classification: antipsychotic (dibenzodiazepine). **Pregnancy risk category:** B.

Mechanism of action

Binds to dopamine receptors in CNS limbic system. It also may interfere with adrenergic, cholinergic, histaminergic, and serotoninergic receptors.

Indications and dosage

• Schizophrenia in patients unresponsive to other therapies. **Adults:** initially, 25 mg P.O. q.i.d. or b.i.d., titrated upward at 25 to 50 mg daily (if tolerated) to 300 to 450 mg daily in 2 weeks. Subsequent dosage increases shouldn't occur more than twice weekly or exceed 100 mg. Maximum dosage is 900 mg daily.

Adverse reactions

Blood: ***leukopenia, granulocytopenia, agranulocytosis.*** **CNS:** *drowsiness, sedation, seizures, dizziness,* syncope, vertigo, tremor, disturbed sleep or nightmares, restlessness, hypokinesia or akinesia, agitation, rigidity, akathisia, confusion, insomnia, hyperkinesia, weakness, lethargy, ataxia, slurred speech, depression, anxiety. **CV:** *tachycardia, hypotension,* hypertension, chest pain, ECG changes. **GI:** *constipation,* nausea, vomiting, *salivation, dry mouth,* heartburn. **GU:** urinary abnormalities, incontinence, abnormal ejaculation, urinary frequency, urgency, or retention. **Skin:** rash. **Other:** fever, muscle pain or spasm, weight gain.

Interactions

Anticholinergics: may potentiate anticholinergic effects of clozapine. **Antihypertensives:** may potentiate hypotensive effects. **Bone marrow suppressants:** potentially increased bone marrow toxicity. **Psychoactive drugs:** possible additive effects. **Warfarin, digoxin, other highly protein-bound drugs:** increased serum levels of these drugs. Monitor closely for adverse reactions.

Nursing diagnoses

• Altered thought processes related to the patient's underlying condition.
• High risk for injury related to adverse reactions.
• Knowledge deficit related to clozapine therapy.

Nursing interventions

• *Contraindicated* in history of clozapine-induced agranulocytosis or severe granulocytopenia; WBC count below 3,500/mm^3; severe CNS depression or coma; myelosuppressive disorders and in those taking drugs that suppress bone marrow function.
• *Use cautiously* in prostatic hypertrophy or glaucoma; clozapine has potent anticholinergic effects.
• Seizures may occur, especially with high doses. Patients should avoid activities requiring alertness.
• Clozapine carries a significant risk of agranulocytosis. If possible, patients should receive at least two trials of a standard antipsychotic drug before clozapine therapy. Baseline WBC and differential counts are required before therapy; monitor WBC counts weekly for at least 4 weeks after clozapine therapy is discontinued.
• If WBC count drops below 3,500/mm^3 after initiating therapy or drops substantially from baseline, monitor patient closely for infection. If WBC count is 3,000 to 3,500/mm^3 and granulocyte count above 1,500/mm^3, perform twice-weekly WBC and differential counts. If WBC count drops below 3,000/mm^3 and granulocyte count below 1,500/mm^3, therapy should be interrupted and patient monitored for signs of infection. May cautiously restart therapy if WBC count returns above 3,000/mm^3; granulocyte count, above 1,500/mm^3. Monitor WBC and differential counts twice weekly until WBC count exceeds 3,500/mm^3.
• If the WBC count drops below 2,000/mm^3 and granulocyte count drops below 1,000/mm^3, the patient may require protective isolation.
• If clozapine must be discontinued, withdraw gradually; changes in patient's condition may require abrupt discontinuation of the drug. Monitor closely for recurrence of psychotic symptoms.
• If therapy reinstated in patient withdrawn from drug, follow usual guidelines for dosage build-up. However, restarting may increase the severity and risk of adverse reactions. If drug was terminated for WBC counts below 2,000/mm^3 or granulocyte counts below 1,000/mm^3, discontinue.

General

Classification: antilipemic (HMG-CoA reductase inhibitor). **Pregnancy risk category:** X.

Mechanism of action

Inhibits the enzyme 3-hydroxy-3-methylglutaryl-coenzyme A (HMG-CoA) reductase. This hepatic enzyme is an early (and rate-limiting) step in the synthetic pathway of cholesterol.

Indications and dosage

• Reduction of low-density lipoprotein and total cholesterol levels in patients with primary hypercholesterolemia (types IIa and IIb). **Adults:** initially, 5 to 10 mg daily h.s. Adjust dosage q 4 weeks based on patient tolerance and response; maximum daily dosage is 40 mg. Most elderly patients respond to a daily dosage of 20 mg or less.

Adverse reactions

CNS: headache, fatigue, dizziness. **CV:** chest pain. **EENT:** rhinitis. **GI:** vomiting, diarrhea, heartburn, nausea. **Respiratory:** cough. **Skin:** rash. **Other:** influenza, localized muscle pain, myalgia, cold.

Interactions

Cholestyramine, colestipol: decreased plasma levels of pravastatin. Administer pravastatin 1 hour before or 4 hours after these drugs. **Drugs that decrease levels or activity of endogenous steroids (such as cimetidine, spironolactone, ketoconazole):** possible increased risk of endocrine dysfunction. No intervention appears necessary; take complete drug history in patients who develop endocrine dysfunction. **Gemfibrozil:** decreased protein-binding and urine clearance of pravastatin. Avoid concomitant use. **Hepatotoxic drugs, chronic alcohol abuse:** increased risk of hepatotoxicity. Avoid concomitant use. **Immunosuppressive agents (such as cyclosporine), fibric acid derivatives (such as clofibrate), high doses of niacin (1 g or more daily), erythromycin:** possible increased risk of rhabdomyolysis. Monitor patient closely if concomitant use can't be avoided.

Nursing diagnoses

• High risk for injury related to the ineffectiveness of pravastatin in lowering cholesterol levels.
• Diarrhea related to adverse drug reaction.
• Knowledge deficit related to pravastatin therapy.

Nursing interventions

• *Contraindicated* in patients with active liver disease or conditions that have unexplained persistent elevations of serum transaminase, in pregnant and breast-feeding women, and in women of childbearing age unless no risk of pregnancy exists.
• Administer the recommended dosage in the evening, preferably at bedtime.
• Initiate drug only after diet and other nondrug therapies have proven ineffective. Patients should continue a cholesterol-lowering diet during therapy.
• Dosage adjustments should be made about every 4 weeks. If cholesterol level falls below the target range, dosage may be reduced.
• Perform liver function tests frequently at the start of therapy and periodically thereafter.
• Liver dysfunction may occur in slightly more than 1% of patients. Discontinue drug and monitor patient closely. A liver biopsy may be performed if enzyme elevations persist.
• Temporarily discontinue drug in any patient with an acute condition that suggests a developing myopathy or in patients with risk factors for renal failure from rhabdomyolysis: severe acute infection; severe endocrine, metabolic, or electrolyte disorders; hypotension; major surgery; or uncontrolled seizures.
• Because of drug's possible impact on liver function, advise patient to restrict alcohol intake.
• Tell the patient to inform the doctor of any adverse reactions, particularly muscle aches and pains.
• Teach the patient to control serum lipids through proper dietary management, weight control, and exercise.

General

Classification: analgesic, antitussive (opioid). **Pregnancy risk category:** C (D for prolonged use or use of high doses at term). **Controlled substance schedule:** II.

Mechanism of action

Binds with opiate receptors at many sites in the CNS (brain, brain stem, and spinal cord), altering both perception of and emotional response to pain through an unknown mechanism. Also suppresses the cough reflex by direct action on the cough center in the medulla.

Indications and dosage

- Mild to moderate pain. **Adults:** 15 to 60 mg P.O. (sulfate) or 15 to 60 mg (phosphate) S.C. or I.M. q 4 hours, p.r.n. or around the clock. **Children:** 3 mg/kg P.O. daily divided q 4 hours, p.r.n. or around the clock.
- Nonproductive cough. **Adults:** 10 to 20 mg P.O. q 4 to 6 hours. Maximum dosage is 120 mg/24 hours. **Children 6 to 12 years:** 5 to 10 mg P.O. q 4 to 6 hours. Maximum dosage is 60 mg/24 hours. **Children 2 to 6 years:** 2.5 to 5 mg P.O. q 4 to 6 hours. Do not exceed 30 mg in 24 hours.

Adverse reactions

CNS: *sedation, clouded sensorium, euphoria,* dizziness, seizures with large doses. **CV:** *hypotension,* bradycardia. **GI:** *nausea, vomiting, constipation, dry mouth,* ileus. **GU:** *urine retention.* **Skin:** pruritus, flushing. **Other:** ***respiratory depression,*** physical dependence.

Interactions

Alcohol, general anesthetics, other narcotic analgesics, tranquilizers, sedatives, hypnotics, alcohol, tricyclic antidepressants, or MAO inhibitors: Use together with extreme caution. Monitor patient response.

Nursing diagnoses

- Pain related to patient's underlying condition.
- Constipation related to binding effect of codeine.
- Knowledge deficit related to codeine therapy.

Nursing interventions

- *Contraindicated* in patients with hypersensitivity to the drug or other opiate analgesics.
- *Use with extreme caution* in head injury, increased intracranial pressure, increased CSF pressure, hepatic or renal disease, hypothyroidism, Addison's disease, acute alcoholism, seizures, severe CNS depression, bronchial asthma, COPD, respiratory depression, and shock and in elderly or debilitated patients.
- Warn ambulatory patient to avoid hazardous activities that require alertness.
- Oral administration may cause GI upset. Advise patient to take the drug with milk or meals to minimize GI distress.
- Opiates may cause constipation. Assess bowel function and need for stool softeners or laxatives. Constipating effect makes codeine useful in treating diarrhea.
- Monitor respiratory and circulatory status and bowel function.
- For full analgesic effect, give before patient has intense pain.
- Codeine and aspirin or acetaminophen are often prescribed together to provide enhanced pain relief.
- Do not administer discolored injection solution.
- An antitussive; don't use when cough is a valuable diagnostic sign or beneficial (as after thoracic surgery).
- Monitor cough type and frequency.
- The abuse potential of codeine is much less than that of morphine.

General

Classification: antihyperthyroid agent, expectorant (electrolyte). **Pregnancy risk category:** D.

Mechanism of action

Inhibits thyroid hormone formation by blocking iodotyrosine and iodothyronine synthesis. It also limits iodide transport into the thyroid gland and blocks thyroid hormone release.

Indications and dosage

• Preparation for thyroidectomy. **Adults and children:** 0.1 to 0.3 ml (strong iodine solution, USP) P.O. t.i.d., or 5 drops (potassium iodide solution, USP) in water P.O. t.i.d. after meals for 2 to 3 weeks before surgery.
• Thyrotoxic crisis. **Adults and children:** 1 ml (strong iodine solution, USP) in water P.O. t.i.d. after meals.
• Radiation protectant for thyroid gland. **Adults:** 100 to 150 mg P.O. 24 hours before and for 3 to 10 days after radiation exposure.
• Expectorant. **Adults:** 0.3 to 0.6 ml saturated potassium iodide solution (SSKI) diluted in water t.i.d. or q.i.d.

Adverse reactions

EENT: acute rhinitis, inflammation of salivary glands, periorbital edema, conjunctivitis, hyperemia. **GI:** burning, irritation, nausea, vomiting, *metallic taste.* **Skin:** acneiform rash, mucous membrane ulceration. **Other:** fever, frontal headache, tooth discoloration, ***hypersensitivity, including symptoms resembling serum sickness.***

Interactions

ACE inhibitors, potassium-sparing diuretics: risk of hyperkalemia. Avoid concomitant use. **Antithyroid drugs:** possible potentiated hypothyroid or goiterogenic effects. Monitor closely. **Lithium carbonate:** possible hypothyroidism. Use with caution.

Nursing diagnoses

• Ineffective airway clearance related to the patient's underlying condition.
• Pain (epigastric) related to adverse GI effects of potassium iodide.
• Knowledge deficit related to potassium iodide therapy.

Nursing interventions

• *Contraindicated* in tuberculosis, iodide hypersensitivity, and hyperkalemia; after meals that contain excessive starch; in laryngeal edema; and in swelling of salivary glands.
• Earliest signs of delayed hypersensitivity caused by iodides are irritation and swelling of the eyelids.
• Dilute oral doses in water, milk, or fruit juice, and give after meals to prevent gastric irritation, to hydrate the patient, and to mask the salty taste.
• Tell the patient to ask the doctor about using iodized salt and eating shellfish during treatment. Iodine-rich foods may not be permitted.
• Warn the patient that sudden withdrawal may precipitate thyroid storm.
• Avoid using enteric-coated tablets, which have been associated with small bowel lesions and can lead to serious complications, including perforation, hemorrhage, or obstruction.
• Store in light-resistant container.
• Give iodides through a straw to avoid tooth discoloration.
• Usually given with other antithyroid drugs.

General

Classification: antigout agent (*Colchicum autumnale* alkaloid). **Pregnancy risk category:** D.

Mechanism of action

As antigout agent, apparently decreases leukocyte motility, phagocytosis, and lactic acid production, thus decreasing urate crystal deposits and reducing inflammation.

Indications and dosage

• Prevention of acute gout attacks. **Adults:** 0.5 or 0.6 mg P.O. daily. Patients who normally have one attack per year or less should receive drug only 3 or 4 days per week. Patients who have more than one attack per year should receive the drug daily. In severe cases, give 1 to 1.8 mg daily.

• Prevention of gout attacks in surgical patients. **Adults:** 0.5 to 0.6 mg P.O. t.i.d. 3 days before and 3 days after surgery.

• Treatment of acute gout, acute gouty arthritis. **Adults:** initially, 1 to 1.2 mg P.O., then 0.5 or 0.6 mg q hour, or 1 to 1.2 mg q 2 hours until pain is relieved; nausea, vomiting, or diarrhea ensues; or maximum dose of 10 mg is reached. Alternatively, give 2 mg I.V. followed by 0.5 mg q 6 hours if necessary. (Some clinicians prefer single I.V. injection of 3 mg.) Total I.V. dosage over 24 hours (one course of treatment) not to exceed 4 mg.

Note: Colchicine overdose can be fatal. After full course of I.V. colchicine (4 mg), don't give additional colchicine by any route for at least 7 days.

Adverse reactions

Blood: ***aplastic anemia and agranulocytosis with prolonged use;*** nonthrombocytopenic purpura. **CNS:** peripheral neuritis. **GI:** *nausea, vomiting, abdominal pain, diarrhea.* **Skin:** urticaria, dermatitis. **Local:** severe local irritation if extravasation occurs. **Other:** alopecia.

Interactions

Alcohol: may impair efficacy of colchicine prophylaxis. **Loop diuretics:** may decrease efficacy of colchicine prophylaxis. **Phenylbutazone:** may increase risk of leukopenia or thrombocytopenia. **Vitamin B_{12}:** impaired absorption of vitamin B_{12}.

Nursing diagnoses

• Pain related to patient's underlying condition.
• High risk for fluid volume deficit related to colchicine-induced adverse GI reactions.
• Knowledge deficit related to colchicine therapy.

Nursing interventions

• *Use cautiously* in hepatic dysfunction, cardiac disease, blood dyscrasias, renal disease, or GI disorders, and in elderly or debilitated patients.
• Reduce dosage if weakness, anorexia, nausea, vomiting, or diarrhea appears. First sign of acute overdosage may be GI effects, followed by vascular damage, weakness, and ascending paralysis. Delirium and seizures may occur without loss of consciousness.
• Discontinue drug as soon as gout pain is relieved or at first GI symptoms.
• **I.V. use:** Give by slow I.V. push over 2 to 5 minutes. Avoid extravasation. Don't dilute colchicine injection with dextrose 5% injection or any other fluid that might change solution pH. If lower concentration of colchicine injection is needed, dilute with 0.9% sodium chloride or sterile water for injection and give over 2 to 5 minutes. Preferably, inject into the tubing of a free-flowing I.V. solution. However, if diluted solution becomes turbid, don't inject.
• Don't give I.M. or S.C.; severe local irritation occurs.
• Baseline laboratory studies, including CBC, should precede therapy and be repeated periodically. Monitor fluid intake and output. Keep output at 2,000 ml daily.
• Store in tightly closed, light-resistant container.

General

Classification: agent for electrolyte balance (potassium supplement). **Pregnancy risk category:** A.

Mechanism of action

Replaces potassium and maintains its level.

Indications and dosage

• Hypokalemia. **Adults:** 40 to 100 mEq P.O. daily in three or four divided doses for treatment; 20 mEq daily for prevention. Further dosage based on serum potassium determinations.

Adverse reactions

The following adverse reactions are signs of hyperkalemia. **CNS:** paresthesia of the extremities, listlessness, confusion, weakness or heaviness of legs, flaccid paralysis. **CV:** ***cardiac arrhythmias,*** ECG changes (prolonged PR interval; wide QRS complex; ST-segment depression; tall, tented T waves). **GI:** *nausea, vomiting, abdominal pain,* diarrhea, GI ulcers with oral products (especially enteric-coated tablets); ulcerations may be accompanied by stenosis, hemorrhage, obstruction, perforation.

Interactions

None significant.

Nursing diagnoses

• Altered nutrition: Less than body requirements, related to the patient's underlying condition.
• High risk for injury related to potassium-induced hyperkalemia.
• Knowledge deficit related to potassium gluconate therapy.

Nursing interventions

• *Contraindicated* in patients with severe renal impairment with oliguria, anuria, or azotemia; in untreated Addison's disease; and in patients with acute dehydration, hyperkalemia, the hyperkalemic form of familial periodic paralysis, or conditions associated with extensive tissue breakdown.
• *Use cautiously* in patients with cardiac disease and in those receiving potassium-sparing diuretics.
• Monitor ECG, serum potassium and creatinine levels, BUN, and intake and output.
• Give oral potassium supplements with extreme caution because their many forms deliver varying amounts of potassium. Never switch products without a doctor's order.
• Don't administer potassium supplements postoperatively until urine flow has been established.
• Have the patient sip liquid potassium slowly to minimize GI irritation.
• Give with or after meals with a full glass of water or fruit juice to lessen GI distress.
• Potassium gluconate does not correct hypokalemic hypochloremic alkalosis.
• Enteric-coated tablets are not recommended because of the potential for GI bleeding and small-bowel ulcerations.

colestipol hydrochloride Colestid

General
Classification: antilipemic (anion exchange resin).
Pregnancy risk category: C.

Mechanism of action
Combines with bile acid to form an insoluble compound that is excreted. The liver must synthesize new bile acid from cholesterol; this leads to reduced low-density-lipoprotein cholesterol levels.

Indications and dosage
• Primary hypercholesterolemia and xanthomas. **Adults:** 5 to 30 g P.O. daily in two to four divided doses.

Adverse reactions
CNS: headache, dizziness. **GI:** *constipation (may require decreasing the dosage),* fecal impaction, hemorrhoids, abdominal discomfort, flatulence, nausea, vomiting, steatorrhea. **Skin:** rashes; irritation of skin, tongue, and perianal area. **Other:** vitamin A, D, and K deficiency from decreased absorption; hyperchloremic acidosis with long-term use or high dosage.

Interactions
Oral antidiabetic agents: may antagonize response to colestipol. Monitor serum lipids. **Orally administered drugs:** absorption may be decreased by colestipol. Separate administration times: other drugs should be taken at least 1 hour before or 4 hours after colestipol.

Nursing diagnoses
• High risk for injury related to the ineffectiveness of colestipol in reducing blood lipid and cholesterol levels.
• Constipation related to adverse drug reactions.
• Knowledge deficit related to colestipol therapy.

Nursing interventions
• *Contraindicated* in patients with hypersensitivity to bile acid sequestering resins and in patients with complete biliary obstruction.
• *Use cautiously* in patients predisposed to constipation and in patients with conditions that may be aggravated by constipation, such as severe, symptomatic coronary artery disease. Long-term use may be associated with deficiency of vitamins A, D, E, and K and folic acid.
• Administer all other medications at least 1 hour before or 4 to 6 hours after colestipol to avoid blocking their absorption.
• Monitor digitalis glycoside levels in patients receiving both medications concurrently. If colestipol therapy is discontinued, digitalis toxicity may result unless dosage is adjusted.
• Watch for signs of vitamin A, D, and K deficiency.
• Lowering dosage, increasing dietary fiber, or adding stool softener may relieve constipation.
• May bind many drugs and cause decreased absorption. Check drug interaction list of individual drugs.
• Administer this drug in at least 3 oz (90 ml) of juice, milk, or water. After drinking this preparation, the patient should swirl a small additional amount of liquid in the same glass and then drink it to ensure ingestion of the entire dose.
• Palatability may be enhanced if the next daily dose is mixed and refrigerated the previous evening.
• Teach patient about proper dietary management (restricting total fat and cholesterol intake), weight control, and exercise. Explain their importance in lowering serum lipid levels.

General

Classification: agent for electrolyte balance (potassium supplement). **Pregnancy risk category:** A.

Mechanism of action

Replaces potassium and maintains its level.

Indications and dosage

• Hypokalemia. **Adults:** 40 to 100 mEq P.O. daily in three or four divided doses for treatment; 20 mEq for prevention. Further dosage based on serum potassium. Use I.V. route when oral replacement isn't feasible or when hypokalemia is life-threatening. Usual dose 20 mEq hourly in concentration of 40 mEq/liter or less. Total daily dosage not to exceed 150 mEq (3 mEq/kg in children). Potassium replacement should be monitored with ECG and frequent serum potassium determinations.

Adverse reactions

The following adverse reactions are signs of hyperkalemia. **CNS:** paresthesia of the extremities, listlessness, confusion, weakness or heaviness of limbs, flaccid paralysis. **CV:** ***peripheral vascular collapse with fall in blood pressure, arrhythmias, heart block, possible cardiac arrest,*** ECG changes (prolonged PR interval; wide QRS; ST-segment depression; tall, tented T waves). **GI:** *nausea, vomiting, abdominal pain,* diarrhea, GI ulcers (possible stenosis, hemorrhage, obstruction, perforation). **GU:** oliguria. **Skin:** cold skin, gray pallor. **Local:** *postinfusion phlebitis.*

Interactions

None significant.

Nursing diagnoses

• Altered nutrition: Less than body requirements, related to the patient's underlying condition.
• High risk for injury related to potassium-induced hyperkalemia.
• Knowledge deficit related to potassium chloride therapy.

Nursing interventions

• *Contraindicated* in severe renal impairment with oliguria, anuria, or azotemia; in untreated Addison's disease; and in acute dehydration, hyperkalemia, the hyperkalemic form of familial periodic paralysis, and conditions associated with extensive tissue breakdown.
• *Use cautiously* in patients with cardiac disease and in those receiving potassium-sparing diuretics.
• Don't give potassium during the immediate postoperative period until urine flow is established.
• Give oral potassium supplements with extreme caution because its many forms deliver varying amounts of potassium. Never switch products without a doctor's order.
• Use a liquid preparation if tablet or capsule passage is likely to be delayed, as in GI obstruction. Have patient sip it slowly to minimize GI irritation.
• Give with or after meals with a full glass of water or fruit juice to lessen GI distress.
• Patient should make sure powders are completely dissolved before ingesting.
• Enteric-coated tablets not recommended due to potential for GI bleeding and small-bowel ulcers.
• Tablets in wax matrix sometimes lodge in esophagus and cause ulcers in cardiac patients who have esophageal compression from enlarged left atrium. In such patients and in those with esophageal stasis or obstruction, use liquid form.
• Often used orally with diuretics that cause potassium excretion. Potassium chloride most useful since diuretics waste chloride ion. Hypokalemic alkalosis treated best with potassium chloride.
• Monitor ECG and serum electrolytes during therapy.
• Don't crush sustained-release products.
• **I.V. use:** Give by infusion only; never I.V. push or I.M. Give slowly as dilute solution; potentially fatal hyperkalemia may result from too-rapid infusion.
• Small amounts of lidocaine injection (1 to 3 ml of the 1% strength) may be added directly to potassium chloride solution to help reverse postinfusion phlebitis.

General

Classification: diagnostic aid, replacement hormone, anti-inflammatory agent, nonsupportive thyroiditis treatment (anterior pituitary hormone).
Pregnancy risk category: C.

Mechanism of action

Stimulates adrenal cortex to secrete its entire spectrum of hormones by replacing the body's own tropic hormone.

Indications and dosage

- Diagnostic test of adrenocortical function. **Adults:** up to 80 units I.M. or S.C. in divided doses; or single dose (repository); or 10 to 25 units (aqueous) in 500 ml D_5W I.V. over 8 hours, between blood samplings.
- Therapeutic use. **Adults:** 40 units S.C. or I.M. in four divided doses (aqueous); 40 units q 12 to 24 hours (repository form).

Adverse reactions

CNS: ***seizures,*** *dizziness,* papilledema, *euphoria, insomnia,* personality changes, depression, psychosis. **EENT:** cataracts, glaucoma. **GI:** peptic ulcer, pancreatitis, abdominal distention, ulcerative esophagitis, nausea, vomiting. **GU:** menstrual irregularities. **Metabolic:** *sodium and fluid retention,* calcium and potassium loss, hypokalemic alkalosis, negative nitrogen balance. **Skin:** impaired wound healing, petechiae, ecchymoses, facial erythema, increased sweating, acne, hyperpigmentation, hirsutism. **Other:** weakness, steroid myopathy, loss of muscle mass, osteoporosis, vertebral compression fractures, cushingoid state, growth suppression in children, activation of latent diabetes mellitus, progressive increase in antibodies, loss of drug's stimulatory effect, ***hypersensitivity.***

Interactions

Anticonvulsants, barbiturates, rifampin: increased metabolism of corticotropin and decreased effectiveness. Monitor for lack of effect. **Estrogens:** may potentiate drug effects. Dosage adjustments may be necessary. **NSAIDs, salicylates:** increased risk of GI bleeding. **Oral anticoagulants:** change in prothrombin time. Monitor and adjust dosage. **Potassium-wasting diuretics:** increased risk of hypokalemia. Monitor serum potassium levels.

Nursing diagnoses

- Activity intolerance related to the patient's underlying condition.
- Fluid volume excess related to corticotropin-induced sodium and fluid retention.
- Knowledge deficit related to corticotropin therapy.

Nursing interventions

- *Contraindicated* in scleroderma, osteoporosis, systemic fungal infections, ocular herpes simplex, recent surgery, peptic ulcer, CHF, hypertension, sensitivity to pork and pork products, adrenocortical hyperfunction or primary insufficiency, or Cushing's syndrome.
- *Use cautiously* in pregnant, breast-feeding, or childbearing-age women, patients being immunized, latent tuberculosis or tuberculin reactivity, hypothyroidism, cirrhosis, infection, acute gouty arthritis, emotional instability or psychotic tendencies, diabetes, abscess, pyogenic infections, renal insufficiency, and myasthenia gravis.
- Before treatment, verify adrenal responsiveness and test for hypersensitivity and allergic reactions.
- Corticotropin should be adjunctive, not sole therapy. Oral agents preferred for long-term therapy.
- Unusual stress may require additional use of rapidly acting corticosteroids. Gradually reduce to smallest effective dose to minimize induced adrenocortical insufficiency.
- Counteract edema by low-sodium, high-potassium intake; nitrogen loss by high-protein diet; and psychotic changes by reducing dosage or administering sedatives.
- Drug may mask signs of chronic disease, decrease host resistance and ability to localize infection.
- To give gel, warm to room temperature, draw into 21G or 22G needle, and give slowly deep I.M.

General
Classification: agent for electrolyte balance (potassium supplement). **Pregnancy risk category:** A.

Mechanism of action
Replaces potassium and maintains its level.

Indications and dosage
• Hypokalemia. **Adults:** 25 to 50 mEq dissolved in one-half to a full glass of water (120 to 240 ml) once daily to q.i.d.

Adverse reactions
CNS: paresthesia of the extremities, listlessness, confusion, weakness or heaviness of legs, flaccid paralysis. **CV:** ***cardiac arrhythmias,*** ECG changes (prolonged PR interval; wide QRS complex; ST segment depression; tall, tented T waves). **GI:** *nausea, vomiting, abdominal pain,* diarrhea, ulcerations, hemorrhage, obstruction, perforation.

Interactions
None significant.

Nursing diagnoses
• Altered nutrition: Less than body requirements, related to the patient's underlying condition.
• High risk for injury related to potassium-induced hyperkalemia.
• Knowledge deficit related to potassium bicarbonate therapy.

Nursing interventions
• *Contraindicated* in patients with severe renal impairment with oliguria, anuria, or azotemia; in untreated Addison's disease; and in patients with acute dehydration, hyperkalemia, the hyperkalemic form of familial periodic paralysis, and conditions associated with extensive tissue breakdown.
• *Use cautiously* in patients with cardiac disease and in those receiving potassium-sparing diuretics.
• Monitor BUN, serum potassium and creatinine, and intake and output.
• Never switch potassium products without a doctor's order.
• Dissolve potassium bicarbonate tablets in 6 to 8 oz of cold water. Dissolve completely to minimize GI irritation.
• Don't administer potassium supplements postoperatively until urine flow has been established.
• Have the patient take with meals and sip slowly over 5 to 10 minutes.
• Potassium bicarbonate cannot be given instead of potassium chloride.
• Potassium bicarbonate doesn't correct hypochloremic alkalosis.
• Available in lime and orange flavors. Ask patient's flavor preference.

cortisone acetate

Cortone Acetate

General

Classification: anti-inflammatory, replacement therapy (glucocorticoid, mineralocorticoid). **Pregnancy risk category:** D.

Mechanism of action

Decreases inflammation, mainly by stabilizing leukocyte lysosomal membranes. Also suppresses immune response, stimulates bone marrow, and influences protein, fat, and carbohydrate metabolism.

Indications and dosage

- Adrenal insufficiency, allergy, inflammation. **Adults:** 25 to 300 mg P.O. or I.M. daily or on alternate days. Dosage reflects severity of disease.

Adverse reactions

Most adverse reactions are dose- or duration-dependent. **CNS:** *euphoria, insomnia,* psychotic behavior, pseudotumor cerebri. **CV:** ***CHF,*** hypertension, edema. **EENT:** cataracts, glaucoma. **GI:** *peptic ulcer,* GI irritation, increased appetite. **Metabolic:** possible hypokalemia, hyperglycemia and carbohydrate intolerance, growth suppression. **Skin:** delayed wound healing, acne, various skin eruptions. **Local:** atrophy at I.M. injection sites. **Other:** weakness, osteoporosis, pancreatitis, hirsutism, susceptibility to infections.

Acute adrenal insufficiency may follow increased stress (infection, surgery, trauma) or abrupt withdrawal after long-term therapy. **Withdrawal symptoms:** rebound inflammation, fatigue, weakness, arthralgia, fever, dizziness, lethargy, depression, fainting, orthostatic hypotension, dyspnea, anorexia, hypoglycemia. ***Sudden withdrawal may be fatal.***

Interactions

Barbiturates, phenytoin, rifampin: decreased corticosteroid effect. **Indomethacin, aspirin, NSAIDs:** increased risk of GI distress and bleeding. **Live attenuated virus vaccines, other vaccines and toxoids:** decreased antibody response and increased risk of neurologic complications. **Oral anticoagulants:** altered dosage requirements. **Potassium-depleting drugs:** enhanced potassium-wasting effects of cortisone. **Skin-test antigens:** reduced response.

Nursing diagnoses

- Fluid volume deficit related to the underlying condition.
- High risk for injury related to cortisone-induced adverse reactions.
- Knowledge deficit related to cortisone therapy.

Nursing interventions

- *Contraindicated* in systemic fungal infection. Injection contraindicated in sulfite sensitivity.
- *Use cautiously* in patients with GI ulceration or renal disease, hypertension, osteoporosis, varicella, vaccinia, exanthema, diabetes mellitus, Cushing's syndrome, thromboembolic disorders, seizures, myasthenia gravis, CHF, tuberculosis, ocular herpes simplex, hypoalbuminemia, emotional instability, and psychotic tendencies.
- Patients receiving long-term therapy should consider exercise or physical therapy. Give vitamin D or calcium supplements as ordered.
- Gradually reduce drug dosage after long-term therapy. Tell patient not to stop drug abruptly or without doctor's consent.
- Always titrate to lowest effective dose.
- Patient may need low-sodium diet and potassium supplement.
- I.M. route has slow onset. Don't use in acute conditions. May use on a twice-daily schedule matching diurnal variation. Rotate injection sites to prevent muscle atrophy.
- Report sudden weight gain or edema to doctor.
- Observe for signs of infection, especially after steroid withdrawal. Tell patient to report slow healing.
- Monitor serum electrolytes and blood glucose.
- Warn patient on long-term therapy about cushingoid effects.
- Give with milk or food to reduce GI irritation.
- Give a daily dose in the morning for better results and less toxicity.

General

Classification: agent for electrolyte balance (potassium supplement). **Pregnancy risk category:** C.

Mechanism of action

Replaces potassium and maintains its level.

Indications and dosage

- Treatment of hypokalemia. **Adults:** Give I.V. for life-threatening hypokalemia or when oral replacement not feasible. Give no more than 20 mEq/hour in concentration of 40 mEq/liter or less. Total 24-hour dosage should not exceed 150 mEq (3 mEq/kg in children). Potassium replacement should be monitored with ECG and frequent serum potassium determinations.
- Prevention of hypokalemia. **Adults:** dosage is individualized according to patient's needs. In most cases, dosage should not exceed 150 mEq/day. Administer as an additive to I.V. infusions. Usual dose is 40 mEq/liter, and solutions are usually infused at a rate not to exceed 20 mEq/hour. **Children:** individualize dose. Usual dose should not exceed 3 mEq/kg/day. Administer as an additive to I.V. infusions.

Adverse reactions

The following adverse reactions are signs of hyperkalemia. **CNS:** paresthesia of the extremities, listlessness, confusion, weakness or heaviness of legs, flaccid paralysis. **CV:** ***peripheral vascular collapse with fall in blood pressure, cardiac arrhythmias,*** heart block, possible cardiac arrest, ECG changes (prolonged PR intervals; wide QRS complex; ST-segment depression; tall, tented T waves). **GI:** nausea, vomiting, abdominal pain, diarrhea, bowel ulceration. **GU:** oliguria. **Skin:** cold skin, gray pallor.

Interactions

None significant.

Nursing diagnoses

- Altered nutrition: Less than body requirements, related to the patient's underlying condition.
- High risk for injury related to potassium-induced hyperkalemia.
- Knowledge deficit related to potassium acetate therapy.

Nursing interventions

- *Contraindicated* in severe renal impairment with oliguria, anuria, or azotemia; in untreated Addison's disease; and in acute dehydration, hyperkalemia, hyperkalemic form of familial periodic paralysis, and conditions associated with extensive tissue breakdown.
- *Use cautiously* in patients with cardiac disease, patients receiving potassium-sparing diuretics, and those with renal impairment.
- During therapy, monitor ECG, renal function, intake and output, and serum potassium, serum creatinine, and BUN levels. Never give potassium postoperatively until urine flow is established.
- Give slowly as diluted solution; potentially fatal hyperkalemia may result from too-rapid infusion.
- **I.V. use:** Parenteral potassium given by I.V. infusion only; never I.V. push or I.M. Observe for pain and redness at infusion site. Large-bore needle reduces local irritation.
- Watch for signs of GI ulceration: obstruction, hemorrhage, pain, distention, severe vomiting, and bleeding.
- Reconstitute potassium acetate powder with liquids; give after meals with a full glass of water or fruit juice to minimize GI irritation.
- To prevent serious hyperkalemia, replace potassium gradually.

General

Classification: diagnostic agent (anterior pituitary hormone). **Pregnancy risk category:** C.

Mechanism of action

By replacing the body's own tropic hormone, cosyntropin stimulates the adrenal cortex to secrete its entire spectrum of hormones.

Indications and dosage

• Diagnostic test of adrenocortical function. **Adults and children:** 0.25 to 1 mg I.M. or I.V. (unless label prohibits I.V. administration) between blood samplings. **Children under 2 years:** 0.125 mg I.M. or I.V.

Adverse reactions

Skin: flushing, pruritus, rash. **Other:** ***hypersensitivity, anaphylaxis*** (rare).

Interactions

None significant.

Nursing diagnoses

• Altered protection related to cosyntropin-induced hypersensitivity.
• Knowledge deficit related to cosyntropin test.

Nursing interventions

• *Use cautiously* in patients with preexisting allergic disease or hypersensitivity to natural corticotropin because of possible hypersensitivity reactions.
• Drug is synthetic duplication of the biologically active part of the corticotropin molecule. It is less likely to produce sensitivity than natural corticotropin from animal sources.
• **I.V. use:** Reconstitute with 1 ml of supplied diluent. For direct injection, administer over at least 2 minutes. The drug may be further diluted with D_5W or 0.9% sodium chloride injection and infused over 6 hours. Solution remains stable for 12 hours at room temperature.
• Monitor the patient for allergic reactions, rashes, dyspnea, wheezing, or any evidence of anaphylaxis.

polythiazide

General
Classification: diuretic, antihypertensive (thiazide). **Pregnancy risk category:** D.

Mechanism of action
Increases urine excretion of sodium and water by inhibiting sodium reabsorption in the cortical diluting site of the nephron.

Indications and dosage
• Hypertension. **Adults:** 2 to 4 mg P.O. daily.
• Edema in heart failure or renal failure. **Adults:** 1 to 4 mg P.O. daily. **Children:** 0.02 to 0.08 mg/kg P.O. daily.

Adverse reactions
Blood: ***aplastic anemia, agranulocytosis,*** leukopenia, thrombocytopenia. **CV:** volume depletion and dehydration, orthostatic hypotension. **GI:** anorexia, nausea, pancreatitis. **Hepatic:** hepatic encephalopathy. **Metabolic:** asymptomatic hyperuricemia, hyperglycemia and impairment of glucose tolerance, fluid and electrolyte imbalances (including dilutional hyponatremia and hypochloremia, hypokalemia, and hypercalcemia), metabolic alkalosis, gout. **Skin:** dermatitis, photosensitivity, rash. **Other:** hypersensitivity reactions, such as pneumonitis and vasculitis.

Interactions
Cholestyramine, colestipol: intestinal absorption of thiazides decreased. Keep doses as separate as possible. **Diazoxide:** increased antihypertensive, hyperglycemic, and hyperuricemic effects. Use together cautiously.

Nursing diagnoses
• Fluid volume excess related to the patient's underlying condition as evidenced by edema.
• Altered urinary elimination related to polythiazide therapy.
• Knowledge deficit related to polythiazide therapy.

Nursing interventions
• *Contraindicated* in anuria or hypersensitivity to thiazides or other sulfonamide-derived drugs.
• *Use cautiously* in severe renal disease, impaired hepatic function, and allergies.
• Monitor intake and output, weight, blood pressure, and serum electrolytes.
• Consult with doctor and dietitian to provide high-potassium diet. Foods rich in potassium include citrus fruits, tomatoes, bananas, dates, and apricots. Watch for signs and symptoms of hypokalemia, such as weakness and cramps.
• Patients receiving a digitalis glycoside may have an increased risk of digitalis toxicity from the potassium-depleting effect of this diuretic. May use with potassium-sparing diuretic to prevent potassium loss.
• Monitor serum uric acid levels, especially in patients with a history of gout.
• Check insulin requirements in patients with diabetes. May treat severe hyperglycemia with oral antidiabetic agents.
• In hypertension, therapeutic response may be delayed several days.
• Give in a.m. to prevent nocturia.
• Elderly patients are especially susceptible to excessive diuresis.
• Thiazides and thiazide-like diuretics should be stopped before tests for parathyroid function are performed.
• Advise patient to avoid sudden posture changes and rise slowly to avoid orthostatic hypotension.
• Advise patient to use a sunscreen.

General

Classification: antibiotic (sulfonamide and folate antagonist). **Pregnancy risk category:** C (D if near term).

Mechanism of action

Sulfamethoxazole inhibits formation of dihydrofolic acid from PABA. Trimethoprim inhibits dihydrofolate reductase. Both decrease bacterial folic acid synthesis.

Indications and dosage

• UTIs, shigellosis. **Adults:** 160 mg trimethoprim/800 mg sulfamethoxazole (double strength [DS] tablet) P.O. q 12 hours for 10 to 14 days in UTIs; 5 days in shigellosis. For simple cystitis or acute urethral syndrome, may give 1 to 3 DS tablets as single dose. If indicated, infuse 8 to 10 mg/kg/day in 2 to 4 divided doses q 6, 8, or 12 hours for up to 14 days. **Children 2 months and over:** 8 mg/kg trimethoprim/40 mg/kg sulfamethoxazole P.O. q 24 hours, in 2 divided doses q 12 hours (10 days, UTIs; 5 days, shigellosis). If indicated, infuse 8 to 10 mg/kg/day in 2 to 4 divided doses q 6, 8, or 12 hours.

• UTIs in prostatitis. **Adults:** 160 mg trimethoprim/800 mg sulfamethoxazole P.O. b.i.d. for 3 to 6 months.

• Prophylaxis of chronic UTIs. **Adults:** 40 mg trimethoprim/200 mg sulfamethoxazole (½ tablet) or 80 mg trimethoprim/400 mg sulfamethoxazole P.O. daily or three times a week for 3 to 6 months.

• Otitis media in penicillin allergy or penicillin-resistant infections. **Children 2 months and over:** 8 mg/kg trimethoprim/40 mg/kg sulfamethoxazole P.O. q 24 hours, in 2 divided doses for 10 days.

• *Pneumocystis carinii* pneumonia. **Adults and children 2 months and over:** 20 mg/kg trimethoprim/100 mg/kg sulfamethoxazole P.O. q 24 hours, in equally divided doses q 6 hours for 14 days. If indicated, infuse 15 to 20 mg/kg/day in 3 or 4 doses q 6 to 8 hours up to 14 days.

• Chronic bronchitis. **Adults:** 160 mg trimethoprim/800 mg sulfamethoxazole P.O. q 12 hours for 10 to 14 days.

• Traveler's diarrhea. **Adults:** For prophylaxis, 160 mg trimethoprim/800 mg sulfamethoxazole P.O. once daily, beginning first day of travel and continuing until 2 days after returning home; maximum of 14 days. For treatment, 160 mg trimethoprim/800 mg sulfamethoxazole P.O. b.i.d. for 3 to 5 days.

Adverse reactions

Blood: ***agranulocytosis, aplastic anemia,*** megaloblastic anemia, thrombocytopenia, leukopenia, ***hemolytic anemia.*** **CNS:** headache, depression, seizures, hallucinations. **GI:** *nausea, vomiting, diarrhea,* abdominal pain, anorexia. **GU:** ***toxic nephrosis,*** crystalluria, hematuria. **Hepatic:** jaundice. **Skin:** ***erythema multiforme,*** *skin eruption,* ***epidermal necrolysis, exfoliative dermatitis,*** photosensitivity, urticaria, pruritus. **Other:** ***hypersensitivity,*** *serum sickness, drug fever,* ***anaphylaxis.***

Interactions

Ammonium chloride, ascorbic acid: possible crystalluria. **Oral anticoagulants:** increased anticoagulant effect. **Oral antidiabetic agents:** increased antidiabetic effect. **Oral contraceptives:** decreased contraceptive effects and possible breakthrough bleeding.

Nursing diagnoses

• High risk for injury related to ineffectiveness of co-trimoxazole to eradicate the infection.
• High risk for fluid volume deficit related to adverse GI reactions to co-trimoxazole.
• Knowledge deficit related to co-trimoxazole.

Nursing interventions

• *Contraindicated* in porphyria, term pregnancy, and megaloblastic anemia from folate deficiency. *Use cautiously* in renal or hepatic impairment, severe allergy, asthma, and blood dyscrasias.
• **I.V. use:** Dilute for infusion with D_5W. Don't mix with other drugs or solutions. Infuse over 90 minutes within 2 hours of mixing.
• "DS" or "DF" product means "double strength."
• Report rash, sore throat, fever, mouth sores (early signs of blood dyscrasia), and superinfection.

General
Classification: antibiotic (polymyxin antibiotic). **Pregnancy risk category:** B.

Mechanism of action
Hinders bacterial cell wall synthesis, damaging the bacterial plasma membrane and making the cell more vulnerable to osmotic pressure (bactericidal).

Indications and dosage
• Acute UTIs or septicemia caused by sensitive *Pseudomonas aeruginosa,* or when other antibiotics are ineffective or contraindicated; bacteremia caused by sensitive *Enterobacter aerogenes* and *Klebsiella pneumoniae,* or acute UTIs caused by *Escherichia coli.* **Adults and children:** 15,000 to 25,000 units/kg daily I.V. infusion, divided q 12 hours; or 25,000 to 30,000 units/kg daily, divided q 4 to 8 hours. I.M. not advised because of severe pain at injection site.
• Meningitis caused by sensitive *P. aeruginosa* or *Haemophilus influenzae* when other antibiotics are ineffective or contraindicated. **Adults and children over 2 years:** 50,000 units intrathecally once daily for 3 to 4 days, then 50,000 units every other day for at least 2 weeks after CSF tests are negative and CSF glucose is normal. **Children under 2 years:** 20,000 units intrathecally once daily for 3 to 4 days, then 25,000 units every other day for at least 2 weeks after CSF tests are negative and CSF glucose is normal.

Adverse reactions
CNS: irritability, drowsiness, facial flushing, weakness, ataxia, headache and meningeal irritation with intrathecal administration, peripheral and perioral paresthesia, ***seizures, coma.*** **EENT:** blurred vision. **GU:** *nephrotoxicity (albuminuria, cylindruria, hematuria, proteinuria, decreased urine output, increased BUN level).* **Skin:** urticaria. **Local:** *pain at I.M. injection site.* **Other:** hypersensitivity reactions with fever, ***anaphylaxis, respiratory paralysis.***

Interactions
Aminoglycosides, amphotericin B, cisplatin, vancomycin, zidovudine: increased risk of nephrotoxicity. Avoid concomitant use. **Neuromuscular blockers:** possible potentiated neuromuscular blockade. Monitor closely.

Nursing diagnoses
• High risk for injury related to the ineffectiveness of polymyxin B sulfate to eradicate the infection.
• Altered urinary elimination related to nephrotoxicity induced by polymyxin B sulfate.
• Knowledge deficit related to polymyxin B sulfate.

Nursing interventions
• *Use cautiously* in impaired renal function or myasthenia gravis.
• Give only to hospitalized patients under constant medical supervision.
• For meningitis, must give intrathecally to achieve adequate CSF levels.
• Give deep I.M. Warn the patient that the injection may be painful.
• Don't give solution containing local anesthetics I.V. or intrathecally.
• Monitor renal function (BUN, serum creatinine, creatinine clearance, urine output) before and during therapy. Intake should be sufficient to maintain output at 1,500 ml/day (between 3,000 and 4,000 ml/day for adults).
• Obtain specimen for culture and sensitivity tests before first dose. Therapy may begin pending test results.
• Notify doctor immediately if patient develops fever, adverse CNS effects, rash, or symptoms of nephrotoxicity.
• If patient is scheduled for surgery, notify anesthesiologist of preoperative treatment with this drug since it may prolong neuromuscular blockade.
• **I.V. use:** When giving I.V., check site daily for phlebitis and irritation. Dilute each 500,000 units in 300 to 500 ml D_5W; infuse over 60 to 90 minutes. Rotate I.V. sites regularly.
• Refrigerate and use parenteral solutions within 72 hours.

General

Classification: mast cell stabilizer, antiasthmatic (chromone derivative). **Pregnancy risk category:** B.

Mechanism of action

Inhibits the degranulation of sensitized mast cells that occurs after a patient's exposure to specific antigens. It also inhibits release of histamine and slow-reacting substance of anaphylaxis (SRS-A).

Indications and dosage

- Adjunct in treatment of severe perennial bronchial asthma. **Adults and children over 5 years:** give 2 metered sprays using inhaler q.i.d. at regular intervals. Also available as aqueous solution administered through a nebulizer.
- Prevention and treatment of allergic rhinitis. **Adults and children over 5 years:** 1 spray in each nostril t.i.d or q.i.d. May give up to 6 times daily.
- Prevention of exercise-induced bronchospasm. **Adults and children over 5 years:** 2 metered sprays inhaled no more than 1 hour before anticipated exercise.
- Allergic ocular disorders. **Adults and children 4 years and older:** 1 to 2 drops in each eye 4 to 6 times daily at regular intervals.
- Systemic mastocytosis. **Adults:** 100 to 200 mg P.O. q.i.d.
- Food allergy. **Adults:** 200 mg P.O. q.i.d. 15 to 20 minutes before meals. Dosage may be doubled in 2 to 3 weeks if results are not satisfactory. **Children 2 to 13 years:** 100 mg P.O. q.i.d. 15 to 20 minutes before meals. Dosage may be doubled in 2 to 3 weeks if results are not satisfactory. Do not exceed 40 mg/kg daily. **Children under 2 years:** up to 20 mg/kg P.O. daily.
- Inflammatory bowel disease. **Adults:** 200 mg P.O. q.i.d. 15 to 20 minutes before meals. **Children 2 to 14 years:** 100 mg P.O. q.i.d. 15 to 20 minutes before meals.

Adverse reactions

CNS: dizziness, headache. **EENT:** *tracheal and throat irritation, cough,* ***bronchospasm after inhalation of dry powder;*** esophagitis; nasal congestion; pharyngeal irritation; wheezing. **GI:** nausea. **GU:** dysuria, urinary frequency. **Skin:** rash, urticaria. **Other:** joint swelling and pain, lacrimation, swollen parotid gland, ***angioedema,*** *eosinophilic pneumonia.*

Interactions

None significant.

Nursing diagnoses

- Ineffective breathing pattern related to underlying condition.
- High risk for impaired skin integrity because of adverse drug effects.
- Knowledge deficit related to cromolyn therapy.

Nursing interventions

- *Contraindicated* in acute asthma attacks and status asthmaticus because the drug is useful only in preventing attacks.
- *Use cautiously* in coronary artery disease or history of cardiac arrhythmias.
- Should be discontinued if patient develops eosinophilic pneumonia.
- Watch for recurrence of asthmatic symptoms when dosage is decreased, especially when corticosteroids are also used.
- Use only when acute episode has been controlled; airway is cleared; and patient is able to inhale.
- Store capsules for inhalation at room temperature in tightly closed container; protect from moisture and temperatures higher than 104° F (40° C).
- Instruct patient to avoid excessive handling of capsule for inhalation.
- Esophagitis may be relieved by antacids or a glass of milk.
- Powder in capsules for oral dose must be dissolved in hot water. May be further diluted with cold water before ingestion. Do not mix with fruit juice, milk, or food.
- Use of oral forms is still investigational.

General

Classification: viral vaccine (vaccine). **Pregnancy risk category:** C.

Mechanism of action

Promotes immunity to poliomyelitis by inducing humoral antibodies and antibodies in the lymphatic tissue.

Indications and dosage

• Poliovirus immunization. **Children and nonimmunized adults:** 0.5 ml P.O. (trivalent oral live vaccine, or TOPV), followed by a second dose of 0.5 ml in 6 to 8 weeks. Give third 0.5-ml dose 6 to 12 months after second dose. A reinforcing dose of 0.5 ml should be given before entry to school. **Infants:** administer 0.5 ml P.O. at 2, 4, and 18 months. Optional dose may be given at 6 months.
• Poliovirus immunization in persons who cannot receive TOPV. **Adults:** 0.5 ml (inactivated vaccine, or IPV) S.C., followed by a second dose in 4 to 8 weeks. Administer a third dose in 6 to 12 months. **Children:** 0.5 ml S.C. at 2 and 4 months. Administer a third dose at 15 to 18 months. A reinforcing dose of 0.5 ml should be given before entry into school.

Adverse reactions

Systemic: ***paralytic poliomyelitis.***

P

Interactions

Immune serum globulin, whole blood, plasma: antibodies in serum may interfere with immune response. Don't use vaccine within 3 months of transfusion. **Tuberculin skin test:** possible suppression of test. Don't test for 6 weeks.

Nursing diagnoses

• Altered protection related to a lack of immunity to poliovirus.
• High risk for injury related to vaccine-induced paralytic poliomyelitis.
• Knowledge deficit related to poliovirus vaccine.

Nursing interventions

• Oral vaccine is *contraindicated* in immunosuppression, cancer, and immunoglobulin abnormalities and in radiation, antimetabolite, alkylating agent, or corticosteroid therapy. These patients should receive IPV.
• Injectable vaccine is *contraindicated* in patients with hypersensitivity to neomycin or streptomycin.
• Should not be administered to neonates under 6 weeks.
• *Use cautiously* in siblings of a child with known immunodeficiency syndrome. IPV is preferred.
• Defer oral vaccines in patients with vomiting or diarrhea. Defer both forms of vaccine in acute illness.
• Patients with immunodeficiency or altered immune status may be at risk for developing the disease if live vaccine is administered. These patients should receive parenteral form.
• The highest risk of poliovirus infection occurs after the first dose of the oral vaccine.
• Adults at high risk for exposure who have completed a primary course may receive another dose.
• This vaccine is not effective in modifying or preventing existing or incubating poliomyelitis.
• Check the parents' immunization history when they bring in child for vaccine; this is an excellent time for parents to receive booster immunizations.
• Keep frozen until used. Once thawed, if unopened, vaccine may be refrigerated for up to 30 days. Opened vials may be refrigerated up to 7 days. Thaw before administration.
• Color change from pink to yellow has no effect on efficacy of the vaccine. Yellow color results from vaccine being stored at low temperatures.
• Obtain history of allergies and reaction to immunization.
• Don't give oral vaccine parenterally.
• An information booklet describes the risks and benefits of this vaccine. Be sure parents read and understand this information before vaccine is administered.

General

Classification: antispasmodic, vasodilator (mandelic acid derivative). **Pregnancy risk category:** C.

Mechanism of action

Drug directly relaxes smooth muscle because of the inhibition of phosphodiesterase, resulting in increased concentrations of cyclic adenosine monophosphate.

Indications and dosage

- Adjunctive treatment of intermittent claudication, arteriosclerosis obliterans, vasospasm and muscular ischemia associated with thrombophlebitis, nocturnal leg cramps, Raynaud's phenomenon, selected cases of ischemic cerebrovascular disease. **Adults:** initially, 1.2 to 1.6 g P.O. daily, in divided doses before meals and h.s. For maintenance, decrease the dosage by 200 mg/day to the lowest effective level. Maintenance dosage is usually 400 to 800 mg daily given in 2 to 4 divided doses.

Adverse reactions

CNS: *headache, tingling of the extremities, dizziness.* **CV:** *mild flushing,* tachycardia. **GI:** pyrosis, eructation, nausea, heartburn. **Other:** *sweating.*

Interactions

None significant.

Nursing diagnoses

- Impaired tissue integrity related to the patient's underlying condition.
- Pain related to adverse drug reactions.
- Knowledge deficit related to cyclandelate therapy.

Nursing interventions

- *Use with extreme caution* in patients with severe obliterative coronary artery or cerebrovascular disease because circulation to these diseased areas may be compromised by the vasodilatory effects of the drug elsewhere (coronary steal syndrome).
- *Use cautiously* in patients with glaucoma or hypotension.
- Give the drug with food or antacids to lessen GI distress.
- Use with, not as a substitute for, appropriate medical or surgical therapy for peripheral or cerebrovascular disease.
- Short-term therapy is of little benefit. Instruct patient to expect long-term treatment and to continue to take medication.
- Tell the patient that adverse reactions usually disappear after several weeks of therapy.

General

Classification: nonnarcotic analgesic, antipyretic, anti-inflammatory (NSAID). **Pregnancy risk category:** C.

Mechanism of action

Produces analgesic, antipyretic, and anti-inflammatory effects, possibly through inhibition of prostaglandin synthesis.

Indications and dosage

- Osteoarthritis and rheumatoid arthritis. **Adults:** 20 mg P.O. daily. If desired, the dose may be divided.

Adverse reactions

Blood: prolonged bleeding time, anemia. **CNS:** headache, drowsiness, dizziness. **CV:** peripheral edema. **GI:** *epigastric distress, nausea, occult blood loss,* ***peptic ulceration, severe GI bleeding.*** **GU:** ***nephrotoxicity.*** **Hepatic:** elevated enzymes. **Skin:** pruritus, rash, urticaria, *photosensitivity.*

Interactions

Alcohol, corticosteroids: increased risk of GI toxicity. Avoid concomitant use. **Aspirin:** decreased plasma levels of piroxicam. Avoid concomitant use. **Lithium:** increased plasma lithium levels. Monitor for toxicity. **Oral anticoagulants:** enhanced risk of bleeding. Monitor patient closely. **Oral antidiabetic agents:** enhanced hypoglycemic effects. Monitor patient closely.

Nursing diagnoses

- Pain related to the patient's underlying condition.
- High risk for impaired skin integrity related to piroxicam-induced photosensitivity.
- Knowledge deficit related to piroxicam therapy.

Nursing interventions

- *Contraindicated* in patients with hypersensitivity to NSAIDs or aspirin.
- *Use cautiously* in elderly patients and in patients with angioedema, GI disorders, history of renal or peptic ulcer disease, or cardiac disease.
- Serious GI toxicity can occur at any time in patients taking long-term NSAID therapy. Teach the patient signs and symptoms of GI bleeding, and tell him to report these immediately.
- Tell him that the full therapeutic effect may be delayed for 2 to 4 weeks.
- Piroxicam causes skin reactions more often than other drugs in its class. Photosensitivity reactions are the most common.
- Check renal, hepatic, and auditory function and CBC periodically during prolonged therapy. Drug should be discontinued if abnormalities occur.
- If adverse GI reactions occur, give the drug with milk, antacids, or meals.
- Because of their antipyretic and anti-inflammatory actions, NSAIDs may mask the signs and symptoms of infection.

General

Classification: antiemetic, antivertigo agent (piperazine derivative antihistamine). **Pregnancy risk category:** B.

Mechanism of action

May affect neural pathways originating in the labyrinth to inhibit nausea and vomiting, but the drug's exact mechanism of action is unknown.

Indications and dosage

• Prevention and treatment of motion sickness. **Adults:** 50 mg P.O. (hydrochloride) one half hour before travel, then q 4 to 6 hours, p.r.n., to maximum of 200 mg daily; or 50 mg I.M. (lactate) q 4 to 6 hours, p.r.n.
• Prevention of postoperative vomiting. **Adults:** 50 mg I.M. (lactate) preoperatively or 20 to 30 minutes before expected termination of surgery; then postoperatively 50 mg I.M. (lactate) q 4 to 6 hours, p.r.n.
• Motion sickness and postoperative vomiting. **Children 6 to 12 years:** 3 mg/kg (lactate) I.M. divided t.i.d., or 25 mg (hydrochloride) P.O. q 4 to 6 hours p.r.n. to a maximum of 75 mg daily.

Adverse reactions

CNS: *drowsiness,* dizziness, auditory and visual hallucinations. **CV:** hypotension. **EENT:** blurred vision. **GI:** dry mouth, constipation. **GU:** urine retention. **Other:** may mask symptoms of ototoxicity, brain tumor, or intestinal obstruction.

Interactions

Alcohol, other CNS depressants: additive CNS depression. Avoid concomitant use.

Nursing diagnoses

• High risk for fluid volume deficit related to nausea and vomiting induced by motion sickness.
• Sensory/perceptual alterations (visual or auditory) related to cyclizine-induced hallucinations.
• Knowledge deficit related to cyclizine therapy.

Nursing interventions

• *Contraindicated* in patients with hypersensitivity to the drug.
• *Use cautiously* in glaucoma, GU or GI obstruction, heart failure and in elderly males with possible prostatic hypertrophy.
• Warn patient against driving and other activities that require alertness until CNS effects of the drug are known.
• Store in cool place. When stored at room temperature, injection may turn slightly yellow, but this color change does not indicate loss of potency.

General

Classification: bronchodilator (beta-adrenergic agonist). **Pregnancy risk category:** C.

Mechanism of action

Relaxes bronchial smooth muscle by acting on beta$_2$-adrenergic receptors.

Indications and dosage

- Prevention and reversal of bronchospasm, asthma. **Adults:** 1 or 2 inhalations (0.2 to 0.4 mg) repeated q 4 to 6 hours. Not to exceed 12 inhalations daily.

Adverse reactions

CNS: tremor, nervousness, dizziness, insomnia, headache. **CV:** tachycardia, palpitations, increased blood pressure. **EENT:** drying or irritation of throat.

Interactions

Propranolol and other beta-adrenergic blockers: decreased bronchodilating effects.

Nursing diagnoses

- Ineffective airway clearance related to the patient's underlying condition.
- Sleep pattern disturbance related to pirbuterol-induced nervousness and insomnia.
- Knowledge deficit related to pirbuterol therapy.

Nursing interventions

- *Contraindicated* in hypersensitivity to adrenergics and in patients with digitalis toxicity or cardiac arrhythmias associated with tachycardia.
- Tell the patient to call the doctor if he experiences increased bronchospasm after using the drug.
- Teach him how to use a metered-dose inhaler correctly: He should clear his nasal passages and throat, then breathe out, expelling as much air from lungs as possible. He should next place the mouthpiece well into his mouth as the dose from the inhaler is released and inhale deeply. After he holds his breath for several seconds, he should remove the mouthpiece and exhale slowly.
- If more than one inhalation is ordered, tell the patient to wait at least 2 minutes before repeating the procedure for a second dose.
- Instruct the patient who is also using a steroid inhaler to use the bronchodilator first, then to wait about 5 minutes before using the steroid. This allows the bronchodilator to open air passages for maximum effectiveness.
- Advise the patient to seek medical attention if a previously effective dosage doesn't control symptoms because this may signify a worsening of the disease.

cyclobenzaprine hydrochloride Flexeril

General
Classification: skeletal muscle relaxant (tricyclic antidepressant). **Pregnancy risk category:** B.

Mechanism of action
Drug's precise mechanism is unknown; reduces transmission of impulses from the spinal cord to skeletal muscle.

Indications and dosage
- Short-term treatment of muscle spasm. **Adults:** 10 mg P.O. t.i.d. for 7 days. Maximum dosage is 60 mg daily for 2 to 3 weeks.

Adverse reactions
CNS: *drowsiness,* euphoria, weakness, headache, insomnia, nightmares, paresthesia, dizziness, depression, visual disturbances, ***precipitation of seizures.*** **CV:** tachycardia. **EENT:** blurred vision. **GI:** dry mouth, abdominal pain, dyspepsia, peculiar taste, constipation. **GU:** urine retention. **Skin:** rash, urticaria, pruritus. **Other:** in high doses, watch for adverse reactions like those of other tricyclic antidepressants.

Interactions
Alcohol, CNS depressants: may cause additive CNS depression. Avoid concomitant use. **MAO inhibitors:** can exacerbate CNS depression or anticholinergic effects. Don't give within 14 days after discontinuing MAO inhibitors.

Nursing diagnoses
- Pain related to underlying condition.
- High risk for injury related to cyclobenzaprine-induced drowsiness.
- Knowledge deficit related to cyclobenzaprine therapy.

Nursing interventions
- *Contraindicated* in patients who have received MAO inhibitors within 14 days; during acute recovery phase of MI; and in heart block, arrhythmias, conduction disturbances, or CHF.
- *Use cautiously* in urine retention, narrow-angle glaucoma, increased intraocular pressure, CV disease, impaired hepatic function, and seizures and in elderly or debilitated patients.
- Nausea, headache, and malaise may occur if drug is stopped abruptly after long-term use.
- Watch for symptoms of overdose, including possible cardiotoxicity. Notify the doctor immediately and have physostigmine available.
- Advise the patient to report urinary hesitancy or urine retention. If constipation is a problem, increase fluid intake and suggest a stool softener.
- Warn the patient to avoid activities that require alertness until the CNS effects of the drug are known.
- Tell the patient that dry mouth may be relieved with sugarless gum or candy.

General

Classification: antineoplastic agent (alkylating agent). **Pregnancy risk category:** D.

Mechanism of action

Although classified as an alkylating agent, the exact mechanism of action is unknown.

Indications and dosage

Dosage and indications may vary. Check current literature for recommended protocol.

- Polycythemia vera. **Adults and children over age 15:** 1 mg/kg P.O. daily for 30 days; may increase to 1.5 to 3 mg/kg P.O. daily until hematocrit reduced to 50% to 55%, then 0.1 to 0.2 mg/kg daily maintenance.
- Chronic granulocytic leukemia. **Adults and children over age 15:** 1.5 to 2.5 mg/kg P.O. daily until WBC count drops to 10,000/mm^3; then start maintenance 7 to 175 mg daily. Stop drug if WBC count falls below 3,000/mm^3 or platelet count falls below 150,000/mm^3.

Adverse reactions

Blood: leukopenia, anemia, ***thrombocytopenia.*** **GI:** nausea, vomiting, abdominal cramps, diarrhea. **Skin:** rash.

Interactions

Anticoagulants: increased risk of bleeding. Avoid concomitant use.

Nursing diagnoses

- Altered nutrition related to GI disturbances and resulting electrolyte imbalances.
- Knowledge deficit related to pipobroman therapy.

Nursing interventions

- *Contraindicated* in patients with bone marrow depression resulting from radiation or cytotoxic chemotherapy because of potential for additive bone marrow depression; in pregnant women because of potential teratogenic effects; and in lactating women because it is not known whether this drug is excreted in breast milk.
- Drug is not recommended for children under age 15.
- Administer in divided doses daily.
- Before therapy begins and periodically thereafter, perform liver and kidney function tests.
- Obtain CBCs once or twice a week and leukocyte counts every other day until desired result is obtained or toxic effects appear.
- Bone marrow studies should be performed before treatment and at time of maximal hematologic response. Bone marrow depression may not occur for 4 weeks or more after initiation of treatment. Leukocyte count is the most reliable index of bone marrow activity, but platelet count is also a helpful guide. Temporarily discontinue treatment if leukocyte count is less than 3,000/mm^3 or if platelet count is less than 150,000/mm^3. Treatment may be reinstated cautiously once counts rise.
- Many patients develop dose-dependent anemia. Dosage reduction and blood transfusions usually reverse the anemia. Anemia caused by a hemolytic process is marked by a rapid drop in hemoglobin, increased bilirubin levels, and reticulocytosis. In this case, the drug should be discontinued.
- Caution patient to call doctor if nausea, vomiting, diarrhea, abdominal cramps, or rash becomes pronounced.
- Because of the possible teratogenic effects, advise patient to use contraceptive measures during therapy.
- The breast-feeding patient should weigh the drug's potential risks to the infant against its importance to her treatment before deciding to continue the therapy or discontinue breast-feeding.

General

Classification: antineoplastic (alkylating agent).
Pregnancy risk category: D.

Mechanism of action

Cross-links strands of cellular DNA and interferes with RNA transcription, causing an imbalance of growth that leads to cell death. Cell cycle-nonspecific.

Indications and dosage

- Breast, head, neck, lung, ovarian cancers; Hodgkin's disease; chronic lymphocytic leukemia; chronic myelocytic leukemia; acute lymphoblastic leukemia; acute myelocytic leukemia; neuroblastoma; retinoblastoma; malignant lymphomas; multiple myeloma; mycosis fungoides; sarcomas; nephrotic syndrome. **Adults:** initially, 40 to 50 mg/kg I.V. in divided doses over 2 to 5 days; then adjust for maintenance. Or 1 to 5 mg/kg P.O. daily, depending on tolerance. Maintenance dosage is 1 to 5 mg/kg P.O. daily; or 10 to 15 mg/kg q 7 to 10 days I.V.; or 3 to 5 mg/kg I.V. twice weekly. **Children:** 2 to 8 mg/kg daily or 60 to 250 mg/m^2 daily P.O. or I.V. for 6 days (dosage depends on susceptibility of neoplasm). Maintenance: 2 to 5 mg/kg or 50 to 150 mg/m^2 P.O. twice weekly.

Adverse reactions

Blood: ***leukopenia,*** WBC nadir days 8 to 15, recovery 17 to 28 days; ***thrombocytopenia; anemia.*** **CV:** ***cardiotoxicity*** (with high doses and in combination with doxorubicin). **GI:** anorexia; *nausea and vomiting;* stomatitis; mucositis. **GU:** gonadal suppression, ***hemorrhagic cystitis,*** bladder fibrosis, nephrotoxicity. **Metabolic:** hyperuricemia; SIADH secretion (with high doses). **Other:** *reversible alopecia;* secondary malignancies, ***pulmonary fibrosis*** (high doses), ***anaphylaxis.***

Interactions

Barbiturates: increased pharmacologic effect and enhanced cyclophosphamide toxicity. **Cardiotoxic drugs:** additive adverse cardiac effects. **Corticosteroids, chloramphenicol:** reduced activity of cyclophosphamide. **Digoxin:** may decrease serum digoxin levels. Monitor levels closely. **Succinylcholine:** prolonged neuromuscular blockade.

Nursing diagnoses

- High risk for infection related to immunosuppressive adverse reactions.
- Pain related to possible adverse GU reactions as evidenced by cystitis.
- Knowledge deficit related to cyclophosphamide therapy.

Nursing interventions

- *Use cautiously.* Dosage modification may be required in severe leukopenia, thrombocytopenia, malignant cell infiltration of bone marrow, recent radiation therapy or chemotherapy, hepatic or renal disease.
- Advise both male and female patients to practice contraception while taking this drug and for 4 months after; drug is potentially teratogenic.
- Monitor CBC and renal and hepatic functions.
- Encourage intake of 3 liters daily to prevent hemorrhagic cystitis. Don't give drug at bedtime; voiding is too infrequent to avoid cystitis. If hemorrhagic cystitis occurs, discontinue drug. Cystitis can occur months after therapy has been stopped. Encourage patients to void every 1 to 2 waking hours.
- Check reconstituted solution for small particles. Filter solution if necessary.
- Avoid I.M. injections if platelets $< 100,000/mm^3$.
- **I.V. use:** Can be given by direct I.V. push into a running I.V. line or by infusion in 0.9% sodium chloride or D_5W. Lyophilized preparation is much easier to reconstitute; request it when preparing I.V.
- To prevent hyperuricemia with resulting uric acid nephropathy, allopurinol may be used with adequate hydration. Monitor serum uric acid.
- Warn patient that reversible alopecia is likely.
- Monitor for cyclophosphamide toxicity if patient's corticosteroid therapy is discontinued.
- Preparation of parenteral form is associated with carcinogenic, mutagenic, and teratogenic risks. Follow institutional policy to reduce risks.

General

Classification: anthelmintic (piperazine). **Pregnancy risk category:** B.

Mechanism of action

Blocks neuromuscular action, paralyzing the worm and causing its expulsion by normal peristalsis.

Indications and dosage

• Enterobiasis (pinworm). **Adults and children:** 65 mg/kg P.O. daily 7 to 8 days. Maximum daily dosage is 2.5 g. Alternatively, give adults 2 g P.O. daily for 7 days, and give children 1 g/m² daily for 7 days.

Some clinicians order according to body weight. **Children under 7 kg:** 250 mg P.O. daily for 7 days. **Children 7 to 14 kg:** 500 mg P.O. daily for 7 days. **Children 14 to 27 kg:** 1 g P.O. daily for 7 days. **Children over 27 kg and adults:** 2 g P.O. daily for 7 days.

• Ascariasis (roundworm). **Adults:** 3.5 g P.O. in single doses for 2 consecutive days. **Children:** 75 mg/kg or 2 g/m² P.O. daily in single doses for 2 consecutive days. Maximum daily dosage is 3.5 g.

Alternatively, give according to body weight. **Children under 14 kg:** 1 g P.O. daily for 2 days. **Children 14 to 23 kg:** 2 g P.O. daily for 2 days. **Children 23 to 45 kg:** 3 g P.O. daily for 2 days. **Children over 45 kg and adults:** 3.5 g P.O. daily for 2 days. Some clinicians continue treatment for 4 days in patients with massive infestation. May repeat in 1 week if necessary.

Adverse reactions

CNS: ataxia, tremor, choreiform movements, muscular weakness, myoclonus, hyporeflexia, paresthesia, seizures, sense of detachment, EEG abnormalities, memory defect, *headache, vertigo.* **EENT:** nystagmus, blurred vision, paralytic strabismus, cataracts with visual impairment, lacrimation, difficulty in focusing, rhinorrhea. **GI:** *nausea, vomiting,* diarrhea, abdominal cramps. **Skin:** urticaria, photodermatitis, ***erythema multiforme,*** purpura, eczematous skin reactions. **Other:** arthralgia, fever, bronchospasm, ***hemolytic anemia.***

Interactions

Pyrantel pamoate: possible antagonism. Don't administer together.

Nursing diagnoses

• Altered health maintenance related to ineffectiveness of piperazine.
• Pain related to headache caused by piperazine.
• Knowledge deficit related to piperazine therapy.

Nursing interventions

• *Contraindicated* in hepatic or renal impairment or seizure disorders.
• *Use cautiously* in severe malnutrition or anemia.
• Discontinue if CNS or significant GI reactions occur.
• Because of potential neurotoxicity, avoid prolonged or repeated treatment, especially in children.
• No dietary restrictions, laxatives, or enemas are necessary.
• Drug may be taken with food; but, for best absorption, tell the patient to take it on an empty stomach.
• Mix powder for oral suspension in 57 ml of water, milk, or fruit juice.
• Treat all family members.
• Teach the patient about the need for good personal hygiene, especially good handwashing technique. To avoid reinfection, teach him to wash perianal area, to change undergarments and bedclothes daily, and to wash hands and clean fingernails before meals and after bowel movements. Advise the patient to refrain from preparing food during infestation.

General

Classification: antitubercular agent (isoxizolidone). **Pregnancy risk category:** C.

Mechanism of action

Inhibits bacterial cell wall biosynthesis by interfering with the use of amino acids.

Indications and dosage

- Adjunctive treatment in pulmonary or extrapulmonary tuberculosis. **Adults:** initially, 250 mg P.O. q 12 hours for 2 weeks; then, if blood levels are below 25 to 30 mcg/ml and no signs of toxicity appear, dosage is increased to 250 mg q 8 hours for 2 weeks. If optimum blood levels are still not achieved and no signs of toxicity appear, then dosage is increased to 250 mg q 6 hours. Maximum dosage is 1 g/day. If CNS toxicity occurs, drug is discontinued for 1 week, then resumed at 250 mg daily for 2 weeks. If no serious toxic effects occur, dosage is increased by 250-mg increments q 10 days until blood level of 25 to 30 mcg/ml is obtained.

Adverse reactions

CNS: ***seizures,*** drowsiness, headache, tremor, dysarthria, vertigo, confusion, loss of memory, ***possible suicidal tendencies*** and other psychotic symptoms, *nervousness, hallucinations, depression,* hyperirritability, paresthesia, paresis, hyperreflexia. **Other:** hypersensitivity (allergic dermatitis).

Interactions

Ethanol or ethionamide: increased risk of CNS toxicity (seizures). **Isoniazid:** monitor for CNS toxicity (dizziness or drowsiness).

Nursing diagnoses

- High risk for infection related to ineffectiveness of cycloserine to eradicate the infection.
- Altered thought processes related to cycloserine-induced adverse CNS reactions.
- Knowledge deficit related to cycloserine therapy.

Nursing interventions

- *Contraindicated* in patients with seizure disorders, depression or severe anxiety, severe renal insufficiency, or chronic alcoholism.
- *Use cautiously* in patients with impaired renal function; reduced dosage is required.
- Considered a "second-line" drug in the treatment of tuberculosis.
- Obtain specimen for culture and sensitivity tests before therapy and periodically thereafter to detect possible resistance.
- Serious neurologic effects can be precipitated by ingestion of alcohol; warn patient to avoid alcohol.
- Toxic reactions may occur with blood levels above 30 mcg/ml.
- Pyridoxine, anticonvulsants, tranquilizers, or sedatives may help to relieve adverse reactions.
- Observe for psychotic symptoms, hallucinations, and possible suicidal tendencies.
- Monitor hematologic tests and renal and liver function studies.
- Instruct the patient to take the drug exactly as prescribed. Warn against discontinuing its use without the doctor's approval.

General

Classification: antibiotic (extended-spectrum penicillin). **Pregnancy risk category:** B.

Mechanism of action

Bactericidal against microorganisms by inhibiting cell wall synthesis during active multiplication. Bacteria resist penicillins by producing penicillinases—enzymes that convert penicillin to inactive penicilloic acid.

Indications and dosage

• Systemic infections caused by susceptible strains of gram-positive and especially gram-negative organisms (including *Proteus* and *Pseudomonas aeruginosa*). **Adults and children over 12 years:** 100 to 300 mg/kg daily divided q 4 to 6 hours I.V. or I.M. Doses for children under 12 years not established.

• Prophylaxis of surgical infections. **Adults:** 2 g I.V., given 30 to 60 minutes before surgery. Depending on type of surgery, dose may be repeated during surgery and once or twice more after surgery.

Adverse reactions

Blood: *bleeding with high doses,* neutropenia, eosinophilia, leukopenia, *thrombocytopenia.* **CNS:** neuromuscular irritability, seizures, headache, dizziness. **GI:** nausea, diarrhea. **Local:** pain at injection site, vein irritation, phlebitis. **Metabolic:** *hypokalemia.* **Other:** hypersensitivity (edema, fever, chills, rash, pruritus, urticaria, ***anaphylaxis***), overgrowth of nonsusceptible organisms.

Interactions

Aminoglycoside antibiotics (such as gentamicin and tobramycin): chemically incompatible. Don't mix in the same I.V. container. **Probenecid:** increased blood levels of piperacillin. Probenecid may be used for this purpose.

Nursing diagnoses

• High risk for injury related to the ineffectiveness of piperacillin to eradicate the infection.

• Altered protection related to piperacillin-induced allergic reaction.

• Knowledge deficit related to piperacillin therapy.

Nursing interventions

• *Use cautiously* in patients with hypersensitivity to cephalosporins (possible cross-hypersensitivity) and those with bleeding tendencies, uremia, or hypokalemia.

• Cystic fibrosis patients tend to be most susceptible to fever or rash.

• Obtain specimen for culture and sensitivity tests before first dose. Therapy may begin pending test results.

• Before giving piperacillin, ask patient if he's had any allergic reactions to penicillin. A negative history of penicillin allergy, however, is no guarantee against future allergic reaction.

• Dosage should be altered in patients with impaired renal function.

• Check CBC and platelets frequently. Drug may cause thrombocytopenia.

• Monitor serum potassium level.

• Patient with high serum level of this drug may have seizures. Institute seizure precautions.

• Almost always used with another antibiotic, such as gentamicin.

• With large doses and prolonged therapy, bacterial and fungal superinfections may occur, especially in elderly, debilitated, or immunosuppressed patients. Monitor patient closely.

• Drug may be better suited to patients on sodium-free diets than carbenicillin and ticarcillin (contains 1.85 mEq sodium/g of piperacillin).

• Piperacillin has shown greater activity against *Pseudomonas aeruginosa* than carbenicillin, ticarcillin, or mezlocillin.

• Give piperacillin at least 1 hour before bacteriostatic antibiotics.

• **I.V. use:** Give I.V. intermittently to prevent vein irritation. Change site every 48 hours.

General

Classification: immunosuppressant (polypeptide antibiotic). **Pregnancy risk category:** C.

Mechanism of action

Inhibits the proliferation of T lymphocytes.

Indications and dosage

• Prophylaxis of organ rejection in kidney, liver, bone marrow, and heart transplants. **Adults and children:** 15 mg/kg P.O. (oral solution) 4 to 12 hours before transplantation and once daily postoperatively for 1 to 2 weeks. Then, gradually reduce dosage by 5%/week to maintenance level of 5 to 10 mg/kg/day. Alternatively, give I.V. concentrate 4 to 5 mg/kg 4 to 12 hours before transplantation. Postoperatively, repeat this dosage daily until patient can tolerate oral solution.

Adverse reactions

Blood: anemia, ***leukopenia, thrombocytopenia.*** **CNS:** *tremor,* headache. **CV:** hypertension. **GI:** *gum hyperplasia,* nausea, vomiting, diarrhea, oral thrush. **GU:** ***nephrotoxicity.*** **Hepatic:** ***hepatotoxicity.*** **Skin:** *hirsutism,* acne. **Other:** sinusitis, flushing, increased LDL cholesterol levels, ***infections.***

Interactions

Aminoglycosides, amphotericin B, co-trimoxazole, NSAIDs: increased risk of nephrotoxicity. Avoid concomitant use. **Azathioprine, corticosteroids, cyclophosphamide, verapamil:** increased immunosuppression. **Carbamazepine, isoniazid, phenobarbital, phenytoin, rifampin:** possible decreased immunosuppressant effect. **Ketoconazole, amphotericin B, cimetidine, diltiazem, erythromycin, imipenem/cilastatin, metoclopramide, prednisolone:** may increase blood levels of cyclosporine. Monitor serum levels.

Nursing diagnoses

• Altered protection related to threat of organ rejection.
• High risk for injury related to cyclosporine-induced nephrotoxicity.
• Knowledge deficit related to cyclosporine therapy.

Nursing interventions

• *Contraindicated* in hypersensitivity to the drug. Injectable form contains polyoxyethylated castor oil (Cremophor EL), which may provoke hypersensitivity reactions. Closely monitor patients receiving I.V. infusion for hypersensitivity reactions.
• Cyclosporine may cause nephrotoxicity. Monitor BUN and serum creatinine levels. Nephrotoxicity may develop 2 to 3 months after transplant surgery. Report these findings to doctor. He may reduce the dosage.
• Monitor liver function tests for hepatotoxicity, which usually occurs during first month after organ transplant.
• Always give cyclosporine with adrenal corticosteroids.
• Absorption of cyclosporine oral solution can be erratic. Monitor cyclosporine levels regularly.
• Measure oral doses carefully in an oral syringe. To increase palatability, mix with whole milk, chocolate milk, or fruit juice. Use a glass container to minimize adherence to container walls.
• Give dosage once daily in the morning. Urge patient to take drug at same time each day.
• Patient may take with meals if drug causes nausea. Anorexia, nausea, and vomiting are usually transient and occur during initiation of therapy.
• Stress to patient that therapy should not be stopped without doctor's approval.
• To prevent thrush, patient should swish and swallow nystatin four times daily.
• **I.V. use:** Usually reserved for patients who can't tolerate oral form. I.V. concentrate is given at one-third the oral dose. Dilute each ml of concentrate in 20 to 100 ml of D_5W or 0.9% sodium chloride injection. Dilute immediately before administration; infuse over 2 to 6 hours.
• If hirsutism occurs, tell patient she may use a depilatory.
• Cyclosporine has been used for various conditions, such as psoriatic arthritis or ulcerative colitis.

General

Classification: skeletal muscle relaxant (nondepolarizing neuromuscular blocker). **Pregnancy risk category:** C.

Mechanism of action

Competes with acetylcholine for receptor sites at motor end-plate. Because this action may be antagonized by cholinesterase inhibitors, pipecuronium is considered a competitive antagonist.

Indications and dosage

• Skeletal muscle relaxation during surgery as adjunct to general anesthesia. **Adults and children:** dosage highly individualized. Initially, 70 to 85 mcg/kg I.V. allows for endotracheal intubation and maintains paralysis for 1 to 2 hours. If succinylcholine is used for endotracheal intubation, initial doses of 50 mcg/kg I.V. provide good relaxation for 45 minutes or more. Maintenance doses of 10 to 15 mcg/kg provide relaxation for about 50 minutes.

Adverse reactions

CV: hypotension, bradycardia, hypertension, myocardial ischemia, ***CVA,*** thrombosis, atrial fibrillation, ***ventricular extrasystole.*** **GU:** anuria. **Metabolic:** increased creatinine levels. **Respiratory:** dyspnea, respiratory depression, ***respiratory insufficiency or apnea.*** **Other:** prolonged weakness.

Interactions

Aminoglycosides, bacitracin, colistin, polymyxin B, colistimethate, tetracyclines: increased weakness. **Magnesium salts:** possible enhanced neuromuscular blockade. **Quinidine, inhalational anesthetics:** enhanced activity (or prolonged action) of nondepolarizing neuromuscular blockers.

Nursing diagnoses

• Self-care deficit related to prolonged musculoskeletal effects.
• Ineffective breathing pattern related to adverse drug reaction.
• Knowledge deficit related to pipecuronium.

Nursing interventions

• *Contraindicated* in patients requiring prolonged mechanical ventilation, before or after other nondepolarizing neuromuscular blockers, and in cesarean section.
• *Use cautiously* in patients with renal failure. No information is available regarding the use of the drug in patients with hepatic disease.
• Give drug only under direct supervision by persons familiar with the use of neuromuscular blockers and airway maintenance techniques. Don't use unless emergency resuscitation equipment is nearby.
• Neuromuscular blockers don't dull consciousness or alter the pain threshold; give sedatives or general anesthetics before neuromuscular blockers are administered.
• Patients with myasthenia gravis or myasthenic syndrome are particularly sensitive to the effects of nondepolarizing relaxants. Shorter-acting agents are recommended for use in such patients.
• Not recommended for use in neonates and infants younger than 3 months.
• Dosage should be adjusted to ideal body weight in obese patients (30% or more over their ideal weight) because prolonged neuromuscular blockade has been reported in such patients.
• A nerve stimulator and train-of-four monitoring are recommended to document antagonism of neuromuscular blockade and recovery of muscle strength. Before attempting pharmacologic reversal with neostigmine, some evidence of spontaneous recovery should be evident.
• Because of its prolonged duration of action, pipecuronium is recommended only for procedures that take 90 minutes or longer.
• Monitor respirations closely until patient is fully recovered from neuromuscular blockade.
• **I.V. use:** Reconstitute with 10 ml solution before use to yield a solution of 1 mg/ml. Large volumes of diluent or addition of the drug to a hanging I.V. solution is not recommended.

cyproheptadine hydrochloride Periactin

General
Classification: antihistamine (histamine$_1$-receptor antagonist), antipruritic (piperidine derivative). **Pregnancy risk category:** B.

Mechanism of action
Competes with histamine for H_1-receptor sites on effector cells. Prevents but does not reverse histamine-mediated responses.

Indications and dosage
• Allergy symptoms, pruritus. **Adults:** 4 mg P.O. t.i.d. or q.i.d. Maximum dosage is 0.5 mg/kg daily. **Children 7 to 14 years:** 4 mg P.O. b.i.d. or t.i.d. Maximum dosage is 16 mg daily. **Children 2 to 6 years:** 2 mg P.O. b.i.d. or t.i.d. Maximum dosage is 12 mg daily. *Note:* Children under 14 years should use only as directed by a doctor.

Adverse reactions
CNS: (especially in elderly patients) *drowsiness,* dizziness, headache, fatigue. **GI:** nausea, vomiting, epigastric distress, *dry mouth.* **GU:** urine retention. **Skin:** rash. **Other:** weight gain.

Interactions
CNS depressants: increased sedation. Use together cautiously. **MAO inhibitors:** increased anticholinergic effects. Don't use together.

Nursing diagnoses
• Ineffective airway clearance related to the patient's underlying condition.
• High risk for injury related to the adverse CNS effects of cyproheptadine.
• Knowledge deficit related to cyproheptadine therapy.

Nursing interventions
• *Contraindicated* in acute asthmatic attacks.
• *Use cautiously* in elderly patients and in patients with increased intraocular pressure, hyperthyroidism, CV or renal disease, hypertension, bronchial asthma, urine retention, prostatic hypertrophy, bladder-neck obstruction, and stenotic peptic ulcers.
• Warn the patient against drinking alcohol during therapy and against driving or performing other activities that require alertness until CNS response to drug is determined.
• Reduce GI distress by giving the drug with food or milk.
• Advise the patient to drink coffee or tea to reduce drowsiness.
• Suggest sugarless gum, sour hard candy, or ice chips for relieving dry mouth.
• If tolerance develops, another antihistamine may be substituted.
• Warn the patient to stop taking the drug 4 days before allergy skin tests to promote accurate results.
• Antihistamines are not recommended for use by women who are breast-feeding because small amounts of drug are excreted in breast milk.

General

Classification: antihypertensive (beta-adrenergic blocker). **Pregnancy risk category:** B.

Mechanism of action

Blocks response to beta stimulation.

Indications and dosage

• Hypertension. **Adults:** initially, 5 mg P.O. b.i.d. Dosage may be increased by 10 mg/day q 2 to 3 weeks up to a maximum of 60 mg/day.

Adverse reactions

CNS: *insomnia, fatigue, dizziness, nervousness,* vivid dreams, hallucinations, lethargy. **CV:** *edema,* bradycardia, ***CHF,*** peripheral vascular disease, hypotension. **EENT:** visual disturbances. **GI:** *nausea,* vomiting, diarrhea. **Metabolic:** hypoglycemia without tachycardia. **Skin:** rash. **Other:** *increased airway resistance, muscle pain, joint pain,* chest pain.

Interactions

Digitalis glycosides: excessive bradycardia and increased depressant effect on myocardium. Use together cautiously. **Epinephrine:** severe vasoconstriction. Monitor blood pressure and observe patient carefully. **Indomethacin:** decreased antihypertensive effect. Monitor blood pressure and adjust dosage. **Insulin, oral antidiabetic drugs:** possible altered requirements for these drugs in previously stabilized diabetics. Monitor for hypoglycemia.

Nursing diagnoses

• Altered tissue perfusion (renal, cerebral, cardiopulmonary, peripheral) related to the patient's underlying condition.
• Fatigue related to adverse CNS reactions to pindolol.
• Knowledge deficit related to pindolol therapy.

Nursing interventions

• *Contraindicated* in diabetes mellitus, asthma, and allergic rhinitis; during ethyl ether anesthesia; in sinus bradycardia and heart block greater than first degree; in cardiogenic shock; and in right ventricular failure secondary to pulmonary hypertension.
• *Use cautiously* in CHF or respiratory disease and in patients taking other antihypertensives.
• Always check the patient's apical pulse rate before giving this drug. If you detect extremes in pulse rates, hold the drug and call the doctor immediately.
• Monitor blood pressure frequently. If the patient develops severe hypotension, notify doctor. He may prescribe a vasopressor.
• Teach the patient about his disease and therapy. Explain the importance of taking this drug as prescribed, even when he's feeling well. Tell the outpatient not to discontinue this drug suddenly; abrupt discontinuation can exacerbate angina and MI. Tell him to call the doctor if adverse reactions occur.
• Instruct the patient to check with the doctor or pharmacist before taking OTC medications.
• Keep in mind that pindolol masks common signs of shock and hypoglycemia.
• Give drug without any special regard for meals.
• Many patients respond favorably to a dose of 5 mg t.i.d.
• Drug may be advantageous for patients who develop bradycardia with other beta blockers.
• Withdraw drug over 1 to 2 weeks after long-term administration.
• The first commercially available beta-adrenergic blocker with partial beta-agonist activity: Pindolol *stimulates* beta-adrenergic receptors as well as blocks them. Therefore, it decreases cardiac output less than other beta-adrenergic blockers.

General

Classification: antineoplastic (antimetabolite).
Pregnancy risk category: D.

Mechanism of action

Inhibits DNA synthesis.

Indications and dosage

- Acute myelocytic and other acute leukemias, malignant lymphomas. **Adults and children:** 200 mg/m^2 daily by continuous I.V. infusion for 5 days. Repeat q 2 weeks.
- Meningeal leukemias and meningeal neoplasms. **Adults and children:** 10 to 30 mg/m^2 intrathecally once q 4 days.

Adverse reactions

Blood: ***leukopenia,*** *WBC nadir 7 to 9 days after drug stopped;* anemia, reticulocytopenia; ***thrombocytopenia,*** platelet nadir occurring on day 10; *megaloblastosis.* **CNS:** neurotoxicity with high doses. **EENT:** *keratitis.* **GI:** *nausea, vomiting,* diarrhea, dysphagia; reddened area at juncture of lips, followed by sore mouth, oral ulcers in 5 to 10 days; projectile vomiting (possible with high dose given by rapid I.V.). **Hepatic:** hepatotoxicity (usually mild and reversible). **Metabolic:** hyperuricemia. **Skin:** rash. **Other:** flulike syndrome.

Interactions

Digoxin: possible decrease in serum digoxin levels. Monitor closely.

Nursing diagnoses

- Altered protection related to cytarabine-induced myelosuppression and immunosuppression.
- Altered oral mucous membrane related to cytarabine-induced stomatitis.
- Knowledge deficit related to cytarabine therapy.

Nursing interventions

- *Contraindicated* in patients with hypersensitivity to the drug.
- *Use cautiously.* Dosage modification may be required in thrombocytopenia, leukopenia, and renal or hepatic disease and after other chemotherapy or radiation therapy.
- Watch for signs of infection (cough, fever, and sore throat) and bleeding (easy bruising, nosebleeds, and bleeding gums). Monitor CBC.
- Provide excellent mouth care to help prevent stomatitis.
- **I.V. use:** Nausea and vomiting occur more frequently when large doses are administered rapidly by I.V. push. These reactions occur less frequently with infusion. To reduce nausea, give antiemetic before cytarabine administration.
- Steroid eye drops are prescribed to prevent drug-induced keratitis.
- Also known as ara-C.
- Monitor intake and output carefully. Maintain high fluid intake and give allopurinol, if ordered, to avoid urate nephropathy in leukemia induction therapy. Monitor serum uric acid.
- Monitor hepatic and renal function.
- Use preservative-free 0.9% sodium chloride or Elliot's B solution for intrathecal use.
- Reconstituted solution is stable for 48 hours. Discard cloudy reconstituted solution.
- Avoid I.M. injections in patients with thrombocytopenia to prevent bleeding.
- Warn patient to watch for signs of infection and bleeding. Instruct him to take his temperature daily.
- Modify or discontinue therapy if polymorphonuclear granulocyte count is below 1,000/mm^3 or if platelet count is below 50,000/mm^3.
- Assess patients receiving high doses for neurotoxicity. May first appear as nystagmus, but can progress to ataxia and cerebellar dysfunction.
- Preparation of parenteral form has carcinogenic, mutagenic, and teratogenic risks for personnel. Follow institutional policy to reduce risks.

General

Classification: antipsychotic (diphenylbutylpiperidine). **Pregnancy risk category:** C.

Mechanism of action

Blocks dopaminergic receptors.

Indications and dosage

- Suppression of severe motor and phonic tics in patients with Tourette syndrome. **Adults and children over 12 years:** initially, 1 to 2 mg P.O. daily in divided doses. Then, increase dosage every other day. Maintenance dosage ranges from 7 to 16 mg daily.

Adverse reactions

CNS: *parkinsonian symptoms,* other extrapyramidal symptoms (dystonia, akathisia, hyperreflexia, opisthotonos, oculogyric crisis), *tardive dyskinesia, sedation.* **CV:** *ECG changes (prolonged QT interval),* hypotension. **EENT:** visual disturbances. **GI:** *dry mouth, constipation.* **GU:** impotence. **Other:** rarely, ***neuroleptic malignant syndrome*** (fever, tachycardia, tachypnea, profuse diaphoresis), muscle tightness.

Interactions

Alcohol, other CNS depressants: increased CNS depression. **Phenothiazines, TCAs, antiarrhythmics:** increased incidence of ECG abnormalities.

Nursing diagnoses

- Impaired thought processes related to the patient's underlying condition.
- High risk for injury related to the drug's adverse reactions.
- Knowledge deficit related to pimozide therapy.

Nursing interventions

- *Contraindicated* in congenital long QT syndrome or history of cardiac arrhythmias, severe toxic CNS depression, or coma.
- *Use cautiously* in hepatic or renal dysfunction, glaucoma, and prostatic hypertrophy.
- Tardive dyskinesia may occur after prolonged use. It may not appear until months or years later and may disappear spontaneously or persist for life despite discontinuation of the drug.
- Neuroleptic malignant syndrome, a rare but frequently fatal reaction, isn't necessarily related to the length of drug use or the type of neuroleptic. However, more than 60% of affected patients are men. Watch for symptoms.
- Acute dystonic reactions may be treated with I.V. diphenhydramine.
- Pimozide is not recommended for treating simple tics except those associated with Tourette syndrome. Don't use in drug-induced motor and phonic tics.
- Avoid concurrent administration of other drugs that prolong the QT interval, such as antiarrhythmics.
- Perform an ECG before treatment and periodically thereafter. Monitor for prolonged QT interval.
- Monitor patients who are also taking anticonvulsants for increased seizure activity. Pimozide may lower the seizure threshold.
- Because pimozide may cause serious adverse effects, the patient and his family should be thoroughly informed before deciding whether he should take the drug. Pimozide is indicated only in patients who have failed to respond satisfactorily to standard treatment.
- Warn the patient not to stop taking drug abruptly and not to exceed prescribed dose.
- Tell him to use sugarless hard candy, gum, and liquids, as needed, to relieve dry mouth.

General
Classification: antiestrogen, androgen (androgen). **Pregnancy risk category:** X.

Mechanism of action
Gonadotropin inhibitor that suppresses the pituitary-ovarian axis. Also acts on estrogen receptors to inhibit estrogenic effects.

Indications and dosage
- Mild endometriosis. **Women:** initially, 100 to 200 mg P.O. b.i.d. Subsequent dosage based upon patient response.
- Moderate to severe endometriosis. **Women:** 400 mg P.O. b.i.d. uninterrupted for 3 to 6 months; may continue for 9 months.
- Fibrocystic breast disease. **Women:** 100 to 400 mg P.O. daily in 2 divided doses uninterrupted for 2 to 6 months.
- Prevention of hereditary angioedema. **Adults:** 200 mg P.O. 2 to 3 times a day, continued until favorable response is achieved. Then dosage should be decreased by half at 1- to 3-month intervals.

Adverse reactions
Androgenic: in women—acne, edema, *weight gain, hirsutism,* hoarseness, clitoral enlargement, *decrease in breast size,* changes in libido, male pattern baldness, *oiliness of skin or hair.* **Blood:** thrombocytopenia. **CNS:** dizziness, headache, sleep disorders, fatigue, tremor, irritability, excitation, lethargy, mental depression, chills, paresthesia. **CV:** elevated blood pressure. **EENT:** visual disturbances. **GI:** gastric irritation, nausea, vomiting, diarrhea, constipation, change in appetite. **GU:** hematuria. **Hepatic:** reversible jaundice. **Hypoestrogenic:** flushing; sweating; vaginitis, including itching, dryness, burning, and vaginal bleeding; nervousness, emotional lability, menstrual irregularities. **Other:** muscle cramps or spasms.

Interactions
None significant.

Nursing diagnoses
- Pain related to implantation of endometrial tissue outside the uterine cavity.
- Body image disturbance related to adverse androgenic reactions associated with danazol.
- Knowledge deficit related to danazol therapy.

Nursing interventions
- *Contraindicated* in undiagnosed abnormal genital bleeding; impaired renal, cardiac, or hepatic function; during pregnancy; and in breast-feeding women.
- *Use cautiously* in seizure disorder or migraine headache.
- Avoid use in women of childbearing age until pregnancy is ruled out. Be sure they understand the importance of effective nonhormonal contraception.
- Use with diet high in calories and protein unless contraindicated.
- Monitor closely for signs of virilization. Some androgenic effects, such as deepening of voice, may not be reversible upon discontinuation of drug.
- Periodically evaluate hepatic function.
- Periodic dosage decreases or gradual drug withdrawal should be considered.
- Advise patient who is taking danazol for fibrocystic disease to examine breasts regularly and to call doctor immediately if breast nodule enlarges during treatment.
- Advise washing after intercourse to decrease the risk of vaginitis. Instruct patient to wear only cotton underwear.
- Has been used investigationally with impressive results in treating hemophilia and Christmas disease; also used to decrease symptoms of systemic lupus erythematosus in women and to treat gynecomastia in men.

General

Classification: miotic (cholinergic agonist). **Pregnancy risk category:** C.

Mechanism of action

Causes contraction of the sphincter muscles of the iris, resulting in miosis. Also produces ciliary spasm, deepening of the anterior chamber, and vasodilation of conjunctival vessels of the outflow tract.

Indications and dosage

- Primary open-angle glaucoma. **Adults and children:** instill 1 to 2 drops (hydrochloride, nitrate) in eye once daily to q.i.d., as directed by doctor. Or, may apply 4% gel (Pilopine HS) once daily. Alternatively, apply one Ocusert Pilo system (20 or 40 mcg/hour) q 7 days.
- Emergency treatment of acute narrow-angle glaucoma. **Adults and children:** 1 drop of 2% solution (hydrochloride, nitrate) q 5 minutes for three to six doses, followed by 1 drop q 1 to 3 hours until pressure is controlled.

Adverse reactions

Eye: suborbital headache, *myopia,* ciliary spasm, *blurred vision,* conjunctival irritation, lacrimation, changes in visual field, *brow pain.* **GI:** nausea, vomiting, abdominal cramps, diarrhea, salivation.

Other: bronchiolar spasm, pulmonary edema, hypersensitivity.

Interactions

Carbachol, echothiophate: additive effect. Don't use together. **Ophthalmic belladonna alkaloids (such as atropine, scopolamine), cyclopentolate:** decreased antiglaucoma effects of pilocarpine; mydriatic effects of these agents blocked by pilocarpine. **Phenylephrine:** decreased dilation by phenylephrine. Don't use together.

Nursing diagnoses

- Sensory/perceptual alterations (visual) related to the patient's underlying condition.
- Pain related to the pilocarpine-induced brow discomfort.
- Knowledge deficit related to pilocarpine therapy.

Nursing interventions

- *Contraindicated* in acute iritis, acute inflammatory disease of the anterior segment of the eye, and secondary glaucoma.
- *Use cautiously* in bronchial asthma and hypertension.
- Miosis starts within 30 minutes and usually lasts 4 to 8 hours.
- Warn patient that vision will be temporarily blurred. Also warn him to avoid hazardous activities until this effect subsides.
- Transient brow pain and myopia are common at first; these symptoms usually disappear in 10 to 14 days.
- Teach the patient how to instill the drug. Advise him to wash his hands before and after administering gel or solution and to apply light finger-pressure on the lacrimal sac for 1 minute after instillation of drops. Warn him not to touch dropper to eye or surrounding tissue.
- Widely used drug to treat primary open-angle glaucoma.
- Used to counteract effects of mydriatics and cycloplegics after surgery or ophthalmoscopic examination.
- May be used alternately with atropine to break adhesions.
- In acute narrow-angle glaucoma before surgery, pilocarpine may be used alone or with mannitol, urea, glycerol, or acetazolamide.
- If the Ocusert Pilo system falls out of the eye during sleep, the patient should wash his hands, rinse the system in cool tap water, and reposition it in the eye. Tell patient not to use it if deformed.
- Instruct him to apply the gel at bedtime, as it will blur vision.

General

Classification: skeletal muscle relaxant (hydantoin derivative). **Pregnancy risk category:** C.

Mechanism of action

Acts directly on skeletal muscle to interfere with intracellular calcium movement.

Indications and dosage

- Spasticity and sequelae of severe chronic disorders (multiple sclerosis, cerebral palsy, spinal cord injury, CVA). **Adults:** 25 mg P.O. daily. Increase gradually in increments of 25 mg at 4- to 7-day intervals, up to 100 mg b.i.d. to q.i.d., to maximum of 400 mg daily. **Children:** 1 mg/kg daily P.O. b.i.d. to q.i.d. Increase gradually p.r.n. by 1 mg/kg daily to maximum of 100 mg q.i.d.
- Management of malignant hyperthermia. **Adults and children:** 1 mg/kg I.V. initially; may repeat up to cumulative dose of 10 mg/kg.
- Prevention or attenuation of malignant hyperthermia in susceptible patients who require surgery. **Adults:** 4 to 8 mg/kg P.O. daily in 3 to 4 divided doses for 1 to 2 days before procedure. Give final dose 3 to 4 hours before procedure.
- Prevention of malignant hyperthermia recurrence. **Adults:** 4 to 8 mg/kg/day P.O. in 4 divided doses for up to 3 days after hyperthermic crisis.

Adverse reactions

CNS: *weakness, drowsiness,* dizziness, light-headedness, malaise, headache, confusion, nervousness, insomnia, ***precipitation of seizures.*** **CV:** tachycardia, blood pressure changes. **EENT:** excessive tearing, visual disturbances. **GI:** anorexia, constipation, cramping, dysphagia, metallic taste, severe diarrhea. **GU:** urinary frequency, incontinence, nocturia, dysuria, crystalluria, difficulty achieving erection. **Hepatic:** hepatitis. **Skin:** eczematous eruption, pruritus, urticaria, photosensitivity. **Other:** abnormal hair growth, drooling, sweating, pleural effusion, myalgia, chills, fever.

Interactions

Alcohol, CNS depressants: increased CNS depression. **Verapamil (I.V.):** possible CV collapse. Stop drug before giving I.V. dantrolene.

Nursing diagnoses

- Hyperthermia related to the patient's underlying condition.
- High risk for injury related to drug-induced drowsiness.
- Knowledge deficit related to dantrolene therapy.

Nursing interventions

- *Contraindicated* when spasticity maintains motor function; for spasms in rheumatic disorders; in hepatic disease; and during breast-feeding.
- *Use cautiously* in severely impaired cardiac or pulmonary function or preexisting hepatic disease; in women; and in those over age 35.
- Don't use more than 45 days if no benefits obtained.
- Patients may have trouble swallowing during therapy. Advise caution when eating to avoid choking.
- Give with meals or milk to prevent GI distress.
- To prepare P.O. suspension for single dose: dissolve capsule contents in juice or other suitable liquid. Multiple doses: use acid vehicle, such as citric acid in USP syrup.
- Amount of relief determines if dosage (and drowsiness) can be reduced.
- Perform liver function tests at start of therapy.
- Watch for hepatitis, severe diarrhea, severe weakness, or sensitivity reactions.
- Warn patient to avoid driving and other hazardous activities until drug's CNS effects are known.
- Tell patient to avoid photosensitivity reactions by using sunscreen and protective clothing, and to report abdominal pain or GI problems promptly.
- **I.V. use:** Give as soon as malignant hyperthermia is recognized. Reconstitute each vial with 60 ml of sterile water for injection and shake until clear. Don't use diluent containing bacteriostatic agent.
- Has been used to treat neuroleptic malignant syndrome.

General

Classification: antimuscarinic antidote (cholinesterase inhibitor). **Pregnancy risk category:** C.

Mechanism of action

Inhibits the destruction of acetylcholine released from the parasympathetic and somatic efferent nerves. Acetylcholine accumulates, promoting increased stimulation of the receptor.

Indications and dosage

• Reversal of CNS toxicity associated with tricyclic antidepressant (TCA) and anticholinergic poisoning. **Adults:** 0.5 to 2 mg I.M. or I.V. (1 mg/minute I.V.) repeated q 20 minutes as necessary if life-threatening signs recur (coma, seizures, arrhythmias). Additional doses of 1 to 4 mg I.M. or I.V. q 30 to 60 minutes may be given. **Children:** 0.02 mg/kg I.M. or I.V. Repeat q 5 to 10 minutes until response is obtained. Maximum dose to 2 mg.

Adverse reactions

CNS: ***seizures,*** hallucinations, twitching, weakness, ataxia, *restlessness, excitability, sweating.* **CV:** irregular pulse, palpitations. **EENT:** miosis. **GI:** nausea, vomiting, epigastric pain, *diarrhea, excessive salivation.* **Other:** ***bronchospasm,*** bronchial constriction, dyspnea.

Interactions

Atropine, anticholinergic agents, procainamide, quinidine: possible reversed cholinergic effects. Observe for lack of drug effect.

Nursing diagnoses

• Anxiety related to the patient's underlying condition.
• Diarrhea related to adverse reaction of the drug.
• Knowledge deficit related to physostigmine therapy.

Nursing interventions

• *Contraindicated* in patients with mechanical obstruction of the intestine or urogenital tract, bronchial asthma, gangrene, diabetes, CV disease, or vagotonia.
• *Use cautiously* in patients with bradycardia, hypotension, seizure disorder, Parkinson's disease, hyperthyroidism, and peptic ulcer.
• Watch closely for adverse reactions, particularly CNS disturbances. Use side rails if patient becomes restless or hallucinates. Adverse reactions may indicate drug toxicity.
• Monitor vital signs frequently, being especially careful to check respirations. Position patient to make breathing easier. Always have atropine injection readily available and be prepared to give atropine 0.5 mg S.C. or slow I.V. push as ordered, and provide respiratory support as needed. Best administered in presence of doctor.
• Use only clear solution. Darkening may indicate loss of potency.
• **I.V. use:** Give I.V. at a controlled rate; use slow, direct injection at no more than 1 mg/minute.
• Physostigmine is the only cholinergic that crosses the blood-brain barrier; therefore, it's the only one useful for treating CNS effects of anticholinergic or TCA toxicity.
• Drug's effectiveness is often immediate and dramatic but may be transient and may require repeat dose.
• Drug is used investigationally to improve cognitive function in patients with Alzheimer's disease. Investigators have used 0.5 mg P.O. q 2 hours, increasing to 2 to 2.5 mg P.O. q 2 hours, six or seven times a day. Maximum dose is 16 mg/day.

demeclocycline hydrochloride

Declomycin

General

Classification: antibiotic (tetracycline). **Pregnancy risk category:** D.

Mechanism of action

Exerts bacteriostatic effect by binding to the 30S ribosomal subunit of microorganisms, thus inhibiting protein synthesis.

Indications and dosage

- Infections caused by susceptible gram-negative and gram-positive organisms, psittacosis, lymphogranuloma venereum, granuloma inguinale, relapsing fever, *Mycoplasma pneumoniae,* trachoma, rickettsiae. **Adults:** 150 mg P.O. q 6 hours or 300 mg q 12 hours. **Children over 8 years:** 6 to 12 mg/kg P.O. daily, divided q 6 to 12 hours.
- Gonorrhea. **Adults:** initially, 600 mg P.O., then 300 mg q 12 hours for 4 days (total 3 g).
- Uncomplicated urethral, endocervical, or rectal infection caused by *Chlamydia trachomatis.* **Adults:** 300 mg P.O. q.i.d. for at least 7 days.
- SIADH (a hyposmolar state). **Adults:** 600 to 1,200 mg P.O. daily in divided doses q 6 to 8 hours.

Adverse reactions

Blood: neutropenia, eosinophilia, thrombocytopenia, *hemolytic anemia.* **CNS:** pseudotumor cerebri. **CV:** pericarditis. **EENT:** dysphagia, glossitis. **GI:** anorexia, *nausea, vomiting, diarrhea,* enterocolitis, anogenital inflammation. **Metabolic:** *increased BUN,* diabetes insipidus syndrome (polyuria, polydipsia, weakness). **Skin:** *rash, increased pigmentation, urticaria.* **Other:** ***hypersensitivity,*** *photosensitivity.*

Interactions

Antacids and laxatives containing aluminum, magnesium, or calcium; food, milk, or other dairy products: decreased antibiotic absorption. Give antibiotic 1 hour before or 2 hours after any of these. **Ferrous sulfate and other iron products, zinc:** reduced antibiotic absorption. Give demeclocycline 3 hours after or 2 hours before iron administration. **Methoxyflurane:** may cause nephrotoxicity. Monitor carefully. **Oral anticoagulants:** increased anticoagulant effect. Monitor prothrombin times and adjust dosage. **Oral contraceptives:** decreased contraceptive effects and increased risk of breakthrough bleeding.

Nursing diagnoses

- High risk for infection related to ineffectiveness of demeclocycline to eradicate the infection.
- High risk for fluid volume deficit related to adverse GI reactions to demeclocycline therapy.
- Knowledge deficit related to demeclocycline therapy.

Nursing interventions

- *Use with extreme caution* in renal or hepatic impairment. Use during last half of pregnancy and in children under 8 years may permanently discolor teeth, cause enamel defects, and retard bone growth.
- Obtain specimen for culture and sensitivity tests. Therapy may begin pending test results.
- Check expiration date. Deteriorated demeclocycline has been linked to reversible nephrotoxicity.
- Don't expose drug to light or heat; store in tight container.
- With large doses or prolonged therapy, monitor for superinfection, especially in high-risk patients.
- Check patient's tongue for signs of monilia infection. Stress good oral hygiene.
- Warn patient to avoid sunlight and ultraviolet light. Sunscreen may help prevent photosensitivity reactions. Photosensitivity persists after drug discontinuation.
- Tell patient not to take drug with milk, other dairy products, food, antacids, or iron products. Tell him to take each dose with a full glass of water on an empty stomach, at least 1 hour before meals or 2 hours afterward and remain standing for 90 seconds after ingestion. Give at least 1 hour before bedtime to avoid esophagitis.
- May cause false-negative Clinistix or Tes-Tape test.

General

Classification: anticonvulsant (hydantoin derivative). **Pregnancy risk category:** D.

Mechanism of action

Stabilizes neuronal membranes and limits seizure activity by either increasing efflux or decreasing influx of sodium ions across cell membranes in motor cortex during generation of nerve impulses. Produces antiarrhythmic effect by normalizing sodium influx to Purkinje fibers when used to treat digitalis glycoside-induced arrhythmias.

Indications and dosage

- Generalized tonic-clonic seizures, status epilepticus. **Adults:** loading dose is 900 mg to 1.5 g I.V. or P.O. divided t.i.d., then start maintenance dosage of 300 mg P.O. daily as a single dose (extended only) or divided t.i.d. **Children:** loading dose is 15 mg/kg I.V. or P.O. divided q 8 to 12 hours, then start maintenance dosage of 5 to 7 mg/kg P.O. or I.V. daily, divided q 12 hours.
- If patient has not received phenytoin previously or has no detectable blood level, use loading dose. **Adults:** 900 mg to 1.5 g I.V. divided into t.i.d. Do not exceed 500 mg each dose. **Children:** 15 mg/kg I.V.
- If patient has been receiving phenytoin but has missed one or more doses and has subtherapeutic levels. **Adults:** 100 to 300 mg I.V. **Children:** 5 to 7 mg/kg I.V. May repeat lower dose in 30 minutes if needed.
- Neuritic pain (migraine, trigeminal neuralgia, Bell's palsy). **Adults:** 200 to 400 mg P.O. daily.
- Ventricular arrhythmias unresponsive to lidocaine or procainamide; supraventricular and ventricular arrhythmias induced by digitalis glycosides. **Adults:** loading dose is 1 g P.O. divided over first 24 hours, followed by 500 mg daily for 2 days, then maintenance dose of 300 mg daily; or 250 mg I.V. over 5 minutes until arrhythmias subside, adverse reactions develop, or 1 g has been given.

Adverse reactions

Blood: ***thrombocytopenia, leukopenia, agranulocytosis, pancytopenia,*** macrocytosis, megaloblastic anemia. **CNS:** *ataxia, slurred speech, confusion,* dizziness, insomnia, nervousness, twitching, headache. **CV:** hypotension, ***ventricular fibrillation.*** **EENT:** *nystagmus, diplopia,* blurred vision. **GI:** *nausea, vomiting, gingival hyperplasia (especially children).* **Hepatic:** ***toxic hepatitis.*** **Skin:** scarlatiniform or morbilliform rash; bullous, *exfoliative,* or purpuric dermatitis; ***Stevens-Johnson syndrome;*** lupus erythematosus; *hirsutism;* ***toxic epidermal necrolysis;*** photosensitivity. **Local:** pain, necrosis, and inflammation at injection site; purple glove syndrome. **Other:** periarteritis nodosa, lymphadenopathy, hyperglycemia, osteomalacia, hypertrichosis.

Interactions

Alcohol, dexamethasone, folic acid: decreased phenytoin activity. **Oral anticoagulants, antihistamines, amiodarone, chloramphenicol, cimetidine, cycloserine, diazepam, diazoxide, disulfiram, influenza vaccine, isoniazid, phenylbutazone, salicylates, sulfamethizole, valproate:** increased phenytoin activity and toxicity. **Oral tube feedings with Osmolite or Isocal:** possible interference with absorption of oral phenytoin.

Nursing diagnoses

- High risk for injury related to patient's underlying seizure activity.
- Altered oral mucous membrane related to phenytoin-induced gingival hyperplasia.

Nursing interventions

- *Contraindicated* in phenacemide or hydantoin hypersensitivity, bradycardia, SA and AV block, or Stokes-Adams syndrome.
- *Use cautiously* in hepatic or renal dysfunction, hypotension, myocardial insufficiency, and respiratory depression; in elderly or debilitated patients; and in those receiving other hydantoin derivatives.
- **I.V. use:** Don't mix drug with D_5W because it will precipitate, and never give faster than 50 mg/minute. Continuous cardiac monitoring during infusion is recommended.
- Therapeutic blood level is 10 to 20 mcg/ml.

General
Classification: antidepressant, anxiolytic (tricyclic dibenzazepine). **Pregnancy risk category:** C.

Mechanism of action
Increases the amount of norepinephrine or serotonin, or both, in the CNS by blocking their reuptake by presynaptic neurons. This allows these neurotransmitters to accumulate.

Indications and dosage
• Depression. **Adults:** 75 to 150 mg P.O. daily in divided doses, increasing to maximum of 300 mg daily. Or give entire dose h.s. **Elderly patients and adolescents:** 25 to 50 mg P.O. daily, increasing slowly to maximum of 100 mg daily.

Adverse reactions
CNS: *drowsiness, dizziness,* excitation, tremor, weakness, confusion, headache, nervousness, EEG changes, ***seizures,*** extrapyramidal reactions. **CV:** orthostatic hypotension, *tachycardia, ECG changes,* hypertension. **EENT:** *blurred vision,* tinnitus, mydriasis. **GI:** *dry mouth, constipation,* nausea, vomiting, anorexia, paralytic ileus. **GU:** *urine retention.* **Skin:** rash, urticaria, photosensitivity. **Other:** *sweating,* allergy. **After abrupt withdrawal of long-term therapy:** nausea, headache, malaise. (Does not indicate addiction.)

Interactions
Alcohol: antagonized desipramine effects. **Barbiturates:** decreased desipramine levels. Monitor for decreased antidepressant effect. **Cimetidine:** possible increased desipramine levels. Monitor for increased adverse reactions. **Epinephrine, norepinephrine:** increased hypertensive effect. Use with caution. **MAO inhibitors:** possible severe excitation, hyperpyrexia, or seizures, usually with high dose. Use together cautiously. **Methylphenidate:** increased desipramine levels. Monitor for enhanced antidepressant effect.

Nursing diagnoses
• Ineffective individual coping related to the patient's underlying condition.
• High risk for injury related to desipramine-induced adverse reactions.
• Knowledge deficit related to desipramine.

Nursing interventions
• *Contraindicated* during acute recovery from MI, in seizure disorders, and in prostatic hypertrophy.
• *Use cautiously* in CV or thyroid disease, urine retention, narrow-angle glaucoma, blood dyscrasias, or hepatic dysfunction; in patients at risk for suicide; and in those receiving electroshock therapy, thyroid drugs, or elective surgery.
• Do not withdraw drug abruptly.
• If psychotic signs increase, dosage should be decreased. Record mood changes. Watch for suicidal tendencies. To lessen suicide risk, allow minimum supply of tablets.
• Drug has low potential for anticholinergic effects; it produces less sedation than amitriptyline or doxepin and does not usually cause orthostatic hypotension.
• Desipramine causes fewer adverse cardiac effects than other tricyclic antidepressants (TCAs).
• Check for urine retention and constipation. Increase fluids to lessen constipation. Suggest stool softener and high-fiber diet, if needed.
• Warn patient to avoid hazardous activities that require alertness and good coordination until drug's CNS effects are known. Drowsiness and dizziness usually subside after a few weeks.
• Expect delay of 2 weeks or more before noticeable effect; 4 weeks or more before full effect.
• When possible, have patient take full dose at bedtime.
• Advise patient not to take any other drugs without first consulting the doctor.
• Hypertensive episodes have occurred during surgery in patients receiving TCAs. Discontinue these drugs several days before surgery.
• Some patients may experience photosensitivity reactions. Advise patient to use a sunscreen, wear protective clothing, and avoid prolonged exposure to strong sunlight.

General
Classification: vasoconstrictor (adrenergic). **Pregnancy risk category:** C.

Mechanism of action
Predominantly stimulates alpha-adrenergic receptors in the sympathetic nervous system.

Indications and dosage
- Hypotensive emergencies during spinal anesthesia. **Adults:** initially, 0.2 mg I.V., then subsequent doses of 0.1 to 0.2 mg.
- Maintenance of blood pressure during spinal or inhalation anesthesia. **Adults:** 2 to 3 mg S.C. or I.M. 3 to 4 minutes before anesthesia. **Children:** 0.04 mg to 0.088 mg/kg S.C. or I.M.
- Mild to moderate hypotension. **Adults:** 2 to 5 mg S.C. or I.M.; repeat in 1 to 2 hours as needed and tolerated. Initial dose should not exceed 5 mg. Alternatively, give 0.1 to 0.5 mg I.V., not to be repeated more often than 10 to 15 minutes. **Children:** 0.1 mg/kg I.M. or S.C.; repeat in 1 to 2 hours as needed and tolerated.
- Paroxysmal supraventricular tachycardia. **Adults:** initially, 0.5 mg rapid I.V.; subsequent doses should not exceed preceding dose by more than 0.1 to 0.2 mg and should not exceed 1 mg.
- Prolongation of spinal anesthesia. **Adults:** 2 to 5 mg added to anesthetic solution.
- Severe hypotension and shock (including drug-induced). **Adults:** 10 mg in 250 ml to 500 ml D_5W or 0.9% sodium chloride injection. Start 100 to 180 mcg/minute I.V. infusion, then decrease to a maintenance infusion of 40 to 60 mcg/minute when blood pressure stabilizes.
- Vasoconstrictor for regional anesthesia. **Adults:** 1 mg phenylephrine added to 20 ml local anesthetic.

Adverse reactions
CNS: *headache, restlessness, light-headedness, weakness.* **CV:** palpitations, bradycardia, ***arrhythmias,*** hypertension, anginal pain. **EENT:** blurred vision. **Skin:** goose bumps, feeling of coolness. **Local:** tissue sloughing with extravasation. **Other:** tachyphylaxis possible with continued use.

Interactions
MAO inhibitors: may cause severe hypertension (hypertensive crisis). Don't use together. **Oxytocics, tricyclic antidepressants:** increased pressor response. Observe patient.

Nursing diagnoses
- Altered tissue perfusion (cardiopulmonary, cerebral, renal, gastrointestinal, peripheral) related to the patient's underlying condition.
- Pain related to adverse drug reaction.
- Knowledge deficit related to phenylephrine therapy.

Nursing interventions
- *Contraindicated* in narrow-angle glaucoma, hypotension, ventricular tachycardia, severe coronary disease, and CV disease.
- *Use with extreme caution* in heart disease, hyperthyroidism, diabetes, bradycardia, partial heart block, sulfite sensitivity, and in elderly patients.
- Causes little or no CNS stimulation.
- Monitor blood pressure frequently. Avoid excessive rise in blood pressure. Maintain at slightly below patient's normal level. In previously normotensive patients, maintain systolic pressure at 80 to 100 mm Hg; in previously hypertensive patients, maintain systolic pressure from 30 to 40 mm Hg below usual level.
- May reverse severe increase in blood pressure with phentolamine.
- **I.V. use:** Use a central venous catheter or large vein, as in the antecubital fossa, to reduce risk of extravasation. Use infusion pump to regulate flow. Avoid abrupt withdrawal.

desmopressin acetate

DDAVP, Stimate

General

Classification: antidiuretic, hemostatic agent (posterior pituitary hormone). **Pregnancy risk category:** B.

Mechanism of action

Increases permeability of renal tubular epithelium to adenosine monophosphate and water; the epithelium promotes reabsorption of water and concentrates urine (antidiuretic hormone effect). Desmopressin also increases Factor VIII activity by releasing endogenous Factor VIII from plasma storage sites.

Indications and dosage

- Nonnephrogenic diabetes insipidus, temporary polyuria and polydipsia associated with pituitary trauma. **Adults:** 0.1 to 0.4 ml intranasally daily in 1 to 3 doses. Adjust morning and evening doses separately for adequate diurnal rhythm. Alternatively, may give injectable form in dosage of 0.5 to 1 ml I.V. or S.C. daily, usually in two divided doses. **Children 3 months to 12 years:** 0.05 to 0.3 ml intranasally daily in 1 or 2 doses.
- Hemophilia A and von Willebrand's disease. **Adults and children:** 0.3 mcg/kg diluted in 0.9% sodium chloride solution and infused slowly over 15 to 30 minutes. May repeat dose if indicated by laboratory studies and patient's condition.
- Primary nocturnal enuresis. **Children 5 years and over:** initially, 20 mcg intranasally h.s. (half in each nostril). Adjust dose according to response. Maximum recommended dose is 40 mcg daily.

Adverse reactions

CNS: headache. **CV:** slight rise in blood pressure (with high dosage). **EENT:** nasal congestion, rhinitis. **GI:** nausea, abdominal cramps. **GU:** vulval pain. **Other:** flushing.

Interactions

Demeclocycline, ethanol, epinephrine, heparin, lithium: increased risk of adverse reactions.

Nursing diagnoses

- Fluid volume deficit related to the patient's underlying condition.
- Pain related to desmopressin-induced headache.
- Knowledge deficit related to desmopressin therapy.

Nursing interventions

- *Contraindicated* in patients with type IIb von Willebrand's disease and in children under age 3 months.
- *Use cautiously* in coronary artery insufficiency or hypertension.
- Adjust fluid intake to reduce risk of water intoxication and sodium depletion, especially in children or elderly patients.
- Overdose may cause oxytocic or vasopressor activity. Withhold drug until effects subside. Furosemide may be used if fluid retention is excessive.
- Some patients may have difficulty measuring and inhaling drug into nostrils. Instruct patient to clear nasal passages before administering drug.
- Nasal congestion, allergic rhinitis, or upper respiratory infections may impair drug absorption. Advise patient to report such conditions because they may require dosage adjustment.
- Intranasal use can cause changes in the nasal mucosa resulting in erratic, unreliable absorption. Doctor may prescribe injectable DDAVP.
- Teach patients using S.C. desmopressin to rotate injection sites to prevent tissue damage.
- Avoid desmopressin injection in hemophilia A with Factor VIII levels up to 5% and in severe von Willebrand's disease.
- In patients treated for hemophilia A and von Willebrand's disease, use of desmopressin may avoid the hazards of using blood products.
- Has been used successfully to reduce blood loss during cardiac surgery.

General

Classification: nonnarcotic analgesic, antipyretic (NSAID). **Pregnancy risk category:** D.

Mechanism of action

Produces anti-inflammatory, analgesic, and antipyretic effects, possibly through inhibition of prostaglandin synthesis.

Indications and dosage

- Pain, inflammation in arthritis, bursitis, acute superficial thrombophlebitis. **Adults:** initially, 100 to 200 mg P.O. t.i.d. or q.i.d. Maximum dosage is 600 mg daily. When improvement is obtained, decrease dosage to 100 mg t.i.d. or q.i.d.
- Acute, gouty arthritis. **Adults:** 400 mg P.O. initially as single dose, then 100 mg q 4 hours for 4 days or until relief is obtained.

Note: Do not continue therapy for longer than 1 week.

Adverse reactions

Blood: ***bone marrow suppression (fatal aplastic anemia, agranulocytosis, thrombocytopenia), hemolytic anemia,*** leukopenia. **CNS:** agitation, confusion, lethargy. **CV:** hypertension, edema, pericarditis, myocarditis, ***cardiac decompensation.*** **EENT:** optic neuritis, blurred vision, retinal hemorrhage or detachment, hearing loss. **GI:** *nausea, vomiting, diarrhea,* ***peptic ulceration,*** *occult blood loss.* **GU:** proteinuria, hematuria, glomerulonephritis, nephrotic syndrome, ***renal failure.*** **Hepatic:** ***hepatitis.*** **Metabolic:** hyperglycemia, toxic and nontoxic goiter, respiratory alkalosis, metabolic acidosis. **Skin:** petechiae, pruritus, purpura, various dermatoses from rash to ***toxic necrotizing epidermolysis.***

Interactions

Alcohol: increased risk of toxicity. Avoid concomitant use. **Antihypertensives:** decreased effectiveness. Monitor blood pressure closely. **Cholestyramine:** may alter phenylbutazone absorption. Give 1 hour before cholestyramine. **Insulin, oral antidiabetics:** enhanced hypoglycemic effect. Monitor patient closely. **Oral anticoagulants:** enhanced risk of bleeding. Monitor patient closely. **Phenytoin, lithium:** increased plasma levels after phenylbutazone administration. Monitor for toxicity.

Nursing diagnoses

- Pain related to the patient's underlying condition.
- High risk for trauma related to GI reactions to phenylbutazone therapy.

Nursing interventions

- *Contraindicated* in patients with hypersensitivity to the drug, other NSAIDs, or aspirin; in children under age 14; and in patients with senility, GI ulcer, blood dyscrasias, or moderate to severe renal, hepatic, cardiac, or thyroid disease.
- *Use cautiously* in patients with mild cardiac, renal, hepatic, or thyroid disease; in GI disorders or a history of peptic ulcer disease; and in patients who may be predisposed to fluid retention.
- Should not be used in patients receiving long-term anticoagulant therapy, hepatotoxic or nephrotoxic drugs, or thrombolytic therapy.
- This drug should be used only if less toxic alternatives are ineffective or contraindicated.
- Warn patient to stop taking drug and notify doctor immediately if fever, sore throat, mouth ulcers, GI discomfort, black or tarry stools, bleeding, bruising, rash, or weight gain occur.
- Give with food, milk, or antacids.
- Complete physical examination and laboratory evaluation are recommended before therapy.
- Monitor hepatic, renal, and thyroid function and CBC before therapy. Check CBC again after 3 days and assess for bleeding.
- Record patient's weight and intake and output daily. May cause sodium retention and edema.
- Response should be seen in 3 to 4 days. Discontinue drug if no response within 1 week.
- This drug has limited use because it produces severe adverse reactions in up to 45% of patients.
- Phenylbutazone may interfere with thyroid function studies by competing for thyroxine binding sites and blocking uptake of iodine into the thyroid.
- May mask signs and symptoms of infection.

General
Classification: anti-inflammatory agent (glucocorticoid). **Pregnancy risk category:** C.

Mechanism of action
Decreases inflammation, mainly by stabilizing leukocyte lysosomal membranes. Also suppresses immune response, stimulates bone marrow, influences protein, fat, and carbohydrate metabolism.

Indications and dosage
- Cerebral edema. **Adults:** initially, 10 mg (sodium phosphate) I.V., then 4 to 6 mg I.M. q 6 hours for 2 to 4 days, then tapered over 5 to 7 days. **Children:** initially, 0.5 to 1.5 mg/kg daily; then 0.2 to 0.5 mg/kg daily in divided doses q 6 hours.
- Inflammatory conditions, allergic reactions, neoplasias. **Adults:** 0.25 to 4 mg P.O. b.i.d., t.i.d., or q.i.d.; or 4 to 16 mg (acetate) I.M. into joint or soft tissue q 1 to 3 weeks; or 0.8 to 1.6 mg (acetate) into lesions q 1 to 3 weeks.
- Shock. **Adults:** 1 to 6 mg/kg (sodium phosphate) I.V. single dosage; or 40 mg I.V. q 2 to 6 hours, p.r.n.
- Dexamethasone suppression test. **Adults:** 0.5 mg P.O. q 6 hours for 48 hours.

Adverse reactions
CNS: *euphoria, insomnia,* psychotic behavior, pseudotumor cerebri. **CV:** ***CHF,*** hypertension, edema. **EENT:** cataracts, glaucoma. **GI:** *peptic ulcer,* GI irritation, increased appetite. **Metabolic:** hypokalemia, hyperglycemia, and carbohydrate intolerance, growth suppression. **Skin:** delayed healing, acne, skin eruptions. **Local:** atrophy at I.M. injection sites. **Other:** weakness, osteoporosis, pancreatitis, hirsutism, susceptibility to infections. Acute adrenal insufficiency may follow increased stress or abrupt withdrawal after chronic therapy. **Withdrawal symptoms:** inflammation, fatigue, arthralgia, fever, dizziness, depression, fainting, orthostatic hypotension, dyspnea, anorexia, hypoglycemia. ***Sudden withdrawal may be fatal.***

Interactions
Barbiturates, phenytoin, rifampin: decreased corticosteroid effect. **Indomethacin, aspirin, NSAIDs:** increased risk of GI distress and bleeding. **Oral anticoagulants:** altered dosage requirements. **Potassium-depleting drugs such as thiazide diuretics:** enhanced potassium-wasting effects of dexamethasone. **Skin-test antigens:** decreased response. **Vaccines and toxoids:** decreased antibody response and increased risk of neurologic complications.

Nursing diagnoses
- Impaired tissue integrity related to the underlying condition.
- High risk for injury related to dexamethasone-induced adverse reactions.

Nursing interventions
- *Contraindicated* in systemic fungal infections and for alternate-day therapy.
- *Use cautiously* in GI ulcers, renal disease, hypertension, osteoporosis, varicella, vaccinia, exanthema, diabetes mellitus, Cushing's syndrome, thromboembolic disorders, seizures, myasthenia gravis, metastatic cancer, CHF, tuberculosis, ocular herpes simplex, hypoalbuminemia, emotional instability, and psychotic tendencies and in children.
- Most adverse reactions dose- or duration-dependent. Always titrate to lowest effective dose.
- Give a daily dose in the morning for less toxicity.
- Teach patient signs of early adrenal insufficiency.
- May mask or exacerbate infections.
- Watch for depression or psychotic episodes.
- Inspect patient's skin for petechiae.
- Monitor growth in infants and children on long-term therapy. Patients receiving long-term therapy should have periodic ophthalmic examinations.
- **I.V. use:** Give direct injection undiluted over at least 1 minute. Dilute solution for infusion and administer as prescribed. For continuous infusion, change solution q 24 hours. Avoid S.C. administration.
- Warn patients on long-term therapy about cushingoid symptoms.

General

Classification: antihypertensive for pheochromocytoma, cutaneous vasodilator (alpha-adrenergic blocker). **Pregnancy risk category:** C.

Mechanism of action

Competitively blocks the effects of catecholamines on alpha-adrenergic receptors.

Indications and dosage

• Diagnostic aid for pheochromocytoma; control or prevention of hypertension before or during pheochromocytomectomy. **Adults:** I.V. diagnostic dose is 5 mg, with close monitoring of blood pressure. Before surgical removal of tumor, give 2 to 5 mg I.M. or I.V. During surgery, patient may need small I.V. doses (1 mg) or small I.M. doses (3 mg). **Children:** I.V. diagnostic dose is 0.1 mg/kg or 3 mg/m^2 as single dose, with close monitoring of blood pressure. Before surgical removal of tumor, give 1 mg I.V. or 3 mg I.M. During surgery, patient may need small I.V. doses (1 mg).

• Treatment of extravasation. **Adults and children:** infiltrate area with 5 to 10 mg phentolamine in 10 ml 0.9% sodium chloride solution or give half the dosage through the infiltrated I.V. and the other half around the site. Must be done within 12 hours.

Adverse reactions

CNS: *dizziness, weakness, flushing.* **CV:** *hypotension,* shock, *arrhythmias,* palpitations, *tachycardia,* angina pectoris. **GI:** *diarrhea,* abdominal pain, *nausea, vomiting,* hyperperistalsis. **Other:** *nasal stuffiness,* hypoglycemia.

Interactions

Epinephrine: excessive hypotension. Don't use together.

Nursing diagnoses

• Altered tissue perfusion (renal, cerebral, cardiopulmonary, peripheral) related to the patient's underlying condition.

• High risk for injury related to adverse reactions to phentolamine.

• Knowledge deficit related to phentolamine therapy.

Nursing interventions

• *Contraindicated* in patients with angina, coronary artery disease, or a history of MI.

• *Use cautiously* in patients with gastritis or peptic ulcer and in patients receiving other antihypertensives.

• Don't administer epinephrine to treat phentolamine-induced hypotension. May cause additional fall in blood pressure ("epinephrine reversal"). Use norepinephrine instead.

• When this drug is given as a diagnostic test for pheochromocytoma, check the patient's blood pressure first. Then check blood pressure frequently during administration.

• Test is positive for pheochromocytoma if I.V. test dose causes severe hypotension.

• Don't give sedatives or narcotics 24 hours before diagnostic test. Rauwolfia alkaloids should be withdrawn at least 4 weeks before such testing.

• Phentolamine has been used experimentally, alone or with papaverine, to treat impotence. Patients are taught to give themselves this drug by intercavernosal injection.

dexchlorpheniramine maleate

Dexchlor, Poladex TD, Polaramine*, Polaramine Repetabs

General

Classification: antihistamine (H_1-receptor antagonist), antipruritic (propylamine derivative). **Pregnancy risk category:** B.

Mechanism of action

Competes with histamine for H_1-receptor sites on effector cells. Prevents but does not reverse histamine-mediated responses.

Indications and dosage

- Rhinitis, allergy symptoms, contact dermatitis, pruritus. **Adults:** 2 mg P.O. q 4 to 6 hours, not to exceed 12 mg/day; or (timed-release tablet) 4 to 6 mg b.i.d. or t.i.d. **Children 6 to 12 years:** 1 mg P.O. q 4 to 6 hours, not to exceed 6 mg/day; or 4 mg (timed-release tablet) h.s. **Children 2 to 6 years:** 0.5 mg P.O. q 4 to 6 hours, not to exceed 3 mg/day.

Note: Children under 6 years should use only as directed by a doctor. Do not use timed-release tablets for children under 6 years.

Adverse reactions

CNS: (especially in elderly patients) *drowsiness,* dizziness, *stimulation.* **GI:** nausea, *dry mouth.* **GU:** polyuria, dysuria, urine retention.

Interactions

CNS depressants: increased sedation. Use together cautiously. **MAO inhibitors:** increased anticholinergic effects. Don't use together.

Nursing diagnoses

- Ineffective airway clearance related to the patient's underlying condition.
- High risk for injury related to dexchlorpheniramine-induced adverse CNS reactions.
- Knowledge deficit related to dexchlorpheniramine therapy.

Nursing interventions

- *Contraindicated* in acute asthmatic attacks.
- *Use cautiously* in elderly patients and in increased intraocular pressure, hyperthyroidism, CV or renal disease, hypertension, bronchial asthma, urine retention, prostatic hypertrophy, bladder-neck obstruction, and stenosing peptic ulcers.
- Warn patient against drinking alcoholic beverages during therapy and against driving or other activities that require alertness until CNS response to drug is determined.
- Coffee or tea may reduce drowsiness. Sugarless gum, sour hard candy, or ice chips may relieve dry mouth.
- If tolerance develops, another antihistamine may be substituted.
- Warn patient to stop taking drug 4 days before allergy skin tests to preserve accuracy of tests.
- Antihistamines are not recommended for use by women who are breast-feeding because small amounts of drug are excreted in breast milk.

General

Classification: anticonvulsant (succinimide derivative). **Pregnancy risk category:** D.

Mechanism of action

Increases seizure threshold. Reduces the paroxysmal spike-and-wave pattern of absence seizures by depressing nerve transmission in the motor cortex.

Indications and dosage

- Absence seizures. **Adults and children:** 500 mg to 1 g P.O. b.i.d. to t.i.d.

Adverse reactions

Blood: transient leukopenia, ***pancytopenia, agranulocytosis.*** **CNS:** muscular weakness, *drowsiness,* dizziness, ataxia, headache. **GI:** nausea, vomiting, anorexia. **GU:** urinary frequency, renal damage, hematuria. **Skin:** pruritus, eruptions, erythema. **Other:** lupus-like syndrome.

Interactions

None significant.

Nursing diagnoses

- High risk for injury related to the patient's underlying seizure disorder.
- Altered protection related to drug-induced bleeding.
- Knowledge deficit related to phensuximide therapy.

Nursing interventions

- *Contraindicated* in hypersensitivity to succinimide derivatives.
- *Use cautiously* in patients with hepatic or renal disease.
- Never withdraw the drug suddenly. Abrupt withdrawal may precipitate absence seizures. Call the doctor immediately if the patient develops adverse reactions.
- Warn the patient to avoid hazardous activities that require alertness and good coordination until CNS effects of the drug are known.
- Obtain CBC every 3 to 4 months; urinalysis and liver function tests every 6 months.
- Tell the patient to report lupus-like symptoms immediately.
- Tell him that the drug may turn his urine pink or red to reddish brown.
- Therapeutic blood level of phensuximide is 40 to 80 mcg/ml.
- Phensuximide may increase the incidence of generalized tonic-clonic seizures if it's used alone to treat patients with mixed seizure types.

General

Classification: nonnarcotic antitussive (levorphanol derivative). **Pregnancy risk category:** C.

Mechanism of action

Suppresses the cough reflex by direct action on the cough center in the medulla (brain).

Indications and dosage

- Nonproductive cough. **Adults:** 10 to 20 mg P.O. q 4 hours, or 30 mg q 6 to 8 hours. Or the controlled-release liquid 60 mg b.i.d. Maximum 120 mg daily. **Children 6 to 12 years:** 5 to 10 mg P.O. q 4 hours, or 15 mg q 6 to 8 hours. Or the controlled-release liquid 30 mg b.i.d. Maximum 60 mg daily. **Children 2 to 6 years:** 2.5 to 5 mg P.O. q 4 hours, or 7.5 mg q 6 to 8 hours. Maximum 30 mg daily.

Adverse reactions

CNS: drowsiness, dizziness. **GI:** nausea, vomiting, stomach pain.

Interactions

MAO inhibitors: hypotension, coma, hyperpyrexia, and death have occurred. Do not use together.

Nursing diagnoses

- Ineffective airway clearance related to the patient's underlying condition producing cough.
- High risk for injury related to dextromethorphan-induced CNS reactions.
- Knowledge deficit related to dextromethorphan therapy.

Nursing interventions

- *Contraindicated* in patients currently taking or within 2 weeks of discontinuing MAO inhibitors.
- Produces no analgesia or addiction and little or no CNS depression.
- An antitussive; don't use when cough is valuable diagnostic sign or beneficial (as after thoracic surgery).
- Use with percussion and chest vibration.
- Monitor cough type and frequency.
- Dose of 15 to 30 mg dextromethorphan is equivalent to 8 to 15 mg codeine as an antitussive.

phenoxybenzamine hydrochloride
Dibenzyline

General
Classification: antihypertensive for pheochromocytoma, cutaneous vasodilator (alpha-adrenergic blocking agent). **Pregnancy risk category:** C.

Mechanism of action
Noncompetitively blocks the effect of catecholamines on alpha-adrenergic receptors.

Indications and dosage
• Hypertension and sweating caused by pheochromocytoma; may be used with propranolol to control excessive tachycardia. **Adults:** initially, 10 mg P.O. daily. Increase daily dosage by 10 mg q 4 days. Maintenance dosage is 20 to 60 mg daily. **Children:** initially, 0.2 mg/kg or 6 mg/m² P.O. daily in a single dose. Maintenance dosage is 12 to 36 mg/m² daily as a single dose or in divided doses.
• Raynaud's disease, frostbite, acrocyanosis. **Adults:** initially, 10 mg P.O., then increase by 10 mg q 4 days to a maximum of 60 mg daily.

Adverse reactions
CNS: lethargy, drowsiness. **CV:** *orthostatic hypotension, tachycardia,* shock. **EENT:** *nasal stuffiness, miosis.* **GI:** *dry mouth,* vomiting, abdominal distress. **Other:** *impotence, inhibition of ejaculation.*

Interactions
Antihypertensives: excessive hypotension. Use together cautiously.

Nursing diagnoses
• Altered tissue perfusion (renal, cerebral, cardiopulmonary, peripheral) related to the patient's underlying condition.
• High risk for injury related to phenoxybenzamine-induced orthostatic hypotension and adverse CNS reactions to the drug.
• Knowledge deficit related to phenoxybenzamine therapy.

Nursing interventions
• *Use cautiously* in cerebrovascular or coronary insufficiency, advanced renal disease, or respiratory disease.
• Watch patient closely for adverse reactions, and call the doctor promptly if they occur. If severe hypotension develops, the patient may require norepinephrine to counteract effect.
• Nasal congestion, inhibition of ejaculation, and impotence usually decrease with continued therapy.
• Monitor the patient's heart rate and blood pressure frequently.
• Patient with tachycardia may require concurrent propranolol therapy.
• This drug may take several weeks to achieve optimal effect.
• Monitor respiratory status carefully. This drug may aggravate symptoms of pneumonia and asthma.
• Teach the patient about his disease and therapy. Explain the importance of taking this drug as prescribed, even when he's feeling well. Tell outpatient not to discontinue the drug suddenly, but to call the doctor if adverse reactions occur.
• Instruct the patient to check with the doctor or pharmacist before taking OTC medications.
• Inform the patient that orthostatic hypotension can be minimized by rising slowly and avoiding sudden position changes.
• Dry mouth can be relieved with sugarless chewing gum, sour hard candy, or ice chips. GI distress can be relieved by taking the drug in divided doses or with milk.
• Used investigationally to treat chronic urine retention.
• Small initial doses are increased gradually until desired effect is obtained. Don't increase dosage more frequently than every 4 days.

dextrothyroxine sodium

Choloxin**

General

Classification: antilipemic (thyroid hormone). **Pregnancy risk category:** C.

Mechanism of action

Accelerates hepatic catabolism of cholesterol and increases bile secretion to lower cholesterol levels.

Indications and dosage

• Hyperlipidemia in euthyroid patients, especially when cholesterol and triglyceride levels are elevated. **Adults:** initial dose 1 to 2 mg P.O. daily, increased by 1 to 2 mg daily at monthly intervals to a total of 4 to 8 mg daily. **Children:** initial dose 0.05 mg/kg P.O. daily, increased by 0.05 mg/kg daily at monthly intervals to a maximum of 4 mg daily. Alternatively, give 1.5 mg/m^2 daily, increased by 1.5 mg/m^2 daily at monthly intervals. Maximum daily dose is 4 mg. The usual maintenance dose is 0.1 mg/kg or 3 mg/m^2 daily in euthyroid children.

Adverse reactions

CV: palpitations, angina pectoris, ***arrhythmias,*** ischemic myocardial changes on ECG, ***MI.*** **EENT:** visual disturbances, ptosis. **GI:** nausea, vomiting, diarrhea, constipation, decreased appetite. **Metabolic:** *insomnia, weight loss, sweating,* flushing, hyperthermia. **Other:** hair loss, menstrual irregularities.

Interactions

Digitalis glycosides: dextrothyroxine may enhance clinical effect. Use together cautiously. **Oral anticoagulants:** dextrothyroxine may potentiate the anticoagulant effect of warfarin or dicumarol. **Sympathomimetics:** dextrothyroxine may precipitate arrhythmias or coronary insufficiency in patients with cardiac disease.

Nursing diagnoses

• High risk for injury related to the patient's elevated blood lipid and cholesterol levels.
• Constipation related to adverse drug reaction.
• Knowledge deficit related to dextrothyroxine therapy.

Nursing interventions

• *Contraindicated* in hepatic or renal disease or iodism. Patients with history of cardiac disease, including arrhythmias, hypertension, or angina pectoris, should receive very small doses.
• May increase need for insulin, diet therapy, or oral antidiabetic agents in patients with diabetes.
• If the use of anticoagulants is being considered, discontinue drug 2 weeks before surgery to avoid possible potentiation of anticoagulant effect.
• Observe patient for signs of hyperthyroidism, such as nervousness, insomnia, and weight loss. If these occur, dosage should be decreased or drug discontinued.
• Teach patient about proper dietary management (restricting total fat and cholesterol intake), weight control, and exercise. Explain their importance in controlling elevated serum lipids.

General

Classification: stimulant laxative (anthraquinone derivative). **Pregnancy risk category:** C.

Mechanism of action

Increases peristalsis by direct effect on the smooth muscle of the intestine. Thought either to irritate the musculature or to stimulate the colonic intramural plexus. Also promotes fluid accumulation in the colon and small intestine.

Indications and dosage

- Constipation. **Adults and children over 12 years:** 30 to 270 mg P.O., preferably h.s. **Children 6 to 12 years:** 30 to 60 mg P.O. h.s. **Children 2 to 5 years:** 15 to 30 mg P.O. h.s.

Adverse reactions

GI: diarrhea; *colic in large doses;* factitious nausea; vomiting; loss of normal bowel function in excessive use; *abdominal cramps,* especially in severe constipation; malabsorption of nutrients; "cathartic colon" (syndrome resembling ulcerative colitis radiologically and pathologically) in chronic misuse; reddish discoloration in alkaline feces or urine. **Skin:** dermatitis, pruritus, rash, pigmentation. **Other:** laxative dependence in long-term or excessive use, ***hypersensitivity.***

Interactions

None significant.

Nursing diagnoses

- Constipation related to interruption of normal pattern of elimination characterized by infrequent or absent stools.
- Pain related to phenolphthalein-induced abdominal cramping.
- Knowledge deficit related to phenolphthalein therapy.

Nursing interventions

- *Contraindicated* in abdominal pain, nausea, vomiting, or other symptoms of appendicitis or acute surgical abdomen; fecal impaction; or intestinal obstruction or perforation.
- *Use cautiously* in rectal bleeding.
- Laxative effect may last up to 3 to 4 days.
- Produces semisolid stool within 8 hours. Time administration so that the drug doesn't interfere with scheduled activities or sleep.
- Warn the patient with a rash to avoid sunlight and discontinue use of the drug. Also warn him not to use any other product containing phenolphthalein.
- Before giving drug, determine if the patient has adequate fluid intake, exercise, and diet. Tell him that dietary sources of bulk include bran and other cereals, fresh fruit, and vegetables.
- Drug may turn alkaline urine red-pink and acidic urine yellow-brown.
- Drug is available in many dosage forms. Most popular OTC laxative.
- Children may mistake the drug for candy. Keep it out of their reach.
- Yellow phenolphthalein is reported to be two to three times as potent as white phenolphthalein, but this has not been proven in clinical studies.

General

Classification: analgesic (opiate agonist-antagonist). **Pregnancy risk category:** C.

Mechanism of action

Produces postoperative analgesia qualitatively similar to morphine.

Indications and dosage

• Management of moderate to severe pain. **Adults:** 5 to 20 mg I.M. q 3 to 6 hours or 2.5 to 10 mg I.V. q 2 to 4 hours. Maximum recommended single I.M. dose is 20 mg, with maximum daily dosage 120 mg. Maximum dosage for I.V. use not determined. **Dosage in renal and hepatic failure:** Limited studies suggest that drug should be used with caution and in lower doses. The half-life increases hepatic failure. Primary means of drug elimination is renal excretion of metabolite.

Adverse reactions

Blood: low hemoglobin. **CNS:** *sedation, dizziness, vertigo,* anxiety, mood disorders, sleep disturbances, headache, slurred speech. **CV:** edema, hypotension, irregular heartbeat, hypertension, chest pain. **GI:** *nausea, vomiting,* dry mouth, constipation, diarrhea, abdominal distress. **Skin:** rash, pruritus, *local irritation at injection site.* **Other:** sweating, chills, flushing, pallor, thrombophlebitis.

Interactions

Alcohol or other CNS depressants: may increase the risk of CNS depression. **Opiates:** patients receiving chronic opioid therapy (opioid-dependent patients) may experience withdrawal symptoms after receiving dezocine. May increase the risk of CNS depression.

Nursing diagnoses

• Pain related to patient's underlying condition.
• Ineffective breathing pattern related to dezocine-induced respiratory depression.
• Knowledge deficit related to dezocine therapy.

Nursing interventions

• *Contraindicated* in hypersensitivity to drug.
• *Use with extreme caution* in patients with head injury because drug's CNS depressant effects may obscure clinical signs. Related drugs have caused elevations of CSF pressure in head injury patients.
• *Use cautiously* and in lower doses in patients with chronic respiratory disease and in patients undergoing biliary surgery. Related drugs have caused significant increases in pressure within the common bile duct.
• Like other potent analgesics, dezocine should be administered with caution to elderly patients.
• Drug produces a dose-dependent respiratory depression similar to that of morphine, usually peaking within 15 minutes of administration. Use only in clinical settings where adequate respiratory support and opiate antagonist (naloxone) are available to reverse respiratory depressant effects.
• Use not recommended for patients with chronic pain because of limited experience and because drug can precipitate an abstinence syndrome in patients with substantial tolerance to opiates.
• **I.V. use:** When giving by direct injection, infuse over at least 5 minutes. Note that the injection contains sulfite preservatives, which may cause allergic reactions in certain sensitive patients.
• Plasma concentrations higher than 45 ng/ml are associated with an increased incidence of adverse reactions.
• Warn patient to avoid driving and other hazardous activities that require alertness until adverse CNS effects of the drug are known. Advise patient to move about cautiously because drug may cause dizziness.
• Although currently not a controlled substance, dezocine will replace morphine in animal drug-dependence studies. However, tolerance or physical dependence has not been reported in humans. Nevertheless, in patients with a history of opiate use or dependence, abuse of this drug is a potential risk.
• Because it is not known if dezocine is excreted in breast milk, breast-feeding is not recommended during therapy.

General

Classification: anticonvulsant, sedative-hypnotic (barbiturate). **Pregnancy risk category:** D. **Controlled substance schedule:** IV.

Mechanism of action

Depresses monosynaptic and polysynaptic transmission in the CNS and increases the threshold for seizure activity in the motor cortex. As a sedative, probably interferes with transmission of impulses from the thalamus to the cortex of the brain.

Indications and dosage

- All forms of seizure disorder, febrile seizures in children. **Adults:** 100 to 200 mg P.O. daily, divided t.i.d. or given as single dosage h.s. **Children:** 4 to 6 mg/kg P.O. daily, usually divided q 12 hours. May be administered once daily, usually h.s.
- Status epilepticus. **Adults:** 10 mg/kg as I.V. infusion (sodium) no faster than 50 mg/minute. May give up to 20 mg/kg total. Administer in acute care or emergency area only. **Children:** 5 to 10 mg/kg I.V. May repeat q 10 to 15 minutes up to total of 20 mg/kg. I.V. injection rate should not exceed 50 mg/minute.
- Sedation. **Adults:** 30 to 120 mg P.O. daily in two or three divided doses. **Children:** 6 mg/kg P.O. divided t.i.d.

- Insomnia. **Adults:** 100 to 320 mg P.O. or I.M. **Children:** 3 to 6 mg/kg.
- Preoperative sedation. **Adults:** 100 to 200 mg I.M. 60 to 90 minutes before surgery. **Children:** 16 to 100 mg I.M. 60 to 90 minutes before surgery.
- Hyperbilirubinemia. **Neonates:** 7 mg/kg daily P.O. from first to fifth day of life; or 5 mg/kg daily I.M. on first day, repeated P.O. on second to seventh days.
- Chronic cholestasis. **Adults and children 12 years and older:** 90 to 180 mg P.O. daily in two or three divided doses. **Children under 12 years:** 3 to 12 mg/kg daily P.O. in two or three divided doses.

Adverse reactions

CNS: *drowsiness, lethargy, hangover,* paradoxical excitement in elderly patients. **GI:** nausea, vomiting. **Skin:** rash, ***Stevens-Johnson syndrome,*** urticaria. **Local:** pain, swelling, thrombophlebitis, necrosis, nerve injury. **Other:** ***angioedema.***

Interactions

Alcohol and other CNS depressants, including narcotic analgesics: excessive CNS depression. Use cautiously. **Diazepam:** increased effects of both drugs. Use together cautiously. **Griseofulvin:** decreased absorption of griseofulvin. **MAO inhibitors:** potentiated barbiturate effect. Monitor for increased CNS and respiratory depression. **Oral anticoagulants, estrogens and oral contraceptives, doxycycline, corticosteroids:** may enhance the metabolism of these drugs. Monitor for decreased effect. **Primidone:** monitor for excessive phenobarbital blood levels. **Rifampin:** may decrease barbiturate levels. **Valproic acid:** increased phenobarbital levels. Monitor for toxicity.

Nursing diagnoses

- High risk for trauma related to patient's underlying seizure disorder.
- Noncompliance related to need for long-term use of phenobarbital therapy.
- Knowledge deficit related to phenobarbital.

Nursing interventions

- *Contraindicated* in barbiturate hypersensitivity, porphyria, hepatic dysfunction, respiratory disease with dyspnea or obstruction, and nephritis and in breast-feeding women.
- *Use cautiously* in hyperthyroidism, diabetes mellitus, anemia and in elderly or debilitated patients.
- **I.V. use:** Reserve for emergency treatment and give slowly under close supervision.
- Give I.M. injection deeply. Superficial injection may cause pain, sterile abscess, tissue sloughing.
- Do not use injectable or parenteral forms if they contain precipitates.
- Watch for signs of barbiturate toxicity.
- Don't stop drug abruptly.
- Full therapeutic effects not seen for 2 to 3 weeks, except when loading dose is used.
- Therapeutic blood levels are 15 to 40 mcg/ml.

General

Classification: antianxiety agent (benzodiazepine). **Pregnancy risk category:** D. **Controlled substance schedule:** IV.

Mechanism of action

Depresses CNS at limbic and subcortical levels of brain. As anticonvulsant, suppresses spread of seizure activity produced by epileptogenic foci in cortex, thalamus, and limbic structures.

Indications and dosage

- Tension, anxiety, adjunct in seizure disorders or skeletal muscle spasm. **Adults:** 2 to 10 mg P.O. t.i.d. or q.i.d. Or, 15 to 30 mg extended-release capsule once daily. **Children over 6 months:** 1 to 2.5 mg P.O. t.i.d. or q.i.d.
- Endoscopic procedures, seizures. **Adults:** 5 to 10 mg I.V. initially, up to 30 mg in 1 hour or possibly more for cardioversion or status epilepticus, depending on response. **Children 5 years and older:** 1 mg I.V. or I.M. slowly q 2 to 5 minutes to maximum of 10 mg. Repeat q 2 to 4 hours. **Children 30 days to 5 years:** 0.2 to 0.5 mg I.V. or I.M. slowly q 2 to 5 minutes to maximum of 5 mg. Repeat q 2 to 4 hours.

Adverse reactions

CNS: *drowsiness, lethargy, hangover, ataxia,* fainting, slurred speech, tremor. **CV:** transient hypotension, bradycardia, ***cardiovascular collapse.*** **EENT:** diplopia, blurred vision, nystagmus. **GI:** nausea, vomiting, abdominal discomfort. **Skin:** rash, urticaria. **Local:** desquamation, *pain, phlebitis at injection site.* **Other:** respiratory depression.

Interactions

Alcohol, other CNS depressants: increased CNS depression. Avoid concomitant use. **Cigarette smoking:** increased clearance of benzodiazepines. Monitor for lack of effect. **Cimetidine:** increased sedation. Monitor carefully. **Digoxin:** benzodiazepines may increase serum levels of digoxin, increasing risk of toxicity. Monitor closely. **Phenobarbital:** increased effects of both drugs. Use together cautiously.

Nursing diagnoses

- Anxiety related to the patient's underlying condition.
- Altered cardiopulmonary tissue perfusion related to adverse drug reactions.
- Knowledge deficit related to diazepam therapy.

Nursing interventions

- *Contraindicated* in shock, coma, acute alcohol intoxication, acute narrow-angle glaucoma, psychoses, myasthenia gravis; in oral form for children under 6 months.
- *Use cautiously* in blood dyscrasia, hepatic or renal damage, depression, open-angle glaucoma; in elderly and debilitated patients; and in those with limited pulmonary reserve.
- Don't withdraw drug abruptly after long-term use; withdrawal symptoms may occur.
- Warn patient to avoid activities that require alertness and good psychomotor coordination until CNS effects of the drug are known.
- Warn patient not to combine drug with alcohol or other depressants.
- **I.V. use:** Give I.V. slowly, at rate not exceeding 5 mg/minute. When injecting I.V., best to administer directly into the vein. If this is not possible, inject slowly through the infusion tubing as close as possible to the vein insertion site. Watch daily for phlebitis at injection site. Do not mix injectable form with other drugs.
- Avoid extravasation. Don't inject into small veins.
- Monitor respirations every 5 to 15 minutes and before each repeated I.V. dose. Have emergency resuscitation equipment and oxygen at bedside.
- If diazepam overdose occurs, flumazenil (a specific benzodiazepine antagonist) may be useful. Know that the duration of action of diazepam is longer than that of flumazenil, and resedation is possible.

General

Classification: antidepressant (MAO inhibitor).
Pregnancy risk category: C.

Mechanism of action

Promotes accumulation of neurotransmitters by inhibiting MAO.

Indications and dosage

- Depression. **Adults:** 45 mg P.O. daily in divided doses, increasing rapidly to 60 mg daily. Then dosage can usually be reduced to 15 mg daily. Maximum is 90 mg daily.

Adverse reactions

CNS: *dizziness*, vertigo, headache, overactivity, hyperreflexia, tremor, muscle twitching, mania, jitters, *insomnia*, confusion, memory impairment, drowsiness, weakness, fatigue. **CV:** paradoxical hypertension, *orthostatic hypotension*, ***arrhythmias***. **GI:** dry mouth, *anorexia*, nausea, constipation. **Other:** peripheral edema, ***suicidal ideation***, sweating, weight changes.

Interactions

Alcohol, barbiturates, other sedatives; narcotics; dextromethorphan; TCAs: unpredictable interaction. Use with caution and in reduced dosage. **Amphetamines, antihistamines, ephedrine, levodopa, meperidine, metaraminol, methotrimeprazine, methylphenidate, phenylephrine, phenylpropanolamine, sympathomimetics:** enhanced pressor effects. Avoid concomitant use. **Insulin, oral antidiabetics:** altered requirements for antidiabetic drugs. **Spinal anesthetics:** increased risk of hypotension.

Nursing diagnoses

- Ineffective individual coping related to the patient's underlying condition.
- High risk for injury related to adverse CNS and CV reactions to phenelzine.
- Knowledge deficit related to phenelzine therapy.

Nursing interventions

- *Contraindicated* in elderly or debilitated patients; in hepatic impairment, CHF, pheochromocytoma, hypertension, CV or cerebrovascular disease, or severe or frequent headaches; with foods containing tryptophan or tyramine; during therapy with other MAO inhibitors or within 10 days of such therapy; within 10 days of elective surgery requiring general anesthetic, cocaine, or local anesthetic containing sympathomimetic vasoconstrictors; and in hyperactive, agitated, or schizophrenic patients.
- *Use cautiously* in patients at risk for suicide or with diabetes, seizure disorders, or Parkinson's disease.
- Because MAO inhibitors may alleviate anginal pain, warn patient to limit activities to avoid overexertion.
- If patient has symptoms of overdose (severe hypotension, palpitations, or frequent headaches), hold dose and notify doctor.
- Dosage is usually reduced to maintenance level as soon as possible.
- Keep drug in tight container, away from heat and light.
- Have phentolamine (Regitine) available to combat severe hypertension.
- Warn patient to avoid foods high in trytophan or tyramine and large amounts of caffeine.
- Warn patient not to take any drugs without checking with doctor. Severe effects can occur if MAO inhibitors are taken with cold, hay fever, or diet preparations.
- Monitor blood pressure and heart rate. Incidence of orthostatic hypotension is high. Monitor walking. Have patient rise from bed slowly and sit up for 1 minute.
- Continue precautions 10 days after stopping drug because of long-lasting effects.
- Expect delay of 2 weeks or more before noticeable effect; 4 weeks or more before full effect.
- Obtain blood pressure, CBC, and liver function tests before therapy, and monitor throughout treatment.
- In most patients, stop MAO inhibitors 14 days before elective surgery to avoid interactions during anesthesia.

General
Classification: antihypertensive (peripheral vasodilator). **Pregnancy risk category:** C.

Mechanism of action
Directly relaxes arteriolar smooth muscle.

Indications and dosage
- Hypertensive crisis. **Adults and children:** 1 to 3 mg/kg I.V. bolus (up to a maximum of 150 mg) q 5 to 15 minutes until adequate response is seen. Repeat at intervals q 4 to 24 hours p.r.n.

Adverse reactions
CNS: *headache,* dizziness, light-headedness, euphoria. **CV:** *sodium and water retention, orthostatic hypotension,* sweating, flushing, warmth, angina, myocardial ischemia, arrhythmias, ECG changes. **GI:** *nausea, vomiting,* abdominal discomfort. **Local:** inflammation and pain from extravasation. **Metabolic:** *hyperglycemia,* hyperuricemia.

Interactions
Hydralazine: may cause severe hypotension. Use together cautiously. **Thiazide diuretics:** may increase the effects of diazoxide. Use together cautiously.

Nursing diagnoses
- Altered tissue perfusion (renal, cerebral, cardiopulmonary, peripheral) related to the patient's underlying condition.
- Fluid volume excess related to diazoxide-induced adverse reactions.
- Knowledge deficit related to diazoxide therapy.

Nursing interventions
- *Use cautiously* in patients with impaired cerebral or cardiac function, diabetes, or uremia and in those taking other antihypertensives.
- **I.V. use:** Monitor blood pressure and ECG continuously. Patient should be supine or in Trendelenburg's position during and for 1 hour after infusion. Notify doctor immediately if severe hypotension develops. Keep norepinephrine available.
- Monitor patient's intake and output carefully. If fluid or sodium retention develops, doctor may want to order diuretics.
- Check patient's standing blood pressure before discontinuing close monitoring for hypotension.
- Take care to avoid extravasation.
- This drug may alter requirements for insulin, diet, or oral antidiabetic agents in previously controlled diabetic patients. Monitor blood glucose daily.
- Weigh patient daily. Notify doctor of any weight increase.
- Watch diabetic patients closely for signs of severe hyperglycemia or hyperosmolar nonketotic syndrome. Insulin may be needed.
- Check patient's uric acid levels frequently. Report abnormalities to doctor.
- Inform patient that orthostatic hypotension can be minimized by rising slowly and avoiding sudden position changes. Instruct patient to remain supine for 30 minutes after injection.
- Infusion of diazoxide has been shown to be as effective as a bolus in some patients.
- Protect I.V. solutions from light. Darkened I.V. solutions of diazoxide are subpotent and should not be used.

phenazopyridine hydrochloride

Azo-Standard◇, Baridium◇, Eridium◇, Geridium◇, Pyridium, Urodine◇, Urogesic◇

General

Classification: urinary analgesic (azo dye). **Pregnancy risk category:** B.

Mechanism of action

Exerts a local anesthetic action on the urinary tract mucosa through an unknown mechanism.

Indications and dosage

- Pain with urinary tract irritation or infection. **Adults:** 100 to 200 mg P.O. t.i.d. **Children:** 100 mg P.O. t.i.d.

Adverse reactions

CNS: headache, vertigo. **GI:** nausea. **Skin:** rash.

Interactions

None significant.

Nursing diagnoses

- Pain related to the patient's underlying condition.
- High risk for injury related to phenazopyridine-induced vertigo.
- Knowledge deficit related to phenazopyridine therapy.

Nursing interventions

- *Contraindicated* in patients with renal or hepatic insufficiency.
- Tell the patient that the drug may turn his urine red or orange. Inform him that it may stain fabrics.
- Advise taking the drug with meals to help minimize GI distress.
- Institute safety measures, such as supervising the patient's activities and keeping the bed's side rails raised, if he experiences vertigo.
- Warn the patient to avoid activities that require alertness and psychomotor coordination if he develops vertigo.
- Collect samples for urinalysis and urine culture and sensitivity tests to detect infection.
- Use phenazopyridine only as an analgesic. Use with antibiotic to treat urinary tract infection.
- Inform the patient that the drug may be stopped in 3 days if pain is relieved.
- Drug may alter Clinistix or Tes-Tape results. Substitute Clinitest for accurate urine glucose test results.
- Stop the drug if skin or sclera becomes yellow-tinged. This effect may indicate drug accumulation caused by impaired renal excretion.
- Most forms of the drug are available without a prescription.

General
Classification: analgesic, antiarthritic (NSAID).
Pregnancy risk category: B.

Mechanism of action
Produces anti-inflammatory, analgesic, and antipyretic effects, possibly through inhibition of prostaglandin synthesis.

Indications and dosage
- Ankylosing spondylitis. **Adults:** 25 mg P.O. q.i.d. and h.s.
- Osteoarthritis. **Adults:** 50 mg P.O. b.i.d. or t.i.d., or 75 mg b.i.d.
- Rheumatoid arthritis. **Adults:** 75 to 100 mg P.O. b.i.d., or 50 to 100 mg P.R. h.s. as substitute for last oral dose of the day. Don't exceed 200 mg daily.

Adverse reactions
CNS: anxiety, depression, drowsiness, insomnia, irritability, *headache*. **CV:** ***CHF***, hypertension. **EENT:** *tinnitus*, laryngeal edema, swelling of the lips and tongue. **GI:** *abdominal pain or cramps, constipation, diarrhea, indigestion, nausea,* abdominal distention, flatulence, peptic ulceration, ***GI bleeding,*** melena, bloody diarrhea, appetite change, colitis. **GU:** azotemia, proteinuria, acute renal failure, oliguria, interstitial nephritis, papillary necrosis, ***nephrotic syndrome,*** *fluid retention.* **Hepatic:** elevated hepatic enzymes, jaundice, hepatitis, ***hepatotoxicity.*** **Respiratory:** asthma. **Skin:** rash, pruritus, urticaria, eczema, dermatitis, alopecia, photosensitivity, bullous eruption, ***Stevens-Johnson syndrome (rare),*** allergic purpura. **Other:** ***anaphylaxis,*** angioedema.

Interactions
Anticoagulants (including warfarin): possible increased incidence of bleeding. Monitor patient. **Aspirin:** avoid concomitant use. **Cyclosporine, digoxin, lithium, methotrexate:** diclofenac may reduce renal clearance of these drugs and increase risk of toxicity. Monitor patient. **Diuretics:** diclofenac may decrease effectiveness of diuretics. **Insulin, oral antidiabetic agents:** diclofenac may alter requirements for antidiabetic agents. Monitor patient. **Potassium-sparing diuretics:** diclofenac may enhance potassium retention and increase serum potassium levels.

Nursing diagnoses
- Pain related to the patient's underlying condition.
- Constipation related to diclofenac-induced GI reactions.
- Knowledge deficit related to diclofenac therapy.

Nursing interventions
- *Contraindicated* in patients with hypersensitivity to diclofenac, aspirin, or other NSAIDs and in those with history of asthma, urticaria, or other allergic reactions to these drugs. Not recommended for use during pregnancy or breast-feeding.
- *Use cautiously* in patients with a history of peptic ulcer disease, hepatic dysfunction, cardiac disease, or other conditions associated with fluid retention or impaired renal function.
- Elevations of liver enzymes may occur during therapy. Measure serum transaminase, especially ALT (SGPT), periodically in patients undergoing longterm therapy. The first serum transaminase measurement should be made no later than 8 weeks after initiation of therapy.
- Tell patient to take diclofenac with milk or meals to minimize GI distress.
- Peptic ulceration and GI bleeding have occurred in patients taking NSAIDs despite the absence of GI symptoms. Teach patient the signs and symptoms of GI bleeding, and tell him to contact the doctor promptly if these symptoms appear.
- Teach patient the signs and symptoms of hepatotoxicity, including nausea, fatigue, lethargy, pruritus, jaundice, right upper quadrant tenderness, and flulike symptoms. Tell him to contact doctor immediately if these symptoms appear.
- Tablets are enteric-coated. Don't crush, break, or chew them.
- Because of their antipyretic and anti-inflammatory actions, NSAIDs may mask the signs and symptoms of infection.

General

Classification: anticonvulsant (hydantoin derivative). **Pregnancy risk category:** D.

Mechanism of action

Stabilizes neuronal membranes and limits seizure activity by either increasing efflux or decreasing influx of sodium ions across cell membranes in the motor cortex during generation of nerve impulses.

Indications and dosage

• Refractory, complex-partial, generalized tonic-clonic, absence, and atypical absence seizures. **Adults:** 500 mg P.O. t.i.d. May increase by 500 mg weekly up to 5 g daily, p.r.n. **Children 5 to 10 years:** 250 mg P.O. t.i.d. May increase by 250 mg weekly, up to 1.5 g daily, p.r.n.

Adverse reactions

Blood: *aplastic anemia, agranulocytosis,* leukopenia. **CNS:** drowsiness, dizziness, insomnia, headaches, paresthesia, *depression, suicidal tendencies,* aggressiveness. **GI:** anorexia, weight loss. **GU:** nephritis with marked albuminuria. **Hepatic:** hepatitis, jaundice. **Skin:** rashes.

Interactions

Ethotoin: paranoia. Use together cautiously. **Other anticonvulsants:** enhanced risk of toxicity.

Nursing diagnoses

• High risk for injury related to patient's underlying seizure activity.
• Knowledge deficit related to phenacemide therapy.

Nursing interventions

• *Contraindicated* in patients with preexisting personality disturbances and in patients who gain satisfactory control of seizures with other anticonvulsants.
• *Use cautiously* in patients with hepatic dysfunction or history of allergy and when a hydantoin derivative is used concomitantly.
• Because phenacemide is extremely toxic, use drug only when other anticonvulsants are ineffective.
• Obtain liver function tests, CBCs, and urinalyses before and at monthly intervals during therapy.
• Tell the patient to report sore throat or fever to the doctor immediately.
• Warn him to avoid activities that require alertness or good psychomotor coordination until the CNS effects of the drug are known.
• Never withdraw the drug suddenly. Call the doctor at once if adverse reactions develop.
• Tell the patient's family to watch for personality or psychological changes and to report them to doctor at once.
• When phenacemide replaces another anticonvulsant, the phenacemide dosage should be increased slowly while the dosage of the drug being discontinued is decreased slowly to maintain adequate seizure control.
• Notify the doctor if the patient develops jaundice or other signs of hepatitis, abnormal urine findings, or a WBC count below 4,000/mm^3.

General

Classification: antibiotic (pencillinase-resistant penicillin). **Pregnancy risk category:** B.

Mechanism of action

A penicillinase-resistant penicillin that is bactericidal against microorganisms by inhibiting cell wall synthesis during active multiplication. Bacteria resist penicillins by producing penicillinases—enzymes that convert penicillins to inactive penicilloic acid. Dicloxacillin resists these enzymes.

Indications and dosage

• Systemic infections caused by penicillinase-producing staphylococci. **Adults:** 1 to 2 g daily P.O., divided into doses given q 6 hours. **Children:** 25 to 50 mg/kg P.O. daily, divided into doses given q 6 hours.

Adverse reactions

Blood: eosinophilia. **CNS:** neuromuscular irritability, seizures. **GI:** *nausea,* vomiting, *epigastric distress,* flatulence, *diarrhea.* **Skin:** *rash.* **Other:** hypersensitivity (pruritus, urticaria, rash, ***anaphylaxis***), overgrowth of nonsusceptible organisms.

Interactions

Probenecid: increases blood levels of dicloxacillin and other penicillins. Probenecid may be used for this purpose.

Nursing diagnoses

• High risk for injury related to ineffectiveness of dicloxacillin to eradicate the infection.
• High risk for fluid volume deficit related to dicloxacillin-induced adverse GI reactions.
• Knowledge deficit related to dicloxacillin therapy.

Nursing interventions

• *Use cautiously* in patients allergic to cephalosporins (possible cross-allergenicity).
• Obtain specimen for culture and sensitivity tests before first dose. Therapy may begin pending test results.
• Before giving dicloxacillin, ask patient if he's had any allergic reactions to penicillin. However, a negative history of penicillin allergy is no guarantee against a future allergic reaction.
• Tell patient to take medication exactly as prescribed, even if he feels better. Entire quantity prescribed should be taken.
• Tell patient to call the doctor if rash, fever, or chills develop. A rash is the most common allergic reaction.
• Drug may cause GI disturbances. Food may interfere with absorption, so give 1 to 2 hours before meals or 2 to 3 hours after.
• With large doses and prolonged therapy, bacterial and fungal superinfections may occur, especially in elderly, debilitated, or immunosuppressed patients. Close observation is essential.
• Periodic assessments of renal, hepatic, and hematopoietic function should be made when therapy is prolonged.
• Warn patient never to use leftover dicloxacillin for a new illness or to share it with family and friends.
• Give dicloxacillin at least 1 hour before bacteriostatic antibiotics.

General

Classification: antipsychotic (antiemetic). **Pregnancy risk category:** C.

Mechanism of action

Blocks postsynaptic dopamine receptors in brain and inhibits medullary chemoreceptor trigger zone.

Indications and dosage

• Psychosis in hospitalized patients. **Adults:** initially, 8 to 16 mg P.O. b.i.d., t.i.d., or q.i.d., increasing to 64 mg daily. **Children over 12 years:** 6 to 12 mg P.O. daily in divided doses.
• Mental disturbances, acute alcoholism, nausea, vomiting, hiccups. **Adults and children over 12 years:** 5 to 10 mg I.M. p.r.n. Maximum 15 mg daily in ambulatory patients, 30 mg daily in hospitalized patients.

Adverse reactions

Blood: transient leukopenia, ***agranulocytosis.*** **CNS:** *extrapyramidal reactions, tardive dyskinesia,* sedation, pseudoparkinsonism, dizziness. **CV:** *orthostatic hypotension,* tachycardia. **EENT:** ocular changes, *blurred vision.* **GI:** *dry mouth, constipation.* **GU:** *urine retention,* dark urine, menstrual irregularities, gynecomastia, inhibited ejaculation. **Hepatic:** cholestatic jaundice, abnormal liver function tests. **Metabolic:** hyperprolactinemia. **Skin:** *mild photosensitivity,* allergic reactions. **Local:** pain at I.M. site, sterile abscess. **Other:** weight gain; increased appetite; rarely, ***neuroleptic malignant syndrome.*** **After abrupt withdrawal of long-term therapy:** gastritis, nausea, vomiting, dizziness, tremor, sweating, tachycardia, headache, insomnia.

Interactions

Alcohol, other CNS depressants: increased CNS depression. **Antacids:** inhibited absorption of oral phenothiazines. **Barbiturates:** possible decreased phenothiazine effect. **Spinal, epidural anesthetics; adrenergic blockers:** avoid use together.

Nursing diagnoses

• Altered health maintenance related to the patient's underlying condition.
• High risk for injury related to extrapyramidal reactions to drug.
• Knowledge deficit related to perphenazine.

Nursing interventions

• *Contraindicated* in coma, CNS depression, bone marrow suppression, or subcortical damage.
• *Use cautiously* in elderly or debilitated patients; in acutely ill or dehydrated children; and in hepatic or CV disease, extreme heat or cold, respiratory disorders, hypocalcemia, seizures, severe reactions to insulin or electroshock, suspected brain tumor or intestinal obstruction, glaucoma, or prostatic hypertrophy.
• Tardive dyskinesia may occur after prolonged use, sometimes months or years later; may stop spontaneously or last for life.
• Give I.V. diphenhydramine for acute dystonia.
• Hold dose and tell doctor if patient develops blood dyscrasias, jaundice, persistent extrapyramidal reactions.
• Monitor therapy by weekly bilirubin tests during first month; periodic blood tests (CBC and liver function); and ophthalmic tests (long-term use).
• Have patient report urine retention or constipation.
• Monitor blood pressure before and during therapy. Watch for orthostatic hypotension, especially with parenteral administration. Keep patient in supine position for 1 hour afterward. Advise him to change positions slowly.
• Give deep I.M. in upper outer quadrant of buttocks.
• Don't stop drug abruptly unless reactions are severe.
• Protect drug from light. Slight yellowing doesn't alter potency.
• Avoid contact dermatitis by keeping drug off skin and clothes.
• Dilute liquid with fruit juice, milk, carbonated beverage, or semisolid food. However, don't mix with grape or apple juice, colas, black coffee, or tea.

General
Classification: oral anticoagulant (coumarin derivative). **Pregnancy risk category:** D.

Mechanism of action
Inhibits vitamin K-dependent activation of clotting factors II, VII, IX, and X.

Indications and dosage
• Prophylaxis and treatment of pulmonary emboli; prevention and treatment of emboli associated with deep vein thrombosis, MI, rheumatic heart disease with heart valve damage, prosthetic heart valves, atrial arrhythmias. **Adults:** 200 to 300 mg P.O. on first day, 25 to 200 mg daily thereafter, based on PT.

Adverse reactions
Blood: ***hemorrhage with excessive dosage,*** eosinophilia, leukopenia, ***agranulocytosis.*** **GI:** anorexia, nausea, vomiting, cramps, *diarrhea,* mouth ulcers. **GU:** hematuria. **Skin:** dermatitis, urticaria, alopecia, *rash.* **Other:** *fever,* hepatitis, jaundice.

Interactions
Acetaminophen: increased bleeding possible with chronic (>2 weeks) therapy with acetaminophen. Monitor carefully. **Allopurinol, amiodarone, cephalosporins, chloramphenicol, ciprofloxacin, clofibrate, diflunisal, thyroid drugs, heparin, anabolic steroids, cimetidine, disulfiram, glucagon, methimazole, metronidazole, propylthiouracil, sulindac, sulfinpyrazone, sulfonamides, tricyclic antidepressants, vitamin E:** increased PT. Monitor patient for bleeding. Consider anticoagulant dosage reduction. **Barbiturates:** inhibition of hypoprothrombinemic effect of anticoagulants. If barbiturates are withdrawn, reduce anticoagulant dosage; inhibition may last weeks after withdrawal, but fatal hemorrhage can occur when inhibiting effect disappears. **Cholestyramine:** decreased response when administered too close together. Administer 6 hours after oral anticoagulants. **Glutethimide, chloral hydrate, sulfinpyrazone, triclofos sodium:** increased or decreased PT. Avoid use if possible. **Griseofulvin, ethchlorvynol, carbamazepine, rifampin:** decreased PT with reduced anticoagulant effect. **Hydantoins:** increased serum levels of hydantoin. **Indomethacin, mefenamic acid, oxyphenbutazone, phenylbutazone, salicylates:** increased PT; ulcerogenic effects. Don't use together. **Sulfonylureas (oral antidiabetic agents):** increased hypoglycemic response. Monitor blood glucose levels.

Nursing diagnoses
• Altered tissue perfusion (renal, cerebral, cardiopulmonary, gastrointestinal, peripheral) related to the patient's underlying condition.
• High risk for fluid volume deficit related to adverse effects of dicumarol therapy.
• Knowledge deficit related to dicumarol therapy.

Nursing interventions
• *Contraindicated* in hemophilia; thrombocytopenic purpura; polycythemia vera; leukemia with pronounced bleeding tendency; open wounds or ulcers; GI, GU, or respiratory tract ulcers; cerebrovascular hemorrhage; aneurysms; pericarditis; pericardial effusions; vasculitis; diverticulitis; pregnancy; impaired hepatic or renal function; severe hypertension; acute nephritis; subacute bacterial endocarditis; recent eye, CNS, or spinal cord surgery.
• *Use with extreme caution* (if at all) in psychiatric, debilitated, or cachectic patients.
• *Use cautiously* in breast-feeding women. Monitor infants for bleeding. Also use cautiously during menses, during use of any drainage tube, and in any patient in whom slight bleeding is dangerous.
• Use caution when adding or stopping any drug for patient receiving anticoagulants. May change the clotting status and result in hemorrhage.
• Stop drug and call doctor if fever or rash develops.
• **I.V. use:** Onset of action is delayed, so heparin sodium is often given during first few days of treatment. Dose given depends on PT. Doctors usually try to maintain PT at 1.5 to 2 times normal.

General

Classification: antiparkinsonian agent (dopaminergic agonist). **Pregnancy risk category:** B.

Mechanism of action

Directly stimulates dopamine receptors in the nigrostriatal system.

Indications and dosage

• Adjunctive treatment to carbidopa-levodopa in managing symptoms associated with Parkinson's disease. **Adults:** initially, 0.05 mg P.O. daily for the first 2 days. Gradually increase dosage by 0.1 to 0.15 mg q third day over the next 12 days of therapy. Subsequent dosage can be increased by 0.25 mg q third day until optimum response is seen. The drug is usually given in divided doses t.i.d. Gradual reductions in carbidopa-levodopa dosage may be made during dosage titration.

Adverse reactions

CNS: headache, asthenia, *dyskinesia, dizziness, hallucinations,* dystonia, confusion, *somnolence,* insomnia, anxiety, depression, tremor, abnormal dreams, personality disorder, psychosis, abnormal gait, akathisia, extrapyramidal syndrome, incoordination, paresthesia, akinesia, hypertonia, neuralgia, speech disorder. **CV:** *orthostatic hypotension,* vasodilation, palpitations, hypotension, syncope, hypertension, ***arrhythmias, MI.*** **EENT:** *rhinitis,* epistaxis, abnormal vision, diplopia, eye disorder. **GI:** abdominal pain, *nausea, constipation,* diarrhea, dyspepsia, anorexia, vomiting, dry mouth, taste alteration. **GU:** urinary frequency, urinary tract infection, hematuria. **Skin:** rash, sweating. **Other:** chest, neck, and back pain; flulike syndrome; chills; infection; facial, peripheral, or generalized edema; weight gain; arthralgia; bursitis; myalgia; twitching.

Interactions

Phenothiazines, butyrophenones, metoclopramide, thioxanthines, and other dopamine antagonists: may antagonize the effects of pergolide.

Nursing diagnoses

• Impaired physical mobility related to underlying parkinsonian syndrome.
• Altered thought processes related to CNS reactions to pergolide.
• Knowledge deficit related to pergolide therapy.

Nursing interventions

• *Contraindicated* in patients allergic to the drug or to ergot alkaloids. Symptomatic orthostatic or sustained hypotension may occur in some patients, especially at the start of therapy.
• Hallucinations may occur in some patients. Tolerance to this adverse reaction was not seen in early clinical trials.
• In premarketing trials, over 140 of approximately 2,300 patients died while taking pergolide. However, the drug did not appear to be responsible for these deaths because the affected patients were elderly, ill, and at high risk for death.
• In early clinical trials, 27% of the patients who attempted pergolide therapy did not finish the trial because of adverse reactions (primarily hallucinations and confusion). Inform patients of the potential adverse reactions. Warn them to avoid activities that could expose them to injury as a result of orthostatic hypotension and syncope.

General

Classification: antimuscarinic, GI antispasmodic (anticholinergic). **Pregnancy risk category:** B.

Mechanism of action

Exerts a nonspecific, direct spasmolytic action on smooth muscle. Also possesses local anesthetic properties that may be partly responsible for spasmolysis.

Indications and dosage

• Adjunctive therapy for peptic ulcers and other functional GI disorders. **Adults:** 10 to 20 mg P.O. t.i.d. or q.i.d.; 20 mg I.M. q 6 hours.

Always adjust dosage according to patient's needs and response. Doses up to 40 mg P.O. q.i.d. have been used, but safety and efficacy of their dosage for more than 2 weeks has not been established.

Adverse reactions

CNS: *headache,* insomnia, drowsiness, *dizziness.* **CV:** *palpitations,* tachycardia. **GI:** nausea, *constipation,* vomiting, *paralytic ileus.* **GU:** *urinary hesitancy, urine retention, impotence.* **Skin:** urticaria, decreased sweating or possible anhidrosis, other dermal manifestations. **Other:** fever, allergic reactions.

Overdosage may cause curare-like symptoms.

Interactions

Amantadine, antihistamines, antiparkinsonian agents, disopyramide, glutethimide, meperidine, phenothiazines, procainamide, quinidine: additive adverse effects. Avoid concomitant use. **Ketoconazole:** anticholinergics may interfere with ketoconazole absorption. Avoid concomitant use. **Methotrimeprazine:** anticholinergics may enhance risk of extrapyramidal reactions. Avoid concomitant use.

Nursing diagnoses

• Pain related to the patient's underlying condition.
• Urinary retention related to adverse drug reactions.
• Knowledge deficit related to dicyclomine therapy.

Nursing interventions

• *Contraindicated* in obstructive uropathy, obstructive disease of GI tract, severe ulcerative colitis, myasthenia gravis, hypersensitivity to anticholinergics, paralytic ileus, intestinal atony, unstable CV status in acute hemorrhage, or toxic megacolon.
• *Use cautiously* in autonomic neuropathy, narrow-angle glaucoma, hyperthyroidism, coronary artery disease, cardiac arrhythmias, CHF, hypertension, hiatal hernia associated with reflux esophagitis, hepatic or renal disease, and ulcerative colitis. Also use cautiously in hot or humid environments. Drug-induced heatstroke can develop.
• Give 30 minutes to 1 hour before meals and at bedtime. Bedtime dose can be larger and should be given at least 2 hours after last meal of day.
• Monitor patient's vital signs and urine output carefully.
• Instruct patient to avoid driving and other hazardous activities if he is drowsy, dizzy, or has blurred vision; to drink plenty of fluids to help prevent constipation; and to report any rash or skin eruption.
• Gum or sugarless hard candy may relieve dry mouth.
• A synthetic tertiary derivative that may have fewer atropine-like adverse reactions.
• Do not use I.V.

General

Classification: hemorrheologic agent (xanthine derivative). **Pregnancy risk category:** C.

Mechanism of action

Improves capillary blood flow by increasing the flexibility of erythrocytes and lowering blood viscosity.

Indications and dosage

- Intermittent claudication caused by chronic occlusive vascular disease. **Adults:** 400 mg P.O. t.i.d. with meals.

Adverse reactions

CNS: headache, dizziness. **GI:** dyspepsia, nausea, vomiting.

Interactions

Anticoagulants: increased anticoagulant effect. **Antihypertensives:** increased hypotensive effect. Dosage adjustments may be necessary.

Nursing diagnoses

- Activity intolerance related to the patient's underlying condition.
- Pain related to headache brought on by pentoxifylline.
- Knowledge deficit related to pentoxifylline therapy.

Nursing interventions

- *Contraindicated* in patients who can't tolerate methylxanthines, such as caffeine, theophylline, and theobromine.
- Pentoxifylline should be taken for a minimum of 8 weeks to achieve clinical effects. Tell the patient not to discontinue the drug during this period unless directed by doctor.
- Advise the patient to take the drug with meals to minimize GI upset.
- Instruct patient to report any adverse GI or CNS reactions. If he experiences these reactions, the doctor may reduce the dosage.
- Pentoxifylline therapy is useful in patients who are not good surgical candidates.
- If the patient smokes, explain to him that nicotine causes vasoconstriction, which can worsen his condition. Suggest that he try a nicotine substitute and encourage his participation in a behavior modification program.
- Tell him to swallow the medication whole, without breaking, crushing, or chewing.
- Monitor the drug's effectiveness by evaluating the patient's leg pain, especially with activity.
- Elderly patients may be more sensitive to the drug's effects.

General

Classification: antiviral (purine analogue). **Pregnancy risk category:** B

Mechanism of action

After didanosine enters the cell, it's converted to its active form, dideoxyadenosine triphosphate (ddATP), which inhibits replication of human immunodeficiency virus (HIV) by preventing DNA replication. In addition, ddATP inhibits the enzyme HIV-RNA dependent DNA polymerase.

Indications and dosage

• Advanced HIV infection in patients who cannot tolerate or who no longer respond to zidovudine. **Adults 75 kg and over:** 300 mg (two 150-mg tablets) P.O. q 12 hours; or 375 mg buffered powder q 12 hours. **Adults 50 to 74 kg:** 200 mg (two 100-mg tablets) P.O. q 12 hours; or 250 mg powder q 12 hours. **Adults 35 to 49 kg:** 125 mg (one 100-mg and one 25-mg tablet) P.O. q 12 hours; or 167 mg powder q 12 hours. **Children:** 200 mg/m^2 P.O. daily in divided doses q 12 hours.

Adverse reactions

CNS: *headache,* insomnia, dizziness, ***seizures,*** confusion, anxiety, nervousness, hypertonia, abnormal thinking. **CV:** hypertension. **GI:** *diarrhea, nausea, vomiting, abdominal pain,* ***pancreatitis,*** dry mouth, dyspepsia, flatulence. **Hepatic:** liver abnormalities. **Skin:** rash, pruritus. **Other:** *peripheral neuropathy,* asthenia, pain, myalgia, arthritis, pneumonia, infection, cough, myopathy.

Interactions

Antacids containing magnesium or aluminum hydroxides: enhanced adverse effects of the antacid component when administered with didanosine tablets or pediatric suspension. Avoid concomitant use. **Ketoconazole, dapsone, drugs that require gastric acid for adequate absorption:** buffering action of didanosine can decrease absorption. Administer these drugs 2 hours before didanosine. **Tetracyclines, fluoroquinolones:** decreased absorption because of buffering agents in tablets or antacids in pediatric suspension.

Nursing diagnoses

• High risk for injury related to ineffectiveness of didanosine to prevent or eradicate the infection.
• Noncompliance (medication administration) related to prolonged therapy.
• Knowledge deficit related to didanosine therapy.

Nursing interventions

• *Use cautiously* in history of pancreatitis. In early studies, drug caused pancreatitis in about 9% of all patients; fatalities have occurred. Also use cautiously in peripheral neuropathy, renal or hepatic impairment, or hyperuricemia.
• Patients receiving a sodium-restricted diet should know that each two-tablet dose contains 529 mg of sodium; each single packet of buffered powder for oral solution contains 1.38 g of sodium.
• Administer didanosine on an empty stomach, regardless of the dosage form used. Studies have shown that administering the drug with meals can result in a 50% decrease in absorption.
• Most patients should receive two tablets per dose.
• Because tablets contain buffers that raise stomach pH to levels that prevent degradation of the active drug, they should be thoroughly chewed before swallowing, and the patient should drink at least 1 oz of water with each dose. If tablets are manually crushed, stir them thoroughly in 1 oz of water to disperse the particles uniformly, then have patient drink the mixture immediately. Single-dose packets contain buffered powder.
• Children over 1 year should receive a two-tablet dose; children under 1 year, a one-tablet dose.
• The pediatric powder for oral solution must be prepared by a pharmacist before dispensing. It must be constituted with Purified Water, USP, then diluted with an antacid (either Mylanta Double Strength Liquid or Maalox TC Suspension) to a final concentration of 10 mg/ml. The admixture is stable for 30 days if refrigerated (at 36° to 46° F [2° to 8° C]). Be sure to shake the solution well before measuring the dose.

General

Classification: anticonvulsant, sedative-hypnotic (barbiturate). **Pregnancy risk category:** D. **Controlled substance schedule:** II (suppositories III).

Mechanism of action

Probably interferes with transmission of impulses from the thalamus to the cortex of the brain.

Indications and dosage

• Sedation. **Adults:** 20 to 40 mg P.O. b.i.d., t.i.d., or q.i.d. **Children:** 6 mg/kg daily P.O. in divided doses.

• Insomnia. **Adults:** 100 to 200 mg P.O. h.s. or 150 to 200 mg deep I.M. (sodium); 100 mg initially, I.V., then additional doses up to 500 mg; 120 to 200 mg P.R. **Children:** 3 to 5 mg/kg I.M. Maximum dosage is 100 mg. Rectal dosages: 2 months to 1 year, 30 mg; 1 to 4 years, 30 to 60 mg; 5 to 12 years, 60 mg; 12 to 14 years, 60 to 120 mg.

• Preanesthetic medication. **Adults:** 150 to 200 mg I.M. or P.O. in two divided doses.

Adverse reactions

CNS: *drowsiness, lethargy, hangover,* paradoxical excitement in elderly patients. **GI:** nausea, vomiting. **Skin:** rash, urticaria. **Other:** ***Stevens-Johnson syndrome, angioedema,*** exacerbation of porphyria.

Interactions

Alcohol or other CNS depressants, including narcotic analgesics: excessive CNS, respiratory depression. **Griseofulvin:** decreased absorption of griseofulvin. **MAO inhibitors:** inhibit barbiturate metabolism; possible prolonged CNS depression. Reduce barbiturate dosage. **Oral anticoagulants, estrogens and contraceptives, doxycycline, corticosteroids:** pentobarbital may enhance metabolism of these drugs. Monitor for decreased effect. **Rifampin:** may decrease barbiturate levels.

Nursing diagnoses

• Sleep pattern disturbance related to underlying patient problem.

• High risk for trauma related to adverse CNS reactions to pentobarbital.

Nursing interventions

• *Contraindicated* in uncontrolled severe pain, respiratory disease with dyspnea or obstruction, previous addiction to sedatives, or porphyria.

• *Use cautiously* in hepatic or renal impairment.

• Use injection solution within 30 minutes after opening container to minimize deterioration. Don't use cloudy solution.

• **I.V. use:** I.V. injection should be reserved for emergency treatment and should be given under close supervision. Administer slowly at a rate not exceeding 50 mg/minute.

• I.V. administration may cause severe respiratory depression, laryngospasm, or hypotension. Have emergency resuscitation equipment readily available.

• Parenteral solution is alkaline. Local tissue reactions and pain at the injection site have followed I.V. use. Avoid extravasation. Assess patency of I.V. site before and during administration.

• Prolonged administration is not recommended. Drug loses efficacy in promoting sleep after 14 days of continued use. Long-term high dosage may cause drug dependence, and patient may experience withdrawal symptoms if drug is suddenly discontinued. Withdraw barbiturates gradually.

• Take precautions to prevent hoarding or self-overdosing by patients who are depressed, suicidal, drug-dependent, or with a history of drug abuse.

• No analgesic effect. May cause restlessness or delirium in presence of pain.

• Watch for signs of barbiturate toxicity: coma, pupillary constriction, cyanosis, clammy skin, and hypotension. Overdose can be fatal.

• Skin eruptions may precede potentially fatal reactions to barbiturate therapy. Discontinue drug when skin reactions occur. In some patients, high fever, stomatitis, headache, or rhinitis may precede skin reactions.

• Don't divide suppositories to ensure accuracy.

• Morning "hangover" common after hypnotic dose.

• Hypnotic doses suppress REM sleep. Patient may experience increased dreaming after drug is discontinued.

General
Classification: topical estrogen (estrogen). **Pregnancy risk category:** X.

Mechanism of action
Increases the synthesis of DNA, RNA, and protein in responsive tissues. Also reduces follicle-stimulating hormone and luteinizing hormone release from the pituitary.

Indications and dosage
• Atrophic vaginitis and kraurosis vulvae. **Postmenopausal women:** 1 to 2 intravaginal applications of vaginal cream daily for 1 to 2 weeks (as directed), then half that dose for the same period. A maintenance dosage of 1 applicatorful one to three times a week may be ordered.

Adverse reactions
GU: vaginal discharge; with excessive use, uterine bleeding. **Local:** increased discomfort, burning sensation. **Other:** breast tenderness. Systemic effects possible.

Interactions
Bromocriptine: may cause amenorrhea, interfering with the effects of bromocriptine. Avoid concomitant use. **Carbamazepine, phenobarbital, rifampin:** decreased effectiveness of estrogen therapy. Monitor closely. **Corticosteroids:** possible enhanced effects. Monitor closely. **Cyclosporine:** increased risk of toxicity. Use together with caution and frequently monitor cyclosporine levels. **Dantrolene, other hepatotoxic medications:** increased risk of hepatotoxicity. Monitor closely. **Oral anticoagulants:** dosage adjustments may be necessary. Monitor prothrombin time. **Tamoxifen:** estrogens may interfere with the effectiveness of tamoxifen. Avoid concomitant use.

Nursing diagnoses
• Impaired tissue integrity related to the underlying condition.
• Pain related to local discomfort or burning sensation caused by dienestrol therapy.
• Knowledge deficit related to therapy with dienestrol.

Nursing interventions
• *Contraindicated* in thrombophlebitis or thromboembolic disorders; cancer of breast, reproductive organs, or genitals; undiagnosed abnormal genital bleeding; and pregnancy.
• *Use cautiously* in menstrual irregularities or endometriosis.
• Patients should have a thorough physical examination before initiating estrogen therapy. Patients receiving long-term therapy should have repeat examinations yearly. Periodically monitor body weight, blood pressure, hepatic function, and serum lipid levels.
• Instruct patient to apply drug at bedtime to increase effectiveness.
• Patient package insert that describes estrogen's adverse reactions is available. However, provide verbal explanation also.
• Systemic reactions possible with normal intravaginal use. Monitor closely.
• Warn patient not to exceed the prescribed dose.
• Withdrawal bleeding may occur if estrogen is suddenly stopped.
• Patient shouldn't wear tampon while receiving vaginal therapy. She may need to wear sanitary pad to protect clothing.
• Teach patient how to insert suppositories or cream. Wash vaginal area with soap and water before application.
• Instruct patient to remain recumbent for 30 minutes after administration to prevent loss of drug.
• Instruct patient to report breast pain or tenderness, vaginal discharge or bleeding, or swelling of the hands or feet.
• Teach patient how to perform breast self-examination.

General

Classification: analgesic, adjunct to anesthesia (opioid partial agonist, narcotic agonist-antagonist). **Pregnancy risk category:** B (D for prolonged use or use of high doses at term). **Controlled substance schedule:** IV (pentazocine hydrochloride amd naloxone hydrochloride, pentazocine lactate).

Mechanism of action

Binds with opiate receptors at many sites in the CNS (brain, brain stem, and spinal cord), altering both the perception of pain and the emotional response to it through an unknown mechanism.

Indications and dosage

- Moderate to severe pain. **Adults:** 50 to 100 mg (hydrochloride) P.O. q 3 to 4 hours, p.r.n. or around the clock. Maximum oral dosage is 600 mg daily. Alternatively, may give 30 mg (lactate) I.M., I.V., or S.C. q 3 to 4 hours, p.r.n. or around the clock. Maximum parenteral dosage is 360 mg daily. Single doses above 30 mg I.V. or 60 mg I.M. or S.C. not recommended.

Adverse reactions

CNS: *sedation,* visual disturbances, *hallucinations,* drowsiness, *dizziness, light-headedness,* confusion, euphoria, headache, *psychotomimetic effects.* **GI:** *nausea, vomiting,* dry mouth, constipation. **GU:** *urine retention.* **Local:** induration, nodules, sloughing, and sclerosis of injection site. **Other:** ***respiratory depression,*** physical and psychological dependence.

Interactions

Alcohol, CNS depressants: additive effects. Use together cautiously. **Narcotic analgesics:** possible decreased analgesic effect. Avoid concomitant use.

Nursing diagnoses

- Pain related to the patient's underlying condition.
- Ineffective breathing pattern related to pentazocine-induced respiratory depression.
- Knowledge deficit related to pentazocine therapy.

Nursing interventions

- *Contraindicated* in patients with hypersensitivity to the drug, emotional instability, drug abuse, head injury, and increased intracranial pressure. Injectable form contains sulfites, which may precipitate allergic reactions in patients with hypersensitivity.
- *Use cautiously* in hepatic or renal disease and in patients with acute MI.
- Psychological and physical dependence may occur.
- Respiratory depression can be reversed with naloxone.
- Do not mix in same syringe with soluble barbiturates.
- Warn ambulatory patient to avoid activities that require alertness.
- Pentazocine may interfere with certain laboratory tests for urinary 17-hydroxycorticosteroids.
- Talwin Nx, the oral pentazocine available in the U.S., contains the narcotic antagonist naloxone. This is designed to prevent illicit I.V. use.

General
Classification: Short-term adjunctive anorexigenic agent, sympathomimetic amine (amphetamine). **Pregnancy risk category:** B. **Controlled substance schedule:** IV.

Mechanism of action
Main site of activity appears to be the cerebral cortex and the reticular activating system. Promotes nerve impulse transmission by releasing stored norepinephrine from nerve terminals in the brain.

Indications and dosage
- Short-term adjunct in exogenous obesity. **Adults:** 25 mg P.O. before meals, t.i.d.; or 75 mg controlled-release tablet P.O. in midmorning.

Adverse reactions
CNS: headache, *nervousness,* dizziness. **CV:** *tachycardia, palpitations,* rise in blood pressure. **EENT:** blurred vision. **GI:** nausea, abdominal cramps, dry mouth, diarrhea, constipation. **Skin:** urticaria. **Other:** impotence, altered libido, menstrual changes.

Interactions
MAO inhibitors: hypertension; possible hypertensive crisis. Don't use together or within 14 days after MAO inhibitor has been discontinued.

Nursing diagnoses
- Ineffective individual coping related to patient's underlying disorder.
- Knowledge deficit related to diethylpropion hydrochloride therapy.

Nursing interventions
- *Contraindicated* in hyperthyroidism, hypertension, angina pectoris, severe CV disease, glaucoma, or history of drug abuse.
- *Use cautiously* in seizure disorder, diabetes mellitus, and hyperexcitability states.
- May alter insulin requirements. Monitor blood and urine glucose levels.
- When tolerance to anorexigenic effect develops, dosage should not be increased, but drug discontinued.
- Habituation or psychic dependence may occur.
- Be sure patient is also on a weight-reduction program.
- Can be used to stop nighttime eating. Rarely causes insomnia.
- Fatigue may result as drug effects wear off. Patient will need more rest.
- Tell patient to avoid drinks containing caffeine, which increase the effects of amphetamines and related amines.
- Have patient report signs of excessive stimulation.
- Urine acidification enhances renal excretion; urine alkalinization enhances renal reabsorption and recycling.
- Use as analeptic is usually discouraged, since CNS stimulation superimposed on CNS depression can lead to neuronal instability and seizures.
- Give at least 6 hours before bedtime to avoid sleep interference.

General

Classification: antiprotozoal (diamidine derivative). **Pregnancy risk category:** C.

Mechanism of action

Interferes with biosynthesis of DNA, RNA, phospholipids, and proteins in susceptible organisms.

Indications and dosage

- Treatment of pneumonia caused by *Pneumocystis carinii*. **Adults and children:** 4 mg/kg I.V. or I.M. once daily for 14 days.
- Prevention of *Pneumocystis carinii* pneumonia in high-risk individuals. **Adults:** 300 mg by inhalation (using a Respirgard II nebulizer) once q 4 weeks.

Adverse reactions

Blood: *leukopenia,* thrombocytopenia, anemia.
CNS: confusion, hallucinations. **CV:** ***hypotension,*** tachycardia. **Endocrine:** ***hypoglycemia,*** hyperglycemia, hypocalcemia. **GI:** nausea, anorexia, metallic taste. **GU:** *elevated serum creatinine,* renal toxicity. **Hepatic:** elevated liver enzymes. **Local:** *sterile abscess, pain or induration at injection site.* **Skin:** rash, facial flushing, pruritus. **Other:** fever.

Interactions

Aminoglycosides, amphotericin B, cisplatin, vancomycin, zidovudine: increased risk of nephrotoxicity.

Nursing diagnoses

- Impaired gas exchange related to the ineffectiveness of pentamidine in correcting pneumonia caused by *Pneumocystis carinii.*
- Altered cerebral tissue perfusion related to pentamidine-induced hypotension.
- Knowledge deficit related to pentamidine therapy.

Nursing interventions

- After the diagnosis of *Pneumocystis carinii* pneumonia has been firmly established, pentamidine has no absolute contraindications.
- *Use cautiously* in hypertension, hypotension, hypoglycemia, hypocalcemia, leukopenia, thrombocytopenia, anemia, and hepatic or renal dysfunction.
- Keep patient lying down during drug adminsitration because sudden, severe hypotension may develop. Monitor blood pressure during administration and several times thereafter until it's stable.
- Monitor blood glucose, serum calcium, serum creatinine, and BUN levels daily. After parenteral administration, blood glucose level may decrease initially; hypoglycemia may be severe in 5% to 10% of patients. This may be followed by hyperglycemia and insulin-dependent diabetes mellitus (which may be permanent).
- Pain and induration occur universally with I.M. injection. Administer by deep I.M. injection.
- In patients with AIDS, pentamidine may produce less severe adverse reactions than the alternative treatment co-trimoxazole. Therefore, in some AIDS patients, pentamidine is considered the treatment of choice.
- Give aerosol form only by the Respirgard II nebulizer manufactured by Marquest. Dosage recommendations are based on the particle size and delivery rate of this device. To administer aerosol form, mix the contents of one vial in 6 ml of sterile water for injection. Do not use saline because this will cause the drug to precipitate. Do not mix with other drugs.
- Avoid using low pressure (< 20 psi) compressors. The flow rate should be 5 to 7 liters/minute from a 40 to 50 psi air or oxygen source.
- Instruct the patient to use the aerosol device until the chamber is empty. This may take up to 45 minutes.
- **I.V. use:** Give I.V. intermittently to prevent vein irritation. Change site every 48 hours.

General

Classification: estrogen replacement, antineoplastic (estrogen). **Pregnancy risk category:** X.

Mechanism of action

Increases DNA, RNA, and protein tissue synthesis. Reduces pituitary release of follicle-stimulating hormone and luteinizing hormone.

Indications and dosage

- Postcoital contraception ("morning-after pill"). **Women:** 25 mg P.O. b.i.d. for 5 days, starting within 72 hours after coitus.
- Prostatic cancer. **Men:** initially, 1 to 3 mg P.O. daily; may be reduced to 1 mg P.O. daily, or 5 mg I.M. twice weekly initially, followed by up to 4 mg I.M. twice weekly. Or 50 to 200 mg (diphosphate) P.O. t.i.d.; or 0.25 to 1 g I.V. daily for 5 days, then once or twice weekly.
- Breast cancer. **Men and postmenopausal women:** 15 mg P.O. daily.

Adverse reactions

CNS: headache, dizziness, chorea, depression, lethargy. **CV:** thrombophlebitis; ***thromboembolism;*** hypertension; edema; ***increased risk of stroke, pulmonary embolism, and myocardial infarction.*** **EENT:** worsening of myopia or astigmatism, intolerance to contact lenses. **GI:** *nausea,* vomiting, abdominal cramps, bloating, diarrhea, constipation, anorexia, increased appetite, excessive thirst, weight changes, pancreatitis. **GU:** in women—breakthrough bleeding, altered menstrual flow, dysmenorrhea, amenorrhea, cervical erosion, altered cervical secretions, enlargement of uterine fibromas, vaginal candidiasis, loss of libido. In men—gynecomastia, testicular atrophy, impotence. **Hepatic:** cholestatic jaundice. **Metabolic:** hyperglycemia, hypercalcemia, folic acid deficiency. **Skin:** melasma, urticaria, acne, seborrhea, oily skin, hirsutism or loss of hair. **Other:** leg cramps, breast tenderness or enlargement.

Interactions

Bromocriptine: may cause amenorrhea, interfering with the effects of bromocriptine. **Carbamazepine, phenobarbital, rifampin:** decreased effectiveness of estrogen therapy. Monitor closely. **Corticosteroids:** possible enhanced effects. **Cyclosporine:** increased risk of toxicity. Monitor cyclosporine levels. **Dantrolene, other hepatotoxic medications:** increased risk of hepatotoxicity. **Oral anticoagulants:** may require dosage adjustments. Monitor PT. **Tamoxifen:** may interfere with the effectiveness of tamoxifen.

Nursing diagnoses

- Sexual dysfunction related to the patient's underlying condition.
- Altered tissue perfusion (cerebral, peripheral, cardiopulmonary) related to thromboembolism caused by diethylstilbestrol.
- Knowledge deficit related to drug therapy.

Nursing interventions

- *Contraindicated* in thrombophlebitis or thromboembolic disorders, undiagnosed abnormal genital bleeding, and pregnancy.
- *Use cautiously* in hypertension, asthma, mental depression, bone disease, migraine, seizures, blood dyscrasias, diabetes mellitus, gallbladder disease, amenorrhea, heart failure, hepatic or renal dysfunction, and family history of breast or genital tract cancer.
- Advise patient to report immediately abdominal pain; pain, numbness, or stiffness in legs or buttocks; pressure or pain in chest; shortness of breath; severe headache; visual disturbances, such as blind spots, flashing lights, or blurriness; vaginal bleeding or discharge; breast lumps; sudden weight gain; swelling of hands or feet; yellow sclera or skin; dark urine; or light-colored stools.
- **I.V. use:** Mix ordered dose in 250 to 500 ml of D_5W or 0.9% sodium chloride injection. Infuse slowly at 1 to 2 ml/minute for the first 15 minutes; if no adverse reactions occur, administer entire dose within 1 hour.
- To administer I.M., give by deep injection. Rotate injection sites to prevent muscle atrophy.

pentaerythritol tetranitrate

Dilar, Duotrate, Naptrate, Pentritol, Pentylan, Peritrate, Peritrate Forte†, Peritrate SA, PETN

General

Classification: antianginal, vasodilator (nitrate).
Pregnancy risk category: C.

Mechanism of action

Reduces cardiac oxygen demand by decreasing left ventricular end-diastolic pressure (preload) and, to a lesser extent, systemic vascular resistance (afterload). Also increases blood flow through the collateral coronary vessels.

Indications and dosage

- Prophylaxis against angina pectoris. **Adults:** 10 to 20 mg P.O. q.i.d.; may be titrated upward to 40 mg P.O. q.i.d. 30 minutes before or 1 hour after meals and h.s.; or 30 to 80 mg sustained-release preparation P.O. b.i.d.

Adverse reactions

CNS: *headache, sometimes with throbbing; dizziness;* weakness. **CV:** *orthostatic hypotension, tachycardia, flushing, palpitations,* fainting. **GI:** nausea, vomiting. **Skin:** cutaneous vasodilation. **Other:** hypersensitivity reactions.

Interactions

None significant.

Nursing diagnoses

- Pain related to the ineffectiveness of pentaerythritol therapy.
- High risk for injury related to adverse CNS reactions to pentaerythritol and drug-induced orthostatic hypotension.
- Knowledge deficit related to pentaerythritol therapy.

Nursing interventions

- *Contraindicated* in patients with head trauma, cerebral hemorrhage, or severe anemia.
- *Use cautiously* in patients with hypotension or glaucoma.
- Monitor blood pressure and the intensity and duration of response to the drug.
- Drug may cause headaches, especially at first. Treat with aspirin or acetaminophen. Dosage may need to be reduced temporarily, but tolerance usually develops.
- Drug should be taken regularly, even long-term, if ordered. Physiologically necessary but not habit-forming.
- Additional doses may be taken before anticipated stress or at bedtime for nocturnal angina.
- Not to be used for relief of acute anginal attacks.
- Drug may cause orthostatic hypotension. To minimize it, tell patient to change to upright position slowly, to go up and down stairs carefully, and to lie down at the first sign of dizziness.
- Advise the patient to avoid alcoholic beverages; they may exacerbate hypotension.
- Drug should not be discontinued abruptly—coronary vasospasm may occur.
- Store drug in a cool place, in a tightly covered container away from light.

difenoxin hydrochloride

Motofen

General

Classification: antidiarrheal (opioid agonist). **Pregnancy risk category:** C.

Mechanism of action

Exerts a direct effect on the intestinal wall to slow motility.

Indications and dosage

• Adjunct in acute nonspecific diarrhea, and acute exacerbations of chronic functional diarrhea. **Adults:** initially, 2 mg P.O., then 1 mg P.O. after each loose bowel movement. Total dosage should not exceed 8 mg daily. Not recommended for use longer than 2 days.

Adverse reactions

CNS: dizziness and light-headedness, drowsiness, headache, fatigue, nervousness, insomnia, confusion. **EENT:** burning eyes, blurred vision. **GI:** nausea, vomiting, dry mouth, epigastric distress, constipation.

Interactions

Alcohol, CNS depressants, tranquilizers, narcotics, barbiturates: enhanced CNS depression. Closely monitor patients. **MAO inhibitors:** potential hypertensive crisis. Avoid concomitant use.

Nursing diagnoses

• Diarrhea related to interruption in normal pattern of elimination, characterized by frequent loose stools.
• Altered thought processes related to drug-induced adverse CNS reactions.
• Knowledge deficit related to difenoxin therapy.

Nursing interventions

• *Contraindicated* in patients with hypersensitivity to difenoxin or atropine, in children under 2 years, and in patients with diarrhea from pseudomembraneous colitis associated with antibiotics. Also contraindicated in patients with jaundice, or diarrhea from organisms that may penetrate the intestinal mucosa (including toxigenic *Escherichia coli, Salmonella,* or *Shigella*).
• *Use cautiously* in patients with a history of drug abuse, or in those currently receiving drugs with a high abuse potential.
• Difenoxin is the principal metabolite of diphenoxylate (Lomotil) and is chemically related to meperidine.
• Atropine has been added to difenoxin to prevent abuse. The small dosage of atropine is unlikely to cause any significant clinical problems, but patients may experience dry mouth, tachycardia, urine retention, and flushing. Monitor for these effects.
• Advise patient to avoid hazardous activities that may require mental alertness, such as driving or operating heavy machinery, until the CNS effects of the drug are known.
• Monitor patient closely for fluid and electrolyte imbalance. Difenoxin-induced decreases in peristalsis may result in fluid retention in the colon, with subsequent dehydration and possibly delayed difenoxin intoxication.
• Advise patient to adhere to dosing schedule. Overdose with difenoxin may result in respiratory depression and coma. Encourage proper storage to keep drug out of children's reach.
• Patients who overdose with difenoxin should be observed for at least 48 hours. Respiratory depression may occur up to 30 hours after ingestion. Gastric lavage, establishment of a patent airway, and mechanically assisted ventilation are advised. Naloxone will reverse the respiratory depression. Because difenoxin has a longer duration of action than naloxone, repeated injections of naloxone will be necessary.

General
Classification: antibiotic (natural penicillin).
Pregnancy risk category: B.

Mechanism of action
Bactericidal against microorganisms by inhibiting cell wall synthesis during active multiplication. Bacteria resist penicillin by producing penicillinases – enzymes that convert penicillin to inactive penicilloic acid.

Indications and dosage
• Mild to moderate systemic infections. **Adults:** 250 to 500 mg (400,000 to 800,000 units) P.O. q 6 hours. **Children:** 15 to 50 mg/kg (25,000 to 90,000 units/kg) P.O. daily, divided into doses given q 6 to 8 hours.
• Endocarditis prophylaxis for dental surgery. **Adults:** 2 g P.O. 30 to 60 minutes before procedure, then 1 g 6 hours after. **Children under 30 kg:** half of the adult dose. *Note:* The American Heart Association considers amoxicillin the preferred agent; penicillin V is considered an alternate drug.

Adverse reactions
Blood: eosinophilia, hemolytic anemia, leukopenia, thrombocytopenia. **CNS:** neuropathy. **GI:** *epigastric distress,* vomiting, diarrhea, *nausea.* **Other:** hypersensitivity (rash, urticaria, chills, fever, edema, ***anaphylaxis***), overgrowth of nonsusceptible organisms.

Interactions
Neomycin: decreased absorption of penicillin. Give penicillin by injection. **Probenecid:** increased blood levels of penicillin. Probenecid may be used for this purpose.

Nursing diagnoses
• High risk for injury related to the ineffectiveness of penicillin V in eradicating the infection.
• Altered protection related to an allergic reaction induced by pencillin V.
• Knowledge deficit related to penicillin V therapy.

Nursing interventions
• *Use cautiously* in patients with other drug allergies, especially to cephalosporins (possible cross-allergenicity), and in GI disturbances.
• Obtain specimen for culture and sensitivity tests before first dose. Therapy may begin pending test results.
• Before giving penicillin, ask the patient if he's had any allergic reactions to this drug. However, a negative history of penicillin allergy is no guarantee against a future allergic reaction.
• Tell patient to take the medication exactly as prescribed, even if he feels better, and to take entire quantity prescribed.
• Tell him to call the doctor if rash, fever, or chills develop. A rash is the most common allergic reaction.
• May cause GI disturbances. Food may interfere with absorption, so give drug 1 to 2 hours before meals or 2 to 3 hours after.
• Instruct the patient to take each dose with a full glass of water, not fruit juice or a carbonated beverage, because acid will inactivate the drug.
• With large doses and prolonged therapy, bacterial and fungal superinfections may occur, especially in elderly, debilitated, or immunosuppressed patients. Close observation is essential.
• Periodically monitor renal and hematopoietic function in patients receiving prolonged therapy.
• Warn the patient never to use leftover penicillin for a new illness or to share penicillin with family or friends.
• Give penicillin V at least 1 hour before bacteriostatic antibiotics.

General

Classification: nonnarcotic, nonsteroidal analgesic, antipyretic (salicylic acid derivative). **Pregnancy risk category:** C.

Mechanism of action

Probably related to inhibition of prostaglandin synthesis.

Indications and dosage

• Mild to moderate pain and osteoarthritis. **Adults:** 500 to 1,000 mg P.O. daily in two divided doses, usually q 12 hours. Maximum dosage 1,500 mg daily. **Adults over 65:** Start with one-half the usual adult dose.

Adverse reactions

CNS: *dizziness,* somnolence, insomnia, *headache,* fatigue. **EENT:** *tinnitus, visual disturbances (rare).* **GI:** *nausea, dyspepsia, GI pain, diarrhea,* vomiting, constipation, flatulence. **GU:** renal impairment, hematuria, interstitial nephritis. **Skin:** *rash,* pruritus, sweating, dry mucous membranes, stomatitis.

Interactions

Acetaminophen, hydrochlorothiazide: diflunisal may substantially increase blood levels, increasing the risk of toxicity. Avoid concomitant use. **Aspirin, antacids:** decreased diflunisal blood levels. Monitor for possible decreased therapeutic effect. **Cyclosporine:** diflunisal may enhance the nephrotoxicity of cyclosporine. Avoid concomitant use. **Methotrexate:** diflunisal may enhance the toxicity of methotrexate. Avoid concomitant use. **Oral anticoagulants, thrombolytic agents:** diflunisal may enhance pharmacologic effects of these agents. Use together cautiously. **Sulindac:** diflunisal decreases blood levels of sulindac's active metabolite. Monitor for decreased pharmacologic effect.

Nursing diagnoses

• Pain related to the patient's underlying condition.
• High risk for injury related to adverse CNS effects of diflunisal.
• Knowledge deficit related to diflunisal therapy.

Nursing interventions

• *Contraindicated* in patients for whom acute asthmatic attacks, urticaria, or rhinitis are precipitated by aspirin or other NSAIDs.
• *Use cautiously* in patients with active GI bleeding or history of peptic ulcer disease, renal impairment, liver disease, and compromised cardiac function or in those taking anticoagulants.
• Like aspirin, diflunisal is a salicylic acid derivative but is metabolized differently. Anti-inflammatory, analgesic, and antipyretic effects are comparable to those of aspirin; however, platelet function is not affected. Do not substitute for aspirin during antithrombotic therapy.
• May be administered with water, milk, or meals.
• Avoid the use of diflunisal in children and teenagers with viral illnesses and flu because of possible association with Reye's syndrome.

General

Classification: antibiotic (natural penicillin). **Pregnancy risk category:** B.

Mechanism of action

Bactericidal against microorganisms by inhibiting cell wall synthesis during active multiplication. Bacteria resist penicillin by producing penicillinases—enzymes that convert penicillin to inactive penicilloic acid.

Indications and dosage

- Moderate to severe systemic infections. **Adults:** 1.2 to 24 million units daily I.M. or I.V., divided into doses given q 4 hours. **Children:** 25,000 to 300,000 units/kg daily I.M. or I.V., divided into doses given q 4 hours.
- Endocarditis prophylaxis for dental surgery. **Adults:** 2 million units I.V. or I.M. 30 to 60 minutes before procedure, then 1 million units 6 hours later.

Adverse reactions

Blood: hemolytic anemia, leukopenia, thrombocytopenia. **CNS:** neuropathy, seizures. **CV:** *CHF with high doses.* **Local:** *vein irritation, pain at injection site, thrombophlebitis.* **Other:** arthralgia, hypersensitivity (chills, fever, edema, maculopapular rash, ***exfoliative dermatitis,*** urticaria, ***anaphylaxis***), overgrowth of nonsusceptible organisms.

Interactions

Probenecid: increased blood levels of penicillin. Probenecid may be used for this purpose.

Nursing diagnoses

- High risk for injury related to the ineffectiveness of penicillin G sodium in eradicating the infection.
- Impaired tissue integrity related to thrombophlebitis caused by I.V. administration of penicillin G sodium.
- Knowledge deficit related to penicillin G sodium therapy.

Nursing interventions

- *Contraindicated* in patients with sodium restrictions.
- *Use cautiously* in patients with other drug allergies, especially to cephalosporins (possible cross-allergenicity).
- Obtain specimen for culture and sensitivity tests before first dose. Therapy may begin pending test results.
- Before giving penicillin, ask the patient if he's had any allergic reactions to this drug. However, a negative history of penicillin allergy is no guarantee against a future allergic reaction.
- If the patient has a high blood level of this drug, he may have seizures. Institute seizure precautions.
- With large doses and prolonged therapy, bacterial or fungal superinfections may occur, especially in elderly, debilitated, or immunosuppressed patients. Close observation is essential.
- Give penicillin G sodium at least 1 hour before bacteriostatic antibiotics.
- **I.V. use:** Give I.V. intermittently to prevent vein irritation. Change site every 48 hours.

General

Classification: antiarrhythmic, inotropic agent (digitalis glycoside). **Pregnancy risk category:** C.

Mechanism of action

Promotes movement of calcium from extracellular to intracellular cytoplasm and inhibits sodium-potassium activated adenosine triphosphatase. These actions strengthen myocardial contraction.

Indications and dosage

• CHF, paroxysmal supraventricular tachycardia, atrial fibrillation and flutter. **Adults:** loading dose is 1.2 to 1.6 mg P.O. in divided doses over 24 hours; average maintenance dosage is 0.15 mg daily (range: 0.05 to 0.3 mg daily). **Children 2 to 12 years:** loading dose is 0.03 mg/kg or 0.75 mg/m² P.O. in divided doses over 24 hours; maintenance dosage is 1/10 of loading dose or 0.003 mg/kg or 0.075 mg/m² daily. Monitor for toxicity. **Children 1 to 2 years:** loading dose is 0.04 mg/kg P.O. over 24 hours in divided doses; maintenance dosage is 0.004 mg/kg daily. Monitor closely for toxicity. **Children 2 weeks to 1 year:** loading dose is 0.045 mg/kg P.O. in divided doses over 24 hours; maintenance dosage is 0.0045 mg/kg daily. Monitor closely for toxicity. **Premature infants, neonates, severely ill older infants:** loading dose is 0.022 mg/kg or 0.3 to 0.35 mg/m² P.O. in divided doses over 24 hours; maintenance dosage is 0.0022 mg/kg daily. Monitor for toxicity.

Adverse reactions

The following are signs of toxicity that may occur with all digitalis glycosides: **CNS:** *fatigue, generalized muscle weakness, agitation, hallucinations,* headache, malaise, dizziness, vertigo, stupor, paresthesia. **CV:** ***increased severity of CHF, arrhythmias (most commonly conduction disturbances with or without AV block, premature ventricular contractions, and supraventricular arrhythmias),*** hypotension. **EENT:** *yellow-green halos around visual images, blurred vision,* light flashes, photophobia, diplopia. **GI:** *anorexia, nausea,* vomiting, diarrhea.

Interactions

Amphotericin B, carbenicillin, ticarcillin, corticosteroids, and diuretics (including loop diuretics, chlorthalidone, metolazone, and thiazides): hypokalemia, predisposing patient to digitalis toxicity. Monitor serum potassium. **Antacids, kaolin-pectin:** decreased absorption of oral digitoxin. Schedule doses as far as possible from oral digitoxin administration. **Cholestyramine, colestipol, metoclopramide:** decreased absorption of oral digitoxin. Monitor for decreased effect and low blood levels. Dosage may have to be increased. **Cimetidine:** decreased digitoxin metabolism. Monitor for digitoxin toxicity. **Parenteral calcium, thiazides:** hypercalcemia and hypomagnesemia, predisposing patient to digitalis toxicity. Monitor serum calcium and serum magnesium. **Phenylbutazone, phenobarbital, phenytoin, rifampin:** faster metabolism and shorter duration of digitoxin. Observe for underdigitalization. **Quinidine, verapamil:** possible increased serum digitoxin levels. Monitor patient closely.

Nursing diagnoses

• Decreased cardiac output related to ineffectiveness of digitoxin.
• High risk for injury related to digitalis toxicity caused by digitoxin.
• Knowledge deficit related to digitoxin therapy.

Nursing interventions

• *Contraindicated* in digitalis-induced toxicity, ventricular fibrillation, and ventricular tachycardia unless caused by CHF. Giving calcium salts to digitalized patient is also contraindicated.
• *Use with extreme caution* in elderly patients and in acute MI, incomplete AV block, sinus bradycardia, premature ventricular contractions, chronic constrictive pericarditis, idiopathic hypertrophic subaortic stenosis, severe pulmonary disease, and hypothyroidism.
• Before giving digitoxin, take apical-radial pulse for a full minute. Record and report to doctor any significant changes. Check blood pressure and obtain 12-lead ECG with these changes.

General

Classification: antibiotic (natural penicillin).
Pregnancy risk category: B.

Mechanism of action

Bactericidal against microorganisms by inhibiting cell wall synthesis during active multiplication. Bacteria resist penicillin by producing penicillinases—enzymes that convert penicillin to inactive penicilloic acid.

Indications and dosage

• Moderate to severe systemic infections. **Adults:** 600,000 to 1.2 million units I.M. daily given as a single dose. **Children:** 300,000 units I.M. daily given as a single dose.
• Uncomplicated gonorrhea. **Adults and children over 12 years:** give 1 g probenecid; then 30 minutes later, give 4.8 million units of penicillin G procaine I.M., divided into two injection sites.
• Pneumococcal pneumonia. **Adults and children over 12 years:** 300,000 to 600,000 units I.M. daily q 6 to 12 hours.

Adverse reactions

Blood: thrombocytopenia, hemolytic anemia, leukopenia. **CNS:** seizures. **Other:** arthralgia, hypersensitivity (rash, urticaria, chills, fever, edema, prostration, ***anaphylaxis***), overgrowth of nonsusceptible organisms.

P

Interactions

Probenecid: increased blood levels of penicillin. Probenecid may be used for this purpose.

Nursing diagnoses

• High risk for injury related to the ineffectiveness of penicillin G procaine in eradicating the infection.
• Altered protection related to an allergic reaction induced by penicillin G procaine.
• Knowledge deficit related to penicillin G procaine therapy.

Nursing interventions

• *Contraindicated* in patients with hypersensitivity to procaine.
• *Use cautiously* in patients with other drug allergies, especially to cephalosporins (possible cross-allergenicity).
• Obtain specimen for culture and sensitivity tests before first dose. Therapy may begin pending test results.
• Before giving penicillin, ask patient if he's had any allergic reactions to this drug. However, a negative history of penicillin allergy is no guarantee against a future allergic reaction.
• Because of the drug's slow absorption rate, allergic reactions are hard to treat.
• Tell the patient to call the doctor if rash, fever, or chills develop. A rash is the most common allergic reaction.
• Give deep I.M. in upper outer quadrant of buttocks in adults; in midlateral thigh in small children. Don't give subcutaneously. Don't massage injection site.
• Never give I.V. Inadvertent I.V. administration has caused death because of CNS toxicity from procaine.
• With large doses and prolonged therapy, bacterial and fungal superinfections may occur, especially in elderly, debilitated, or immunosuppressed patients. Close observation is essential.
• Periodically evaluate renal and hematopoietic function.
• Give penicillin G procaine at least 1 hour before bacteriostatic antibiotics.

General

Classification: antiarrhythmic, inotropic agent (digitalis glycoside). **Pregnancy risk category:** C.

Mechanism of action

Promotes movement of calcium from extracellular to intracellular cytoplasm and inhibits sodium-potassium activated adenosine triphosphatase. These actions strengthen myocardial contraction.

Indications and dosage

• CHF, paroxysmal supraventricular tachycardia, atrial fibrillation and flutter. **Adults:** loading dose 0.5 to 1 mg I.V. or P.O. in divided doses over 24 hours; maintenance dosage 0.125 to 0.5 mg I.V. or P.O. daily (average 0.25 mg). Treatment of arrhythmias requires larger doses, depending on patient response. **Adults over 65 years:** 0.125 mg P.O. daily as maintenance dose. Frail or underweight elderly patients may require only 0.0625 mg daily or 0.125 mg every other day. **Children over 2 years:** loading dose 0.02 to 0.04 mg/kg P.O. divided q 8 hours over 24 hours; I.V. loading dose 0.015 to 0.035 mg/kg; maintenance dosage 0.012 mg/kg P.O. daily divided q 12 hours. **Children 1 month to 2 years:** loading dose 0.035 to 0.06 mg/kg P.O. daily divided t.i.d.; I.V. loading dose 0.03 to 0.05 mg/kg; maintenance dosage 0.01 to 0.02 mg/kg P.O. daily divided q 12 hours. **Neonates under 1 month:** loading dose 0.035 mg/kg P.O. divided q 8 hours over 24 hours; I.V. loading dose 0.02 to 0.03 mg/kg; maintenance dosage 0.01 mg/kg P.O. daily divided q 12 hours. **Premature infants:** loading dose 0.025 mg/kg I.V. divided t.i.d. over 24 hours; maintenance dosage 0.01 mg/kg I.V. daily divided q 12 hours.

Adverse reactions

CNS: *fatigue, generalized muscle weakness, agitation, hallucinations,* headache, malaise, dizziness, vertigo, stupor, paresthesia. **CV:** ***increased CHF, arrhythmias,*** hypotension. **EENT:** *yellow-green halos around visual images, blurred vision,* light flashes, photophobia, diplopia. **GI:** *anorexia, nausea,* vomiting, diarrhea.

Interactions

Amiloride: inhibits and increases digoxin excretion. Monitor for altered digoxin effect. **Amphotericin B, carbenicillin, ticarcillin, corticosteroids, and diuretics (including loop diuretics, chlorthalidone, metolazone, and thiazides):** hypokalemia, predisposing patient to digitalis toxicity. Monitor serum potassium. **Antacids, kaolin-pectin:** decreased absorption of oral digoxin. Schedule doses as far as possible from oral digoxin administration. **Anticholinergics:** may increase absorption of oral digoxin. Monitor blood levels and observe for toxicity. **Cholestyramine, colestipol, metoclopramide:** decreased absorption of oral digoxin. Monitor for decreased effect and low blood levels. Dosage may have to be increased. **Parenteral calcium, thiazides:** hypercalcemia and hypomagnesemia, predisposing patient to digitalis toxicity. Monitor serum calcium and serum magnesium. **Quinidine, diltiazem, amiodarone, nifedipine, verapamil:** increased digoxin blood levels. Monitor for toxicity.

Nursing diagnoses

• Decreased cardiac output related to ineffectiveness of digoxin.
• High risk for injury related to digitalis toxicity caused by digoxin.
• Knowledge deficit related to digoxin therapy.

Nursing interventions

• *Contraindicated* in digitalis-induced toxicity, ventricular fibrillation, and ventricular tachycardia unless caused by CHF. Administering calcium salts to digitalized patient is also contraindicated.
• *Use with extreme caution* in elderly patients and in those with acute MI, incomplete AV block, sinus bradycardia, premature ventricular contractions, chronic constrictive pericarditis, idiopathic hypertrophic subaortic stenosis, renal insufficiency, severe pulmonary disease, or hypothyroidism. Reduce dosage in renal impairment.

General

Classification: antibiotic (natural penicillin).
Pregnancy risk category: B.

Mechanism of action

Bactericidal against microorganisms by inhibiting cell wall synthesis during active multiplication. Bacteria resist penicillin by producing penicillinases – enzymes that convert penicillin to inactive penicilloic acid.

Indications and dosage

- Moderate to severe systemic infections. **Adults:** 1.6 to 3.2 million units P.O. daily in divided doses given q 6 hours (1 mg = 1,600 units); or 1.2 to 24 million units I.M. or I.V. daily in divided doses given q 4 hours. **Children:** 25,000 to 100,000 units/kg P.O. daily in divided doses given q 6 hours; or 25,000 to 300,000 units/kg I.M. or I.V. daily in divided doses given q 4 hours.

Adverse reactions

Blood: hemolytic anemia, leukopenia, thrombocytopenia. **CNS:** neuropathy, seizures with high doses. **Metabolic:** possible severe potassium toxicity with high doses (hyperreflexia, seizures, coma). **Local:** *thrombophlebitis, pain at injection site.* **Other:** hypersensitivity (rash, urticaria, maculopapular eruptions, ***exfoliative dermatitis,*** chills, fever, edema, ***anaphylaxis***), overgrowth of nonsusceptible organisms.

Interactions

Probenecid: increased blood levels of penicillin. Probenecid may be used for this purpose.

Nursing diagnoses

- High risk for injury related to the ineffectiveness of penicillin G potassium in eradicating the infection.
- Altered protection related to an allergic reaction to pencillin G potassium.
- Knowledge deficit related to penicillin G potassium therapy.

Nursing interventions

- *Use cautiously* in patients with other drug allergies, especially to cephalosporins (possible cross-allergenicity).
- Obtain specimen for culture and sensitivity tests before first dose. Therapy may begin pending test results.
- Before giving penicillin, ask the patient if he's had any allergic reactions to this drug. However, a negative history of penicillin allergy is no guarantee against a future allergic reaction.
- Tell patient to take the medication exactly as prescribed, even if he feels better, and to take entire amount prescribed.
- Tell him to call the doctor if rash, fever, or chills develop. A rash is the most common allergic reaction.
- When given orally, drug may cause GI disturbances. Food may interfere with absorption, so give 1 to 2 hours before meals or 2 to 3 hours after.
- Extremely painful when given I.M. Inject deep into large muscle.
- Patients with poor renal function are predisposed to high blood levels. Monitor renal function closely.
- If patient has a high blood level of this drug, he may have seizures. Institute seizure precautions.
- With large doses and prolonged therapy, bacterial and fungal superinfections may occur, especially in elderly, debilitated, or immunosuppressed patients. Close observation is essential.
- Warn patient never to use leftover penicillin for a new illness or to share penicillin with family or friends.
- Give penicillin G potassium at least 1 hour before bacteriostatic antibiotics.
- **I.V. use:** When giving I.V., mix with D_5W or a saline solution.
- Give I.V. intermittently to prevent vein irritation. Change site every 48 hours.

General
Classification: antianginal (calcium channel blocker). **Pregnancy risk category:** C.

Mechanism of action
Inhibits calcium ion influx across cardiac and smooth muscle cells, decreasing myocardial contractility and oxygen demand, and dilates coronary arteries and peripheral arterioles.

Indications and dosage
- Management of vasospastic (Prinzmetal's or variant) angina and classic chronic stable angina pectoris. **Adults:** 30 mg P.O. t.i.d. or q.i.d. before meals and at bedtime. Dosage may be gradually increased to maximum 360 mg/day, in divided doses. Alternatively, use 120 or 180 mg (dual-release capsule). Titrate as needed and tolerated to maximum 480 mg daily.
- Hypertension. **Adults:** 60 mg P.O. b.i.d. (extended-release capsule). Titrate dosage to effect. Maximum recommended dosage is 360 mg/day; experience with higher doses is limited. Alternatively, initially use 180 to 240 mg daily (dual-release capsule). Maximum effect is seen within 14 days. Adjust dosage as necessary.
- Atrial fibrillation or flutter; paroxysmal supraventricular tachycardia. **Adults:** 0.25 mg/kg as a bolus injection over 2 minutes. If response is inadequate, a dose of 0.35 mg/kg may be given after 15 minutes and followed with a continuous infusion of 10 mg/hour. Some patients may respond to infusion rates of 5 mg/hour; do not exceed the maximum dose of 15 mg/hour. Infusions lasting longer than 24 hours are not recommended.

Adverse reactions
CNS: *headache, fatigue, drowsiness,* dizziness, nervousness, depression, insomnia, confusion. **CV:** *edema,* ***arrhythmias,*** flushing, bradycardia, hypotension, conduction abnormalities, ***CHF.*** **GI:** *nausea,* vomiting, diarrhea. **GU:** nocturia, polyuria. **Hepatic:** transient elevation of liver enzymes. **Skin:** *rash,* pruritus. **Other:** photosensitivity.

Interactions
Cimetidine: may inhibit diltiazem metabolism. Monitor for toxicity. **Cyclosporine:** diltiazem may increase serum cyclosporine levels, possibly by decreasing its metabolism, leading to increased risk of cyclosporine toxicity. Avoid concomitant use. **Digoxin:** diltiazem may increase serum levels of digoxin. Monitor for toxicity. **Furosemide:** forms a precipitate when mixed with diltiazem injection. Administer through separate I.V. lines. **Propranolol (and other beta blockers):** may prolong cardiac conduction time. Use together cautiously.

Nursing diagnoses
- Pain related to ineffectiveness of diltiazem therapy.
- Altered protection related to diltiazem-induced arrhythmia.
- Knowledge deficit related to diltiazem therapy.

Nursing interventions
- *Contraindicated* in sick sinus syndrome, unless a functioning ventricular pacemaker is present; hypotension when systolic blood pressure is less than 90 mm Hg; and second- or third-degree AV block.
- *Use cautiously* in elderly patients because duration of action may be prolonged, in impaired ventricular function or conduction abnormalities, and in impaired hepatic or renal function.
- Monitor blood pressure during initiation of therapy and dosage adjustments. Assist patients with ambulation because dizziness may occur.
- If systolic pressure is less than 90 mm Hg, or heart rate is less than 60 beats/minute, withhold dose and notify doctor.

General

Classification: antibiotic (natural penicillin).
Pregnancy risk category: B.

Mechanism of action

Bactericidal against microorganisms by inhibiting cell wall synthesis during active multiplication. Bacteria resist penicillin by producing penicillinases—enzymes that convert penicillin to inactive penicilloic acid.

Indications and dosage

- Congenital syphilis. **Children under age 2:** 50,000 units/kg I.M. as a single dose.
- Group A streptococcal upper respiratory infections. **Adults:** 1.2 million units I.M. in a single injection. **Children over 27 kg:** 900,000 units I.M. in a single injection. **Children under 27 kg:** 300,000 to 600,000 units I.M. in a single injection.
- Prophylaxis of poststreptococcal rheumatic fever. **Adults and children:** 1.2 million units I.M. once a month or 600,000 units twice a month.
- Syphilis of less than 1 year's duration. **Adults:** 2.4 million units I.M. in a single dose.
- Syphilis of more than 1 year's duration. **Adults:** 2.4 million units I.M. weekly for 3 successive weeks.

Adverse reactions

Blood: eosinophilia, hemolytic anemia, thrombocytopenia, leukopenia. **CNS:** neuropathy, seizures with high doses. **Local:** pain and sterile abscess at injection site. **Other:** hypersensitivity (maculopapular and ***exfoliative dermatitis,*** chills, fever, edema, ***anaphylaxis***).

Interactions

Probenecid: increased blood levels of penicillin. Probenecid may be used for this purpose.

Nursing diagnoses

- High risk for injury related to the ineffectiveness of penicillin G benzathine in eradicating the infection.
- Altered protection related to allergic reactions to pencillin G benzathine.
- Knowledge deficit related to penicillin G benzathine therapy.

Nursing interventions

- *Use cautiously* in patients with other drug allergies, especially to cephalosporins (possible cross-allergenicity).
- Obtain specimen for culture and sensitivity tests before first dose. Therapy may begin pending test results.
- Before giving penicillin, ask the patient if he's had any allergic reactions to this drug. However, a negative history of penicillin allergy is no guarantee against a future allergic reaction.
- Very slow absorption time makes allergic reactions difficult to treat.
- Tell the patient to call the doctor if rash, fever, or chills develop. Fever and eosinophilia are the most common allergic reactions.
- With large doses and prolonged therapy, bacterial and fungal superinfections may occur, especially in elderly, debilitated, or immunosuppressed patients. Close observation is essential.
- Shake the medication well before injection.
- Inject deeply into upper outer quadrant of buttocks in adults; in midlateral thigh in infants and small children.
- Give penicillin G benzathine at least 1 hour before bacteriostatic antibiotics.
- Never give I.V. Inadvertent I.V. administration has caused cardiac arrest and death.

General

Classification: antihistamine, antiemetic, antivertigo agent (H_1-receptor antagonist). **Pregnancy risk category:** B.

Mechanism of action

Unknown. May affect neural pathways originating in the labyrinth to inhibit nausea and vomiting.

Indications and dosage

- Nausea, vomiting, dizziness of motion sickness (treatment and prevention). **Adults:** 50 mg P.O. q 4 hours, or 100 mg q 4 hours if drowsiness is not objectionable; or 50 mg I.M., p.r.n.; or 50 mg I.V. diluted in 10 ml sodium chloride solution, injected over 2 minutes. Maximum dose is 400 mg/day. **Children:** 5 mg/kg P.O. or I.M., divided q.i.d. Maximum dosage is 300 mg daily. Don't use in children under 2 years.

Adverse reactions

CNS: *drowsiness,* headache, incoordination, dizziness. **CV:** palpitations, hypotension. **EENT:** blurred vision, tinnitus. **GI:** dry mouth and respiratory passages.

Interactions

Alcohol, CNS depressants: additive CNS depression. Avoid concomitant use.

Nursing diagnoses

- High risk for fluid volume deficit related to nausea and vomiting induced by motion sickness.
- Pain related to dimenhydrinate-induced headache.
- Knowledge deficit related to dimenhydrinate therapy.

Nursing interventions

- *Contraindicated* in patients with hypersensitivity to the drug.
- *Use cautiously* in seizures, narrow-angle glaucoma, and enlargement of prostate gland.
- Be alert for signs of sclerosis. Undiluted solution is irritating to veins.
- Warn patient against driving and other activities that require alertness until CNS effects of the drug are known.
- Dimenhydrinate may mask ototoxicity of aminoglycoside antibiotics.
- Avoid mixing parenteral preparation with other drugs; dimenhydrinate is incompatible with many solutions.
- Be aware that dimenhydrinate may mask symptoms of ototoxicity, brain tumor, or intestinal obstruction.

General

Classification: antihypertensive (beta-adrenergic blocker). **Pregnancy risk category:** C.

Mechanism of action

Blocks both $beta_1$- and $beta_2$-adrenergic receptors.

Indications and dosage

• Mild to moderate hypertension. **Adults:** 20 mg P.O. once daily. Usually given with other antihypertensive drugs, such as thiazide diuretics.

Adverse reactions

CNS: syncope, *dizziness,* vertigo, headache, fatigue, depression, paresthesia, hypoesthesia or hyperesthesia, lethargy, anxiety, diminished concentration, sleep disturbances, nightmares, bizarre or frequent dreams, sedation, changes in behavior, catatonia, hallucinations, alteration of time perception, memory loss, light-headedness. **CV:** *bradycardia,* chest pain, ***CHF,*** asymptomatic hypotension, peripheral ischemia, worsening of angina or arterial insufficiency, peripheral vascular insufficiency, claudication, edema, ***pulmonary edema,*** vasodilation, symptomatic postural hypotension, tachycardia, palpitations, conduction disturbances, first-degree and third-degree heart block, intensification of AV block. **EENT:** eye discomfort. **GI:** gastric pain, flatulence, dry mouth, nausea, constipation, heartburn, vomiting, taste alteration. **GU:** impotence, nocturia, urine retention. **Metabolic:** hyperglycemia, hypoglycemia. **Respiratory:** pharyngitis, laryngospasm, respiratory distress, shortness of breath. **Skin:** pallor, flushing, rash. **Other:** allergic reactions, decreased libido.

Interactions

Clonidine: possible paradoxical hypertension. Also, beta blockers may enhance rebound hypertension when clonidine is withdrawn. **Insulin, oral antidiabetic agents:** altered antidiabetic response. Monitor patient closely. **NSAIDs:** possibly decreased antihypertensive effects. **Prazosin, terazosin:** possibly enhanced "first dose" orthostatic hypotension. **Sympathomimetics, including isoproterenol, dopamine, or dobutamine:** reduced antihypertensive response. **Theophylline:** possibly decreased bronchodilator effect.

Nursing diagnoses

• Altered tissue perfusion (renal, cerebral, cardiopulmonary, peripheral) related to the patient's underlying condition.
• Potential for injury related to adverse CNS reactions to penbutolol.
• Knowledge deficit related to penbutolol therapy.

Nursing interventions

• *Contraindicated* in patients with sinus bradycardia, cardiogenic shock, CHF, or overt cardiac failure; in patients with greater than first-degree heart block; in patients with pheochromocytoma unless alpha-adrenergic blockers are also used; and in those with chronic airway disease.
• *Use cautiously* in patients with a history of CHF controlled by digitalis glycosides and diuretics or those with a history of bronchospastic disease.
• Advise patients not to discontinue the drug abruptly, because sudden withdrawal of other beta blockers has precipitated angina and MI. However, withdrawal of beta blockers in patients who've had an MI doesn't present major problems.
• Teach patient the signs and symptoms of CHF (edema and pulmonary congestion). Advise him to contact the doctor if these effects occur.
• Always check patient's apical pulse before giving this drug. If you detect extremes in pulse rates, withhold drug and call doctor immediately.
• Monitor blood pressure, ECG, and heart rate and rhythm frequently.
• Explain to patient the importance of taking this drug regularly, even when he's feeling well. Tell him to call doctor if adverse reactions occur.
• Advise the patient to check with his doctor or pharmacist before taking OTC medications.

General

Classification: oxytocic (prostaglandin). **Pregnancy risk category:** not applicable.

Mechanism of action

Produces strong, prompt contractions of uterine smooth muscle, possibly mediated by calcium and cAMP.

Indications and dosage

• Abort second trimester pregnancy, evacuate uterus in cases of missed abortion, intrauterine fetal deaths up to 28 weeks of gestation, or benign hydatidiform mole. **Adults:** insert 20-mg suppository high into posterior vaginal fornix. Repeat q 3 to 5 hours until abortion is complete.

Adverse reactions

CNS: headache, *dizziness*. **CV:** hypotension (in large doses). **GI:** *nausea, vomiting, diarrhea.* **GU:** vaginal pain, vaginitis. **Other:** *fever, shivering, chills, joint inflammation, nocturnal leg cramps, bronchospasm.*

Interactions

Alcohol: high doses may decrease effectiveness.

Nursing diagnoses

• High risk for fluid volume deficit related to possible dinoprostone-induced vomiting and diarrhea.
• High risk for altered body temperature related to possible dinoprostone-induced fever.
• Knowledge deficit related to dinoprostone therapy.

Nursing interventions

• *Contraindicated* in pelvic inflammatory disease or history of pelvic surgery, incisions, uterine fibroids, or cervical stenosis.
• *Use cautiously* in asthma, seizure disorder, anemia, diabetes, hypertension or hypotension, jaundice, and cardiovascular, renal, or hepatic disease.
• Administer only when critical care facilities are readily available.
• Replace fluids if nausea or diarrhea occurs. Keep in mind that patient may be pretreated with an antiemetic and an antidiarrheal agent.
• Store suppositories in freezer at temperature of − 4° F (− 20° C). Just before use, warm dinoprostone suppositories in their wrapping to room temperature.
• After administration, have patient remain supine for 10 minutes.
• Be aware that dinoprostone-induced fever is self-limiting and transient and occurs in approximately 50% of all patients. Treat with water or alcohol sponging and increased fluid intake rather than with aspirin.
• Check vaginal discharge daily.
• Keep in mind that abortion should be complete within 30 hours.
• Know that dinoprostone is being investigated as an agent that promotes cervical inducibility (cervical "ripening") before induction of labor with oxytocin.

General

Classification: analeptic (oxazolidinedione derivative, CNS stimulant). **Pregnancy risk category:** B. **Controlled substance schedule:** IV.

Mechanism of action

Main site of activity appears to be the cerebral cortex and the reticular activating system. Promotes nerve impulse transmission by releasing stored norepinephrine from nerve terminals in the brain.

Indications and dosage

• Attention deficit disorder with hyperactivity. **Children 6 years and older:** initially, 37.5 mg P.O. given in the morning. Daily dose can be raised by 18.75 mg weekly. The effective dosage range is 56.25 to 75 mg daily; the maximum dosage is 112.5 mg daily.

Adverse reactions

CNS: *insomnia,* malaise, irritability, fatigue, mild depression, dizziness, headache, drowsiness, hallucinations, nervousness (with large doses), ***seizures,*** *Tourette syndrome, psychosis.* **CV:** *tachycardia (with large doses).* **GI:** anorexia, abdominal pain, nausea, diarrhea. **Hepatic:** elevated liver enzymes. **Skin:** rash.

Interactions

Insulin, oral antidiabetics: pemoline may alter requirements of antidiabetic agents.

Nursing diagnoses

• High risk for injury related to the patient's underlying disorder.
• Sleep pattern disturbance related to pemoline-induced insomnia.
• Knowledge deficit related to pemoline therapy.

Nursing interventions

• *Contraindicated* in patients with hepatic dysfunction and in children under age 6.
• *Use cautiously* in patients with impaired renal function or a history of Tourette syndrome. Drug may accumulate.
• May precipitate Tourette syndrome in children. Monitor especially at the start of therapy.
• Closely monitor patients on long-term therapy for possible blood or hepatic abnormalities and for growth suppression.
• Drug is structurally dissimilar to amphetamines or methylphenidate. However, it may produce similar adverse reactions, including lowered seizure threshold. Also, the drug has a greater potential for abuse and dependence than previously thought.
• Therapeutic effects may not be evident for up to 4 weeks.
• Give the drug at least 6 hours before bedtime to avoid insomnia.

General

Classification: antihistamine, antiemetic, antivertigo agent, antitussive, sedative-hypnotic, topical anesthetic, antidyskinetic (H_1-receptor antagonist). **Pregnancy risk category:** B.

Mechanism of action

Competes with histamine for H_1-receptor sites on effector cells. Prevents but does not reverse histamine-mediated responses, particularly histamine's effects on the smooth muscle of the bronchial tubes, GI tract, uterus, and blood vessels. Structurally related to local anesthetics, diphenhydramine provides local anesthesia by preventing initiation and transmission of nerve impulses. Also suppresses the cough reflex by a direct effect in the medulla of the brain.

Indications and dosage

- Rhinitis, allergy symptoms, motion sickness, Parkinson's disease. **Adults:** 25 to 50 mg P.O. t.i.d. or q.i.d.; or 10 to 50 mg deep I.M. or I.V. Maximum I.M. or I.V. dosage is 400 mg daily. **Children under 12 years:** 5 mg/kg daily P.O., deep I.M., or I.V. divided q.i.d. Maximum dosage is 300 mg daily.
- Sedation. **Adults:** 25 to 50 mg P.O., or deep I.M., p.r.n.
- As a nighttime sleep aid. **Adults:** 50 mg P.O. at bedtime.
- Nonproductive cough. **Adults:** 25 mg P.O. q 4 hours (not to exceed 150 mg daily). **Children 6 to 12 years:** 12.5 mg P.O. q 4 hours (not to exceed 75 mg daily). **Children 2 to 6 years:** 6.25 mg P.O. q 4 hours (not to exceed 37.5 mg daily).

Note: Children under 12 years should use only as directed by a doctor.

Adverse reactions

CNS: (especially in elderly patients) *drowsiness,* confusion, insomnia, headache, vertigo. **CV:** palpitations. **EENT:** diplopia, nasal stuffiness. **GI:** *nausea,* vomiting, diarrhea, *dry mouth,* constipation. **GU:** dysuria, urine retention. **Skin:** urticaria, photosensitivity.

Interactions

Alcohol, CNS depressants: increased sedation. Use together cautiously. **MAO inhibitors:** increased anticholinergic effects. Don't use together.

Nursing diagnoses

- Ineffective airway clearance related to the patient's underlying condition.
- High risk for injury related to diphenhydramine-induced drowsiness.
- Knowledge deficit related to diphenhydramine therapy.

Nursing interventions

- *Contraindicated* in acute asthmatic attacks.
- *Use cautiously* in narrow-angle glaucoma, prostatic hypertrophy, pyloroduodenal and bladder-neck obstruction, and stenosing peptic ulcers; in newborns; and in asthmatic, hypertensive, or cardiac patients. Antihistamines are not recommended for use by women who are breast-feeding because small amounts of drug are excreted in breast milk.
- Alternate injection sites to prevent irritation. Administer deep I.M. into large muscle.
- Warn patient to avoid alcoholic beverages and driving or other hazardous activities during therapy.
- Give with food or milk to reduce GI distress. Tell patient to take coffee or tea to reduce drowsiness. Sugarless gum, sour hard candy, or ice chips may relieve dry mouth.
- When used to prevent motion sickness, instruct patient to take 30 minutes before travel.
- Tell patient to stop taking drug 4 days before allergy skin tests to preserve accuracy.
- Inform patient of possible photosensitivity. Advise use of a sunscreen.

General

Classification: antidepressant (serotonin uptake inhibitor). **Pregnancy risk category:** B.

Mechanism of action

• Blocks the reuptake of serotonin (5-HT) into nerve terminals within the CNS.

Indications and dosage

• Depression. **Adults:** initially, 20 mg P.O. daily, preferably in the morning. As indicated, increase dosage in 10-mg/day increments, at 1-week intervals, to a maximum of 50 mg daily. **Elderly or debilitated patients; patients with severe hepatic or renal disease:** initially, 10 mg P.O. daily, preferably in the morning. Increase dosage as above to a maximum of 40 mg daily.

Adverse reactions

CNS: blurred vision, *somnolence, dizziness, insomnia, tremor, nervousness,* anxiety, paresthesia, decreased libido. **CV:** palpitations, vasodilation, postural hypotension. **EENT:** lump or tightness in throat. **GI:** *nausea, dry mouth, constipation, diarrhea, decreased appetite,* flatulence, vomiting, dyspepsia, increased appetite. **GU:** *ejaculatory disturbances, male genital disorders,* urinary disorders, female genital disorders. **Skin:** *sweating,* rash. **Other:** asthenia, hyponatremia, myopathy, myalgia, myasthenia, taste perversion.

Interactions

Cimetidine: decreased hepatic metabolism of paroxetine, leading to risk of toxicity. Dosage adjustments may be necessary. **Digoxin:** paroxetine may decrease digoxin levels. Monitor closely. **MAO inhibitors:** concomitant use may increase risk of serious, sometimes fatal, adverse reactions. Don't administer paroxetine (or MAO inhibitors) within 14 days of discontinuing MAO inhibitor (or paroxetine) therapy. **Phenobarbital, phenytoin:** possible altered pharmacokinetics of both drugs. Dosage adjustments may be necessary. **Procyclidine:** paroxetine may increase procyclidine levels. Monitor for excessive anticholinergic effects. **Tryptophan:** may increase incidence of adverse reactions, such as sweating, headache, nausea, and dizziness. Avoid concomitant use. **Warfarin:** increased risk of bleeding. Avoid concomitant use.

Nursing diagnoses

• Ineffective individual coping related to the patient's underlying condition.
• Sleep pattern disturbance related to paroxetine-induced insomnia and drowsiness.
• Knowledge deficit related to paroxetine therapy.

Nursing interventions

• *Use cautiously* in patients with a history of seizure disorders or mania; hepatic or renal impairment; or severe, concomitant systemic illness.
• Several cases of hyponatremia have been reported, usually in elderly patients; some were taking diuretics or were otherwise volume depleted. Therefore, use cautiously in patients at risk for volume depletion and monitor appropriately.
• Because drug is excreted in breast milk, also use cautiously in breast-feeding women.
• Closely supervise high-risk suicidal patients during initial drug therapy. Such patients should receive prescriptions for a limited number of tablets to reduce the risk of overdose.
• Expect a delay before maximum clinical benefits of drug are seen. Typically, full effects of antidepressant therapy are seen after 4 weeks or more of therapy. Clinical trials with paroxetine have demonstrated clinical efficacy for periods of 1 year at average doses of 30 mg daily.
• Overdose is usually associated with nausea, vomiting, drowsiness, sinus tachycardia, and dilated pupils. There is no specific antidote for the drug; forced diuresis, dialysis, hemoperfusion, and exchange transfusion are believed to be of little benefit. Establish and maintain an airway, and perform gastric evacuation. Activated charcoal (20 to 30 g) may be administered every 4 to 6 hours for the first 24 to 48 hours after ingestion.

diphenidol hydrochloride Vontrol**

General
Classification: antiemetic and antivertigo agent.
Pregnancy risk category: C.

Mechanism of action
Influences the chemoreceptor trigger zone to inhibit nausea and vomiting.

Indications and dosage
- Peripheral (labyrinthine) dizziness. **Adults:** 25 to 50 mg P.O. q 4 hours, p.r.n.
- Nausea and vomiting. **Adults:** 25 to 50 mg P.O. q 4 hours, p.r.n. **Children over 23 kg:** 0.88 mg/kg P.O. q 4 hours, not to exceed 5.5 mg/kg/24 hours. Usual dosage is 25 mg.

Adverse reactions
CNS: *drowsiness,* dizziness, sleep disturbances, *confusion;* auditory and visual hallucinations, disorientation occur within 3 days of starting drug, subside within 3 days after stopping drug. **CV:** transient hypotension. **GI:** dry mouth, nausea, indigestion, heartburn. **Skin:** urticaria. **Other:** antiemetic effect may mask symptoms of ototoxicity, brain tumor, intestinal obstruction, or other conditions.

Interactions
None significant.

Nursing diagnoses
- High risk for fluid volume deficit related to nausea and vomiting induced by motion sickness.
- Knowledge deficit related to diphenidol therapy.

Nursing interventions
- *Contraindicated* in anuria.
- *Use cautiously* in glaucoma, pyloric stenosis, pylorospasm, obstructive lesions of GI or GU tract, prostatic hypertrophy, or organic cardioaspasm.
- Be aware that this drug is used in Ménière's disease, following middle and inner ear surgery, labyrinthine disturbances, and to control nausea and vomiting associated with infectious diseases, cancers, radiation sickness, general anesthetics, and antineoplastic agents.
- Expect to discontinue drug if auditory or visual hallucinations or disorientation or confusion occurs.
- Closely supervise patient. Patients are usually hospitalized when receiving this drug. Monitor intake and output; report any changes.
- Be aware that treatment of toxicity is symptomatic and supportive.

General
Classification: amebicide (aminoglycoside). **Pregnancy risk category:** C.

Mechanism of action
Acts as an intestinal amebicide. Drug's specific mechanism of action is unknown.

Indications and dosage
- Acute and chronic intestinal amebiasis. **Adults and children:** 25 to 35 mg/kg P.O. daily in three doses for 5 to 10 days after meals.
- Tapeworms (fish, beef, pork, dog). **Adults:** 1 g P.O. q 15 minutes for four doses. **Children:** 11 mg/kg P.O. q 15 minutes for four doses.

Adverse reactions
Blood: eosinophilia. **CNS:** headache, vertigo. **EENT:** ototoxicity. **GI:** anorexia, *nausea, vomiting, epigastric pain and burning, abdominal cramps,* diarrhea, constipation, increased motility, steatorrhea, pruritus ani, malabsorption syndrome. **GU:** hematuria, nephrotoxicity. **Skin:** rash, exanthema, pruritus. **Other:** overgrowth of nonsusceptible organisms.

Interactions
None significant.

Nursing diagnoses
- High risk for injury related to dosage regimen inadequate to relieve infection.
- Altered nutrition: Less than body requirements, related to nausea, vomiting, epigastric pain and burning, and abdominal cramps.
- Knowledge deficit related to paromomycin therapy.

Nursing interventions
- *Contraindicated* in patients with impaired renal function or intestinal obstruction.
- *Use cautiously* in patients with ulcerative lesions of the bowel to avoid inadvertent absorption and resulting renal toxicity. Drug is poorly absorbed orally, but will accumulate with renal impairment or ulcerative lesions.
- Ask the patient about a history of sensitivity to drug before the first dose.
- Administer the drug with or after meals.
- To help prevent reinfestation, teach the patient about the need for good personal hygiene, especially proper hand-washing technique. Tell him to refrain from preparing food until stools are negative.
- Criterion for cure is the absence of amebae in stools, which are examined weekly for 6 weeks after treatment and thereafter at monthly intervals for 2 years. Examine the feces of family members or suspected contacts.
- Avoid high doses or prolonged therapy.
- Watch for signs of superinfection, such as continued fever and other signs of new infections, especially monilial infections.

General

Classification: antidiarrheal (opiate). **Pregnancy risk category:** C. **Controlled substance schedule:** V.

Mechanism of action

Increases smooth-muscle tone in the GI tract, inhibits motility and propulsion, and diminishes secretions.

Indications and dosage

- Acute, nonspecific diarrhea. **Adults:** initially, 5 mg P.O. q.i.d., then adjust dosage. **Children 2 to 12 years:** 0.3 to 0.4 mg/kg P.O. daily in 4 divided doses (liquid form). For maintenance, initial dose may be reduced by as much as 75%.

Don't use in children under 2 years.

Adverse reactions

CNS: *sedation, dizziness,* headache, drowsiness, lethargy, restlessness, depression, euphoria. **CV:** tachycardia. **EENT:** mydriasis. **GI:** *dry mouth,* nausea, vomiting, abdominal discomfort or distention, ***paralytic ileus,*** anorexia, fluid retention in bowel (may mask depletion of extracellular fluid and electrolytes, especially in young children treated for acute gastroenteritis). **GU:** urine retention. **Skin:** pruritus, giant urticaria, rash. **Other:** physical dependence in long-term use, ***angioedema, respiratory depression.***

Interactions

Alcohol, CNS depression, tranquilizers, narcotics, barbiturates: enhanced CNS depression. Closely monitor patients. **MAO inhibitors:** potential hypertensive crisis. Avoid concomitant use.

Nursing diagnoses

- Diarrhea related to interruption of normal elimination pattern characterized by frequent loose stools.
- Altered thought processes related to drug-induced CNS adverse reactions.
- Knowledge deficit related to diphenoxylate therapy.

Nursing interventions

- *Contraindicated* in acute diarrhea resulting from poison until toxic material is eliminated from GI tract; acute diarrhea caused by organisms that penetrate intestinal mucosa; diarrhea resulting from antibiotic-induced pseudomembranous enterocolitis; and in jaundiced patients.
- *Use cautiously* in children, in hepatic disease, in narcotic dependence, in pregnant women, and in acute ulcerative colitis. Stop therapy immediately if abdominal distention or other signs of toxic megacolon develop.
- Correct fluid and electrolyte disturbances before starting drug. Dehydration, especially in young children, may increase risk of delayed toxicity.
- Advise patient to avoid hazardous activities such as driving until the adverse CNS effects of the drug are known.
- The risk of physical dependence increases with high dosage and long-term use. Atropine sulfate is included to discourage abuse.
- Know that drug is not likely to be effective if no response occurs within 48 hours.
- Tell patient not to use this drug to treat acute diarrhea for longer than 2 days and to seek medical attention if diarrhea continues.
- Warn patient not to exceed recommended dosage. Naloxone may be used to treat respiratory depression resulting from overdose. A dose of 2.5 mg of diphenoxylate is as effective as 5 ml camphorated tincture of opium.
- This drug is not indicated in the treatment of antibiotic-induced diarrhea.

General

Classification: anti-inflammatory agent (glucocorticoid). **Pregnancy risk category:** C.

Mechanism of action

Decreases inflammation, mainly by stabilizing leukocyte lysosomal membranes. Also suppresses the immune response, stimulates bone marrow, and influences protein, fat, and carbohydrate metabolism.

Indications and dosage

• Inflammatory conditions. **Adults:** 0.5 to 6 mg P.O. t.i.d. or q.i.d. **Children:** 58 to 800 mcg/kg P.O. daily, divided t.i.d. or q.i.d.

Adverse reactions

Most adverse reactions are dose- or duration-dependent. **CNS:** *euphoria, insomnia,* psychotic behavior, pseudotumor cerebri. **CV:** edema, ***CHF,*** hypertension. **EENT:** cataracts, glaucoma. **GI:** *peptic ulcer,* GI irritation, increased appetite. **Metabolic:** hypokalemia, hyperglycemia, carbohydrate intolerance, growth suppression. **Skin:** delayed wound healing, acne, skin eruptions. **Other:** weakness, osteoporosis, pancreatitis, hirsutism, susceptibility to infections. Acute adrenal insufficiency may occur with increased stress (infection, surgery, or trauma) or abrupt withdrawal after long-term therapy. **Withdrawal symptoms:** rebound inflammation, fatigue, weakness, arthralgia, fever, dizziness, lethargy, depression, fainting, orthostatic hypotension, dyspnea, anorexia, hypoglycemia. ***Sudden withdrawal may be fatal.***

Interactions

Barbiturates, phenytoin, rifampin: decreased corticosteroid effect. Corticosteroid dose may need to be increased. **NSAIDs, indomethacin, aspirin:** increased risk of GI distress and bleeding. Combine cautiously. **Oral anticoagulants:** altered dosage requirements. Monitor prothrombin times closely. **Potassium-depleting drugs such as thiazide diuretics:** enhanced potassium-wasting effects of paramethasone. Monitor serum potassium levels. **Skin-test antigens:** decreased response. Defer testing until after therapy. **Vaccines and toxoids:** reduced antibody response and increased risk of neurologic complications. Avoid concomitant use.

Nursing diagnoses

• Altered protection related to inflammation.
• High risk for injury related to the adverse effects of paramethasone.
• Knowledge deficit related to paramethasone therapy.

Nursing interventions

• *Contraindicated* in systemic fungal infections and alternate-day therapy.
• *Use cautiously* in GI ulceration or renal disease, hypertension, osteoporosis, varicella, vaccinia, exanthema, diabetes mellitus, Cushing's syndrome, thromboembolic disorders, seizures, myasthenia gravis, metastatic cancer, CHF, tuberculosis, ocular herpes simplex, hypoalbuminemia, emotional instability, and psychotic tendencies.
• Tell patient receiving long-term therapy to exercise or have physical therapy. Give vitamin D or calcium supplements as ordered.
• Gradually lower dosage after lengthy therapy, titrating to lowest effective dose.
• Monitor patient's weight, blood pressure, and serum electrolytes.
• Drug may mask or exacerbate infections.
• Give a daily dose in the morning for better results and less toxicity.
• Watch for signs of early adrenal insufficiency.
• Instruct patient to carry a card identifying his need for supplemental systemic glucocorticoids.
• Watch for depression or psychosis with high doses.
• Recommend periodic ophthalmic examinations for patients receiving long-term therapy.
• Unless contraindicated, give low-sodium diet high in potassium and protein.
• Warn patients on long-term therapy about cushingoid symptoms.

General
Classification: diphtheria and tetanus prophylaxis (toxoid). **Pregnancy risk category:** C.

Mechanism of action
Promotes immunity to diphtheria and tetanus by inducing production of antitoxins.

Indications and dosage
- Primary immunization. **Adults and children over 7 years:** use adult strength; 0.5 ml I.M. 4 to 6 weeks apart for two doses and a third dose 1 year later. Booster is 0.5 ml I.M. q 10 years. **Children 1 to 6 years:** use pediatric strength; 0.5 ml I.M. at least 4 weeks apart for two doses. Give booster dosage 6 to 12 months after the second injection. If the final immunizing dose is given after the 7th birthday, use the adult strength. **Infants 6 weeks to 1 year:** use pediatric strength; 0.5 ml I.M. at least 4 weeks apart for three doses. Give booster dose 6 to 12 months after third injection.

Adverse reactions
Systemic: chills, fever, malaise, ***anaphylaxis.*** **Local:** stinging, edema, erythema, pain, induration.

Interactions
None significant.

Nursing diagnoses
- Altered protection related to lack of immunity to diphtheria and tetanus toxoids.
- Ineffective breathing pattern related to possible diphtheria and tetanus toxoids-induced anaphylaxis.
- Knowledge deficit related to diphtheria and tetanus toxoids.

Nursing interventions
- *Contraindicated* in immunosuppression, radiation, or corticosteroid therapy. Defer in respiratory illness or polio outbreaks, or acute illness except in emergency. Use single antigen during polio risks. In children under 6 years, use only when diphtheria, tetanus, and pertussis combination is contraindicated because of pertussis component.
- Verify strength (pediatric or adult) of toxoids used.
- Obtain history of allergies and reaction to immunization.
- Keep epinephrine 1:1,000 available.
- Give in site not recently used for vaccines or toxoids.

General

Classification: anticonvulsant (oxazolidinedione).
Pregnancy risk category: D.

Mechanism of action

Raises the threshold for cortical seizures but does not modify seizure pattern. Decreases projection of focal activity and reduces both repetitive spinal-cord transmission and spike-and-wave patterns of absence (petit mal) seizures.

Indications and dosage

- Refractory absence seizures. **Adults:** initially, 300 mg P.O. t.i.d. May increase by 300 mg weekly, up to 600 mg q.i.d., if needed. **Children over 6 years:** 0.9 g P.O. daily in divided doses t.i.d. or q.i.d. **Children 2 to 6 years:** 0.6 g P.O. daily in divided doses t.i.d. or q.i.d. **Children under 2 years:** 0.3 g P.O. daily in divided doses b.i.d.

Adverse reactions

Blood: ***neutropenia, leukopenia,*** eosinophilia, ***thrombocytopenia, pancytopenia, agranulocytosis, hypoplastic and aplastic anemia.*** **CNS:** *drowsiness,* fatigue, vertigo, headache, paresthesia, irritability. **CV:** hypertension, hypotension. **EENT:** photophobia, diplopia, epistaxis, retinal hemorrhage. **GI:** nausea, vomiting, abdominal pain, weight loss, bleeding gums. **GU:** albuminuria, vaginal bleeding. **Hepatic:** abnormal liver function tests. **Skin:** acneiform or morbilliform rash, ***exfoliative dermatitis, erythema multiforme,*** petechiae, alopecia, photosensitivity. **Other:** lymphadenopathy, lupus-like syndrome.

P

Interactions

None significant.

Nursing diagnoses

- Altered thought processes related to the patient's underlying condition.
- Altered protection related to drug-induced blood disorders.
- Knowledge deficit related to paramethadione therapy.

Nursing interventions

- *Contraindicated* in patients with renal or hepatic dysfunction or severe blood dyscrasia.
- *Use cautiously* in patients with retinal or optic nerve diseases.
- Nausea, dizziness, and visual disturbances can be signs of overdose. If the patient experiences these symptoms, he should call the doctor at once.
- Never withdraw the drug suddenly. Call the doctor immediately if adverse reactions develop.
- Discontinue the drug if scotomata, signs of hepatitis or lupus-like syndrome, lymphadenopathy, rash, nephrosis, hair loss, or generalized tonic-clonic seizures occur.
- Monitor CBC. Discontinue the drug if neutrophil count falls below 2,500/mm^3.
- Obtain liver function studies and urinalysis before therapy, then monthly during therapy.
- Tell the patient to report sore throat, fever, malaise, bruises, petechiae, or epistaxis to the doctor immediately.
- Advise him to wear dark glasses if photosensitivity occurs.
- Warn him not to drive a car or operate machinery until the CNS effects of the drug are known.
- Dilute oral solution with water before giving because it contains 65% alcohol.
- Give the drug with food or milk to minimize GI upset.

General

Classification: diphtheria, tetanus, and pertussis prophylaxis (toxoid and vaccine). **Pregnancy risk category:** D.

Mechanism of action

Promotes active immunity to diphtheria, tetanus, and pertussis by inducing production of antitoxins and antibodies.

Indications and dosage

- Primary immunization. **Children 6 weeks to 6 years:** 0.5 ml I.M. 2 months apart for three doses and a fourth dose 1 year later. Booster is 0.5 ml I.M. when starting school.

Not advised for adults or children over 6 years. The acellular vaccine may be used only for the fourth or fifth dose in children 17 months to 7 years who have previously been immunized with three or four doses of the whole-cell vaccine.

Adverse reactions

Systemic: slight fever, chills, malaise, ***seizures, encephalopathy, anaphylaxis,*** anorexia, vomiting. **Local:** *soreness, redness,* expected nodule remaining several weeks. **Other:** ***sudden infant death syndrome.***

Interactions

Immunosuppressive therapy: may reduce response to diphtheria and tetanus toxoids and pertussis (DTP) vaccine. Avoid if possible.

Nursing diagnoses

- Altered protection related to lack of immunity to diphtheria, tetanus, and pertussis.
- High risk for injury related to DTP-induced seizures.
- Knowledge deficit related to DTP vaccine.

Nursing interventions

- *Contraindicated* in corticosteroid therapy, immunosuppression, and history of seizures. Defer in acute febrile illness.
- Obtain history of allergies and reaction to immunization.
- Do not administer the pertussis component to children with preexisting neurologic disorders or to children who reacted to previous DTP injection by exhibiting neurologic signs. Give diphtheria and tetanus toxoids (DT) instead.
- Give parents information booklet describing the risks and benefits of this vaccine. Be sure parents read and understand the information before vaccine is administered.
- Administer DTP injection at same time as trivalent oral polio vaccine.
- Keep epinephrine 1:1,000 available.
- Keep vaccine refrigerated until ready to administer. Shake before using.
- Do not give subcutaneously. Administer only by deep I.M. injection, preferably in thigh or deltoid muscle.
- Do not use DTP vaccine for active infection.
- The acellular vaccine may have a lower incidence of local pain and fever.
- Also known as DPT.

para-aminosalicylate sodium

Sodium P.A.S.

General

Classification: antitubercular (aminobenzoic acid analogue). **Pregnancy risk category:** C.

Mechanism of action

Inhibits the enzymes responsible for folic acid biosynthesis (bacteriostatic).

Indications and dosage

- Adjunctive treatment of tuberculosis. **Adults:** 14 to 16 g P.O. daily, divided t.i.d. or q.i.d. **Children:** 240 to 360 mg/kg P.O. daily, divided t.i.d. or q.i.d.

Adverse reactions

Blood: ***leukopenia, agranulocytosis,*** eosinophila, thrombocytopenia, hemolytic anemia. **CNS:** encephalopathy. **CV:** vasculitis. **GI:** *nausea, vomiting,* diarrhea, *abdominal pain.* **GU:** albuminuria, hematuria, crystalluria. **Hepatic:** *jaundice, hepatitis.* **Metabolic:** acidosis, hypokalemia. **Skin:** rash. **Other:** infectious mononucleosis-like syndrome, fever, lymphadenopathy.

Interactions

Ascorbic acid, ammonium chloride: increasing urine acidity, increasing possibility of para-aminosalicylate crystalluria. Avoid concomitant use if possible. **Probenecid:** may increase levels of para-aminosalicylate. Use together cautiously. **Diphenhydramine:** inhibits absorption of para-aminosalicylate. Monitor for decreased para-aminosalicylate effect.

Nursing diagnoses

- Altered protection related to potential for tuberculosis recurrence and possible transmission of mycobacterial foci to other areas of the body.
- Impaired gas exchange related to changes in pulmonary tissue.
- Knowledge deficit related to para-aminosalicylate therapy.

Nursing interventions

- Contraindicated in patients on sodium-restricted diets. A 15-g dose provides 1.6 g sodium.
- *Use cautiously* in patients with impaired renal function, decreased hepatic function, or gastric ulcers.
- Give with meals or antacid to reduce GI distress. Tell patient to swallow enteric-coated tablets whole and not with antacids.
- Tell patient to notify doctor at once if fever, sore throat, rash, or symptoms of hepatic impairment (loss of appetite, fatigue, malaise, jaundice, dark urine) occur.
- Warn patient not to discontinue this drug without the doctor's consent.
- Concomitant administration of at least one other effective antitubercular drug is recommended.

General

Classification: coronary vasodilator, platelet aggregation inhibitor (pyrimidine analogue). **Pregnancy risk category:** C.

Mechanism of action

Inhibits platelet adhesion. Also inhibits the enzymes adenosine deaminase and phosphodiesterase.

Indications and dosage

- Inhibition of platelet adhesion in prosthetic heart valves, in combination with warfarin or aspirin. **Adults:** 75 to 100 mg P.O. q.i.d.
- Transient ischemic attack. **Adults:** 400 to 800 mg P.O. daily in divided doses.
- As an alternative to exercise in the evaluation of coronary artery disease during thallium myocardial perfusion imaging. **Adults:** 0.57 mg/kg as an I.V. infusion at a constant rate over 4 minutes (0.142 mg/kg/minute). Do not give more than 60 mg.

Adverse reactions

CNS: *headache, dizziness,* weakness. **CV:** flushing, fainting, *hypotension; chest pain,* ***ECG abnormalities,*** *blood pressure lability, hypertension* (with I.V. infusion). **GI:** *nausea,* vomiting, diarrhea. **Local:** irritation (with undiluted injection). **Skin:** rash.

Interactions

None significant.

Nursing diagnoses

- Altered cardiopulmonary tissue perfusion related to the patient's underlying condition.
- Pain related to adverse drug reactions.
- Knowledge deficit related to dipyridamole therapy.

Nursing interventions

- *Use cautiously* in hypotension and in patients receiving anticoagulant therapy.
- Observe for adverse reactions, especially with large doses. Monitor blood pressure.
- Administer 1 hour before meals. May administer with meals if patient develops GI distress.
- Watch for signs of bleeding or prolonged bleeding time, especially if patient is receiving large doses or long-term therapy.
- **I.V. use:** When given as a diagnostic agent, dilute in 0.45% or 0.9% sodium chloride solution or D_5W in a ratio of at least 1:2 for a total volume of 20 to 50 ml. Inject thallium-201 within 5 minutes of completing the 4-minute dipyridamole infusion.
- Use dipyridamole with oral anticoagulants to prevent thromboembolism in postoperative prosthetic valve patients. Do not use dipyridamole alone. Its value as part of an antithrombotic regimen is controversial; it may not be significantly better than using aspirin alone.

General

Classification: peripheral vasodilator (benzylisoquinolone derivative, opiate alkaloid). **Pregnancy risk category:** C.

Mechanism of action

Directly relaxes smooth muscle from the inhibition of phosphodiesterase, resulting in increased concentrations of cAMP.

Indications and dosage

- Relief of cerebral and peripheral ischemia associated with arterial spasm and myocardial ischemia; treatment of smooth muscle spasm (coronary occlusion, angina pectoris, sequelae of peripheral and pulmonary embolism, certain cerebral angiospastic states) and visceral spasms (biliary, ureteral, or GI colic). **Adults:** 60 to 300 mg P.O. 1 to 5 times daily; or 150- to 300-mg sustained-release preparations q 8 to 12 hours; or 30 to 120 mg I.M. or I.V. q 3 hours, as indicated.

Adverse reactions

CNS: *headache.* **CV:** *increased heart rate, increased blood pressure* (with parenteral use), depressed AV and intraventricular conduction, hypotension, ***arrhythmias.*** **GI:** constipation, *nausea.* **Other:** *sweating, flushing,* malaise, ***hepatic damage,*** increased depth of respiration.

Interactions

Levodopa: possible interference with the therapeutic effects of levodopa in patients with Parkinson's disease.

Nursing diagnoses

- Altered cerebral and peripheral tissue perfusion related to the patient's underlying condition.
- Pain related to adverse CV drug reactions.
- Knowledge deficit related to papaverine therapy.

Nursing interventions

- *Contraindicated* for I.V. use in patients with Parkinson's disease or complete AV block.
- *Use cautiously* in patients with glaucoma.
- Monitor blood pressure and heart rate and rhythm, especially in cardiac disease. Withhold dose and notify doctor immediately if changes occur.
- Not often used parenterally, except when immediate effect is desired.
- Give I.V. slowly (over 1 to 2 minutes) to avoid serious adverse reactions.
- Most effective when given early in the course of a disorder.
- Tell the patient to take his medication regularly; long-term therapy is required.
- Monitor for adverse hepatic reactions in patients receiving long-term therapy.
- Do not add lactated Ringer's solution to the injectable form; it will precipitate.
- Advise the patient to avoid tasks that require alertness (such as driving or operating heavy machinery) until CNS effects of the drug are known.
- Instruct him to avoid sudden posture changes to minimize the risks of orthostatic hypotension.
- The FDA has announced that this drug may not be effective for disease states indicated.
- Papaverine has been used experimentally, alone or with phenoxybenzamine, to treat impotence in males. Patients are taught to give the drug to themselves by intercavernosal injection.

General

Classification: antiarrhythmic (pyridine derivative). **Pregnancy risk category:** C.

Mechanism of action

A class Ia antiarrhythmic that depresses phase 0. It prolongs the action potential. All class I drugs have membrane stabilizing effects.

Indications and dosage

• Premature ventricular contractions (unifocal, multifocal, or coupled); ventricular tachycardia not severe enough to require electrocardioversion; to convert atrial fibrillation or flutter to normal sinus rhythm. **Adults:** usual maintenance dosage 150 to 200 mg P.O. q 6 hours; for patients who weigh less than 50 kg or those with renal, hepatic, or cardiac impairment – 100 mg P.O. q 6 hours. May give sustained-release capsule q 12 hours. **Children 12 to 18 years:** 6 to 15 mg/kg P.O. daily. **Children 4 to 12 years:** 10 to 15 mg/kg P.O. daily. **Children 1 to 4 years:** 10 to 20 mg/kg P.O. daily. **Children under 1 year:** 10 to 30 mg/kg P.O. daily. All children's dosages should be divided into equal amounts and given q 6 hours.

Recommended dosages in advanced renal insufficiency: if creatinine clearance is 30 to 40 ml/minute, dosing interval is q 8 hours; if creatinine clearance is 15 to 30 ml/minute, dosing interval is q 12 hours; if creatinine clearance is less than 15 ml/minute, dosing interval is q 24 hours.

Adverse reactions

CNS: dizziness, agitation, depression, fatigue, muscle weakness, syncope. **CV:** *hypotension,* ***CHF, heart block,*** edema, weight gain, ***arrhythmias.*** **EENT:** *blurred vision, dry eyes, dry nose.* **GI:** nausea, vomiting, anorexia, bloating, abdominal pain, *constipation, dry mouth.* **GU:** urine retention and urinary hesitancy. **Hepatic:** cholestatic jaundice. **Metabolic:** hypoglycemia. **Skin:** rash.

Interactions

Antiarrhythmics: possible additive or antagonized antiarrhythmic effects. **Phenytoin:** increases disopyramide's metabolism. Monitor for decreased antiarrhythmic effect.

Nursing diagnoses

• Decreased cardiac output related to ineffectiveness of disopyramide.
• Altered protection related to disopyramide-induced proarrhythmias.
• Knowledge deficit related to disopyramide therapy.

Nursing interventions

• *Contraindicated* in cardiogenic shock or second- or third-degree heart block with no pacemaker. Avoid if possible, or use very cautiously in CHF.
• *Use cautiously* in underlying conduction abnormalities, urinary tract diseases (especially prostatic hypertrophy), hepatic or renal impairment, myasthenia gravis, or narrow-angle glaucoma. Adjust dosage in renal insufficiency.
• Check apical pulse before administering drug. Notify doctor if pulse rate is slower than 60 beats/minute or faster than 120 beats/minute.
• Don't give sustained-release capsule for rapid control of ventricular arrhythmias; when therapeutic blood levels must be rapidly attained; in cardiomyopathy or possible cardiac decompensation; or in severe renal impairment.
• When transferring patient from immediate-release to sustained-release capsules, advise him to begin a sustained-release capsule 6 hours after taking the last immediate-release capsule.
• Discontinue if heart block develops, if QRS complex widens by more than 25%, or if Q-T interval lengthens by more than 25% above baseline.
• Pharmacist may prepare disopyramide suspension from 100-mg capsules using cherry syrup. Protect suspension from light.

General

Classification: skeletal muscle relaxant (nondepolarizing neuromuscular blocking agent). **Pregnancy risk category:** C.

Mechanism of action

Prevents acetylcholine from binding to receptors on muscle end plate, thus blocking depolarization.

Indications and dosage

• Adjunct to anesthesia to induce skeletal muscle relaxation, facilitate intubation, lessen muscle contractions in seizures, and assist with mechanical ventilation. Dosage depends on anesthetic, individual needs, and response. Dosages are representative and must be adjusted. **Adults:** initially, 0.04 to 0.1 mg/kg I.V., then 0.01 mg/kg q 30 to 60 minutes. **Children over 10 years:** initially, 0.04 to 0.1 mg/kg I.V., then ⅕ initial dose q 30 to 60 minutes.

Adverse reactions

CV: tachycardia, hypertension. **Skin:** transient rashes. **Local:** burning sensation. **Other:** excessive sweating and salivation, ***prolonged dose-related apnea,*** wheezing, residual weakness, allergic or idiosyncratic hypersensitivity reactions.

Interactions

Aminoglycoside antibiotics; polymyxin antibiotics (polymyxin B sulfate, colistin); clindamycin; quinidine; general anesthetics (such as halothane): potentiated neuromuscular blockade, leading to increased skeletal muscle relaxation and possible respiratory paralysis. Use cautiously during surgical and postoperative periods. **Lithium, narcotic analgesics:** potentiated neuromuscular blockade, leading to increased skeletal muscle relaxation and possible respiratory paralysis. Use with extreme caution, and reduce dose of pancuronium.

Nursing diagnoses

• Ineffective breathing pattern related to the patient's underlying condition.
• Impaired verbal communication related to drug-induced paralysis.
• Knowledge deficit related to pancuronium therapy.

Nursing interventions

• *Contraindicated* in hypersensitivity to bromides, preexisting tachycardia, and in patients for whom even a minor increase in heart rate is undesirable.
• *Use cautiously* in elderly or debilitated patients; renal, hepatic, or pulmonary impairment; respiratory depression; myasthenia gravis; myasthenic syndrome of lung cancer or bronchogenic carcinoma; dehydration; thyroid disorders; collagen diseases; porphyria; electrolyte disturbances; hyperthermia; toxemic states; and (in large doses) cesarean section.
• Pancuronium should be used only by personnel experienced in airway management.
• Keep emergency respiratory equipment handy.
• Neuromuscular blockers do not obtund consciousness or alter the pain threshold. Patients should receive sedatives or general anesthetics before neuromuscular blockers are administered.
• Drug doesn't cause histamine release or hypotension but may raise heart rate and blood pressure.
• Dose of 1 mg is the approximate therapeutic equivalent of 5 mg tubocurarine chloride.
• Monitor electrolytes and vital signs, and measure intake and output.
• A nerve stimulator and train-of-four monitoring are recommended to confirm antagonism of neuromuscular blockade and recovery of muscle strength. Look for evidence of spontaneous recovery, before attempting reversal with neostigmine.
• Once spontaneous recovery starts, pancuronium-induced neuromuscular blockade may be reversed with an anticholinesterase agent. Usually given with an anticholinergic.
• Monitor respirations closely until patient is fully recovered from neuromuscular blockade.
• Allow succinylcholine effects to subside before giving pancuronium.
• **I.V. use:** Don't mix with barbiturate solutions (precipitate will form); use only fresh solutions.

General

Classification: inotropic agent (beta-adrenergic agonist). **Pregnancy risk category:** C.

Mechanism of action

An analog of isoproterenol that directly stimulates $beta_1$ receptors of the heart to increase myocardial contractility and stroke volume, resulting in increased cardiac output.

Indications and dosage

• Refractory heart failure and as adjunct in cardiac surgery. **Adults:** 2.5 to 10 mcg/kg/minute as an I.V. infusion. Rarely, infusion rates up to 40 mcg/kg/minute may be needed.

Adverse reactions

CNS: headache. **CV:** *increased heart rate,* ***hypertension, premature ventricular contractions,*** angina, nonspecific chest pain. **GI:** nausea, vomiting. **Other:** shortness of breath.

Interactions

Beta blockers: may antagonize dobutamine effects. Do not use together. **General anesthetics:** greater incidence of ventricular arrhythmias.

Nursing diagnoses

• Decreased cardiac output related to the patient's underlying condition.
• Ineffective breathing pattern related to adverse drug reactions.
• Knowledge deficit related to dobutamine therapy.

Nursing interventions

• *Contraindicated* in idiopathic hypertrophic subaortic stenosis and in patients with hypersensitivity to the drug or any component of the formulation. Contains sulfites, which may cause an allergic response in sensitive patients.
• *Use cautiously* in patients with a history of hypertension. Drug may precipitate an exaggerated pressor response.
• Because drug increases AV conduction, patients with atrial fibrillation may develop a rapid ventricular rate. Administer a digitalis glycoside before dobutamine as ordered.
• Correct hypovolemia with plasma volume expanders before initiating dobutamine therapy.
• Continuously monitor ECG, blood pressure, pulmonary artery wedge pressure, and cardiac output. Also monitor urine output.
• Monitor serum electrolytes. Drug may lower serum potassium levels.
• **I.V. use:** Administer using a central venous catheter or large peripheral vein. Titrate infusion according to doctor's orders and patient's condition. Use an infusion pump.
• Concentrate for injection must be diluted before administration. Compatible solutions include D_5W, 0.45% sodium chloride solution, 0.9% sodium chloride solution, and lactated Ringer's injection. The contents of one vial (250 mg) diluted with 1,000 ml of solution yields a concentration of 250 mcg/ml; diluted with 500 ml, a concentration of 500 mcg/ml; diluted with 250 ml, a concentration of 1,000 mcg/ml. Maximum concentration should not exceed 5 mg/ml. I.V. solutions remain stable for 24 hours.
• Incompatible with alkaline solutions. Do not mix with sodium bicarbonate injection. Infusions for up to 72 hours produce no more adverse effects than shorter infusions.
• Avoid extravasation, which may cause an inflammatory response. Change I.V. sites regularly to avoid phlebitis.
• Know that oxidation of drug may slightly discolor admixtures containing dobutamine. This does not indicate a significant loss of potency.

General

Classification: digestant (pancreatic enzyme).
Pregnancy risk category: C.

Mechanism of action

Replaces endogenous exocrine pancreatic enzymes and aids in the digestion of starches, fats, and proteins.

Indications and dosage

• Exocrine pancreatic secretion insufficiency, cystic fibrosis in adults and children, steatorrhea and other disorders of fat metabolism secondary to insufficient pancreatic enzymes. **Adults and children:** dosage ranges from 1 to 3 capsules or tablets P.O. before or with meals and 1 capsule or tablet with snack; or 1 to 2 powder packets before meals or snacks. Dosage must be titrated to patient's response.

Adverse reactions

GI: *nausea*, diarrhea with high doses.

Interactions

Antacids: may negate pancrelipase's beneficial effect. Don't use together.

Nursing diagnoses

• Altered nutrition: Less than body requirements, related to the patient's underlying condition.
• Noncompliance with drug therapy related to long-term regimen.
• Knowledge deficit related to pancrelipase therapy.

Nursing interventions

• *Contraindicated* in patients with severe pork hypersensitivity.
• Use only after confirmed diagnosis of exocrine pancreatic insufficiency. Not effective in GI disorders unrelated to pancreatic enzyme deficiency.
• Lipase activity greater than with other pancreatic enzymes.
• For infants, mix powder with applesauce and give with meals. Avoid contact with or inhalation of powder because it may be irritating. Older children may take capsules with food.
• Dosage varies with degree of maldigestion and malabsorption, amount of fat in diet, and enzyme activity of individual preparations.
• Adequate replacement decreases the number of bowel movements and improves stool consistency.
• Enteric coating on some products may reduce the availability of enzyme in the upper portion of the jejunum.
• Crushing or chewing of capsule interferes with the enteric coating.
• Minimal USP standards dictate that each milligram of pancrelipase contains 24 units lipase, 100 units protease, and 100 units amylase.
• Cotazym Capsules contain 8,000 units lipase, 30,000 units protease, 30,000 units amylase, and 25 mg calcium carbonate.
• Cotazym-S Capsules contain 5,000 units lipase, 20,000 units protease, and 20,000 units amylase.
• Creon Capsules contain 8,000 units lipase, 13,000 units protease, and 30,000 units amylase.
• Festal II Tablets contain 6,000 units lipase, 20,000 units protease, and 30,000 units amylase.
• Ilozyme Tablets contain 11,000 units lipase, 30,000 units protease, and 30,000 units amylase.
• Ku-Zyme HP Capsules contain 8,000 units lipase, 30,000 units protease, and 30,000 units amylase.
• Pancrease Capsules contain 4,000 units lipase, 25,000 units protease, and 20,000 units amylase.
• Pancrease MT4 contains 4,000 units lipase, 12,000 units protease, and 30,000 units amylase.
• Pancrease MT10 contains 10,000 units lipase, 30,000 units protease, and 30,000 units amylase.
• Pancrease MT16 contains 16,000 units lipase, 48,000 units protease, and 48,000 units amylase.
• Viokase Powder contains 16,800 units lipase, 70,000 units protease, and 70,000 units amylase.
• Viokase Tablets contain 8,000 units lipase, 30,000 units protease, and 30,000 units amylase.

General

Classification: emollient laxative (surfactant).
Pregnancy risk category: C.

Mechanism of action

Reduces surface tension of interfacing liquid contents of the bowel. This detergent activity promotes incorporation of additional liquid into the stool, forming a softer mass.

Indications and dosage

• Stool softener. **Adults and older children:** 50 to 300 mg (sodium) of tablets, capsules, oral liquid, or syrup P.O. daily; or 50 to 300 mg (calcium or potassium) of capsules P.O. daily until bowel movements are normal. Alternatively, give enema (where available). Dilute 1:24 with sterile water before administration, and give 100 to 150 ml (retention enema), 300 to 500 ml (evacuation enema), or 0.5 to 1.5 liters (flushing enema). **Children 6 to 12 years:** 40 to 120 mg (sodium) P.O. daily. **Children 3 to 6 years:** 20 to 60 mg (sodium) P.O. daily. **Children under 3 years:** 10 to 40 mg (sodium) P.O. daily.

Higher dosages are for initial therapy. Adjust dosage to individual response. Usual dosage in children and adults with minimal needs is 50 to 150 mg (calcium) P.O. daily.

Adverse reactions

EENT: throat irritation. **GI:** bitter taste, mild abdominal cramping, diarrhea. **Other:** laxative dependence in long-term or excessive use.

Interactions

Mineral oil: may increase mineral oil absorption and cause lipoid pneumonia. Don't administer together.

Nursing diagnoses

• Constipation related to interruption of normal pattern of elimination.
• Diarrhea related to prolonged or excessive use of docusate.
• Knowledge deficit related to docusate therapy.

Nursing interventions

• *Contraindicated* in patients with hypersensitivity to the drug and in those with intestinal obstruction, undiagnosed abdominal pain, vomiting or other signs of appendicitis, fecal impaction, or acute surgical abdomen.
• Administer docusate as ordered. Many doctors feel that the minimum effective dosage is 300 mg daily. A lower dosage may not produce satisfactory results. Do not give docusate for more than 1 week without doctor's knowledge.
• Docusate prevents but does not treat constipation.
• Know that docusate is the laxative of choice in patients who should not strain during defecation, such as those recovering from MI or rectal surgery; in disease of rectum and anus that makes passage of firm stool difficult; or in postpartum constipation. Drug acts within 24 to 48 hours to produce firm, semisolid stool.
• Give liquid in milk, fruit juice, or infant formula to mask bitter taste.
• To prevent constipation, teach patient that dietary sources of bulk include bran and other cereals, fresh fruit, and vegetables.
• Discontinue if severe abdominal cramping occurs; docusate doesn't stimulate intestinal peristaltic movements.
• Store at 59° to 86° F (15° to 30° C). Protect liquid from light.

General

Classification: digestant (pancreatic enzyme).
Pregnancy risk category: C.

Mechanism of action

Replaces endogenous exocrine pancreatic enzymes and aids in the digestion of starches, fats, and proteins.

Indications and dosage

• Exocrine pancreatic secretion insufficiency, digestive aid in diseases associated with the deficiency of pancreatic enzymes, such as cystic fibrosis. **Adults and children:** 1 to 3 tablets P.O. with meals.

Adverse reactions

GI: nausea, diarrhea with high doses. **Other:** hyperuricosuria with high doses.

Interactions

Antacids: may negate pancreatin's beneficial effect. Don't use together.

Nursing diagnoses

• Altered health maintenance related to the patient's underlying condition.
• Noncompliance with drug therapy related to a long-term regimen.
• Knowledge deficit related to pancreatin therapy.

Nursing interventions

• *Use cautiously* in patients who are hypersensitive to pork. Bovine preparations are available for these patients, but they are less effective.
• Balance fat, protein, and starch intake properly to avoid indigestion. Dosage varies according to the degree of maldigestion and malabsorption, the amount of fat in diet, and the enzyme activity of individual preparations.
• Adequate replacement decreases the number of bowel movements and improves stool consistency.
• Not effective in GI disorders unrelated to pancreatic enzyme deficiency.
• For infants, mix the powder with applesauce and give with meals. Avoid inhalation of powder. Older children may swallow capsules with food.
• Enteric coating on some products may reduce the availability of pancreatic enzymes in the upper portion of the jejunum.
• Store drug in airtight containers at room temperature.
• Don't crush or chew the enteric-coated forms.
• Minimal USP standards dictate that each milligram of bovine or porcine pancreatin contains 2 units lipase, 25 units protease, and 25 units amylase.
• Dizymes contains 250 mg pancreatin, 6,750 units lipase, 41,250 units protease, and 43,750 units amylase.
• Hi-Vegi-Lip contains 2,400 mg pancreatin, 12,000 units lipase, 60,000 units protease, and 60,000 units amylase.
• Pancreatin Enseals contain 1,000 mg pancreatin, 2,000 units lipase, 25,000 units protease, and 25,000 units amylase.
• Pancreatin Tablets contain 325 mg pancreatin, 650 units lipase, 8,125 units protease, and 8,125 units amylase.

General

Classification: inotropic agent, vasopressor (adrenergic). **Pregnancy risk category:** C.

Mechanism of action

Stimulates dopaminergic, beta-adrenergic, and alpha-adrenergic receptors of the sympathetic nervous system.

Indications and dosage

• Shock, hemodynamic imbalances, decreased perfusion to vital organs, decreased cardiac output; hypotension, acute renal failure. **Adults:** 2 to 5 mcg/kg/minute I.V. infusion, up to 50 mcg/kg/minute.

Titrate the dosage to the desired hemodynamic or renal response.

Adverse reactions

CNS: headache. **CV:** ***arrhythmias,*** ectopic beats, tachycardia, anginal pain, palpitations, *hypotension,* bradycardia, widening of QRS complex, conduction disturbances, vasoconstriction. **GI:** nausea, vomiting. **Local:** necrosis and tissue sloughing with extravasation. **Other:** piloerection, dyspnea.

Interactions

Beta blockers: may antagonize dopamine's effects. **Ergot alkaloids:** extreme elevations in blood pressure. Don't use together. **Inhalational anesthetics:** increased risk of arrhythmias or hypertension. Monitor closely. **MAO inhibitors:** may cause hypertensive crisis. Avoid if possible. **Phenytoin:** may lower blood pressure of dopamine-stabilized patients. Monitor carefully.

Nursing diagnoses

• Altered tissue perfusion (cerebral, cardiopulmonary, renal) related to patient's underlying condition.
• Impaired tissue integrity related to adverse drug reactions.
• Knowledge deficit related to dopamine therapy.

Nursing interventions

• *Contraindicated* in uncorrected tachyarrhythmias, pheochromocytoma, or ventricular fibrillation.
• *Use cautiously* in patients with occlusive vascular disease, cold injuries, diabetic endarteritis, or arterial embolism; in pregnant patients; and in those taking MAO inhibitors.
• During infusion, frequently monitor ECG, blood pressure, cardiac output, central venous pressure, pulmonary artery wedge pressure, pulse rate, urine output, and color and temperature of extremities. Titrate infusion rate according to findings and doctor's guidelines. Use a continuous infusion pump to regulate flow rate.
• If a disproportionate rise in diastolic pressure occurs, decrease infusion rate and observe for further evidence of predominant vasoconstrictor activity.
• If doses exceed 50 mcg/kg/minute, check urine output often. If urine flow decreases without hypotension, consider reducing dose.
• If drug is stopped, watch closely for sudden drop in blood pressure. Drug should be tapered slowly to evaluate stability of blood pressure.
• **I.V. use:** Use a central line or a large vein, such as in the antecubital fossa, to minimize risk of extravasation. If extravasation occurs, stop infusion immediately and call doctor; he may order infiltration of the area with 5 to 10 mg phentolamine and 10 to 15 ml 0.9% sodium chloride solution.
• Don't mix with alkaline solutions. Use D_5W, 0.9% sodium chloride solution, or a combination of the two. Mix just before use.
• Do not mix other drugs in I.V. container with dopamine. Do not give alkaline drugs through I.V. line containing dopamine.
• Discard dopamine solution after 24 hours or earlier if solution is discolored.

General

Classification: oxytocic, lactation stimulant (posterior pituitary hormone). **Pregnancy risk category:** not applicable.

Mechanism of action

Causes potent and selective stimulation of uterine and mammary gland smooth muscle.

Indications and dosage

- Induction or stimulation of labor. **Adults:** initially, 1-ml ampule (10 units) in 1,000 ml of D_5W or 0.9% sodium chloride solution infused at 1 to 2 milliunits/minute. Increase rate at 15- to 30-minute intervals until normal contraction pattern is established. Maximum is 1 to 2 ml (20 milliunits)/minute. Decrease rate when labor is firmly established.
- Reduction of postpartum bleeding after expulsion of placenta. **Adults:** 10 to 40 units added to 1,000 ml of D_5W or 0.9% sodium chloride solution infused at rate necessary to control bleeding, usually 10 to 20 milliunits/minute. Also, 1 ml (10 units) can be given I.M. after delivery of placenta.
- Incomplete or inevitable abortion. **Adults:** I.V. infusion with 10 units of oxytocin in 500 ml of 0.9% sodium chloride solution or dextrose 5% in 0.9% sodium chloride solution. Infuse at rate of 10 to 20 milliunits/minute.

Adverse reactions

Maternal—**Blood:** afibrinogenemia (may be related to postpartum bleeding). **CNS:** ***subarachnoid hemorrhage*** resulting from hypertension; ***seizures or coma*** resulting from water intoxication. **CV:** ***hypertension;*** increased heart rate, systemic venous return, and cardiac output; ***arrhythmias.*** **GI:** nausea, vomiting. **Other:** ***hypersensitivity,*** tetanic contractions, ***abruptio placentae, impaired uterine blood flow,*** pelvic hematoma, ***increased uterine motility, anaphylaxis.***

Fetal—**Blood:** hyperbilirubinemia. **CV:** bradycardia, tachycardia, ***premature ventricular contractions.*** **Other:** ***anoxia, asphyxia.***

Interactions

Cyclopropane anesthetics: less pronounced bradycardia; hypotension. **Thiopental anesthetics:** delayed induction reported. **Vasoconstrictors:** severe hypertension.

Nursing diagnoses

- Fluid volume deficit related to postpartum bleeding.
- Fluid volume excess related to oxytocin-induced antidiuretic effect.
- Knowledge deficit related to oxytocin therapy.

Nursing interventions

- *Contraindicated* in cephalopelvic disproportion or when delivery requires conversion, as in transverse lie; fetal distress, when delivery isn't imminent; severe toxemia; partial placenta previa; prematurity; and other obstetric emergencies.
- *Use with extreme caution* during first two stages of labor; cervical laceration, uterine rupture, and maternal and fetal death have been reported.
- *Use cautiously* in history of cervical or uterine surgery, grand multiparity, uterine sepsis, traumatic delivery, or overdistended uterus and in primiparas over 35 years.
- **I.V. use:** Administer by piggyback infusion only so the drug may be discontinued without interrupting the I.V. line. Use an infusion pump.
- Used to induce or reinforce labor only when pelvis is known to be adequate, when vaginal delivery is indicated, when fetal maturity is assured, and when fetal position is favorable. Should be used only in hospital where critical care facilities and doctor are immediately available.
- Never give simultaneously by more than one route.
- Monitor and record uterine contractions, heart rate, blood pressure, intrauterine pressure, fetal heart rate, and character of blood loss every 15 minutes.
- If contractions occur less than 2 minutes apart, are above 50 mm Hg, or last 90 seconds or longer, stop infusion, turn patient on her side, and notify doctor.
- Not recommended for routine I.M. use. However, 10 units may be given I.M. after delivery of placenta to control postpartum uterine bleeding.
- Have magnesium sulfate (20% solution) available for relaxation of the myometrium.

General

Classification: antihypertensive (alpha-adrenergic blocker). **Pregnancy risk category:** B.

Mechanism of action

Acts on the peripheral vasculature to produce vasodilation.

Indications and dosage

• Essential hypertension. **Adults:** initiate dosage at 1 mg P.O. daily and determine effect on standing and supine blood pressure at 2 to 6 hours and 24 hours after dosing. If necessary, increase dose to 2 mg daily. To minimize adverse reactions, titrate dosage slowly (usually increase dosage only q 2 weeks). Increase to a daily dose of 4 mg, then 8 mg if necessary. Maximum daily dosage is 16 mg, but dosage that exceeds 4 mg daily is associated with a greater incidence of adverse reactions.

Adverse reactions

CNS: dizziness, vertigo, headache, somnolence, drowsiness, fatigue, malaise, syncope, paresthesia. **CV:** *orthostatic hypotension,* hypotension, edema, palpitations, ***arrhythmias,*** tachycardia, peripheral ischemia. **Skin:** rash, pruritus. **Other:** arthralgia, myalgia, muscle weakness, rhinitis.

Interactions

None reported.

Nursing diagnoses

• Altered tissue perfusion (renal, cerebral, cardiopulmonary, peripheral) related to the patient's underlying condition.
• Decreased cardiac output related to doxazosin-induced adverse reactions.
• Knowledge deficit related to doxazosin therapy.

Nursing interventions

• *Contraindicated* in patients with hypersensitivity to the drug and quinazoline derivatives (including prazosin and terazosin).
• *Use cautiously* in patients with impaired hepatic function.
• Titrate dosage increase gradually, with adjustments every 2 weeks. The 2-, 4- and 8-mg tablets are not indicated for initial therapy.
• Patients taking doxazosin are susceptible to a "first-dose" effect similar to that produced by other alpha-adrenergic blocking agents; marked orthostatic hypotension may be accompanied by dizziness or syncope. Orthostatic hypotension is most common after the first dose, but can also occur when therapy is interrupted for a few days and during periods of dosage adjustment. Warn the patient that dizziness or fainting may occur.
• If syncope occurs, place patient in a recumbent position and treat supportively. A transient hypotensive response is not considered a contraindication to continued therapy.
• Warn patient that the drug may cause drowsiness. Tell patient to avoid driving and other hazardous activities that require alertness until the adverse CNS effects of the drug are known.

General
Classification: antibiotic (tetracycline). **Pregnancy risk category:** D.

Mechanism of action
Exerts bacteriostatic effect by binding to the 30S ribosomal subunit of microorganisms, thus inhibiting protein synthesis.

Indications and dosage
- Infections caused by sensitive gram-negative and gram-positive organisms. **Adults:** 250 mg P.O. q 6 hours; 100 mg I.M. q 8 to 12 hours; 250 mg I.M. as a single dose. **Children over 8 years:** 25 to 50 mg/kg P.O. daily, divided q 6 hours; 15 to 25 mg/kg I.M. daily, divided q 8 to 12 hours.
- Brucellosis. **Adults:** 500 mg P.O. q.i.d. for 3 weeks with streptomycin 1 g I.M. q 12 hours first week, once daily second week.
- Syphilis in patients sensitive to penicillin. **Adults:** 30 to 40 g total dosage P.O., divided equally over 10 to 15 days.
- Gonorrhea in patients sensitive to penicillin. **Adults:** initially, 1.5 g P.O., followed by 0.5 g q.i.d. for a total of 9 g.
- Uncomplicated urethral, endocervical, or rectal infections caused by *Chlamydia trachomatis*. **Adults:** 500 mg. P.O. q.i.d. for at least 7 days.

Adverse reactions
Blood: neutropenia, eosinophilia. **CNS:** ***intracranial hypertension.*** **CV:** pericarditis. **EENT:** dysphagia, glossitis. **GI:** *anorexia, nausea,* vomiting, *diarrhea,* enterocolitis, anogenital inflammation. **Metabolic:** *increased BUN levels.* **Skin:** *maculopapular and erythematous rashes, urticaria, photosensitivity, increased pigmentation.* **Local:** *irritation after I.M. injection, thrombophlebitis.* **Other:** ***hypersensitivity.***

Interactions
Antacids (including sodium bicarbonate) and laxatives containing aluminum, magnesium, or calcium; food, milk, or other dairy products: decrease antibiotic absorption. Give antibiotic 1 hour before or 2 hours after. **Ferrous sulfate and other iron products, zinc:** decrease antibiotic absorption. Give tetracyclines 3 hours after or 2 hours before iron administration. **Methoxyflurane:** may cause severe nephrotoxicity with tetracyclines. **Oral contraceptives:** decreased contraceptive effectiveness and increased risk of breakthrough bleeding.

Nursing diagnoses
- High risk for infection related to ineffectiveness of oxytetracycline in eradicating the infection.
- High risk for fluid volume deficit related to adverse GI reactions.

Nursing interventions
- *Use with extreme caution* in patients with impaired renal or hepatic function. Use during last half of pregnancy and in children under 8 years may cause permanent discoloration of teeth, enamel defects, and retardation of bone growth.
- Obtain specimen for culture and sensitivity tests before first dose. Therapy may begin pending test results.
- Check expiration date. Outdated or deteriorated oxytetracycline has been associated with reversible nephrotoxicity (Fanconi's syndrome).
- Inject I.M. dose deeply, rotating sites. I.M. preparations contain a local anesthetic; ask patient about hypersensitivity to local anesthetics.
- With large doses or prolonged therapy, monitor for superinfections.
- Check patient's tongue for signs of monilia infection. Stress good oral hygiene.
- Warn patient to avoid direct sunlight and ultraviolet light. A sunscreen may help prevent photosensitivity reactions. Photosensitivity persists for considerable time after discontinuation of drug.
- Give drug at least 1 hour before bedtime to prevent esophagitis.
- Tell patient to take medication exactly as precribed, even if he feels better, and to take entire quantity prescribed.

doxepin hydrochloride

Adapin**, Sinequan, Triadapin†

General

Classification: antidepressant (tricyclic). **Pregnancy risk category:** C.

Mechanism of action

Increases the amount of norepinephrine or serotonin, or both, in the CNS by blocking their reuptake by the presynaptic neurons. This allows these neurotransmitters to accumulate.

Indications and dosage

• Depression. **Adults:** initially, 50 to 75 mg (tablets or oral concentrate) P.O. daily in divided doses, to maximum of 300 mg daily. Alternatively, entire dosage may be given at bedtime.

Adverse reactions

CNS: *drowsiness, dizziness,* excitation, tremors, weakness, confusion, headache, nervousness, EEG changes, ***seizures,*** extrapyramidal reactions. **CV:** *orthostatic hypotension, tachycardia, ECG changes,* hypertension. **EENT:** *blurred vision,* tinnitus, glossitis, mydriasis. **GI:** *dry mouth, constipation,* nausea, vomiting, anorexia, paralytic ileus. **GU:** *urine retention.* **Skin:** rash, urticaria, photosensitivity. **Other:** *sweating,* allergy. **After abrupt withdrawal of long-term therapy:** nausea, headache, malaise (does not indicate addiction).

Interactions

Alcohol or other depressants: increased CNS depression. Avoid concomitant use. **Barbiturates:** decrease TCA blood levels. Monitor for decreased antidepressant effect. **Cimetidine:** may increase doxepin serum levels. Monitor for increased adverse reactions. **MAO inhibitors:** may cause severe excitation, hyperpyrexia, or seizures, usually with high dose. Use together cautiously. **Methylphenidate:** increases TCA blood levels. Monitor for enhanced antidepressant effect.

Nursing diagnoses

• Ineffective individual coping related to the patient's underlying condition.
• High risk for injury related to doxepin-induced CNS and CV adverse reactions.
• Knowledge deficit related to doxepin therapy.

Nursing interventions

• *Contraindicated* in patients with narrow-angle glaucoma, prostatic hypertrophy, or history of seizures or during the acute recovery phase of MI.
• *Use cautiously* in patients with urine retention or thyroid, cardiovascular, or hepatic disease and in patients at risk for suicide.
• Dilute oral concentrate with 120 ml water, milk, or juice (not carbonated beverages).
• Tell patient to take full dose at bedtime whenever possible. Warn patient about the possibility of morning orthostatic hypotension.
• Reduce dose in elderly or debilitated patients, adolescents, and those receiving other medications (especially anticholinergics). Tell patient not to take any other drugs without first consulting the doctor.
• Decrease dose if psychotic symptoms increase. Record mood changes. Watch for suicidal tendencies.
• Warn patient to avoid hazardous activities that require alertness and good psychomotor coordination until CNS effects of the drug are known.
• Offer sugarless hard candy or gum to relieve dry mouth. Saliva substitutes may be necessary.
• Check for urine retention and constipation. Increase fluids to lessen constipation. Suggest stool softener or a high-fiber diet, if needed.
• Advise patient to use a sunscreen, wear protective clothing, and avoid prolonged exposure to strong sunlight.
• Expect delay of 2 weeks or more before noticeable effect occurs; 4 weeks or more before full effect.

General

Classification: spasmolytic (sodium channel blocker). **Pregnancy risk category:** C.

Mechanism of action

Exerts a nonspecific, direct spasmolytic action on smooth muscle. Also possesses local anesthetic properties that may be partly responsible for spasmolysis.

Indications and dosage

- Adjunctive treatment of peptic ulcer. **Adults:** 10 mg P.O. b.i.d. in the morning and h.s., or 5 mg b.i.d. or t.i.d.

Adverse reactions

CNS: *headache,* insomnia, drowsiness, *dizziness.* **CV:** *palpitations,* tachycardia. **EENT:** *blurred vision,* mydriasis, increased intraocular pressure, cycloplegia, photophobia. **GI:** *constipation,* dry mouth, nausea, vomiting, *paralytic ileus.* **GU:** *urinary hesitancy, urine retention, impotence.* **Skin:** urticaria, decreased sweating or anhidrosis, other dermal manifestations. **Other:** fever, allergic reactions. **Overdose:** possible curare-like symptoms.

Interactions

Amantadine, antihistamines, antiparkinsonian agents, disopyramide, glutethimide, meperidine, phenothiazines, procainamide, quinidine: additive adverse effects. Avoid concomitant use. **Ketoconazole:** anticholinergics may interfere with ketoconazole absorption. Avoid concomitant use. **Methotrimeprazine:** anticholinergics may enhance risk of extrapyramidal reactions. Avoid concomitant use.

Nursing diagnoses

- Pain related to the patient's underlying condition.
- High risk for injury related to adverse CNS reactions to oxyphencyclimine.
- Knowledge deficit related to oxyphencyclimine therapy.

Nursing interventions

- *Contraindicated* in narrow-angle glaucoma, obstructive uropathy, obstructive disease of GI tract, severe ulcerative colitis, myasthenia gravis, hypersensitivity to anticholinergics, paralytic ileus, intestinal atony, unstable cardiovascular status in acute hemorrhage, or toxic megacolon.
- *Use cautiously* in autonomic neuropathy, hyperthyroidism, coronary artery disease, cardiac arrhythmias, CHF, hypertension, hiatal hernia associated with reflux esophagitis, hepatic or renal disease, and ulcerative colitis, and in patients over age 40 because of increased incidence of glaucoma. Also use cautiously in hot or humid environments. Drug-induced heatstroke can develop.
- Give 30 minutes to 1 hour before breakfast and at bedtime.
- Monitor patient's vital signs and urine output carefully.
- Instruct patient to avoid driving and other hazardous activities if he is drowsy, dizzy, or has blurred vision; to drink plenty of fluids to help prevent constipation; and to report any rash or skin eruption.
- Gum or sugarless hard candy may relieve dry mouth.
- May cause fewer atropine-like adverse reactions than other commonly used spasmolytics.

General

Classification: antibiotic (tetracycline). **Pregnancy risk category:** D.

Mechanism of action

Exerts bacteriostatic effect by binding to the 30S ribosomal subunit of microorganisms, thus inhibiting protein synthesis.

Indications and dosage

- Infections caused by sensitive gram-negative and gram-positive organisms, trachoma, rickettsiae, *Mycoplasma,* or *Chlamydia;* trachoma; Lyme disease. **Adults:** 100 mg P.O. q 12 hours on first day, then 100 mg P.O. daily; or 200 mg I.V. on first day in one or two infusions, then 100 to 200 mg I.V. daily. **Children over 8 years (under 45 kg):** 4.4 mg/kg P.O. or I.V. daily, divided q 12 hours first day, then 2.2 to 4.4 mg/kg daily. For children over 45 kg, dosage is same as adults.
- Gonorrhea in patients allergic to penicillin. **Adults:** 200 mg P.O. initially, followed by 100 mg P.O. at bedtime, and 100 mg P.O. b.i.d. for 3 days; or 300 mg P.O. initially and repeat dose in 1 hour.
- Primary or secondary syphilis in patients allergic to penicillin. **Adults:** 300 mg P.O. daily in divided doses for at least 10 days.
- Uncomplicated urethral, endocervical, or rectal infections caused by *Chlamydia trachomatis* or *Ureaplasma urealyticum.* **Adults:** 100 mg P.O. b.i.d. for at least 7 days.
- To prevent "traveler's diarrhea" commonly caused by enterotoxigenic *Escherichia coli.* **Adults:** 100 mg P.O. daily.

Adverse reactions

Blood: neutropenia, eosinophilia. **CNS:** ***intracranial hypertension.*** **CV:** pericarditis. **EENT:** sore throat, glossitis, dysphagia. **GI:** anorexia, *epigastric distress, nausea,* vomiting, *diarrhea,* enterocolitis, anogenital inflammation. **Skin:** *maculopapular and erythematous rashes, photosensitivity, increased pigmentation, urticaria.* **Local:** thrombophlebitis. **Other:** ***hypersensitivity.***

Interactions

Antacids and laxatives containing aluminum, magnesium, or calcium: decrease antibiotic absorption. Give antibiotic 1 hour before or 2 hours after any of the above. **Ferrous sulfate and other iron products, zinc:** decrease antibiotic absorption. Give doxycycline 3 hours after or 2 hours before iron administration. **Oral contraceptives:** decreased contraceptive effectiveness and increased risk of breakthrough bleeding. **Phenobarbital, carbamazepine, alcohol:** decrease antibiotic effect. Try to avoid concomitant use.

Nursing diagnoses

- High risk for infection related to ineffectiveness of doxycycline in eradicating the infection.
- High risk for fluid volume deficit related to adverse GI reactions to doxycycline therapy.
- Knowledge deficit related to doxycycline therapy.

Nursing interventions

- Obtain specimen for culture and sensitivity tests before first dose.
- With large doses or prolonged therapy, monitor for superinfection.
- Check patient's tongue for signs of monilia infection. Stress good oral hygiene.
- **I.V. use:** Reconstitute powder for injection with sterile water for injection. Use 10 ml in 100-mg vial and 20 ml in 200-mg vial. Dilute solution to 100 to 1,000 ml for I.V. infusion. Give I.V. infusion slowly (minimum 1 hour). Infusion must be completed within 12 hours (within 6 hours in lactated Ringer's solution or dextrose 5% in lactated Ringer's solution). Do not infuse solutions more concentrated than 1 mg/ml. Reconstituted solution is stable for 72 hours refrigerated. Protect from sunlight during infusion. Monitor I.V. site for phlebitis.

General

Classification: analgesic (opioid) **Pregnancy risk category:** B (D for prolonged use or use of high doses at term). **Controlled substance schedule:** II.

Mechanism of action

Binds with opiate receptors at many sites in the CNS (brain, brain stem, and spinal cord), altering both perception of and emotional response to pain through an unknown mechanism.

Indications and dosage

- Moderate to severe pain. **Adults:** 1 to 1.5 mg I.M. or S.C. q 4 to 6 hours, p.r.n. or around the clock; or 0.5 mg I.V. q 4 to 6 hours, p.r.n. or around the clock; or 2.5 to 5 mg P.R. q 4 to 6 hours, p.r.n. or around the clock.

Adverse reactions

CNS: *sedation, somnolence, clouded sensorium, euphoria,* dizziness, seizures with large doses. **CV:** *hypotension,* bradycardia. **GI:** *nausea, vomiting, constipation,* ileus. **GU:** *urine retention.* **Other:** ***respiratory depression,*** physical dependence.

Interactions

Alcohol, CNS depressants, TCAs, MAO inhibitors: additive effects. Reduce oxymorphone dose and monitor closely.

Nursing diagnoses

- Pain related to patient's underlying condition.
- Ineffective breathing pattern related to oxymorphone-induced respiratory depression.
- Knowledge deficit related to oxymorphone therapy.

Nursing interventions

- *Contraindicated* in patients with hypersensitivity to the drug or to other opiate analgesics.
- *Use with extreme caution* in head injury, increased intracranial pressure, seizures, asthma, COPD, alcoholism, increased CSF pressure, acute abdominal conditions, prostatic hyperplasia, severe hepatic or renal disease, urethral stricture, CNS depression, respiratory depression, hypothyroidism, Addison's disease, cardiac arrhythmias, reduced blood volume, and toxic psychosis and in elderly or debilitated patients.
- Warn ambulatory patient to avoid activities that require mental alertness or physical coordination.
- Monitor cardiovascular and respiratory status and bladder and bowel function. Hold dose and notify doctor if respiratory rate drops below 12 breaths/minute.
- Patient may need laxative.
- Well absorbed rectally. Alternative to narcotics with limited dosage forms.
- Keep narcotic antagonist (naloxone) and resuscitative equipment available.
- For better analgesic effect, give before patient has intense pain.
- When used postoperatively, encourage turning, coughing, and deep breathing and use of the incentive spirometer to avoid atelectasis.
- Not intended for mild to moderate pain. May worsen gallbladder pain.

General

Classification: antiemetic (cannabinoid). **Pregnancy risk category:** B. **Controlled substance schedule:** II.

Mechanism of action

A derivative of marijuana. Antiemetic and appetite stimulant effects are produced through an unknown action in the CNS.

Indications and dosage

- Nausea and vomiting associated with cancer chemotherapy. **Adults:** 5 mg/m² P.O. 1 to 3 hours before administration of chemotherapy. Then give same dose q 2 to 4 hours after chemotherapy is administered for a total of four to six doses per day. Dosage may be increased in increments of 2.5 mg/m² to a maximum of 15 mg/m² per dose.
- Anorexia and weight loss in patients with AIDS. **Adults:** 2.5 mg P.O. b.i.d. before lunch and dinner.

Adverse reactions

CNS: *dizziness, ataxia,* depersonalization, disorientation, hallucinations, headache, irritability, memory lapse, muddled thinking, paranoia, perceptual difficulties, weakness, paresthesia. **CV:** tachycardia, orthostatic hypotension. **EENT:** visual distortions. **GI:** *dry mouth.*

Interactions

Alcohol, CNS depressants, sedatives, psychotomimetic substances: additive effects. Don't use together.

Nursing diagnoses

- High risk for fluid volume deficit related to nausea and vomiting induced by chemotherapy.
- Altered thought processes related to dronabinol-induced CNS adverse reactions.
- Knowledge deficit related to dronabinol therapy.

Nursing interventions

- *Contraindicated* for nausea and vomiting from any cause other than cancer chemotherapy, for anorexia and weight loss from any cause other than AIDS, and in patients with hypersensitivity to sesame oil.
- *Use cautiously* in elderly patients and those with hypertension, heart disease, or psychiatric illness.
- Warn patients against hazardous activities that require alertness until CNS effects of the drug are known.
- Drug effects may persist for days after treatment ends. CNS effects are intensified at higher drug dosages. Duration of persistent effect varies greatly among patients. Therefore, patient should be supervised for untoward responses until it's certain that he's no longer experiencing the drug's effects.
- Dronabinol is the principal active substance present in *Cannabis sativa* (marijuana). Be aware of the high potential for physical and psychic dependence and abuse.
- To prevent panic and anxiety, tell patients this drug may induce unusual changes in mood or other adverse behavioral effects.
- Impress upon family members that patient should be under supervision by a responsible person during and immediately after the treatment.

General

Classification: analgesic (opioid). **Pregnancy risk category:** B (D for prolonged use or use of high doses at term). **Controlled substance schedule:** II.

Mechanism of action

Binds with opiate receptors at many sites in the CNS (brain, brain stem, and spinal cord), altering both perception of and emotional response to pain through an unknown mechanism.

Indications and dosage

• Moderate to severe pain. **Adults:** One to 2 tablets P.O. q 6 hours, p.r.n. or around the clock. Or 5 mg (5 ml) of oxycodone oral solution P.O. q 6 hours. Or 1 to 3 suppositories P.R. daily, p.r.n. or around the clock.

Adverse reactions

CNS: *sedation, somnolence, clouded sensorium, euphoria,* dizziness, seizures with large doses. **CV:** *hypotension,* bradycardia. **GI:** *nausea, vomiting, constipation,* ileus. **GU:** *urine retention.* **Other:** ***respiratory depression,*** physical dependence.

Interactions

Alcohol, general anesthetics, other narcotic analgesics, tranquilizers, sedatives, hypnotics, TCAs, or MAO inhibitors: increased CNS depression. Avoid concomitant use. **Anticoagulants:** some oxycodone hydrochloride products contain aspirin and may increase anticoagulant effect. Monitor clotting times. Use together cautiously.

Nursing diagnoses

• Pain related to patient's underlying condition.
• Ineffective breathing pattern related to oxycodone-induced respiratory depression.
• Knowledge deficit related to oxycodone therapy.

Nursing interventions

• *Contraindicated* in patients with hypersensitivity to the drug or to other opiate analgesics.
• *Use with extreme caution* in head injury, increased intracranial pressure, increased CSF pressure, seizures, asthma, COPD, alcoholism, prostatic hyperplasia, severe hepatic or renal disease, acute abdominal conditions, urethral stricture, hypothyroidism, Addison's disease, cardiac arrhythmias, reduced blood volume, and toxic psychosis and in elderly or debilitated patients.
• Warn ambulatory patient to avoid hazardous activities that require mental alertness or physical coordination.
• Monitor circulatory and respiratory status and bladder and bowel function. Hold dose and notify doctor if respirations are shallow or if respiratory rate falls below 12 breaths/minute.
• Because drug has a constipating effect, patient may require a laxative.
• For full analgesic effect, give before patient has intense pain.
• To minimize GI upset, give after meals or with milk.
• Oxycodone is available in combination with other drugs, such as aspirin (Percodan, Percodan-Demi) or acetaminophen (Percocet, Tylox).
• Single-agent oxycodone solution or tablets are especially good for patients who shouldn't take aspirin or acetaminophen.

General

Classification: anticholinergic agonist, diagnostic agent (cholinesterase inhibitor). **Pregnancy risk category:** C.

Mechanism of action

Inhibits the destruction of acetylcholine released from the parasympathetic and somatic efferent nerves. Acetylcholine accumulates, promoting increased stimulation of the receptor. Edrophonium has a very short duration of action.

Indications and dosage

• Curare antagonist (to reverse neuromuscular blocking action). **Adults:** 10 mg I.V. given over 30 to 45 seconds. Dose may be repeated as necessary to 40 mg maximum dosage. Larger dosages may potentiate rather than antagonize effect of curare.
• Diagnostic aid in myasthenia gravis (Tensilon test). **Adults:** 1 to 2 mg I.V. within 15 to 30 seconds, then 8 mg if no response (increase in muscular strength). Alternatively, give 10 mg I.M. If a cholinergic reaction occurs, give 2 mg I.M. 30 minutes later to rule out a false-negative response. **Children over 34 kg:** 2 mg I.V. If no response within 45 seconds, give 1 mg q 45 seconds to maximum of 10 mg. Alternatively, give 5 mg I.M. **Children up to 34 kg:** 1 mg I.V. If no response within 45 seconds, give 1 mg q 45 seconds to maximum of 5 mg. Alternatively, give 2 mg I.M. **Infants:** 0.5 mg to 1 mg I.M. or S.C.
• To differentiate myasthenic crisis from cholinergic crisis. **Adults:** 1 mg I.V. If no response in 1 minute, repeat dose once. Increased muscular strength confirms myasthenic crisis; no increase or exaggerated weakness confirms cholinergic crisis.
• Paroxysmal supraventricular tachycardia. **Adults:** 5 to 10 mg I.V. given over 1 minute or less. Alternatively, give a test dose of 2 mg I.V., followed by 2 mg every minute for a total of 10 mg I.V. If heart rate decreases, infuse at 0.25 mg/minute; increase as needed to a maximum of 2 mg/minute. **Children:** 2 mg I.V. Administer slowly.

Adverse reactions

CNS: ***seizures,*** weakness, dysarthria, dysphagia, sweating. **CV:** hypotension, bradycardia, AV block. **EENT:** excessive lacrimation, diplopia, miosis, conjunctival hyperemia. **GI:** nausea, vomiting, *diarrhea, abdominal cramps,* excessive salivation. **GU:** urinary frequency, incontinence. **Respiratory:** ***paralysis, bronchospasm, laryngospasm,*** increased bronchial secretions. **Other:** muscle cramps, muscle fasciculations.

Interactions

Aminoglycosides, anesthetics: prolonged or enhanced muscle weakness. Monitor closely. **Digitalis glycosides:** may increase the heart's sensitivity to edrophonium. Use together cautiously. **Procainamide, quinidine:** may reverse cholinergic effects. Observe for lack of drug effect.

Nursing diagnoses

• Altered health maintenance related to underlying condition.
• Urinary retention related to adverse effects of edrophonium.
• Knowledge deficit related to edrophonium therapy.

Nursing interventions

• *Contraindicated* in mechanical obstruction of intestine or urinary tract, bradycardia, or hypotension.
• *Use cautiously* in hyperthyroidism, cardiac disease, peptic ulcer, and bronchial asthma.
• **I.V. use:** For easier parenteral administration, use a tuberculin syringe with an I.V. needle. When giving drug to differentiate myasthenic crisis from cholinergic crisis, observe patient's muscle strength closely.

General

Classification: antispasmodic (synthetic tertiary amine). **Pregnancy risk category:** C.

Mechanism of action

Has both a direct spasmolytic effect and an atropine-like effect on urinary tract smooth muscles. It increases urinary bladder capacity and provides some local anesthesia and mild analgesia.

Indications and dosage

• Neurogenic bladder. **Adults:** 5 mg P.O. b.i.d. to t.i.d., to maximum of 5 mg q.i.d. **Children over 5 years:** 5 mg P.O. b.i.d., to maximum of 5 mg t.i.d.

Adverse reactions

CNS: *drowsiness,* dizziness, insomnia, restlessness, flushing. **CV:** *palpitations, tachycardia.* **EENT:** *transient blurred vision,* mydriasis, cycloplegia. **GI:** nausea, vomiting, *constipation, dry mouth,* bloated feeling. **GU:** impotence, *urinary hesitancy or urine retention.* **Skin:** rash, urticaria, allergic reactions in patients with sensitivity to anticholinergics. **Other:** decreased sweating, fever, suppression of lactation.

Interactions

None significant.

Nursing diagnoses

• Pain related to patient's underlying condition.
• High risk for injury related to oxybutynin-induced blurred vision and drowsiness.
• Knowledge deficit related to oxybutynin therapy.

Nursing interventions

• *Contraindicated* in myasthenia gravis, GI obstruction, glaucoma, adynamic ileus, megacolon, severe or ulcerative colitis, and obstructive uropathy and in elderly or debilitated patients with intestinal atony.
• *Use cautiously* in elderly patients and in autonomic neuropathy, reflux esophagitis, and hepatic or renal disease.
• May aggravate symptoms of hyperthyroidism, coronary artery disease, CHF, cardiac arrhythmias, tachycardia, hypertension, or prostatic hyperplasia.
• Therapy should be stopped periodically to determine whether patient can get along without it. Minimizes tendency toward tolerance.
• Rapid onset of action, peaks at 3 to 4 hours, and lasts 6 to 10 hours.
• Neurogenic bladder should be confirmed by cystometry before oxybutynin is given. Evaluate patient response to therapy periodically by cystometry.
• Rule out partial intestinal obstruction in patients with diarrhea, especially those with colostomy or ileostomy, before giving oxybutynin.
• If UTI is present, patient should receive antibiotics concomitantly.
• Warn patient that drug may impair alertness or vision. He should avoid driving and other hazardous activities until the adverse CNS effects of the drug are known.
• Since oxybutynin suppresses sweating, its use during very hot weather may precipitate fever or heatstroke.
• Store at 59° to 86° F (15° to 30° C) in tightly closed containers.

General

Classification: antihypertensive (ACE inhibitor). **Pregnancy risk category:** C (D in 2nd and 3rd trimesters).

Mechanism of action

Prevents conversion of angiotensin I to angiotensin II.

Indications and dosage

- Hypertension. **Adults:** initially, 5 mg P.O. once daily, then adjust according to response. Usual dosage range is 10 to 40 mg daily as a single dose or two divided doses. Alternatively, give by I.V. infusion 1.25 mg q 6 hours over 5 minutes.
- Conversion from I.V. therapy to oral therapy. **Adults:** initially, 5 mg P.O. once a day. Adjust dosage to response.
- Conversion from oral therapy to I.V. therapy. **Adults:** 1.25 mg I.V. over 5 minutes q 6 hours. Higher doses show no greater efficacy.
- Adjunctive treatment of heart failure (with diuretics and digitalis glycosides). **Adults:** initially, 2.5 mg P.O. b.i.d. Adjust dosage based on clinical or hemodynamic response. Usual range is 5 to 20 mg daily in two divided doses; maximum dosage is 40 mg/day.

Adverse reactions

Blood: ***neutropenia, agranulocytosis.*** **CNS:** *headache, dizziness, fatigue,* insomnia. **CV:** *hypotension.* **GI:** diarrhea, nausea. **GU:** decreased renal function (patients with bilateral renal artery stenosis or CHF). **Skin:** rash. **Other:** persistent cough, ***angioedema.***

Interactions

Insulin, oral antidiabetic agents: risk of hypoglycemia, especially at initiation of enalapril therapy. Monitor closely. **Lithium:** lithium toxicity can occur. Monitor lithium levels. **NSAIDs:** may reduce antihypertensive effect. Monitor blood pressure. **Potassium supplements, potassium-sparing diuretics:** increased risk of hyperkalemia. Avoid these agents unless hypokalemic blood levels are confirmed.

Nursing diagnoses

- Altered tissue perfusion (renal, cerebral, cardiopulmonary, peripheral) related to the patient's underlying condition.
- Decreased cardiac output related to enalapril-induced adverse reactions.
- Knowledge deficit related to enalapril therapy.

Nursing interventions

- *Contraindicated* during pregnancy because ACE inhibitors can cause fetal and neonatal injury or death. These problems have not developed when fetal exposure occurs only during the first trimester. When pregnancy is detected, discontinue ACE inhibitors as soon as possible.
- *Use cautiously* in preexisting renal impairment or collagen vascular disease. Diabetic patients, patients with impaired renal function or CHF, and patients taking drugs that can increase serum potassium may develop hyperkalemia. Monitor potassium intake and serum potassium level.
- Discontinue diuretics 2 to 3 days before beginning enalapril therapy, to reduce risk of hypotension. Then, if enalapril does not control blood pressure, diuretic therapy may be added.
- When used to treat heart failure, monitor patient closely for hypotension. Observe patient for at least 2 hours; then, for at least 1 hour after blood pressure has stabilized.
- Explain the importance of taking this drug as prescribed. Tell outpatient not to discontinue drug suddenly, but to call the doctor if unpleasant adverse reactions occur.
- Tell patient to report any swelling of face, eyes, lips, or tongue, or breathing difficulty, which may indicate angioedema (laryngeal edema).
- Also advise patient to report any light-headedness or sign of infection.

General

Classification: bronchodilator (xanthine derivative). **Pregnancy risk category:** C.

Mechanism of action

A soluble salt of theophylline, which inhibits phosphodiesterase, the enzyme that degrades cAMP, resulting in relaxation of smooth muscle of the bronchial airways and pulmonary blood vessels.

Indications and dosage

• Relief of acute bronchial asthma and reversible bronchospasm associated with chronic bronchitis and emphysema. **Adults and children over 12 years:** 200 mg P.O. q 6 hours; or 400 to 600 mg sustained-release form P.O. q 12 hours, then adjust dosage based upon serum theophylline levels. **Children 2 to 12 years:** 4 mg/kg P.O. q 6 hours. Adjust as needed to maintain therapeutic levels of theophylline (10 to 20 mcg/ml).

Adverse reactions

CNS: *restlessness, dizziness,* headache, *insomnia,* light-headedness, *seizures,* muscle twitching. **CV:** *palpitations, sinus tachycardia,* extrasystoles, flushing, marked hypotension, increase in respiratory rate. **GI:** *nausea, vomiting, anorexia,* bitter aftertaste, dyspepsia, heavy feeling in stomach. **Skin:** urticaria.

Interactions

Adenosine: decreased antiarrhythmic effectiveness. Higher doses of adenosine may be necessary. **Barbiturates, carbamazepine, nicotine, phenytoin, rifampin:** enhanced metabolism and decreased theophylline blood levels. Monitor for decreased effect. **Beta-adrenergic blockers:** antagonism. Propranolol and nadolol, especially, may cause bronchospasms in sensitive patients. Use together cautiously. **Cimetidine, influenza virus vaccine, macrolide antibiotics (such as erythromycin), oral contraceptives, quinolone antibiotics (such as ciprofloxacin):** decreased hepatic clearance of theophylline; elevated theophylline levels. Monitor for signs of toxicity.

Nursing diagnoses

• Ineffective airway clearance related to patient's underlying condition.
• High risk for injury related to adverse CNS reactions to oxtriphylline.
• Knowledge deficit related to oxtriphylline therapy.

Nursing interventions

• *Contraindicated* in hypersensitivity to xanthines (caffeine, theobromine) and in preexisting cardiac arrhythmias, especially tachyarrhythmias.
• Monitor effectiveness of therapy by monitoring serum theophylline levels. Therapeutic levels are 10 to 20 mcg/ml, although some patients will respond at lower levels. Toxicity usually occurs with levels above 20 mcg/ml.
• Tell patient to report GI distress, palpitations, irritability, restlessness, nervousness, or insomnia; may indicate excessive CNS stimulation.
• Administer drug after meals and at bedtime.
• Store at 59° to 86° F (15° to 30° C). Protect elixir from light and tablets from moisture.
• Equivalent to 64% anhydrous theophylline.
• Monitor therapy carefully. Individuals metabolize theophyllines at different rates. Dosage adjustments are necessary in elderly patients; in patients with CHF, cor pulmonale, or hepatic disease; and in smokers.
• Combination products that contain ephedrine are not recommended; excessive CNS stimulation may result (nervousness, tremors, akathisia).

enoxaparin sodium
Lovenox

General
Classification: antithrombolytic (synthetic heparin derivative). **Pregnancy risk category:** B.

Mechanism of action
Has a higher ratio of anti-Factor Xa to anti-Factor IIa than heparin and doesn't significantly alter bleeding time, platelet function, PT, or activated partial thromboplastin time (APTT).

Indications and dosage
• Prevention of deep vein thrombosis after hip replacement. **Adults:** 30 mg S.C. b.i.d. Initiate therapy as soon as possible, but no later than 24 hours, after surgery. Most patients receive the drug for 7 to 10 days.

Adverse reactions
Blood: thrombocytopenia, hemorrhage, hypotension, hypochromic anemia. **Local:** mild irritation, pain, hematoma, erythema. **Other:** fever, ecchymosis, peripheral edema, ***anaphylaxis.***

Interactions
Oral anticoagulants: increased risk of bleeding. Use cautiously.

Nursing diagnoses
• High risk for fluid volume deficit related to adverse effects of enoxaparin therapy.
• Knowledge deficit related to enoxaparin therapy.

Nursing interventions
• *Contraindicated* in patients with hypersensitivity to the drug, heparin, or pork products; patients with active major bleeding episodes; or those with thrombocytopenia associated with antiplatelet antibody.
• *Use cautiously* in patients with uncontrolled hypertension, bleeding diathesis, or conditions that increase the risk of hemorrhage, such as bacterial endocarditis; in those with a history of GI ulceration or hemorrhagic stroke; or shortly after brain, eye, or spinal surgery.
• Perform baseline hematologic studies, including CBC and platelet count, and repeat periodically during therapy. Usually there's no need to check hematologic parameters daily in patients with normal baseline studies.
• Alternate injection sites between the left and right anterolateral and posterolateral abdominal wall. Administer with patient lying down.
• If overdose occurs, enoxaparin may be neutralized by protamine sulfate. Give 1 mg of protamine sulfate for each mg of enoxaparin administered. Although hemorrhagic complications may be corrected by such treatment, the APTT may remain prolonged.
• Have resuscitation equipment readily available when administering protamine sulfate because hypotensive and anaphylactic reactions have occurred.

General

Classification: anxiolytic, sedative-hypnotic (benzodiazepine). **Pregnancy risk category:** C. **Controlled substance schedule:** IV.

Mechanism of action

Depresses the CNS at the limbic and subcortical levels of the brain.

Indications and dosage

- Alcohol withdrawal. **Adults:** 15 to 30 mg P.O. t.i.d. or q.i.d.
- Severe anxiety. **Adults:** 15 to 30 mg P.O. t.i.d. or q.i.d.
- Tension, mild to moderate anxiety. **Adults:** 10 to 15 mg P.O. t.i.d. or q.i.d.

Adverse reactions

Blood: ***leukopenia (rare).*** **CNS:** *drowsiness, lethargy, hangover,* syncope. **CV:** transient hypotension. **GI:** nausea, vomiting, abdominal discomfort. **Hepatic:** ***hepatic dysfunction.***

Interactions

Alcohol, other CNS depressants: increased CNS depression. Avoid concomitant use. **Cigarette smoking:** increased clearance of benzodiazepines. Monitor for lack of effect. **Digoxin:** benzodiazepines may increase serum levels of digoxin, increasing risk of toxicity. Monitor closely.

Nursing diagnoses

- Anxiety related to the patient's underlying condition.
- High risk for injury related to drug-induced CNS reactions.
- Knowledge deficit related to oxazepam therapy.

Nursing interventions

- *Contraindicated* in patients with hypersensitivity to the drug and in those with acute narrow-angle glaucoma, depression, or psychoses.
- *Use cautiously* in patients with history of seizure disorders, drug allergies, blood dyscrasias, renal disease, or depression.
- Dosage should be reduced in elderly or debilitated patients.
- Possibility of abuse and addiction exists. Don't stop drug abruptly; withdrawal symptoms may occur.
- Warn patient to avoid hazardous activities that require alertness or good psychomotor coordination until CNS effects of the drug are known.
- Warn patient not to combine drug with alcohol or other depressants.
- Oxazepam has fewer cumulative effects than many other benzodiazepines because of its short half-life.
- Periodic hepatic, renal, and hematopoietic function studies should be performed in patients receiving repeated or prolonged therapy.
- If oxazepam overdose occurs, flumazenil (a specific benzodiazepine antagonist) may be useful. Know that the duration of action of oxazepam is longer than that of flumazenil, and resedation is possible.

General
Classification: bronchodilator, vasopressor, sympathomimetic (adrenergic). **Pregnancy risk category:** C.

Mechanism of action
Both a direct- and indirect-acting sympathomimetic that stimulates alpha- and beta-adrenergic receptors.

Indications and dosage
• Correction of hypotensive states; support ventricular rate in Adams-Stokes syndrome. **Adults:** 25 to 50 mg I.M. or S.C., or 10 to 25 mg I.V. p.r.n. to maximum of 150 mg/24 hours. **Children:** 3 mg/kg S.C. or I.V. daily, in four to six divided doses.
• Bronchodilator or nasal decongestant. **Adults:** 12.5 to 50 mg P.O. b.i.d., t.i.d., or q.i.d. Maximum dosage is 400 mg daily in six to eight divided doses. **Children:** 2 to 3 mg/kg oral solution P.O. daily in four to six divided doses.

Adverse reactions
CNS: *insomnia, nervousness,* dizziness, headache, muscle weakness, sweating, euphoria, confusion, delirium. **CV:** *palpitations,* tachycardia, hypertension. **EENT:** dryness of nose and throat. **GI:** nausea, vomiting, anorexia. **GU:** urine retention, painful urination due to visceral sphincter spasm.

Interactions
Acetazolamide: increased serum ephedrine levels. Monitor for toxicity. **Alpha-adrenergic blocking agents:** unopposed beta-adrenergic effects, resulting in hypotension. **Antihypertensives:** decreased effects. **Beta-adrenergic blocking agents:** unopposed alpha-adrenergic effects, resulting in hypertension. **Digitalis glycosides, general anesthetics (halogenated hydrocarbons):** increased risk of ventricular arrhythmias. **Ergot alkaloids:** enhanced vasoconstrictor activity. **Guanadrel, guanethidine:** enhanced pressor effects of ephedrine. **Levodopa:** enhanced risk of ventricular arrhythmias. **MAO inhibitors, TCAs:** when given with sympathomimetics, may cause severe hypertension (hypertensive crisis). **Methyldopa:** may inhibit effects of ephedrine. Use together cautiously.

Nursing diagnoses
• Decreased cardiac output related to patient's underlying condition.
• Ineffective airway clearance related to patient's underlying condition.
• Knowledge deficit related to ephedrine therapy.

Nursing interventions
• *Contraindicated* in porphyria, severe coronary artery disease, cardiac arrhythmias, narrow-angle glaucoma, or psychoneurosis; and in patients on MAO-inhibitor therapy.
• *Use cautiously* in elderly patients and those with hypertension, hyperthyroidism, nervous or excitable states, cardiovascular disease, or prostatic hypertrophy.
• Be aware that ephedrine is not a substitute for blood or fluid volume deficit. Volume deficit should be replaced before vasopressors are administered.
• Ephedrine administration, identify and correct any hypoxia, hypercapnia, and acidosis, which may reduce effectiveness or increase the incidence of adverse reactions.
• Tell patient that effectiveness decreases after 2 to 3 weeks, at which time increased dosage may be needed. Tolerance develops, but drug is not known to cause addiction.
• Warn patient not to take OTC drugs that contain ephedrine without informing doctor.
• To prevent insomnia, avoid giving within 2 hours before bedtime.
• **I.V. use:** Give I.V. injection slowly.

General

Classification: nonnarcotic analgesic, antipyretic (NSAID). **Pregnancy risk category:** C.

Mechanism of action

Produces anti-inflammatory, analgesic, and antipyretic effects, possibly through inhibition of prostaglandin synthesis.

Indications and dosage

• Acute and long-term management of signs and symptoms of osteoarthritis or rheumatoid arthritis. **Adults:** initially, 1,200 mg P.O. daily. Individualize dosage to the smallest effective dose to minimize adverse reactions. Smaller patients or those with mild symptoms may require only 600 mg daily. Maximum is 1,800 mg or 26 mg/kg, whichever is lower, in divided doses.

Adverse reactions

CNS: depression, sedation, somnolence, confusion, sleep disturbances. **GI:** *nausea, dyspepsia, diarrhea, constipation,* abdominal pain or distress, anorexia, flatulence, vomiting. **GU:** dysuria, urinary frequency. **Skin:** *rash,* photosensitivity. **Other:** tinnitus.

O

Interactions

Alcohol, aspirin, corticosteroids: increased risk of adverse GI reactions. Avoid concomitant use. **Antihypertensives:** decreased antihypertensive effect. Periodically monitor blood pressure and adjust dosage of antihypertensive as ordered. **Aspirin:** oxaprozin displaces salicylates from plasma protein-binding sites, increasing risk of salicylate toxicity. Avoid concomitant use. **Oral anticoagulants:** increased risk of bleeding. Use together cautiously.

Nursing diagnoses

• Pain related to the patient's underlying condition.
• High risk for injury related to oxaprozin-induced gastric ulcerations.
• Knowledge deficit related to oxaprozin therapy.

Nursing interventions

• *Contraindicated* in patients with hypersensitivity to the drug, aspirin, or other NSAIDs.
• *Use cautiously* in patients with a history of peptic ulcer disease or hepatic or renal dysfunction.
• Serious GI toxicity can occur at any time in NSAID therapy. Teach patient signs and symptoms of GI bleeding, and tell him to report these to doctor immediately.
• Because renal prostaglandins play a role in the maintenance of renal perfusion, patients with preexisting conditions that lead to a reduction in renal blood flow may experience renal toxicity with NSAID therapy. Those at greatest risk are elderly patients, patients taking diuretics, and those with impaired renal, hepatic, or cardiac function.
• As with other NSAIDs, elevations of liver function tests can occur after long-term use in up to 15% of patients. Rarely, patients may progress to severe hepatic dysfunction. Periodically monitor liver function tests in patients receiving long-term therapy.
• Tell patient that full therapeutic effect may be delayed for 2 to 4 weeks.
• Give dose 30 minutes before or 2 hours after meals. If adverse GI reactions occur, give with milk or meals.
• Because of their antipyretic and anti-inflammatory actions, NSAIDs may mask the signs and symptoms of infection.
• Oxaprozin has been associated with photosensitivity reactions. Advise patient to use a sunscreen, wear protective clothing, and avoid prolonged exposure to sunlight.

General

Classification: bronchodilator, vasopressor, cardiac stimulant, local anesthetic (adjunct), topical antihemorrhagic (adrenergic). **Pregnancy risk category:** C.

Mechanism of action

Stimulates alpha- and beta-adrenergic receptors within the sympathetic nervous system.

Indications and dosage

- Bronchospasm, hypersensitivity reactions, anaphylaxis. **Adults:** 0.1 to 0.5 ml of 1:1,000 S.C. or I.M. Repeat q 10 to 15 minutes, p.r.n. Or 0.1 to 0.25 ml 1:1,000 I.V. **Children:** 0.01 ml (10 mcg) of 1:1,000/kg S.C. Repeat q 20 minutes to 4 hours, p.r.n.; or 0.005 ml/kg of 1:200 (hydrochloride). Repeat q 8 to 12 hours, p.r.n.
- Hemostasis. **Adults:** 1:50,000 to 1:1,000, applied topically.
- Acute asthmatic attacks (inhalation). **Adults and children:** 1 or 2 inhalations of 1:100 or 2.25% racemic, q 1 to 5 minutes until relief is obtained; 0.2 mg/dose usual content.
- Prolongation of local anesthetic effect. **Adults and children:** 0.2 to 0.4 ml of 1:1,000 intraspinal; or 1:500,000 to 1:50,000 local mixed with local anesthetic.
- Restoration of cardiac rhythm in cardiac arrest. **Adults:** 0.5 to 1 mg I.V. or into endotracheal tube. May be given intracardiac if no I.V. route or intratracheal route available. Some clinicians advocate higher dose (up to 5 mg), especially in patients who don't respond to usual I.V dose. Following initial I.V. administration, may be infused I.V. at a rate of 1 to 4 mcg/minute. **Children:** 10 mcg/kg I.V. or 5 to 10 mcg (0.05 to 0.1 ml of 1:10,000)/kg intracardiac.

Adverse reactions

CNS: *nervousness,* tremor, euphoria, anxiety, coldness of extremities, vertigo, *headache,* sweating, disorientation, agitation. In patients with Parkinson's disease, the drug increases rigidity and tremor. **CV:** *palpitations;* widened pulse pressure; ***hypertension; tachycardia; ventricular fibrillation; CVA;*** anginal pain; ECG changes, including a decrease in the T-wave amplitude. **Metabolic:** hyperglycemia, glycosuria. **Other:** pulmonary edema, dyspnea, pallor.

Interactions

Alpha-adrenergic blockers: hypotension due to unopposed beta-adrenergic effects. **Beta blockers, such as propranolol:** vasoconstriction and reflex bradycardia. Monitor patient carefully. **Digitalis glycosides, general anesthetics (halogenated hydrocarbons):** increased risk of ventricular arrhythmias. **Doxapram, mazindol, methylphenidate:** enhanced CNS stimulation or pressor effects. **Ergot alkaloids:** enhanced vasoconstrictor activity. **Guanadrel, guanethidine:** enhanced pressor effects of epinephrine. **Levodopa:** enhanced risk of cardiac arrhythmias. **MAO inhibitors:** increased risk of hypertensive crisis. **TCAs, antihistamines, thyroid hormones:** may cause severe adverse cardiac effects; avoid giving with sympathomimetics.

Nursing diagnoses

- Ineffective airway clearance related to patient's underlying condition.
- Decreased cardiac output related to epinephrine-induced adverse CV effects.
- Knowledge deficit related to epinephrine therapy.

Nursing interventions

- *Contraindicated* in narrow-angle glaucoma, shock (other than anaphylactic shock), organic brain damage, cardiac dilatation, or coronary insufficiency; during general anesthesia with halogenated hydrocarbons or cyclopropane; and in labor (may delay second stage).
- *Use with extreme caution* in degenerative heart disease secondary to long-standing bronchial asthma or emphysema; in elderly patients; and in hyperthyroidism, angina, hypertension, psychoneurosis, and diabetes.
- **I.V. use:** Don't mix with alkaline solutions. Use D_5W, 0.9% sodium chloride solution, or combination of the two. Mix just before use.

General

Classification: antibiotic (penicillinase-resistant penicillin). **Pregnancy risk category:** B.

Mechanism of action

Bactericidal against microorganisms by inhibiting cell wall synthesis during active multiplication. Bacteria resist penicillins by producing penicillinases—enzymes that convert penicillins to inactive penicilloic acid. Oxacillin resists these enzymes.

Indications and dosage

- Systemic infections caused by penicillinase-producing staphylococci. **Adults:** 2 to 4 g P.O. daily, divided into doses given q 6 hours; or 2 to 12 g I.M. or I.V. daily, divided into doses given q 4 to 6 hours. **Children:** 50 to 100 mg/kg P.O. daily, divided into doses given q 6 hours; or 100 to 200 mg/kg I.M. or I.V. daily, divided into doses given q 4 to 6 hours.

Adverse reactions

Blood: granulocytopenia, thrombocytopenia, eosinophilia, ***hemolytic anemia***, transient neutropenia. **CNS:** seizures, neuropathy, neuromuscular irritability. **GI:** oral lesions. **GU:** interstitial nephritis, transient hematuria, proteinuria. **Hepatic:** hepatitis, elevated enzymes. **Local:** *thrombophlebitis.* **Other:** hypersensitivity (fever, chills, rash, urticaria, ***anaphylaxis***), overgrowth of nonsusceptible organisms.

Interactions

Probenecid: increases blood levels of oxacillin and other penicillins. Probenecid may be used for this purpose.

Nursing diagnoses

- High risk for injury related to the ineffectiveness of oxacillin in eradicating the infection.
- Impaired tissue integrity related to oxacillin-induced thrombophlebitis when administered I.V.
- Knowledge deficit related to oxacillin therapy.

Nursing interventions

- *Use cautiously* in patients with drug allergies, especially to cephalosporins (possible cross-allergenicity); in premature neonates; and in infants.
- Obtain specimen for culture and sensitivity tests before first dose. Therapy may begin pending test results.
- Before giving oxacillin, ask patient if he's had any allergic reactions to penicillin. However, a negative history of penicillin allergy is no guarantee against a future allergic reaction.
- Tell the patient to take medication exactly as prescribed, even if he feels better. The entire quantity prescribed should be taken.
- Instruct him to call the doctor if rash, fever, or chills develop. A rash is the most common allergic reaction.
- When given orally, the drug may cause GI disturbances. Food may interfere with absorption, so give drug 1 to 2 hours before meals or 2 to 3 hours afterward.
- Don't give I.M. or I.V. unless infection is severe or patient can't take oral dose.
- Monitor liver function studies periodically; watch for elevated AST and ALT.
- With large doses and prolonged therapy, bacterial and fungal superinfections may occur, especially in elderly, debilitated, or immunosuppressed patients. Close observation is essential.
- Give oxacillin at least 1 hour before bacteriostatic antibiotics.
- **I.V. use:** When giving I.V., mix with D_5W or a saline solution.
- Give I.V. intermittently to prevent vein irritation. Change site every 48 hours.

General

Classification: antianemic agent (glycoprotein).
Pregnancy risk category: C.

Mechanism of action

Produced by recombinant DNA techniques. Mimics the effects of erythropoietin, a naturally occurring hormone produced by the kidney. It acts on the erythroid tissues in the bone marrow stimulating the mitotic activity of erythroid progenitor cells and early precursor cells, causing them to differentiate into RBCs. It functions as a growth factor and as a differentiating factor.

Indications and dosage

- Anemia due to reduced production of endogenous erythropoietin or end-stage renal disease. **Adults:** dosage is individualized. Starting dose is 50 to 100 units/kg I.V. three times weekly. (Nondialysis patients with chronic renal failure or patients receiving continuous peritoneal dialysis may receive the drug by S.C. injection or I.V.) Reduce dosage when target hematocrit is reached or if hematocrit rises more than 4 points in any 2-week period. Increase dosage if hematocrit does not increase by 5 to 6 points after 8 weeks of therapy. Maintenance dose is usually 25 units/kg three times weekly.
- Adjunctive treatment of HIV-infected patients with anemia secondary to zidovudine therapy. **Adults:** 100 units/kg I.V. or S.C. three times weekly for 8 weeks or until target hemoglobin is reached.

Adverse reactions

Blood: iron deficiency, elevated platelet count. **CNS:** headache, ***seizures.*** **CV:** *hypertension,* decreased plasma volume. **GI:** nausea, vomiting, diarrhea. **Skin:** rash. **Other:** increased clotting of arteriovenous grafts.

Interactions

None reported.

Nursing diagnoses

- Altered protection related to reduced production of endogenous erythropoietin.
- High risk for injury related to epoetin-induced seizures.
- Knowledge deficit related to epoetin therapy.

Nursing interventions

- *Contraindicated* in patients with uncontrolled hypertension. Reduce dosage in patients who exhibit a rapid rise in hematocrit (more than 4 points in any 2-week period) because of the risk of hypertension.
- Patient's response to epoetin is probably dependent on amount of endogenous erythropoietin in the plasma. Patients with levels of 500 units/liter or more usually have transfusion-dependent anemia and will probably not respond to the drug; with levels below 500 units/liter, mild to moderate anemia; and with levels below 100 units/liter, renal failure. Those with levels below 500 units/liter usually respond well.
- Adjust dosage on individual basis according to patient's response in HIV infection. Dosage recommendations are for patients with endogenous erythropoietin levels of 500 units/liter or less and cumulative zidovudine doses of 4.2 g/week or less.
- Monitor blood pressure before initiating therapy. Up to 80% of patients with chronic renal failure have hypertension. Blood pressure may rise, especially when hematocrit is increasing during early therapy. Diet restrictions or drug therapy may be needed to control blood pressure.
- Monitor blood count during therapy. Hematocrit may rise and cause excessive clotting.
- Observe patient for pain or discomfort in long bones and pelvis, chills, and diaphoresis about 2 hours after injection.
- As ordered, give additional heparin to prevent clotting during dialysis treatments.
- Tell patient to avoid hazardous activities, such as driving or operating heavy machinery, during early therapy. Excessively rapid hematocrit rise may be linked to seizures.
- Inform patient that blood samples will be drawn weekly for blood counts; dosage adjustments may be indicated.

General

Classification: skeletal muscle relaxant (diphenhydramine analogue). **Pregnancy risk category:** C.

Mechanism of action

Precise mechanism unknown. Reduces transmission of impulses from the spinal cord to skeletal muscle. May also block central cholinergic receptors in the cerebrum or medulla.

Indications and dosage

- Adjunctive treatment in painful, acute musculoskeletal conditions. **Adults:** 100 mg P.O. b.i.d., or 60 mg I.V. or I.M. q 12 hours p.r.n. For maintenance, switch to oral therapy beginning 12 hours after last parenteral dose.

Adverse reactions

Blood: *aplastic anemia.* **CNS:** disorientation, restlessness, irritability, weakness, *drowsiness,* headache, dizziness. **CV:** palpitations, tachycardia. **EENT:** dilated pupils, blurred vision, difficulty swallowing. **GI:** constipation, *dry mouth,* nausea, vomiting, paralytic ileus, epigastric distress. **GU:** urinary hesitancy or urine retention.

Interactions

Alcohol, other CNS depressants: increased CNS depression. Avoid concomitant use.

Nursing diagnoses

- Pain related to the patient's underlying condition.
- Altered oral mucous membrane related to adverse drug reactions.
- Knowledge deficit related to orphenadrine therapy.

Nursing interventions

- *Contraindicated* in narrow-angle glaucoma; prostatic hyperplasia; pyloric, duodenal, or bladder-neck obstruction; myasthenia gravis; tachycardia; severe hepatic or renal disease; or ulcerative colitis.
- *Use cautiously* in elderly or debilitated patients with cardiac disease, arrhythmias, sulfite sensitivity, and in those exposed to high temperatures.
- Check all dosages carefully. Even a slight overdose can lead to toxicity. Early signs are very dry mouth, dilated pupils, blurred vision, skin flushing, and fever.
- Monitor the patient's vital signs carefully.
- Tell the patient to report urinary hesitancy and urine retention. Have him void before taking the drug.
- Relieve dry mouth with cool drinks, sugarless gum, or hard candy.
- Monitor CBC, hepatic function, and urinalysis in patients receiving long-term therapy.
- Advise patients to avoid tasks that require alertness until the CNS effects of the drug are known.
- **I.V. use:** Inject the drug over approximately 5 minutes while the patient is supine. Wait 5 to 10 minutes and then help patient to sit up.
- When given I.V., drug may cause paradoxical initial bradycardia. This effect usually disappears in 2 minutes.

General

Classification: oxytocic (ergot alkaloid). **Pregnancy risk category:** not applicable.

Mechanism of action

Increases motor activity of the uterus by direct stimulation. Prolonged uterine contraction helps control hemorrhage.

Indications and dosage

- Prevention and treatment of postpartum and postabortion hemorrhage from uterine atony or subinvolution. **Adults:** 0.2 mg I.M. q 2 to 4 hours, maximum of 5 doses; or 0.2 mg I.V. (only for severe uterine bleeding or other life-threatening emergency) over 1 minute while blood pressure and uterine contractions are monitored. I.V. dose may be diluted to 5 ml with injection of 0.9% sodium chloride solution. After initial I.M. or I.V. dose, may give 0.2 to 0.4 mg P.O. q 6 to 12 hours for 2 to 7 days. Decrease dosage if severe uterine cramping occurs.

Adverse reactions

CNS: dizziness, headache. **CV:** ***hypertension,*** chest pain. **EENT:** tinnitus. **GI:** nausea, vomiting. **GU:** uterine cramping. **Other:** sweating, dyspnea, ***hypersensitivity.***

Interactions

Regional anesthetics, dopamine, I.V. oxytocin: excessive vasoconstriction. Use together cautiously.

Nursing diagnoses

- Fluid volume deficit related to postpartum hemorrhage.
- Pain related to ergonovine-induced uterine cramping.
- Knowledge deficit related to ergonovine therapy.

Nursing interventions

- *Contraindicated* for induction or augmentation of labor, before delivery of placenta, in threatened spontaneous abortion, and in patients with allergy or sensitivity to ergot preparations.
- *Use cautiously* in hypertension, cardiac disease, venoatrial shunts, mitral valve stenosis, obliterative vascular disease, sepsis, and hepatic or renal impairment.
- Administer only when meticulous observation is possible. Uterine hyperstimulation during labor may lead to uterine tetany, which may impair placental blood flow and cause amniotic fluid embolism.
- Monitor blood pressure, pulse rate, and uterine response. Report sudden changes in vital signs, frequent periods of uterine relaxation, and character and amount of vaginal bleeding.
- Hypocalcemia may decrease patient response. If patient is not also taking a digitalis glycoside, cautious administration of calcium gluconate I.V. may produce desired oxytocic action.
- Expect contractions to begin 5 to 15 minutes after P.O. administration. May continue 3 hours or more after P.O. or I.M. administration.
- Keep patient warm.
- Store drug in tightly closed, light-resistant container. Discard if discolored.
- **I.V. use:** Contractions begin immediately after I.V. injection and may continue for up to 45 minutes.
- Store I.V. solutions below 46.4° F (8° C). Daily stock may be kept at cool room temperature for 60 days.
- I.V. ergonovine is also used to diagnose coronary artery spasm (Prinzmetal's angina).
- Also known as ergometrine maleate.

General
Classification: antidiarrheal (opiate). **Pregnancy risk category:** B (D for prolonged use or high doses at term). **Controlled substance schedule:** II (III for camphorated opium tincture).

Mechanism of action
Increases smooth muscle tone in the GI tract, inhibits motility and propulsion, and diminishes secretions.

Indications and dosage
• Acute, nonspecific diarrhea. **Adults:** 0.6 ml opium tincture (range 0.3 to 1 ml) P.O. q.i.d. Maximum dosage 6 ml daily; or 5 to 10 ml camphorated opium tincture daily b.i.d., t.i.d., or q.i.d. until diarrhea subsides. **Children:** 0.25 to 0.5 ml/kg camphorated opium tincture P.O. daily, b.i.d., t.i.d., or q.i.d. until diarrhea subsides.

Adverse reactions
GI: nausea, vomiting. **Other:** physical dependence after long-term use.

Interactions
None significant.

Nursing diagnoses
• Diarrhea related to interruption of normal pattern of elimination.
• Altered nutrition: Less than body requirements, related to drug-induced nausea and vomiting.
• Knowledge deficit related to opium tincture therapy.

Nursing interventions
• *Contraindicated* in acute diarrhea resulting from poisoning until toxins are removed from the GI tract, and in diarrhea caused by microorganisms that penetrate the intestinal mucosa.
• *Use cautiously* in patients with asthma, prostatic hyperplasia, hepatic disease, and narcotic dependence.
• Don't use for more than 2 days. Risk of physical dependence increases with long-term use.
• An effective and prompt-acting antidiarrheal; drug dosage can be adjusted precisely to the patient's needs.
• Opium content of opium tincture is 25 times greater than camphorated opium tincture. Camphorated opium tincture is more diluted, and teaspoonful doses are easier to measure than dropper quantities of opium tincture.
• Milky fluid forms when camphorated opium tincture is added to water.
• Camphorated opium tincture dosage of 0.06 to 0.5 ml daily has been used to treat infants with mild narcotic dependence.
• Store in tightly capped, light-resistant container.
• Mix with sufficient water to ensure passage to stomach.
• Narcotic antagonist naloxone can reverse the respiratory depression resulting from overdose.

General

Classification: vasoconstrictor (ergot alkaloid).
Pregnancy risk category: X.

Mechanism of action

Inhibits the effects of epinephrine, norepinephrine, and other sympathomimetic amines. Also has antiserotonin effects.

Indications and dosage

• Vascular or migraine headache. **Adults:** initially, 2 mg P.O. or S.L., then 1 to 2 mg P.O. q hour or S.L. q ½ hour, to maximum of 6 mg daily and 10 mg weekly. Alternatively, use aerosol inhaler: 1 spray (360 mcg) initially, repeated every 5 minutes p.r.n. to a maximum of 6 sprays (2.16 mg) per 24 hours or 15 sprays (5.4 mg) per week.

Patient may also use rectal suppositories. Initially, 2 mg rectally at the onset of the attack, repeated in 1 hour p.r.n. Maximum dose is 2 suppositories per attack or 5 suppositories per week.

Adverse reactions

CV: numbness and tingling in fingers and toes, transient tachycardia or bradycardia, precordial distress and pain, increased arterial pressure, angina pectoris. **GI:** nausea, vomiting, diarrhea, abdominal cramps. **Skin:** itching. **Other:** weakness in legs, muscle pain in extremities, localized edema.

Interactions

Erythromycin, troleandomycin, other macrolides: may cause symptoms of ergot toxicity. Vasopressors (nitroprusside, nifedipine, or prazosin) may be ordered to treat such an attack. Monitor closely. **Propranolol and other beta blockers:** blocked natural pathway for vasodilation in patients receiving ergot alkaloids and thus could result in excessive vasoconstriction. Watch closely if drugs are used together.

Nursing diagnoses

• Pain related to the patient's underlying condition.
• Fluid volume deficit related to adverse GI effects of ergotamine.
• Knowledge deficit related to ergotamine therapy.

Nursing interventions

• *Contraindicated* in pregnancy and in peripheral and occlusive vascular diseases, coronary artery disease, hypertension, hepatic or renal dysfunction, sepsis.
• Avoid prolonged administration; don't exceed recommended dosage.
• Drug is most effective when used during prodromal stage of headache or as soon as possible after onset. Sublingual tablets are preferred during early stage of attack because of their rapid absorption.
• Provide a quiet, low-light environment to help patient relax.
• Help patient evaluate underlying causes of physical or emotional stress, which may precipitate attacks.
• Obtain an accurate dietary history from patient to determine if a relationship exists between certain foods and onset of headache.
• Stress importance of taking drug as prescribed. Warn patient not to increase dosage without first consulting the doctor. Explain that ergotamine rebound, or an increase in frequency and duration of headache, may occur if the drug is stopped.
• Teach patient how to use the inhaler correctly.
• Instruct patient on long-term therapy to check for and report feeling of coldness in extremities or tingling of fingers and toes due to vasoconstriction. Severe vasoconstriction may result in tissue damage.
• Tell patient to avoid prolonged exposure to cold weather whenever possible. Cold may increase many of the drug's adverse reactions.
• Store drug in light-resistant container.

General

Classification: antiemetic serotonin (5-HT_3) antagonist. **Pregnancy risk category:** B.

Mechanism of action

Selectively antagonizes a specific type of serotonin receptor (5-HT_3), which is located in the CNS within the chemoreceptor trigger zone and in the peripheral nervous system on terminals of the vagus nerve. The drug's blocking action may occur at both sites.

Indications and dosage

- Prevention of nausea and vomiting associated with emetogenic chemotherapy. **Adults and children over 12 years:** 8 mg P.O. 30 minutes before the start of chemotherapy. Follow with 8 mg 4 hours and 8 hours after the first dose. Then follow with 8 mg q 8 hours for 1 to 2 days. Alternatively, infuse a single dose of 32 mg over 15 minutes, beginning 30 minutes before chemotherapy. Drug may also be administered in three doses of 0.15 mg/kg I.V. Give first dose 30 minutes before chemotherapy; administer subsequent doses 4 and 8 hours after the first dose. Infuse drug over 15 minutes. **Children ages 4 to 11:** 4 mg P.O. 30 minutes before chemotherapy. Follow with 4 mg 4 hours and 8 hours after the first dose. Then follow with 4 mg q 8 hours for 1 to 2 days. Alternatively, infuse a single dose of 32 mg over 15 minutes, beginning 30 minutes before chemotherapy. Drug may also be administered in three doses of 0.15 mg/kg I.V. Give first dose 30 minutes before chemotherapy; administer subsequent doses 4 and 8 hours after the first dose. Infuse drug over 15 minutes.

Adverse reactions

CNS: headache. **GI:** *diarrhea, constipation.* **Metabolic:** transient elevations in AST and ALT levels. **Skin:** rash. **Other:** ***bronchospasm (rare).***

Interactions

Drugs that alter hepatic drug metabolizing enzymes, such as phenobarbital or cimetidine: may alter pharmacokinetics of ondansetron. No dosage adjustment appears necessary.

Nursing diagnoses

- High risk for fluid volume deficit related to chemotherapy-induced nausea and vomiting.
- Constipation related to infrequent or absent bowel movements induced by ondansetron.
- Knowledge deficit related to ondansetron therapy.

Nursing interventions

- *Contraindicated* in patients hypersensitive to the drug.
- *Use cautiously* in patients with hepatic failure. Limit daily dosage (oral or I.V.) to 8 mg.
- **I.V. use:** Dilute the drug in 50 ml of D_5W or 0.9% sodium chloride solution before administration. The drug is also stable for up to 48 hours after dilution in dextrose 5% in 0.9% sodium chloride injection, dextrose 5% in 0.45% sodium chloride injection, and 3% sodium chloride injection.
- Decreased ondansetron clearance and prolonged half-life are reported in patients over age 75. However, no recommendations exist for reducing dosage because these pharmacokinetic changes haven't been associated with reduced safety or efficacy.

General
Classification: antianginal, vasodilator (nitrate).
Pregnancy risk category: C.

Mechanism of action
Reduces cardiac oxygen demand by decreasing left ventricular end-diastolic pressure (preload) and, to a lesser extent, systemic vascular resistance (afterload). Also increases blood flow through the collateral coronary vessels.

Indications and dosage
• Prophylaxis and long-term management of frequent or recurrent anginal pain, reduced exercise tolerance associated with angina pectoris. **Adults:** 5 mg P.O., S.L., or buccally t.i.d., increasing in 2 to 3 days if needed.

Adverse reactions
CNS: *headache, sometimes with throbbing; dizziness;* weakness. **CV:** *orthostatic hypotension, tachycardia, flushing, palpitations,* fainting. **GI:** nausea, vomiting. **Skin:** cutaneous vasodilation. **Local:** sublingual burning. **Other:** hypersensitivity reactions.

Interactions
None significant.

Nursing diagnoses
• Pain related to ineffectiveness of erythrityl therapy.
• High risk for injury related to erythrityl-induced dizziness or orthostatic hypotension.
• Knowledge deficit related to erythrityl therapy.

Nursing interventions
• *Contraindicated* in hypersensitivity to nitrates, head trauma, cerebral hemorrhage, or severe anemia.
• *Use cautiously* in hypotension.
• Monitor blood pressure and intensity and duration of response to drug.
• If drug causes headache, treat with aspirin or acetaminophen. Dosage may need to be reduced temporarily, but tolerance usually develops.
• Teach patient how to take the drug form prescribed. Stress the importance of taking the drug exactly as prescribed and to keep it easily accessible at all times.
• Tell patient to take an additional dose before anticipated stress or at bedtime if angina is nocturnal.
• Advise patient to avoid alcoholic beverages because they may produce increased hypotension.
• To minimize orthostatic hypotension, have patient change to upright position slowly, go up and down stairs carefully, and lie down at the first sign of dizziness.
• Teach patient to take sublingual tablet at first sign of attack. He should wet the tablet with saliva, place it under the tongue until completely absorbed, and sit down and rest. Dose may be repeated every 10 to 15 minutes for a maximum of three doses. If no relief, patient should call doctor or go to hospital emergency department. If patient complains of tingling sensation with drug placed sublingually, he may try holding tablet in buccal pouch.
• Teach patient to take tablet on empty stomach, either 30 minutes before or 1 to 2 hours after meals, and to swallow tablets whole.
• Warn patient that discontinuing the drug abruptly may cause coronary vasospasm.
• Instruct patient to store drug in cool place, in a tightly closed container from light. To ensure freshness, replace supply every 3 months. Remove cotton from container because it absorbs drug.

General

Classification: gastric acid suppressant (benzimidazole). **Pregnancy risk category:** C.

Mechanism of action

Inhibits activity of the acid (proton) pump, $H+/K+$ ATPase, located at the secretory surface of the gastric parietal cell. This blocks the formation of gastric acid.

Indications and dosage

- Severe erosive esophagitis; symptomatic, poorly responsive gastroesophageal reflux disease (GERD). **Adults:** 20 mg P.O. daily for 4 to 8 weeks. Patients with GERD should have failed initial therapy with a histamine H_2-antagonist.
- Pathologic hypersecretory conditions (such as Zollinger-Ellison syndrome). **Adults:** initially, 60 mg P.O. daily, with dosage titrated according to patient response. Daily dosage exceeding 80 mg should be administered in divided doses. Dosages up to 120 mg t.i.d. have been administered. Therapy should continue as long as clinically indicated.
- Duodenal ulcers. **Adults:** 20 mg P.O. daily for 4 to 8 weeks.

Adverse reactions

CNS: headache, dizziness. **GI:** diarrhea, abdominal pain, nausea, vomiting, constipation, flatulence. **Respiratory:** cough. **Skin:** rash. **Other:** back pain.

Interactions

Diazepam, warfarin, phenytoin: decreased hepatic clearance possibly leading to increased serum levels. Monitor closely. **Ketoconazole, iron derivatives, ampicillin esters:** may exhibit poor bioavailability in patients taking omeprazole because optimal absorption of these drugs requires a low gastric pH.

Nursing diagnoses

- Pain related to the patient's underlying condition.
- Diarrhea related to omeprazole-induced adverse GI reactions.
- Knowledge deficit related to omeprazole therapy.

Nursing interventions

- *Contraindicated* in patients with hypersensitivity to the drug or any component of the enteric formulation.
- Prolonged (2-year) studies in rats revealed a dose-related increase in gastric carcinoid tumors; studies in humans have not detected a risk from short-term exposure to the drug. Further study is needed to assess the impact of sustained hypergastrinemia and hypochlorhydria. The manufacturer recommends that therapy with omeprazole not exceed the indicated duration.
- Capsules should be swallowed whole and not opened or crushed.
- Omeprazole increases its own bioavailability with repeated administration. The drug is labile in gastric acid, and less drug is lost to hydrolysis as the drug increases gastric pH.
- Dosage adjustments are not required for renal or hepatic impairment.
- Most patients with duodenal ulcers heal within 4 weeks. Omeprazole should not be used for maintenance therapy.

General

Classification: antibiotic (macrolide). **Pregnancy risk category:** B.

Mechanism of action

Inhibits bacterial protein synthesis by binding to the 50S subunit of the ribosome.

Indications and dosage

- Acute pelvic inflammatory disease caused by *Neisseria gonorrhoeae.* **Women:** 500 mg I.V. (gluceptate, lactobionate) q 6 hours for 3 days, then 250-mg tablets, capsules, or oral suspension (base, estolate, stearate) or 400 mg tablets (ethylsuccinate) P.O. q 6 hours for 7 days.
- Endocarditis prophylaxis for dental procedures in patients allergic to penicillin. **Adults:** 1 g (base, estolate, stearate) or 800 to 1,600 mg (ethylsuccinate) P.O. 1 hour before procedure, then 500 mg (base, estolate, stearate) or 400 to 800 mg (ethylsuccinate) P.O. 6 hours later.
- Intestinal amebiasis. **Adults:** 250 mg (base, estolate, stearate) or 400 mg (ethylsuccinate) P.O. q 6 hours for 10 to 14 days. **Children:** 30 to 50 mg/kg (base, estolate, ethylsuccinate, stearate) P.O. daily, divided q 6 hours for 10 to 14 days.
- Mild to moderately severe respiratory tract, skin, and soft-tissue infections caused by sensitive group A beta-hemolytic streptococci, *Diplococcus pneumoniae, Mycoplasma pneumoniae, Corynebacterium diphtheriae, Bordetella pertussis, Listeria monocytogenes.* **Adults:** 250 to 500 mg (or base, estolate, stearate) P.O. q 6 hours; or 400 to 800 mg (ethylsuccinate) P.O. q 6 hours; or 15 to 20 mg/kg I.V. daily, as continuous infusion or divided q 6 hours. **Children:** 30 to 50 mg/kg (erythromycin salts) P.O. daily, divided q 6 hours; or 15 to 20 mg/kg I.V. daily, divided q 4 to 6 hours.
- Syphilis. **Adults:** 500 mg (or base, estolate, stearate) P.O. q.i.d. for 15 days.
- Uncomplicated urethral, endocervical, or rectal infections where tetracyclines are contraindicated. **Adults:** 500 mg (base, estolate, stearate) or 800 mg (ethylsuccinate) P.O. q.i.d. for at least 7 days.
- Urogenital *Chlamydia trachomatis* infections during pregnancy. **Adults:** 500 mg (base, estolate, stearate) P.O. q.i.d. for at least 7 days; or 250 mg (base, estolate, stearate) or 400 mg (ethylsuccinate) P.O. q.i.d. for at least 14 days.
- Conjunctivitis caused by *Chlamydia trachomatis* in neonates. **Neonates:** 50 mg/kg P.O. daily in four divided doses for at least 2 weeks.
- Pneumonia of infancy due to *Chlamydia trachomatis.* **Infants:** 50 mg/kg/day in four divided doses for at least 3 weeks.

Adverse reactions

EENT: hearing loss with high I.V. doses. **GI:** *abdominal pain and cramping, nausea, vomiting, diarrhea.* **Hepatic:** cholestatic jaundice (with erythromycin estolate). **Skin:** urticaria, rash. **Local:** *venous irritation, thrombophlebitis after I.V. injection.* **Other:** overgrowth of nonsusceptible bacteria or fungi, ***anaphylaxis,*** fever.

Interactions

Carbamazepine: increased carbamazepine blood levels and increased risk of toxicity. Monitor closely. **Clindamycin, lincomycin:** may be antagonistic. Don't use together. **Oral anticoagulants:** increased anticoagulant effects. Monitor PT closely. **Theophylline:** decreased erythromycin blood level and increased theophylline toxicity. Use together cautiously.

Nursing diagnoses

- High risk for injury related to ineffectiveness of erythromycin in eradicating the infection.
- High risk for fluid volume deficit related to erythromycin-induced adverse GI reactions.
- Knowledge deficit related to erythryomycin therapy.

Nursing interventions

- Estolate salt is *contraindicated* in hepatic disease. *Use* other erythromycin salts *cautiously* in impaired hepatic function.
- **I.V. use:** Administer I.V. dose over 60 minutes. Reconstitute according to manufacturer's directions, and dilute each 250 mg in at least 100 ml 0.9% sodium chloride solution.

General
Classification: anti-inflammatory (salicylate). **Pregnancy risk category:** C.

Mechanism of action
Converted to 5-aminosalicylic acid (5-ASA or mesalamine) in the colon. Acts as a local anti-inflammatory agent in the colon.

Indications and dosage
• Maintenance of remission of ulcerative colitis in patients intolerant of sulfasalazine. **Adults:** 500 mg P.O. b.i.d. with meals.

Adverse reactions
CNS: headache, depression, vertigo, dizziness. **GI:** *diarrhea,* nausea, abdominal pain, heartburn. **Skin:** rash, itching. **Other:** arthralgia.

Interactions
None reported.

Nursing diagnoses
• Pain related to underlying disorder.
• Diarrhea related to olsalazine-induced adverse effects.
• Knowledge deficit related to olsalazine therapy.

Nursing interventions
• *Contraindicated* in patients with hypersensitivity to salicylates.
• *Use cautiously* in patients with preexisting renal disease. Regularly monitor BUN and creatinine levels and urinalysis in these patients. Although problems have not been reported for this drug, the possibility of renal tubular damage from absorbed mesalamine or its metabolites must be considered.
• Clinical trials showed that 17% of all patients reported diarrhea sometime during therapy. Although diarrhea appears dose-related, it is difficult to distinguish from a worsening of the symptoms of the disease. Exacerbation of the disease has been noted with similar drugs.
• Teach the patient to take the drug in evenly divided doses, with food.

esmolol hydrochloride

Brevibloc

General

Classification: antiarrhythmic ($beta_1$-adrenergic blocker). **Pregnancy risk category:** C.

Mechanism of action

A class II antiarrhythmic, esmolol is an ultra-short-acting $beta_1$-selective adrenergic blocker. Decreases heart rate, myocardial contractility, and blood pressure.

Indications and dosage

• Supraventricular tachycardia. **Adults:** loading dose is 500 mcg/kg/minute by I.V. infusion over 1 minute, followed by a 4-minute maintenance infusion of 50 mcg/kg/minute. If adequate response does not occur within 5 minutes, repeat the loading dose followed by a maintenance infusion of 100 mcg/kg/minute for 4 minutes. Maximum maintenance infusion is 200 mcg/kg/minute.

Adverse reactions

CNS: dizziness, somnolence, headache, agitation, fatigue. **CV:** *hypotension* (sometimes with diaphoresis). **GI:** *nausea,* vomiting. **Local:** inflammation and induration at infusion site. **Other:** bronchospasm.

Interactions

Diazepam, furosemide, sodium bicarbonate, and thiopental sodium: may decrease effectiveness of esmolol. Avoid concomitant use. **Digoxin:** esmolol may increase serum digoxin levels by 10% to 20%. **Morphine:** may increase esmolol blood levels. Titrate esmolol carefully. **Reserpine (and other catecholamine-depleting drugs):** may cause additive bradycardia and hypotension. Titrate esmolol carefully. **Succinylcholine:** esmolol may prolong neuromuscular blockade.

Nursing diagnoses

• Decreased cardiac output related to ineffectiveness of esmolol therapy.
• Altered cerebral tissue perfusion related to esmolol-induced hypotension.
• Knowledge deficit related to esmolol therapy.

Nursing interventions

• *Contraindicated* in sinus bradycardia, heart block greater than first degree, cardiogenic shock, or overt heart failure.
• *Use cautiously* in impaired renal function, diabetes, or bronchospasm.
• Esmolol has an extremely short duration of action and can be accurately titrated. This makes it more effective than other beta blockers in treating cardiac arrhythmias.
• Also be aware that esmolol is recommended only for short-term use, no longer than 48 hours.
• **I.V. use:** Don't give esmolol by I.V. push; use a controlled infusion device. Drug must be diluted before infusion.
• Monitor continuous ECG and blood pressure during infusion. Up to 50% of all patients treated with esmolol develop hypotension. Monitor closely, especially if patient's pretreatment blood pressure was low.
• If hypotension develops, decrease the dose or, if necessary, stop the infusion. These interventions usually reverse hypotension within 30 minutes.
• If a local reaction develops at the infusion site, change to another site. Avoid butterfly needles.
• When patient's heart rate becomes stable, expect esmolol to be replaced by alternative (longer-acting) antiarrhythmics, such as propranolol, digoxin, or verapamil. As the replacement drug is started, gradually reduce the esmolol infusion over 1 hour.

ofloxacin

Floxin

General
Classification: antibiotic (fluoroquinolone). **Pregnancy risk category:** C.

Mechanism of action
Bactericidal effects may result from the drug's ability to inhibit bacterial DNA gyrase and to prevent DNA replication in susceptible bacteria.

Indications and dosage
- Lower respiratory tract infections caused by strains of *Haemophilus influenzae* or *Streptococcus pneumoniae*. **Adults:** 400 mg P.O. q 12 hours for 10 days.
- Cervicitis or urethritis caused by *Chlamydia trachomatis* or *Neisseria gonorrhoeae*. **Adults:** 300 mg P.O. q 12 hours for 7 days.
- Acute, uncomplicated gonorrhea. **Adults:** 400 mg P.O. as a single dose.
- Mild-to-moderate skin and skin structure infections caused by *Staphylococcus aureus, S. epidermidis, Streptococcus pyogenes*, or *Proteus mirabilis*. **Adults:** 400 mg P.O. q 12 hours for 10 days.
- Cystitis caused by *Escherichia coli* or *Klebsiella pneumoniae*. **Adults:** 200 mg P.O. q 12 hours for 3 days.
- UTIs caused by *Citrobacter diversus, Enterobacter aerogenes, Escherichia coli, Proteus mirabilis*, or *Pseudomonas aeruginosa*. **Adults:** 200 mg P.O. q 12 hours for 7 to 10 days.
- Prostatitis caused by *E. coli*. **Adults:** 200 mg P.O. q 12 hours for 6 weeks.

Adverse reactions
CNS: headache, dizziness, fatigue, malaise, drowsiness, sleep disorders, nervousness, light-headedness, seizures. **CV:** chest pain. **GI:** nausea, anorexia, abdominal pain, diarrhea, dry mouth, flatulence, dysgeusia. **GU:** vaginitis, genital pruritus. **Skin:** rash, pruritus, photosensitivity. **Other:** ***hypersensitivity reaction***, visual disturbances, fever.

Interactions
Antacids containing aluminum or magnesium hydroxide, iron salts, sucralfate, products containing zinc: may interfere with the GI absorption of ofloxacin. Separate administration by 2 hours. **Anticoagulants:** increased effect. Monitor for bleeding and prothrombin time. **Antineoplastic agents:** may lower serum levels of quinolones. **Theophylline:** some quinolones may decrease clearance of theophylline. Monitor theophylline levels.

Nursing diagnoses
- High risk for injury related to ineffectiveness of ofloxacin to eradicate the infection.
- High risk for fluid volume deficit related to adverse GI reactions caused by ofloxacin.
- Knowledge deficit related to ofloxacin therapy.

Nursing interventions
- *Contraindicated* in children and breast-feeding women because drug has caused arthropathy or osteochondrosis in young animals. Use during pregnancy only when benefits outweigh fetal risks.
- *Use cautiously* in patients with seizure disorders or other CNS diseases. If patient experiences excessive CNS stimulation, discontinue medication and notify doctor. Because the drug is mainly eliminated by renal excretion, adjust dosage in patients with renal failure.
- Advise patients to take the drug with plenty of fluids, but not with meals, and to avoid antacids, sucralfate, and products containing iron or zinc for 2 hours before or after each dose.
- Tell patient to stop drug and notify doctor if rash or other signs of hypersensitivity develop.

General

Classification: hypnotic (benzodiazepine). **Pregnancy risk category:** X. **Controlled substance schedule:** IV.

Mechanism of action

Acts on the limbic system and thalamus of the CNS by binding to specific benzodiazepine receptors.

Indications and dosage

- Adjunctive treatment of insomnia. **Adults:** 1 mg P.O. h.s. Some patients may require 2 mg. **Elderly patients:** 1 mg P.O. h.s. Use higher doses with extreme care. Frail elderly or debilitated patients may take 0.5 mg, but this low dose may be only marginally effective.

Adverse reactions

CNS: fatigue, dizziness, *daytime drowsiness*, headache.

Interactions

Alcohol, CNS depressants including antihistamines, opiate analgesics, and other benzodiazepines: increased CNS depression. Avoid concomitant use. **Cimetidine, oral contraceptives, disulfiram, isoniazid:** may impair the metabolism and clearance of benzodiazepines and prolong their plasma half-life. Monitor for increased CNS depression. **Rifampin, cigarette smoking:** may increase metabolism and clearance and decrease plasma half-life. Monitor for decreased effectiveness. **Theophylline:** pharmacologic antagonism. Monitor for decreased effectiveness.

Nursing diagnoses

- Sleep pattern disturbance related to patient's underlying condition.
- High risk for trauma related to adverse CNS reactions caused by estazolam.
- Knowledge deficit related to estazolam therapy.

Nursing interventions

- *Contraindicated* in patients allergic to the drug or other benzodiazepines, in pregnant patients, and in patients with suspected or confirmed sleep apnea.
- *Use cautiously* in patients with hepatic, renal, or pulmonary disease.
- Consider the possibility of purposeful overdose by patients who are depressed, suicidal, or known users of illegal drugs. Closely monitor drug administration to prevent hoarding of doses.
- Warn patient that additive depressant effects can occur if alcohol is consumed on the day after use of the drug.
- Do not discontinue the drug abruptly after prolonged use (possibly after 6 weeks of continuous therapy) because withdrawal symptoms may occur.
- Check hepatic and renal function and CBC before and periodically during long-term therapy.
- Warn patient about dizziness and drowsiness. Tell him to avoid driving and other hazardous activities that require alertness until the adverse CNS effects of the drug are known. Supervise walking; raise bed rails, especially for elderly patients.
- Tell patient not to increase dosage of the drug but to inform the doctor if he feels that the drug is no longer effective.
- If estazolam overdose occurs, flumazenil (a specific benzodiazepine antagonist) may be useful. The duration of action of flumazenil is shorter than that of estazolam, and resedation is possible.

General

Classification: antifungal (macrolide). **Pregnancy risk category:** B.

Mechanism of action

Probably acts by binding to sterols in the fungal cell membrane, altering cell permeability and allowing leakage of intracellular components.

Indications and dosage

- GI infections. **Adults:** 500,000 to 1 million units as oral tablets, t.i.d.
- Oral, vaginal, and intestinal infections caused by *Candida albicans (Monilia)* and other *Candida* species. **Adults:** 400,000 to 600,000 units oral suspension q.i.d. for oral candidiasis. **Children and infants over 3 months:** 250,000 to 500,000 units oral suspension q.i.d. **Neonates and premature infants:** 100,000 units oral suspension q.i.d.
- Vaginal infections. **Adults:** 100,000 units, as vaginal tablets, inserted high into vagina, daily or b.i.d. for 14 days.

Adverse reactions

GI: transient nausea, vomiting, diarrhea (usually with large oral dosage).

Interactions

None significant.

N

Nursing diagnoses

- Injury related to high risk of ineffectiveness of nystatin to eradicate the fungus infection.
- Fluid volume deficit related to potential nystatin-induced adverse GI reactions.
- Knowledge deficit related to nystatin therapy.

Nursing interventions

- Nystatin is virtually nontoxic and nonsensitizing when used orally, vaginally, or topically, but advise patient to report redness, swelling, or irritation.
- Vaginal tablets can be used by pregnant women up to 6 weeks before term to treat maternal infection that may cause thrush in newborns.
- Continue therapy during menstruation.
- Instruct patient to wash applicator thoroughly after each use.
- Explain that use of antibiotics, oral contraceptives, and corticosteroids; diabetes; reinfection by sexual partner; and tight-fitting panty hose are predisposing factors of vaginal infection. Encourage patient to use cotton (not synthetic) underpants.
- For treatment of oral candidiasis (thrush): Be sure the mouth is clean of food debris before administering drug, then tell patient to hold suspension in mouth for several minutes before swallowing. When treating infants, swab medication on oral mucosa. Instruct patient in good oral hygiene techniques. Tell patient overuse of mouthwash or poorly fitting dentures, especially in older patients, may alter flora and promote infection.
- Advise patient to continue medication for at least 2 days after symptoms disappear to ensure against reinfection. Consult doctor for exact length of therapy.
- Instruct patient in careful hygiene for affected areas, including cleansing perineal area from front to back after defecation.
- Not effective against systemic infections.

General

Classification: estrogen replacement, antineoplastic (estrogen). **Pregnancy risk category:** X.

Mechanism of action

Increases the synthesis of DNA, RNA, and protein in responsive tissues. Also reduces release of follicle-stimulating hormone and luteinizing hormone from the pituitary.

Indications and dosage

- Menopausal symptoms, hypogonadism, female castration, primary ovarian failure. **Women:** 1 to 2 mg P.O. daily, in cycles of 21 days on and 7 days off, or cycles of 5 days on and 2 days off; or 0.2 to 1 mg I.M. weekly. Alternatively, apply one Estraderm transdermal patch twice weekly, in cycles of 21 days on and 7 days off.
- Kraurosis vulvae. **Women:** 1 to 1.5 mg I.M. one or more times weekly.
- Atrophic vaginitis. **Women:** 2 to 4 g intravaginal cream daily for 1 to 2 weeks; maintenance dosage: 1 g one to three times weekly.
- Menopausal symptoms. **Women:** 1 to 5 mg (cypionate) I.M. q 3 to 4 weeks. Or 5 to 20 mg (valerate) I.M., repeated once after 2 to 3 weeks.
- Postpartum breast engorgement. **Women:** 10 to 25 mg (valerate) I.M. at end of first stage of labor.

- Inoperable breast cancer. **Women:** 10 mg P.O. (oral estradiol) t.i.d. for 3 months.
- Inoperable prostatic cancer. **Men:** 30 mg (valerate) I.M. q 1 to 2 weeks. Or, 1 to 2 mg (oral estradiol) t.i.d.

Adverse reactions

CNS: headache, dizziness, chorea, depression, libido changes, lethargy. **CV:** thrombophlebitis, ***thromboembolism,*** hypertension, edema. **EENT:** worsening of myopia or astigmatism, intolerance to contact lenses. **GI:** *nausea,* vomiting, abdominal cramps, bloating, diarrhea, constipation, anorexia, increased appetite, weight changes, pancreatitis. **GU:** in women—breakthrough bleeding, altered menstrual flow, dysmenorrhea, amenorrhea, cervical erosion, altered cervical secretions, enlargement of uterine fibromas, vaginal candidiasis. In men—gynecomastia, testicular atrophy, impotence. **Hepatic:** cholestatic jaundice. **Metabolic:** hyperglycemia, hypercalcemia, folic acid deficiency. **Skin:** melasma, urticaria, acne, seborrhea, oily skin, hirsutism or hair loss. **Other:** breast tenderness, enlargement, secretion; leg cramps.

Interactions

Bromocriptine: may cause amenorrhea, interfering with the effects of bromocriptine. Avoid concomitant use. **Carbamazepine, phenobarbital, rifampin:** decreased effectiveness of estrogen therapy. Monitor closely. **Corticosteroids:** possible enhanced effects. Monitor closely. **Cyclosporine:** increased risk of toxicity. Use together with caution and frequently monitor cyclosporine levels. **Dantrolene, other hepatotoxic medications:** increased risk of hepatotoxicity. Monitor closely. **Oral anticoagulants:** dosage adjustments may be necessary. Monitor PT. **Tamoxifen:** may interfere with effectiveness of tamoxifen. Avoid concomitant use.

Nursing diagnoses

- Sexual dysfunction related to the patient's underlying hormonal deficiency.
- Altered tissue perfusion (cerebral, peripheral, cardiopulmonary) related to estradiol-induced thromboembolism.
- Knowledge deficit related to estradiol therapy.

Nursing interventions

- *Contraindicated* in thrombophlebitis or thromboembolic disorders; cancer of breast or reproductive organs; undiagnosed abnormal genital bleeding; and pregnancy.
- *Use cautiously* in hypertension, mental depression, bone diseases, blood dyscrasias, migraine, seizures, diabetes mellitus, amenorrhea, heart failure, hepatic or renal dysfunction, or family history of breast or genital tract cancer.

General
Classification: peripheral vasodilator (beta-adrenergic receptor). **Pregnancy risk category:** C.

Mechanism of action
Stimulates beta receptors and may directly relax vascular smooth muscle.

Indications and dosage
• Increase of blood supply in vasospastic disorders (arteriosclerosis obliterans, thromboangiitis obliterans, diabetic vascular disease, night leg cramps, Raynaud's phenomenon and disease, ischemic ulcer, frostbite, acrocyanosis, acroparesthesia, sequelae of thrombophlebitis) and in circulatory disturbances of the middle ear (primary cochlear ischemia, cochlear striae, vascular ischemia, macular or ampullar ischemia); other disturbances caused by labyrinth artery spasm or obstruction. **Adults:** 3 to 12 mg P.O. t.i.d. or q.i.d.

Adverse reactions
CNS: trembling, *nervousness,* weakness, *dizziness (not associated with labyrinth artery insufficiency).* **CV:** *palpitations, hypotension,* flushing. **GI:** nausea, vomiting.

Interactions
None significant.

Nursing diagnoses
• Altered tissue perfusion (cerebral, peripheral) related to the patient's underlying condition.
• Knowledge deficit related to nylidrin hydrochloride therapy.

Nursing interventions
• *Contraindicated* in acute MI, paroxysmal tachycardia, angina pectoris, or thyrotoxicosis.
• *Use cautiously* in uncompensated heart disease or peptic ulcer.
• Advise patient to avoid tasks that require mental alertness (such as driving or operating heavy machinery) until CNS effects of the drug are known.
• Instruct patient to avoid sudden posture changes to minimize the risks of orthostasis.

General
Classification: antineoplastic (estrogen, alkylating agent). **Pregnancy risk category:** D.

Mechanism of action
Acts by binding selectively to a protein present in the human prostate.

Indications and dosage
• Palliative treatment of metastatic or progressive cancer of the prostate. **Men:** 10 to 16 mg/kg P.O. in three to four divided doses. Usual dosage is 14 mg/kg daily. Therapy should continue for up to 3 months and, if successful, be maintained as long as the patient responds.

Adverse reactions
Blood: ***leukopenia, thrombocytopenia.*** **CNS:** loss of libido. **CV:** ***myocardial infarction, CVA,*** sodium and fluid retention, ***edema, pulmonary emboli,*** thrombophlebitis, ***CHF,*** hypertension. **GI:** *nausea, vomiting,* diarrhea. **Skin:** rash, pruritus. **Other:** *painful gynecomastia and breast tenderness,* thinning of hair, hyperglycemia, fluid retention.

Interactions
Calcium-rich foods (milk and dairy products): impaired absorption of estramustine.

Nursing diagnoses
• High risk for fluid volume deficit related to drug-induced GI effects.
• High risk for injury related to drug-induced adverse cardiac reactions.
• Knowledge deficit related to estramustine therapy.

Nursing interventions
• *Contraindicated* in patients hypersensitive to estradiol and nitrogen mustard. Also contraindicated in active thrombophlebitis or thromboembolic disorders, except in those cases where the actual tumor mass is the cause of the thromboembolic phenomenon.
• *Use cautiously* in patients with history of thrombophlebitis or thromboembolic disorders and cerebrovascular or coronary artery disease.
• Estramustine is a combination of the estrogen estradiol and a nitrogen mustard. It is effective in patients refractory to estrogen therapy alone.
• Tell the patient to take this drug on an empty stomach (2 hours before or 1 hour after meals) and to avoid taking the drug with milk or dairy products.
• Monitor patient's weight gain because estramustine may exaggerate preexisting peripheral edema or CHF.
• Monitor blood pressure and glucose tolerance periodically throughout therapy.
• Each 140-mg capsule contains 12.5 mg sodium.
• Encourage patients of childbearing age to use contraceptives; drug is known to be teratogenic and mutagenic.
• Tell the patient he may continue therapy as long as he's responding favorably.
• Store capsules in refrigerator.

General

Classification: antidepressant (TCA). **Pregnancy risk category:** D.

Mechanism of action

Increases the amount of norepinephrine or serotonin, or both, in the CNS by blocking their reuptake by the presynaptic neurons. This allows these neurotransmitters to accumulate.

Indications and dosage

- Depression. **Adults:** 25 mg P.O. t.i.d. or q.i.d., gradually increasing to maximum of 150 mg daily. Alternatively, entire dose may be given h.s.

Adverse reactions

CNS: *drowsiness, dizziness,* excitation, ***seizures,*** tremor, weakness, confusion, headache, nervousness, EEG changes, extrapyramidal reactions. **CV:** *tachycardia, ECG changes,* hypertension. **EENT:** *blurred vision,* tinnitus, mydriasis. **GI:** *dry mouth, constipation,* nausea, vomiting, anorexia, paralytic ileus. **GU:** *urine retention.* **Skin:** rash, urticaria, photosensitivity. **Other:** *sweating,* allergy. **After abrupt withdrawal of long-term therapy:** nausea, headache, malaise.

Interactions

Barbiturates: decrease TCA blood levels. Monitor for decreased antidepressant effect. **Cimetidine:** may increase nortriptyline serum levels. Monitor for increased adverse reactions. **Epinephrine, norepinephrine:** increase hypertensive effect. Use with caution. **MAO inhibitors:** may cause severe excitation, hyperpyrexia, or seizures, usually with high dose. Use together cautiously. **Methylphenidate:** increases TCA blood levels. Monitor for enhanced antidepressant effect.

Nursing diagnoses

- Ineffective individual coping related to the patient's underlying condition.
- Constipation related to nortriptyline-induced adverse GI reactions.
- Knowledge deficit related to nortriptyline therapy.

Nursing interventions

- *Contraindicated* during acute recovery phase of MI, in prostatic hypertrophy, and in patients with history of seizure disorders.
- *Use cautiously* in CV disease, urine retention, glaucoma, thyroid disease, impaired hepatic function, or blood dyscrasias; in patients who are at risk for suicide; or in those receiving electroshock therapy, thyroid medication, or elective surgery.
- Drug is similar in anticholinergic effects to other cyclics. Avoid combining with alcohol or other depressants. Do not withdraw drug abruptly. Advise patient not to use other drugs (prescription or OTC) without consulting doctor.
- Check for urine retention and constipation. Increase fluids to lessen constipation.
- Reduce dosage in elderly or debilitated patients and adolescents.
- If psychotic signs increase, dosage should be reduced. Record mood changes. Watch for suicidal tendencies. To lessen suicide risk, allow minimum tablet supply.
- Warn patient to avoid hazardous activities that require alertness and good psychomotor coordination until CNS effects of the drug are known, usually after a few weeks.
- Expect delay of 2 weeks or more before noticeable effect; 4 weeks or more before full effect.
- Patient should take full dose at bedtime.
- Hypertensive episodes have occurred during surgery in patients receiving TCAs; discontinue these drugs several days before surgery.

General
Classification: estrogen replacement, antineoplastic, antiosteoporotic (estrogen). **Pregnancy risk category:** X.

Mechanism of action
Increases DNA, RNA, and protein tissue synthesis. Reduces release of follicle-stimulating hormone and luteinizing hormone.

Indications and dosage
- Abnormal uterine bleeding (hormonal imbalance). **Women:** 25 mg I.V. or I.M. Repeat in 6 to 12 hours.
- Breast cancer (at least 5 years after menopause). **Women:** 10 mg P.O. t.i.d. for 3 months or more.
- Female castration, primary ovarian failure, and osteoporosis. **Women:** 1.25 mg P.O. daily in cycles of 3 weeks on, 1 week off.
- Hypogonadism. **Women:** 2.5 mg P.O. b.i.d. or t.i.d. 20 consecutive days each month.
- Menopausal symptoms. **Women:** 0.3 to 1.25 mg P.O. daily in cycles of 3 weeks on, 1 week off.
- Postpartum breast engorgement. **Women:** 3.75 mg P.O. q 4 hours for five doses or 1.25 mg q 4 hours for 5 days.
- Atrophic vaginitis, kraurosis vulvae related to menopause. **Women:** 2 to 4 g intravaginally in cycles of 3 weeks on, 1 week off.

- Inoperable prostatic cancer. **Men:** 1.25 to 2.5 mg P.O. t.i.d.

Adverse reactions
CNS: headache, dizziness, chorea, depression, libido changes, lethargy. **CV:** thrombophlebitis; ***thromboembolism;*** hypertension; edema; ***increased risk of stroke, pulmonary embolism, and MI.*** **EENT:** worsening of myopia or astigmatism, intolerance to contact lenses. **GI:** *nausea,* vomiting, abdominal cramps, bloating, diarrhea, constipation, anorexia, increased appetite, weight changes, pancreatitis. **GU:** in women—breakthrough bleeding, altered menstrual flow, dysmenorrhea, amenorrhea, cervical erosion, altered cervical secretions, enlargement of uterine fibromas, vaginal candidiasis. In men—gynecomastia, testicular atrophy, impotence. **Hepatic:** cholestatic jaundice. **Metabolic:** hyperglycemia, hypercalcemia, folic acid deficiency. **Skin:** melasma, urticaria, acne, seborrhea, flushing (when given rapidly I.V.), hirsutism or loss of hair. **Other:** breast changes, leg cramps.

Interactions
Bromocriptine: may cause amenorrhea. Avoid concomitant use. **Carbamazepine, phenobarbital, rifampin:** decreased effectiveness of estrogen therapy. Monitor closely. **Corticosteroids:** possible enhanced effects. Monitor closely. **Cyclosporine:** increased risk of toxicity. Use together with caution; frequently monitor cyclosporine levels. **Dantrolene, other hepatotoxic drugs:** increased risk of hepatotoxicity. Monitor closely. **Oral anticoagulants:** may require dosage adjustments. Monitor PT. **Tamoxifen:** may interfere with effectiveness of tamoxifen. Avoid concomitant use.

Nursing diagnoses
- Sexual dysfunction related to hormonal imbalance.
- Altered tissue perfusion (cerebral, peripheral, cardiopulmonary) related to estrogen-induced thromboembolism.
- Knowledge deficit related to therapy with conjugated estrogens.

Nursing interventions
- *Contraindicated* in thrombophlebitis or thromboembolic disorders, undiagnosed abnormal genital bleeding, and pregnancy.
- *Use cautiously* in hypertension, gallbladder disease, bone diseases, blood dyscrasias, migraine, seizures, diabetes mellitus, amenorrhea, heart failure, hepatic or renal dysfunction, or family history (mother, grandmother, sister) of breast or genital tract cancer; may require discontinuation of the drug.

General

Classification: contraceptive (progestin). **Pregnancy risk category:** X.

Mechanism of action

Suppresses ovulation, possibly by inhibiting pituitary gonadotropin secretion. Also forms a thick cervical mucus.

Indications and dosage

- Contraception. **Women:** 0.075 mg P.O. daily.

Adverse reactions

CNS: cerebral thrombosis or hemorrhage, migraine headache, lethargy, depression. **CV:** hypertension, thrombophlebitis, ***pulmonary embolism,*** edema. **GI:** nausea, vomiting, abdominal cramps, gallbladder disease. **GU:** *breakthrough bleeding, change in menstrual flow,* dysmenorrhea, spotting, amenorrhea, cervical erosion, vaginal candidiasis. **Hepatic:** cholestatic jaundice. **Skin:** melasma, rash. **Other:** breast tenderness, enlargement, or secretion.

Interactions

Barbiturates, carbamazepine, rifampin: decreased progestin effects. Monitor for diminished therapeutic response. **Bromocriptine:** may cause amenorrhea, interfering with bromocriptine effects. Avoid concomitant use.

Nursing diagnoses

- High risk for fluid volume deficit related to drug-induced excessive uterine bleeding.
- Altered pulmonary tissue perfusion related to drug-induced thromboembolism.
- Knowledge deficit related to oral contraceptive therapy.

Nursing interventions

- *Contraindicated* in thromboembolic disorders, breast cancer, undiagnosed abnormal vaginal bleeding, severe hepatic disease, or missed abortion and in pregnant women.
- *Use cautiously* in diabetes mellitus, seizure disorder, migraine, cardiac or renal disease, asthma, and mental illness.
- FDA regulations require that, before receiving first dose, patients read package insert explaining possible progestin adverse reactions. Provide verbal explanation also. Patient should report any unusual symptoms immediately and should stop drug and call doctor if visual disturbances, migraine, or numbness or tingling in limbs occurs.
- Tell patient to take pill every day, even if menstruating. Pill should be taken at the same time every day.
- A progestin-only oral contraceptive known as "minipill."
- Teach the patient how to perform a monthly breast self-examination.
- Women using oral contraceptives should be advised of the increased risk of serious adverse CV reactions associated with heavy cigarette smoking (15 or more cigarettes per day). These risks are quite marked in women over 35 years.
- Risk of pregnancy increases with each tablet missed. A patient who misses one tablet should take it as soon as she remembers; she should then take the next tablet at the regular time. A patient who misses two tablets should take one as soon as she remembers and then take the next regular dose at the usual time; she should use a nonhormonal method of contraception in addition to norgestrel until 14 tablets have been taken. A patient who misses three or more tablets should discontinue the drug and use a nonhormonal method of contraception until after her menses. If her menstrual period does not occur within 45 days, pregnancy testing is necessary.
- Instruct the patient to immediately report excessive bleeding or bleeding between menstrual cycles, breast pain or tenderness, vaginal discharge, or swelling of the hands or feet.

General

Classification: estrogen replacement, antineoplastic (estrogen). **Pregnancy risk category:** X.

Mechanism of action

Increases the synthesis of DNA, RNA, and protein in responsive tissues. Also reduces release of follicle-stimulating hormone and luteinizing hormone from the pituitary.

Indications and dosage

- Inoperable prostatic cancer. **Men:** 1.25 to 2.5 mg P.O. t.i.d.
- Breast cancer. **Men and postmenopausal women:** 10 mg P.O. t.i.d. for 3 or more months.
- Hypogonadism, castration, primary ovarian failure. **Women:** 2.5 mg P.O. daily to t.i.d. in cycles of 3 weeks on, 1 week off.
- Menopausal symptoms. **Women:** average 0.3 to 3.75 mg P.O. daily in cycles of 3 weeks on, 1 week off.

Adverse reactions

CNS: headache, dizziness, chorea, depression, libido changes, lethargy. **CV:** thrombophlebitis; ***thromboembolism;*** hypertension; edema; ***increased risk of stroke, pulmonary embolism, and MI.*** **EENT:** worsening of myopia or astigmatism, intolerance to contact lenses. **GI:** *nausea,* vomiting, abdominal cramps, bloating, diarrhea, constipation, anorexia, increased appetite, weight changes, pancreatitis. **GU:** in women – breakthrough bleeding, altered menstrual flow, dysmenorrhea, amenorrhea, cervical erosion, altered cervical secretions, enlargement of uterine fibromas, vaginal candidiasis. In men – gynecomastia, testicular atrophy, impotence. **Hepatic:** cholestatic jaundice. **Metabolic:** hyperglycemia, hypercalcemia, folic acid deficiency. **Skin:** melasma, rash, acne, hirsutism or hair loss, seborrhea, oily skin. **Other:** breast changes (tenderness, enlargement, secretion).

Interactions

Bromocriptine: may cause amenorrhea, interfering with the effects of bromocriptine. Avoid concomitant use. **Carbamazepine, phenobarbital, rifampin:** decreased effectiveness of estrogen therapy. Monitor closely. **Corticosteroids:** possible enhanced effects. Monitor closely. **Cyclosporine:** increased risk of toxicity. Use together with caution and frequently monitor cyclosporine levels. **Dantrolene, other hepatotoxic medications:** increased risk of hepatotoxicity. Monitor closely. **Oral anticoagulants:** dosage adjustments may be necessary. Monitor PT. **Tamoxifen:** may decrease effectiveness of tamoxifen therapy. Avoid concomitant use.

Nursing diagnoses

- Altered protection related to the patient's underlying condition.
- Altered tissue perfusion (cerebral, peripheral, cardiopulmonary) related to estrogen-induced thromboembolism.
- Knowledge deficit related to therapy with esterified estrogens.

Nursing interventions

- *Contraindicated* in thrombophlebitis or thromboembolic disorders, undiagnosed abnormal genital bleeding, and pregnancy.
- *Use cautiously* in patients with history of hypertension, mental depression, gallbladder disease, migraine, seizures, diabetes mellitus, amenorrhea, or family history (mother, grandmother, sister) of breast or genital tract cancer; may require discontinuation of drug.
- Give patient package insert describing adverse effects of esterified estrogens, and provide verbal explanation.
- Warn patient to report immediately abdominal pain; pain, numbness, or stiffness in legs or buttocks; pressure or pain in chest; shortness of breath; severe headaches; visual disturbances, such as blind spots, flashing lights, or blurriness; vaginal bleeding or discharge; breast lumps; swelling of hands or feet; yellow skin or sclera; dark urine; or light-colored stools.

General

Classification: antibiotic (fluoroquinolone). **Pregnancy risk category:** C.

Mechanism of action

Inhibits bacterial DNA synthesis, mainly by inhibiting DNA gyrase. Bactericidal.

Indications and dosage

- Complicated or uncomplicated UTIs caused by susceptible strains of *Escherichia coli, Klebsiella, Enterobacter, Proteus, Pseudomonas aeruginosa, Citrobacter, Staphylococcus aureus* and *S. epidermidis,* and group D streptococci. **Adults:** for uncomplicated infections, 400 mg P.O. b.i.d. for 7 to 10 days. For complicated infections, 400 mg b.i.d. for 10 to 21 days.

Adverse reactions

Blood: eosinophilia. **CNS:** fatigue, somnolence, headache, dizziness. **GI:** nausea, constipation, flatulence, heartburn, dry mouth. **Hepatic:** transient elevations of AST (SGOT) and ALT (SGPT). **Skin:** rash. **Other:** ***hypersensitivity reactions*** (rash, anaphylactic reactions).

Interactions

Antacids, iron products, sucralfate: may hinder absorption. Separate administration times by 2 hours. **Nitrofurantoin:** decreases norfloxacin's effectiveness. Don't use together. **Probenecid:** may increase serum levels of norfloxacin by decreasing its excretion. **Theophylline:** norfloxacin may impair theophylline metabolism, resulting in increased plasma levels and risk of toxicity. Monitor closely.

Nursing diagnoses

- High risk for injury related to ineffectiveness of norfloxacin to eradicate the infection.
- Constipation related to adverse effect of norfloxacin on GI tract.
- Knowledge deficit related to norfloxacin therapy.

Nursing interventions

- *Contraindicated* in patients with hypersensitivity to nalidixic acid and cinoxacin.
- Warn patients not to exceed the recommended dosages. Advise them to drink several glasses of water throughout the day to maintain hydration and adequate urine output.
- Advise patients to take the drug 1 hour before or 2 hours after meals because food, antacids, iron products, and sucralfate may hinder absorption.
- Because norfloxacin may cause dizziness, patients should avoid hazardous activities that require alertness and good coordination until the CNS effects of the drug are known.

General

Classification: estrogen replacement (estrogen). **Pregnancy risk category:** X.

Mechanism of action

Increases DNA, RNA, and protein tissue synthesis; reduces release of follicle-stimulating hormone and luteinizing hormone.

Indications and dosage

- Atrophic vaginitis and menopausal symptoms. **Women:** 0.1 to 0.5 mg I.M. two or three times weekly.
- Female hypogonadism and primary ovarian failure. **Women:** 0.1 to 1 mg I.M. weekly in single or divided doses.
- Inoperable prostatic cancer. **Men:** 2 to 4 mg I.M. two to three times weekly.

Adverse reactions

CNS: headache, dizziness, chorea, depression, libido changes, lethargy. **CV:** thrombophlebitis, ***thromboembolism,*** hypertension, edema. **EENT:** worsening of myopia or astigmatism, intolerance to contact lenses. **GI:** *nausea,* vomiting, abdominal cramps, bloating, diarrhea, constipation, anorexia, increased appetite, weight changes, pancreatitis. **GU:** in women – breakthrough bleeding, altered menstrual flow, dysmenorrhea, amenorrhea, cervical erosion, altered cervical secretions, enlargement of uterine fibromas, vaginal candidiasis. In men – gynecomastia, testicular atrophy, impotence. **Hepatic:** cholestatic jaundice. **Metabolic:** hyperglycemia, hypercalcemia, folic acid deficiency. **Skin:** melasma, urticaria, acne, seborrhea, oily skin, hirsutism or hair loss. **Other:** breast changes, leg cramps.

Interactions

Bromocriptine: may cause amenorrhea, interfering with the effects of bromocriptine. Avoid concomitant use. **Carbamazepine, phenobarbital, rifampin:** decreased effectiveness of estrogen therapy. Monitor closely. **Corticosteroids:** possible enhanced effects. Monitor closely. **Cyclosporine:** increased risk of toxicity. Use together with caution and frequently monitor cyclosporine levels. **Dantrolene, other hepatotoxic medications:** increased risk of hepatotoxicity. Monitor closely. **Oral anticoagulants:** dosage adjustments may be necessary. Monitor PT. **Tamoxifen:** estrogens may interfere with the effectiveness of tamoxifen. Avoid concomitant use.

Nursing diagnoses

- Impaired tissue integrity related to vaginitis.
- Altered tissue perfusion (cerebral, peripheral, cardiopulmonary) related to estrone-induced thromboembolism.
- Knowledge deficit related to estrone therapy.

Nursing interventions

- *Contraindicated* in thrombophlebitis or thromboembolic disorders; cancer of breast or reproductive organs; undiagnosed abnormal genital bleeding; and pregnancy.
- *Use cautiously* in hypertension, mental depression, migraine, seizures, diabetes mellitus, amenorrhea, hepatic or renal dysfunction, or family history (mother, grandmother, sister) of breast or genital tract cancer; may require discontinuation of the drug.
- Rotate injection sites to prevent muscle atrophy.
- Give patient package insert describing adverse effects of estrone, and provide verbal explanation.
- Warn patient to report immediately abdominal pain; pain, numbness, or stiffness in legs or buttocks; pressure or pain in chest; shortness of breath; severe headaches; visual disturbances, such as blind spots, flashing lights, or blurriness; vaginal bleeding or discharge; breast lumps; swelling of hands or feet; yellow skin and sclera; dark urine; or light-colored stools.
- Teach women how to perform routine breast self-examination.

General
Classification: contraceptive (progestin). **Pregnancy risk category:** X.

Mechanism of action
Suppresses ovulation, possibly by inhibiting pituitary gonadotropin secretion. Also forms a thick cervical mucus.

Indications and dosage
- Amenorrhea, abnormal uterine bleeding. **Women:** 2.5 to 10 mg P.O. daily on days 5 to 25 of menstrual cycle.
- Endometriosis. **Women:** 5 mg P.O. daily for 14 days, then increase by 2.5 mg daily q 2 weeks up to 15 mg daily.

Adverse reactions
CNS: dizziness, migraine headache, lethargy, depression. **CV:** hypertension, thrombophlebitis, ***pulmonary embolism***, edema. **GI:** nausea, vomiting, abdominal cramps. **GU:** breakthrough bleeding, dysmenorrhea, amenorrhea, cervical erosion, abnormal secretions, uterine fibromas, vaginal candidiasis. **Hepatic:** cholestatic jaundice. **Metabolic:** hyperglycemia. **Skin:** melasma, rash. **Other:** breast tenderness, enlargement, or secretion; decreased libido.

Interactions
Barbiturates, carbamazepine, rifampin: decreased progestin effects. Monitor for diminished therapeutic response. **Bromocriptine:** may cause amenorrhea, interfering with bromocriptine effects. Avoid concomitant use.

Nursing diagnoses
- High risk for fluid volume deficit related to abnormal uterine bleeding.
- Fluid volume excess related to norethindrone-induced edema.
- Knowledge deficit related to norethindrone therapy.

Nursing interventions
- *Contraindicated* in thromboembolic disorders, breast cancer, undiagnosed abnormal vaginal bleeding, severe hepatic disease, or missed abortion and in pregnant women.
- *Use cautiously* in diabetes mellitus, seizure disorder, migraine, cardiac or renal disease, asthma, and mental illness.
- FDA regulations require that, before receiving first dose, patients read package insert explaining possible progestin adverse reactions. Provide verbal explanation also. Patient should report any unusual symptoms immediately and should stop drug and call doctor if visual disturbances or migraine occur.
- Don't use as test for pregnancy; drug may cause birth defects and masculinization of female fetus.
- Preliminary estrogen treatment is usually needed in menstrual disorders.
- Twice as potent as norethindrone.
- Teach patient how to perform a monthly breast self-examination.

General

Classification: estrogen replacement (estrone conjugate). **Pregnancy risk category:** X.

Mechanism of action

Increases the synthesis of DNA, RNA, and proteins in responsive tissues.

Indications and dosage

- Atrophic vaginitis, kraurosis vulvae, or moderate to severe vasomotor symptoms associated with menopause. **Women:** 0.625 to 5 mg P.O. daily. Dosage is usually given on a cyclical, short-term basis. Alternatively, give 2 to 4 g vaginal cream daily, in cycles of 3 weeks on and 1 week off.
- Primary ovarian failure, female castration, or female hypogonadism. **Women:** 1.25 to 7.5 mg P.O. daily for 3 weeks, followed by a rest period of 8 to 10 days. If bleeding does not occur by the end of the rest period, repeat cycle.
- Prevention of osteoporosis. **Women:** 0.625 mg P.O. daily for 25 days of a 31-day cycle each month.

Adverse reactions

CNS: depression, headache, dizziness, migraine, changes in libido. **CV:** edema, thrombophlebitis; ***increased risk of stroke, pulmonary embolism, and MI.*** **GI:** nausea, vomiting, abdominal cramps, bloating, cholestatic jaundice. **GU:** increased size of uterine fibromyomata, vaginal candidiasis, cystitis-like syndrome, dysmenorrhea, amenorrhea, breakthrough bleeding, premenstrual-like syndrome. **Skin:** hemorrhagic eruption, erythema nodosum, erythema multiforme, hirsutism, chloasma, hair loss. **Other:** breast engorgement or enlargement, weight changes, aggravation of porphyria.

Interactions

Bromocriptine: may cause amenorrhea, interfering with the effects of bromocriptine. Avoid concomitant use. **Carbamazepine, phenobarbital, rifampin:** decreased effectiveness of estrogen therapy. Monitor closely. **Corticosteroids:** possible enhanced effects. Monitor closely. **Cyclosporine:** increased risk of toxicity. Use together with caution and frequently monitor cyclosporine levels. **Dantrolene, other hepatotoxic medications:** increased risk of hepatotoxicity. Monitor closely. **Oral anticoagulants:** dosage adjustments may be necessary. Monitor PT. **Tamoxifen:** may interfere with the effectiveness of tamoxifen. Avoid concomitant use.

Nursing diagnoses

- Impaired tissue integrity related to the patient's underlying condition.
- Fluid volume excess related to estropipate-induced edema.
- Knowledge deficit related to estropipate therapy.

Nursing interventions

- *Contraindicated* in thrombophlebitis or thromboembolic disorders; cancer of the breast, reproductive organs, or genitalia; undiagnosed genital bleeding; and pregnancy.
- *Use cautiously* in hypertension, asthma, mental depression, bone diseases, blood dyscrasias, gallbladder disease, migraine, seizures, diabetes mellitus, amenorrhea, heart failure, hepatic or renal dysfunction, and a family history of breast or genital cancer; may require discontinuation of the drug.
- Give patient package insert describing adverse reactions to estropipate, including the increased risk of endometrial carcinoma, and also provide verbal explanation.
- Warn patient to report immediately abdominal pain; pain, stiffness, or numbness in the legs or buttocks; pressure or pain in the chest; shortness of breath; severe headaches; visual disturbances, such as blind spots or flashing lights; vaginal bleeding or discharge; breast lumps; swelling of the hands or feet; yellow skin or sclera; dark urine; or light-colored stools.

General
Classification: contraceptive (progestin). **Pregnancy risk category:** X.

Mechanism of action
Suppresses ovulation, possibly by inhibiting pituitary gonadotropin secretion. Also forms a thick cervical mucus.

Indications and dosage
- Amenorrhea, abnormal uterine bleeding. **Women:** 5 to 20 mg P.O. daily on days 5 to 25 of menstrual cycle.
- Endometriosis. **Women:** 10 mg P.O. daily for 14 days, then increase by 5 mg P.O. daily q 2 weeks up to 30 mg daily.
- Contraception. **Women:** initiate therapy with 0.35 mg P.O. on the first day of menstruation. Then, 0.35 mg P.O. daily.

Adverse reactions
CNS: dizziness, migraine headache, lethargy, depression. **CV:** hypertension, thrombophlebitis, ***pulmonary embolism,*** edema. **GI:** nausea, vomiting, abdominal cramps. **GU:** breakthrough bleeding, dysmenorrhea, amenorrhea, cervical erosion, or abnormal secretions, uterine fibromas, vaginal candidiasis. **Hepatic:** cholestatic jaundice. **Metabolic:** hyperglycemia. **Skin:** melasma, rash. **Other:** breast tenderness, enlargement, or secretion; decreased libido.

Interactions
Barbiturates, carbamazepine, rifampin: decreased progestin effects. Monitor for diminished therapeutic response.

Nursing diagnoses
- High risk for fluid volume deficit related to abnormal uterine bleeding.
- Fluid volume excess related to norethindrone-induced edema.
- Knowledge deficit related to norethindrone therapy.

Nursing interventions
- *Contraindicated* in thromboembolic disorders, breast cancer, undiagnosed abnormal vaginal bleeding, severe hepatic disease, or missed abortion and in pregnant women.
- *Use cautiously* in diabetes mellitus, seizure disorder, migraine, cardiac or renal disease, asthma, and mental illness.
- Don't use as test for pregnancy; drug may cause birth defects and masculinization of female fetus.
- FDA regulations require that, before receiving first dose, patients read package insert explaining possible progestin adverse reactions. Provide verbal explanation also. Patient should report any unusual symptoms immediately and should stop drug and call doctor if visual disturbances or migraine occur.
- Watch patient carefully for signs of edema.
- Preliminary estrogen treatment is usually needed in menstrual disorders.
- Teach the patient how to perform a monthly breast self-examination.

General

Classification: diuretic (loop diuretic). **Pregnancy risk category:** D.

Mechanism of action

Inhibits sodium and chloride reabsorption at the ascending loop of Henle's proximal portion.

Indications and dosage

- Acute pulmonary edema. **Adults:** 50 to 100 mg I.V. slowly over several minutes.
- Edema. **Adults:** 50 to 200 mg P.O. daily. Refractory cases may require up to 200 mg b.i.d. **Children:** initial dose is 25 mg P.O.; increased in 25-mg increments daily until desired effect is achieved.

Adverse reactions

Blood: ***agranulocytosis,*** neutropenia, thrombocytopenia. **CV:** volume depletion and dehydration, orthostatic hypotension. **EENT:** transient deafness with too-rapid I.V. injection. **GI:** abdominal discomfort and pain, diarrhea. **Metabolic:** hypokalemia; hypochloremic alkalosis; asymptomatic hyperuricemia; fluid and electrolyte imbalances including dilutional hyponatremia, hypocalcemia, hypomagnesemia; hyperglycemia and impairment of glucose tolerance. **Skin:** dermatitis.

Interactions

Aminoglycoside antibiotics: potentiated ototoxic adverse reactions of both ethacrynic acid and aminoglycosides. Use together cautiously. **Antihypertensive agents:** increased risk of hypotension. Use together cautiously. **NSAIDs:** decreased diuretic effectiveness. Use together cautiously. **Warfarin:** potentiated anticoagulant effect. Use together cautiously.

Nursing diagnoses

- Fluid volume excess related to patient's underlying condition.
- Altered urinary elimination related to ethacrynate therapy.
- Knowledge deficit related to ethacrynate therapy.

Nursing interventions

- *Contraindicated* in patients with anuria and in infants.
- *Use cautiously* in patients with electrolyte abnormalities. Development of electrolyte imbalance, azotemia, or oliguria may require discontinuing drug.
- Be aware that ethacrynate is a potent diuretic. Elderly patients are especially susceptible to excessive diuresis. Give P.O. doses in morning to prevent nocturia.
- Monitor intake and output, weight, blood pressure, and serum electrolytes.
- Consult with doctor and dietitian to provide high-potassium diet. Watch for signs of hypokalemia (muscle weakness and cramps).
- In the patient receiving digitalis glycosides, monitor for signs of digitalis toxicity from ethacrynate's potassium-depleting effect.
- Monitor serum uric acid, especially in patients with a history of gout.
- Don't give S.C. or I.M.
- Advise patient to avoid sudden posture changes and rise slowly to avoid orthostatic hypotension.
- Severe diarrhea may necessitate discontinuing drug.
- **I.V. use:** Reconstitute vacuum vial with 50 ml D_5W or 0.9% sodium chloride solution. Discard unused solution after 24 hours. Don't use cloudy or opalescent solutions. Give slowly through tubing of running infusion over several minutes.
- Provide sodium and potassium chloride supplementation, if needed.

General

Classification: vasopressor (adrenergic, direct acting). **Pregnancy risk category:** D.

Mechanism of action

Stimulates alpha- and $beta_1$-adrenergic receptors within the sympathetic nervous system.

Indications and dosage

• Restoration of blood pressure in acute hypotensive states. **Adults:** initially, 8 to 12 mcg/minute I.V. infusion, then adjust to maintain normal blood pressure. Average maintenance dosage is 2 to 4 mcg/minute. **Children:** 2 mcg/m^2 minute I.V. infusion; adjust dosage based upon patient response.

Adverse reactions

CNS: *headache*, anxiety, weakness, dizziness, tremor, restlessness, insomnia. **CV:** bradycardia, ***severe hypertension***, marked increase in peripheral resistance, decreased cardiac output, ***arrhythmias, ventricular tachycardia, fibrillation***, bigeminal rhythm, atrioventricular dissociation, precordial pain. **GU:** decreased urine output. **Metabolic:** metabolic acidosis, hyperglycemia, increased glycogenolysis. **Local:** irritation with extravasation. **Other:** fever, respiratory difficulty.

Interactions

Alpha-adrenergic blockers: may antagonize drug effects. **Antihistamines, ergot alkaloids, guanethidine, methyldopa:** when given with sympathomimetics, may cause severe hypertension. Don't give together. **Inhalational anesthetics:** increased risk of arrhythmias. Monitor closely. **MAO inhibitors:** increased risk of hypertensive crisis.

Nursing diagnoses

• Altered tissue perfusion (cardiopulmonary, renal, GI, peripheral, cerebral) related to the patient's underlying condition.
• Altered urinary elimination related to adverse reaction to norepinephrine.
• Knowledge deficit related to norepinephrine therapy.

Nursing interventions

• *Contraindicated* in mesenteric or peripheral vascular thrombosis, pregnancy, profound hypoxia, hypercarbia, and hypotension from blood volume deficits and during cyclopropane and halothane anesthesia.
• *Use with extreme caution* in patients receiving MAO inhibitors or TCAs.
• *Use cautiously* in hypertension, hyperthyroidism, severe cardiac disease, and sulfite sensitivity.
• Not a substitute for blood or fluid volume deficit. Volume deficit should be replaced before vasopressors are administered.
• **I.V. use:** Use a central venous catheter or a large vein. Administer in dextrose 5% in 0.9% sodium chloride injection.
• Check site frequently for signs of extravasation. If it occurs, stop infusion immediately and call doctor.
• Never leave patient unattended during infusion. Check blood pressure every 2 minutes until stabilized; then every 5 minutes.
• Frequently monitor ECG, blood pressure, cardiac output, central venous pressure, pulmonary capillary wedge pressure, pulse rate, urine output, and color and temperature of extremities. Titrate infusion rate according to findings and doctor's guidelines. Use a continuous infusion pump to regulate flow. In previously hypertensive patients, blood pressure should be raised no higher than 40 mm Hg below preexisting systolic pressure.
• When stopping drug, slow infusion rate gradually. Monitor vital signs, even after drug is stopped. Watch for severe drop in blood pressure.
• Report decreased urine output immediately.

ethambutol hydrochloride

Etibit†, Myambutol

General

Classification: antitubercular agent (semisynthetic antitubercular). **Pregnancy risk category:** B.

Mechanism of action

Interferes with the synthesis of one or more metabolites of susceptible bacteria, altering cellular metabolism during cell division (bacteriostatic).

Indications and dosage

- Adjunctive treatment in pulmonary tuberculosis.

Adults and children over 13 years: initial treatment for patients who have not received previous antitubercular therapy is 15 mg/kg P.O. daily in single dose. **Re-treatment:** 25 mg/kg P.O. daily in single dose for 60 days with at least one other antitubercular drug; then decrease to 15 mg/kg P.O. daily in single dose.

Adverse reactions

CNS: headache, dizziness, mental confusion, possible hallucinations, peripheral neuritis (numbness and tingling of extremities). **EENT:** optic neuritis (vision loss and loss of color discrimination, especially red and green). **GI:** anorexia, nausea, vomiting, abdominal pain. **Metabolic:** *elevated uric acid.* **Other:** ***anaphylactic reactions,*** fever, malaise, bloody sputum.

Interactions

None significant.

Nursing diagnoses

- High risk for injury related to ineffectiveness of ethambutol in eradicating the infection.
- Altered health maintenance related to ethambutol-induced gout caused by elevated uric acid levels.
- Knowledge deficit related to ethambutol therapy.

Nursing interventions

- *Contraindicated* in optic neuritis and in children under 13 years.
- *Use cautiously* in impaired renal function, cataracts, recurrent eye inflammations, gout, and diabetic retinopathy.
- Expect to reduce dosage in patients with renal impairment.
- Perform visual acuity and color discrimination tests before and during therapy.
- Monitor serum uric acid; observe patient for symptoms of gout.
- Reassure patient that visual disturbances will disappear several weeks to months after drug is stopped.

General

Classification: antinuclear agent (H_2-receptor antagonist). **Pregnancy risk category:** C.

Mechanism of action

Competitively inhibits the action of histamine at H_2 receptor sites of the parietal cells, decreasing gastric acid secretion.

Indications and dosage

- Active duodenal ulcer treatment. **Adults:** 300 mg P.O. daily h.s. Alternatively, patient may receive 150 mg b.i.d.
- Maintenance therapy of duodenal ulcer. **Adults:** 150 mg daily h.s.
- Gastroesophageal reflux disease. **Adults:** 150 mg P.O. b.i.d.

Adverse reactions

Blood: ***thrombocytopenia.*** **CNS:** *somnolence.* **CV:** arrhythmias. **Skin:** *sweating,* rash, urticaria, ***exfoliative dermatitis.*** **Other:** hepatic damage, hyperuricemia, gynecomastia.

Interactions

Aspirin: nizatidine may elevate serum salicylate levels in patients taking high doses of aspirin.

Nursing diagnoses

- Pain related to the patient's underlying condition.
- High risk for impaired skin integrity related to nizatidine-induced dermatitis.
- Knowledge deficit related to nizatidine therapy.

Nursing interventions

- *Contraindicated* in patients with hypersensitivity to H_2-receptor antagonists.
- Dosage should be reduced in patients with impaired renal function. Patients with a creatinine clearance of 20 to 50 ml/minute should receive 150 mg daily for treatment of active duodenal ulcer or 150 mg every other day for maintenance therapy. Patients with a creatinine clearance below 20 ml/minute should receive 150 mg every other day for treatment or 150 mg every third day for maintenance.
- False-positive test results for urobilinogen may occur.
- Nizatidine has not been associated with antiandrogenic activity and does not appear to affect hepatic drug-metabolizing enzyme systems.
- Urge patient to avoid cigarette smoking, which will increase gastric acid secretion and worsen disease.
- Capsules may be opened and contents mixed with apple juice. However, drug has been shown to lose some potency when combined with tomato-based mixed-vegetable juices. Check with pharmacist for compatibility.

ethaverine hydrochloride

Ethaquin, Ethatab, Ethavex-100, Isovex

General

Classification: coronary vasodilator (isoquinoline derivative). **Pregnancy risk category:** C.

Mechanism of action

Directly relaxes smooth muscle by inhibiting phosphodiesterase, resulting in increased concentrations of cAMP.

Indications and dosage

- Long-term treatment of peripheral and cerebrovascular insufficiency associated with arterial spasm; spastic conditions of GI and GU tracts. **Adults:** 100 to 200 mg P.O. t.i.d.

Adverse reactions

CNS: *headache,* drowsiness. **CV:** *hypotension, flushing,* sweating, vertigo, cardiac depression, arrhythmias. **GI:** *nausea, anorexia, abdominal distress, dry throat,* constipation, diarrhea. **Hepatic:** jaundice, altered liver function tests. **Skin:** rash. **Other:** respiratory depression, malaise, lassitude.

Interactions

None significant.

Nursing diagnoses

- Altered cerebral and peripheral tissue perfusion related to patient's underlying condition.
- Impaired skin integrity related to adverse reactions.
- Knowledge deficit related to ethaverine therapy.

Nursing interventions

- *Contraindicated* in complete AV dissociation and severe hepatic disease.
- *Use cautiously* in women who are pregnant or of childbearing age and in glaucoma or pulmonary embolus; may precipitate arrhythmias.
- Withhold dose and call doctor if signs of hepatic hypersensitivity develop (GI symptoms, altered liver function tests, jaundice, and eosinophilia).
- The FDA has announced that this drug may not be effective for disease states indicated.

General

Classification: antihypertensive (vasodilator). **Pregnancy risk category:** C.

Mechanism of action

Relaxes arteriolar and venous smooth muscles.

Indications and dosage

• Lowering of blood pressure quickly in hypertensive emergencies, control of hypotension during anesthesia, reduction of preload and afterload in cardiac pump failure or cardiogenic shock; may be used with or without dopamine. **Adults:** 50-mg vial diluted with 2 to 3 ml of D_5W I.V. and then added to 250, 500, or 1,000 ml D_5W. Infuse at 0.5 to 10 mcg/kg/minute. Average dose is 3 mcg/kg/minute. Maximum infusion rate is 10 mcg/kg/minute.

Patients taking other antihypertensives along with nitroprusside are very sensitive to this drug. Adjust dosage accordingly.

Adverse reactions

The following adverse reactions usually indicate overdosage: **CNS:** *headache, dizziness,* ataxia, loss of consciousness, coma, weak pulse, absent reflexes, widely dilated pupils, *restlessness, muscle twitching, diaphoresis.* **CV:** distant heart sounds, palpitations, dyspnea, shallow breathing. **GI:** *vomiting, nausea, abdominal pain.* **Metabolic:** acidosis. **Skin:** pink color.

Interactions

None significant.

Nursing diagnoses

• Altered tissue perfusion (renal, cerebral, cardiopulmonary, peripheral) related to the patient's underlying condition.
• Pain related to nitroprusside-induced adverse reactions such as headache and abdominal discomfort.
• Knowledge deficit related to nitroprusside therapy.

Nursing interventions

• *Use cautiously* in hypothyroidism or hepatic or renal disease and in patients receiving other antihypertensives. Keep patient supine when initiating or titrating nitroprusside therapy.
• Because of light sensitivity, wrap I.V. solution in foil. It's not necessary to wrap the tubing in foil. Fresh solution should have faint brownish tint. Discard after 24 hours.
• Don't use bacteriostatic water for injection or sterile sodium chloride solution for reconstitution.
• Obtain baseline vital signs before giving this drug, and find out what parameters the doctor wants to achieve.
• **I.V. use:** Infuse with a continuous infusion pump. This drug is best run piggyback through a peripheral line with no other medication. Don't adjust rate of main I.V. line while drug is running. Even small bolus of nitroprusside can cause severe hypotension.
• Check blood pressure every 5 minutes at start of infusion and every 15 minutes thereafter. If severe hypotension occurs, turn off I.V. nitroprusside—effects of drug quickly reverse.
• Excessive doses or rapid infusion (greater than 15 mcg/kg/minute) of this drug can cause cyanide toxicity, so check serum thiocyanate levels every 72 hours. Thiocyanate levels of greater than 100 mcg/ml are associated with toxicity. Watch for signs of thiocyanate toxicity: profound hypotension, metabolic acidosis, dyspnea, headache, loss of consciousness, ataxia, vomiting. If these occur, discontinue drug immediately and notify doctor.
• Sometimes used with a direct-acting cardiac stimulant such as dopamine in patients with refractory heart failure.

General

Classification: sedative-hypnotic (chlorinated acetylenic carbinol). **Pregnancy risk category:** C. **Controlled substance schedule:** IV.

Mechanism of action

Unknown.

Indications and dosage

- Sedation. **Adults:** 100 to 200 mg P.O. b.i.d. or t.i.d.
- Insomnia. **Adults:** 500 mg to 1 g P.O. h.s. May repeat 100 to 200 mg if awakened in early morning.

Adverse reactions

Blood: thrombocytopenia. **CNS:** facial numbness, drowsiness, fatigue, nightmares, dizziness, residual sedation, muscular weakness, syncope, ataxia. **CV:** hypotension. **EENT:** unpleasant aftertaste, blurred vision. **GI:** distress, nausea, vomiting. **Skin:** rashes, urticaria.

Interactions

Alcohol or other CNS depressants, including narcotic analgesics, TCAs, and MAO inhibitors: excessive CNS depression. Use together cautiously. **Oral anticoagulants:** ethchlorvynol may enhance the metabolism of coumarin derivatives, decreasing their effectiveness. Monitor closely.

Nursing diagnoses

- Sleep pattern disturbance related to underlying patient problem.
- High risk for trauma related to adverse CNS reactions caused by ethchlorvynol.
- Knowledge deficit related to ethchlorvynol therapy.

Nursing interventions

- *Contraindicated* in patients with hypersensitivity to the drug and in those with uncontrolled pain or porphyria.
- *Use cautiously* in hepatic or renal impairment; in elderly or debilitated patients; in mental depression with suicidal tendencies; and if patient has previously overreacted to barbiturates or alcohol.
- Give with milk or food to minimize transient dizziness or ataxia caused by rapid absorption.
- Do not discontinue drug abruptly. Ethchlorvynol may cause dependence and severe withdrawal symptoms. Withdraw gradually.
- Take precautions to prevent hoarding or self-overdosing by patients who are depressed, suicidal, or drug-dependent or those who have a history of drug abuse. Overdosage is very difficult to treat and has a high mortality.
- Watch for signs of toxicity, such as poor muscle coordination, confusion, hypothermia, speech or vision disturbances, tremor, and weakness.
- Keep in mind that the 750-mg strength contains tartrazine dye. May cause allergic reactions in susceptible patients.
- Warn patient to avoid hazardous activities requiring mental alertness or physical coordination. Supervise walking; raise bed rails, especially for elderly patients.
- Slight darkening of liquid from exposure to air and light doesn't affect safety or potency, but store in tight, light-resistant container to avoid possible deterioration.
- Drug is effective for short-term use only; treatment period should not exceed 1 week.

General

Classification: antianginal, vasodilator (nitrate).
Pregnancy risk category: C.

Mechanism of action

Reduces cardiac oxygen demand by decreasing left ventricular end-diastolic pressure (preload) and, to a lesser extent, systemic vascular resistance (afterload). Also increases blood flow through the collateral coronary vessels.

Indications and dosage

- Prophylaxis against chronic anginal attacks. **Adults:** 2.5 mg sustained-release capsule q 8 to 12 hours. Or 2% ointment (start with ½" [1.25 cm] ointment, increasing by ½" increments until headache occurs, then decreasing to previous dose; usual dose is 1" to 2" [2.5 to 5 cm]). Or transdermal disk or pad applied to hairless site once daily.
- Relief of acute angina pectoris, prophylaxis to prevent or minimize anginal attacks when taken immediately before stressful events. **Adults:** 1 S.L. tablet (gr 1/400, 1/200, 1/150, 1/100) dissolved under the tongue or in the buccal pouch immediately upon indication of anginal attack (may repeat q 5 minutes for 15 minutes); Nitrolingual spray, 1 or 2 sprays onto or under tongue (may repeat q 3 to 5 minutes; maximum of 3 doses in 15 minutes).
- Control of hypertension associated with surgery; treatment of CHF associated with MI; relief of acute angina pectoris; production of controlled hypotension during surgery. **Adults:** initial I.V. infusion rate is 5 mcg/minute. Increase by 5 mcg/minute q 3 to 5 minutes until a response is noted. If a 20 mcg/minute rate doesn't produce a response, increase as much as 20 mcg/minute q 3 to 5 minutes.

Adverse reactions

CNS: *headache, dizziness,* weakness. **CV:** *orthostatic hypotension, tachycardia, flushing, palpitations.* **GI:** nausea, vomiting. **Skin:** cutaneous vasodilation. **Local:** sublingual burning. **Other:** hypersensitivity reactions.

Interactions

Antihypertensives: possibly enhanced hypotensive effect. Monitor closely.

Nursing diagnoses

- Pain related to ineffectiveness of nitroglycerin.
- High risk for injury related to nitroglycerin-induced dizziness or orthostatic hypotension.
- Knowledge deficit related to nitroglycerin therapy.

Nursing interventions

- *Contraindicated* in hypersensitivity to nitrites, head trauma, cerebral hemorrhage, hypertrophic cardiomyopathy, or severe anemia.
- *Use cautiously* in hypotension.
- Monitor blood pressure and intensity and duration of response to drug.
- Minimize tolerance by removing transdermal systems in the evening and applying a new system the next morning or by omitting the last daily dose of a buccal, sustained-release, or ointment form.
- Advise patient to avoid alcoholic beverages; may produce increased hypotension.
- Store drug in cool, dark place in tightly closed, original container. Replace supply of sublingual tablets every 3 months. Remove cotton from container, since it absorbs drug.
- Teach patient to swallow oral tablets whole on empty stomach and to chew chewable tablets thoroughly before swallowing.
- To apply ointment, spread uniform, thin layer on any nonhairy area. Do not rub in; cover with plastic film. Remove all excess ointment from previous site before applying the next dose.
- **I.V. use:** Administer with an infusion pump and titrate to desired response. Mix in glass bottles and avoid use of I.V. filters.

General

Classification: estrogen replacement, antineoplastic (estrogen). **Pregnancy risk category:** X.

Mechanism of action

Increases DNA, RNA, and protein tissue synthesis. Reduces pituitary release of follicle-stimulating hormone and luteinizing hormone.

Indications and dosage

- Breast cancer (5 or more years after menopause). **Women:** 1 mg P.O. t.i.d.
- Hypogonadism. **Women:** 0.05 mg P.O. daily to t.i.d. for 2 weeks a month, followed by 2 weeks progesterone therapy; continue for 3 to 6 monthly dosing cycles, followed by 2 months off.
- Menopausal symptoms. **Women:** 0.02 to 0.05 mg P.O. daily for cycles of 3 weeks on, 1 week off.
- Inoperable prostatic cancer. **Men:** 0.15 to 2 mg P.O. daily.

Adverse reactions

CNS: headache, dizziness, chorea, depression, libido changes, lethargy. **CV:** thrombophlebitis, ***thromboembolism,*** hypertension, edema. **EENT:** worsening of myopia or astigmatism, intolerance to contact lenses. **GI:** *nausea,* vomiting, abdominal cramps, bloating, diarrhea, constipation, anorexia, increased appetite, weight changes. **GU:** in women—breakthrough bleeding, altered menstrual flow, dysmenorrhea, amenorrhea, cervical erosion, altered cervical secretions, enlargement of uterine fibromas, vaginal candidiasis. In men—gynecomastia, testicular atrophy, impotence. **Hepatic:** cholestatic jaundice. **Metabolic:** hyperglycemia, hypercalcemia, folic acid deficiency. **Skin:** melasma, urticaria, acne, seborrhea, oily skin, hirsutism or hair loss. **Other:** breast changes, leg cramps.

Interactions

Bromocriptine: may cause amenorrhea. Avoid concomitant use. **Carbamazepine, phenobarbital, rifampin:** decreased effectiveness of estrogen therapy. Monitor closely. **Corticosteroids:** possible enhanced effects. Monitor closely. **Cyclosporine:** increased risk of toxicity. Use together with caution and frequently monitor cyclosporine levels. **Dantrolene, other hepatotoxic medications:** increased risk of hepatotoxicity. Monitor closely. **Oral anticoagulants:** dosage adjustments may be necessary. Monitor PT. **Tamoxifen:** may interfere with the effectiveness of tamoxifen. Avoid concomitant use.

Nursing diagnoses

- Sexual dysfunction related to the patient's underlying condition.
- Altered tissue perfusion (cerebral, peripheral, cardiopulmonary) related to drug-induced thromboembolism.
- Knowledge deficit related to ethinyl estradiol therapy.

Nursing interventions

- *Contraindicated* in thrombophlebitis or thromboembolic disorders, undiagnosed abnormal genital bleeding, and pregnancy.
- *Use cautiously* in hypertension, mental depression, bone diseases, migraine, seizures, blood dyscrasias, diabetes mellitus, amenorrhea, heart failure, hepatic or renal dysfunction, or family history (mother, grandmother, sister) of breast or genital tract cancer; may require discontinuation of the drug.
- Give patient package insert describing adverse effects of ethinyl estradiol, and provide verbal explanation.
- Warn patient to immediately report abdominal pain; pain, numbness, or stiffness in legs or buttocks; pressure or pain in chest; shortness of breath; severe headaches; visual disturbances, such as blind spots, flashing lights, or blurriness; vaginal bleeding or discharge; breast lumps; swelling of hands or feet; yellow skin or sclera; dark urine; or light-colored stools.

General
Classification: urinary tract antiseptic (nitrofuran). **Pregnancy risk category:** B.

Mechanism of action
Bacteriostatic in low concentration and possibly bactericidal in high concentration. Interferes with bacterial enzyme systems and possibly with bacterial cell wall formation.

Indications and dosage
• Pyelonephritis, pyelitis, and cystitis caused by susceptible *Escherichia coli, Staphylococcus aureus,* enterococci; certain strains of *Klebsiella, Proteus,* and *Enterobacter.* **Adults and children over 12 years:** 50 to 100 mg P.O. q.i.d. with milk or meals. Alternatively, give 100 mg dual-release capsules P.O. q 12 hours for 7 days. **Children 1 month to 12 years:** 5 to 7 mg/kg P.O. daily, divided q.i.d.
• Long-term suppression therapy. **Adults:** 50 to 100 mg P.O. daily h.s. **Children:** 1 to 2 mg/kg P.O. daily h.s.

Adverse reactions
Blood: ***hemolysis in patients with G6PD deficiency, agranulocytosis,*** thrombocytopenia. **CNS:** peripheral neuropathy, headache, dizziness, drowsiness, *ascending polyneuropathy with high doses or renal impairment.* **GI:** *anorexia, nausea, vomiting,* abdominal pain, *diarrhea.* **Hepatic:** hepatitis. **Skin:** maculopapular, erythematous, or eczematous eruption; pruritus; urticaria; ***exfoliative dermatitis; Stevens-Johnson syndrome.*** **Other:** ***asthmatic attacks in patients with history of asthma; anaphylaxis;*** hypersensitivity; transient alopecia; drug fever; overgrowth of nonsusceptible organisms in the urinary tract; ***pulmonary sensitivity reactions*** *(cough, chest pain, fever, dyspnea).*

Interactions
Magnesium-containing antacids: decreased nitrofurantoin absorption. Separate administration times by 1 hour. **Nalidixic acid, norfloxacin:** possible decreased effectiveness. Don't use together. **Probenecid, sulfinpyrazone:** increased blood levels and decreased urine levels. May result in increased toxicity and lack of therapeutic effect. Don't use together.

Nursing diagnoses
• High risk for injury related to ineffectiveness of nitrofurantoin to eradicate the infection.
• High risk for fluid volume deficit related to nitrofurantoin-induced adverse GI reactions.
• Knowledge deficit related to nitrofurantoin therapy.

Nursing interventions
• *Contraindicated* in children 1 month and under and in moderate to severe renal impairment, anuria, oliguria, or creatinine clearance under 40 ml/minute.
• *Use cautiously* in G6PD deficiency.
• Hypersensitivity may develop when used for long-term therapy.
• Obtain specimen for culture and sensitivity tests before starting therapy and repeat p.r.n. Continue treatment for 3 days after sterile urine specimens have been obtained.
• Monitor CBC regularly.
• Monitor intake and output carefully. May turn urine brown or darker.
• Store in amber container. Keep away from metals other than stainless steel or aluminum to avoid precipitate formation. Warn patients not to use pillboxes made of these materials.
• Monitor pulmonary status.
• Monitor for superinfection.
• May cause false-positive results with urine glucose test using copper sulfate reduction method (Clinitest) but not with glucose oxidase tests (Tes-Tape, Diastix, Clinistix).
• Dual-release capsules are formulated to permit twice-daily dosing. This should improve patient compliance. Dual-release capsules contain 25 mg nitrofurantoin macrocrystals and 75 mg nitrofurantoin monohydrate. The macrocrystals have a slower dissolution and absorption than the monohydrate. The monohydrate forms a slow-releasing gel matrix when it contacts fluids in the GI tract.

General

Classification: antitubercular agent (isonicotinic acid derivative). **Pregnancy risk category:** D.

Mechanism of action

Unknown. Probably inhibits peptide synthesis (bacteriostatic).

Indications and dosage

• Adjunctive treatment of pulmonary or extrapulmonary tuberculosis (when primary therapy with streptomycin or isoniazid cannot be used or has failed). **Adults:** 500 mg to 1 g P.O. daily in divided doses. Concomitant administration of other effective antitubercular drugs and pyridoxine recommended. **Children:** 15 to 20 mg/kg P.O. daily in three to four doses. Maximum dosage 1 g.

Adverse reactions

Blood: thrombocytopenia. **CNS:** asthenia, drowsiness, *peripheral neuritis,* psychic disturbances (especially mental depression). **CV:** postural hypotension. **GI:** *anorexia,* metallic taste in mouth, nausea, vomiting, sialorrhea, *epigastric distress,* diarrhea, stomatitis, weight loss. **Hepatic:** jaundice, hepatitis, elevated AST (SGOT) and ALT (SGPT). **Skin:** rash, ***exfoliative dermatitis.***

Interactions

None significant.

Nursing diagnoses

• High risk for infection related to ineffectiveness of ethionamide in eradicating the infection.
• High risk for impaired skin integrity related to ethionamide-induced adverse reactions.
• Knowledge deficit related to ethionamide therapy.

Nursing interventions

• *Contraindicated* in severe hepatic damage.
• *Use cautiously* in diabetes mellitus.
• Perform culture and sensitivity tests before starting therapy. Stop drug if skin rash occurs; may progress to exfoliative dermatitis.
• Monitor hepatic function every 2 to 4 weeks.
• Give with meals or antacids to minimize GI effects. Patient may require antiemetic.
• Pyridoxine may be ordered to prevent neuropathy.
• Instruct patient to take drug exactly as prescribed; warn against discontinuing drug without doctor's consent.
• Warn patient to avoid excess alcohol ingestion because it may make him more vulnerable to liver damage.

General
Classification: cerebral vasodilator (calcium channel blocker). **Pregnancy risk category:** C.

Mechanism of action
Inhibits calcium ion influx across cardiac and smooth muscle cells, thus decreasing myocardial contractility and oxygen demand, and dilates coronary and cerebral arteries and arterioles. Initially thought to relieve vasospasm in patients after subarachnoid hemorrhage, its mechanism of action is not fully known; blockade of calcium influx into cerebral neurons may contribute to drug's effect.

Indications and dosage
- Improvement of neurologic deficits in patients after subarachnoid hemorrhage from ruptured congenital aneurysms. **Adults:** 60 mg P.O. q 4 hours for 21 days. Therapy should begin within 96 hours after subarachnoid hemorrhage.

Adverse reactions
CNS: headaches. **CV:** decreased blood pressure, flushing, edema.

Interactions
Antihypertensives: possible enhanced hypotensive effect. **Calcium channel blockers:** possible enhanced CV effects.

Nursing diagnoses
- Altered health maintenance related to the patient's underlying condition.
- Pain related to adverse drug reaction.
- Knowledge deficit related to nimodipine therapy.

Nursing interventions
- There are no known contraindications to nimodipine therapy, and the drug was relatively well tolerated in clinical trials. Nimodipine should be reserved for patients who are in good neurologic condition postictus (for example, Hunt and Hess grades I to III).
- Patients with hepatic failure should receive lower doses. Begin therapy at 30 mg P.O. every 4 hours, with close monitoring of blood pressure and heart rate.
- Monitor blood pressure and heart rate in all patients, especially at the initiation of therapy.

ethosuximide

Zarontin

General

Classification: anticonvulsant (succinimide derivative). **Pregnancy risk category:** C.

Mechanism of action

Increases seizure threshold. Reduces the paroxysmal spike-and-wave pattern of absence seizures by depressing nerve transmission in the motor cortex.

Indications and dosage

• Absence seizures. **Adults and children over 6 years:** initially, 250 mg capsules or syrup P.O. b.i.d. May increase by 250 mg q 4 to 7 days up to 1.5 g daily. **Children 3 to 6 years:** 250 mg P.O. daily or 125 mg P.O. b.i.d. May increase by 250 mg q 4 to 7 days up to 1.5 g daily.

Adverse reactions

Blood: leukopenia, eosinophilia, ***agranulocytosis,*** pancytopenia, ***aplastic anemia.*** **CNS:** *drowsiness,* headache, *fatigue, dizziness,* ataxia, irritability, hiccups, *euphoria, lethargy.* **EENT:** myopia. **GI:** *nausea, vomiting,* diarrhea, gum hypertrophy, weight loss, cramps, tongue swelling, *anorexia, epigastric and abdominal pain.* **GU:** vaginal bleeding. **Skin:** urticaria, pruritic and erythematous rashes, hirsutism.

Interactions

None significant.

Nursing diagnoses

• Altered thought processes related to patient's underlying seizure disorder.
• Altered protection related to ethosuximide-induced blood disorders.
• Knowledge deficit related to ethosuximide therapy.

Nursing interventions

• *Contraindicated* in hypersensitivity to succinimide derivatives.
• *Use cautiously* in hepatic or renal disease.
• Ethosuximide is currently the drug of choice for treating absence seizures.
• The drug may cause positive direct Coombs' test.
• Regularly assess seizure activity. Keep in mind that drug may increase frequency of generalized tonic-clonic seizures when used alone in patients who have mixed types of seizures.
• Monitor serum blood levels; therapeutic levels range between 40 and 80 mcg/ml.
• Obtain CBC every 3 to 6 months.
• Give drug with food to minimize GI distress.
• Warn patient to avoid activities that require alertness and good psychomotor coordination until CNS effects of the drug are known.
• Never withdraw drug suddenly. Abrupt withdrawal may precipitate absence seizures. Call doctor immediately if adverse reactions develop.

General
Classification: antianginal (calcium channel blocker). **Pregnancy risk category:** C.

Mechanism of action
Inhibits calcium ion influx across cardiac and smooth muscle cells, decreasing myocardial contractility and oxygen demand, and dilates coronary arteries and arterioles.

Indications and dosage
• Management of vasospastic (also called Prinzmetal's or variant) angina and classic chronic stable angina pectoris; Raynaud's disease. **Adults:** Starting dose is 10 mg P.O. t.i.d. Usual effective dose range is 10 to 20 mg t.i.d. Some patients may require up to 30 mg q.i.d. Maximum daily dosage is 180 mg.
• Hypertension. **Adults:** 30 or 60 mg P.O. (sustained-release form only) once daily. Titrate over a 7- to 14-day period.

Adverse reactions
CNS: *dizziness, light-headedness, flushing, headache,* weakness, syncope. **CV:** peripheral edema, hypotension, palpitations. **EENT:** nasal congestion. **GI:** *nausea, heartburn,* diarrhea. **Metabolic:** hypokalemia. **Other:** muscle cramps, dyspnea.

Interactions
Cimetidine, ranitidine: decreased nifedipine metabolism. **Propranolol, other beta blockers:** may cause hypotension and heart failure. Use together cautiously.

Nursing diagnoses
• Pain related to ineffectiveness of nifedipine therapy.
• High risk for injury related to nifedipine-induced CNS reactions.
• Knowledge deficit related to nifedipine therapy.

Nursing interventions
• *Use cautiously* in CHF or hypotension and in elderly patients because duration of action may be prolonged.
• Monitor blood pressure regularly, especially in patients who are also taking beta blockers or antihypertensives.
• Monitor serum potassium level regularly.
• Patient may briefly develop anginal exacerbation when beginning drug therapy or when dosage is increased. Reassure him that this symptom is temporary.
• Although rebound effect hasn't been observed when drug is stopped, dosage should still be reduced slowly under doctor's supervision.
• If patient is kept on nitrate therapy while drug dosage is being titrated, urge him to continue his compliance. Sublingual nitroglycerin, especially, may be taken as needed when anginal symptoms are acute.
• Instruct patient to swallow the capsule whole without breaking, crushing, or chewing it. The sustained-release tablets should never be chewed, crushed, or broken.
• Sublingual form of nifedipine is not available. However, the liquid in the oral capsule can be withdrawn by puncturing the capsule with a needle. Instill the drug into the buccal pouch.
• Sublingual nifedipine may be useful in decreasing blood pressure during hypertensive emergencies. Continuous blood pressure and ECG monitoring is recommended.
• Protect capsules from direct light and moisture and store at room temperature.

ethotoin

Peganone

General

Classification: anticonvulsant (hydantoin derivative). **Pregnancy risk category:** D.

Mechanism of action

Stabilizes neuronal membranes and limits seizure activity by either increasing efflux or decreasing influx of sodium ions across cell membranes in the motor cortex during generation of nerve impulses.

Indications and dosage

• Generalized tonic-clonic or complex-partial seizures. **Adults:** initially, 250 mg P.O. q.i.d. after meals. May increase slowly over several days to 3 g daily divided q.i.d. **Children:** initially, 250 mg P.O. b.i.d. May increase up to 250 mg P.O. q.i.d.

Adverse reactions

Blood: thrombocytopenia, leukopenia, ***agranulocytosis, pancytopenia,*** megaloblastic anemia. **CNS:** fatigue, insomnia, dizziness, headache, numbness. **CV:** chest pain. **EENT:** diplopia, nystagmus. **GI:** *nausea, vomiting, diarrhea,* gingival hyperplasia (rare). **Skin:** rash. **Other:** fever, lymphadenopathy.

Interactions

Alcohol, folic acid: monitor for decreased ethotoin activity. **Oral anticoagulants, antihistamines, chloramphenicol, cimetidine, diazepam, diazoxide, disulfiram, isoniazid, phenylbutazone, salicylates, sulfamethizole, valproate:** monitor for increased ethotoin activity and toxicity. **Phenacemide:** paranoia. Use together cautiously.

Nursing diagnoses

• High risk for injury related to underlying seizure disorder.
• Altered protection related to ethotoin-induced blood disorders.
• Knowledge deficit related to ethotoin therapy.

Nursing interventions

• *Contraindicated* in hydantoin hypersensitivity or hepatic or hematologic disorders.
• *Use cautiously* in patients receiving other hydantoin derivatives.
• Ethotoin is the hydantoin derivative of choice in young adults who are prone to gingival hyperplasia caused by phenytoin. Otherwise, the drug is infrequently used in the treatment of epilepsy.
• Obtain CBC and urinalysis when therapy starts and periodically thereafter. Also, periodically monitor liver function tests on long-term use.
• Ethotoin generally produces milder adverse reactions than phenytoin; however, the large doses required to maintain its therapeutic effect frequently cause GI distress.
• To avoid GI distress, give after meals. Schedule doses as evenly as possible over 24 hours.
• Tell patient to avoid activities that require alertness and good psychomotor coordination until CNS effects of the drug are known.
• Warn patient that heavy use of alcohol may diminish benefits of drug.
• Discontinue drug if lymphadenopathy or lupus-like syndrome (fever, bruising, and sore throat) develops.
• Never withdraw drug suddenly. Call doctor at once if adverse reactions develop.

General
Classification: anthelmintic. **Pregnancy risk category:** B.

Mechanism of action
Inhibits the metabolic process of oxidative phosphorylation in tapeworms.

Indications and dosage
• Tapeworms (fish, beef, and pork). **Adults:** 4 tablets (2 g) chewed thoroughly as a single dose. **Children** (more than 34 kg): 3 tablets (1.5 g) chewed thoroughly as a single dose. **Children** (11 to 34 kg): 2 tablets (1 g) chewed thoroughly as a single dose.
• Dwarf tapeworm. **Adults:** 4 tablets chewed thoroughly as a single dose for 7 days. **Children over 2 years** (more than 34 kg): 3 tablets chewed thoroughly on the first day, then 2 tablets for the next 6 days. **Children over 2 years** (11 to 34 kg): 2 tablets chewed thoroughly on the first day, then 1 tablet daily for the next 6 days.

Adverse reactions
CNS: drowsiness, dizziness, headache. **EENT:** oral irritation. **GI:** *nausea, vomiting, anorexia,* diarrhea, bad taste in mouth. **Skin:** rash, pruritus ani.

Interactions
None reported.

Nursing diagnoses
• Altered health maintenance related to ineffectiveness of niclosamide.
• High risk for fluid volume deficit related to niclosamide-induced GI reactions.
• Knowledge deficit related to niclosamide therapy.

Nursing interventions
• Instruct patient to chew tablets thoroughly and wash down with water; for children, the tablets can be crushed and mixed with water or applesauce.
• Tablets should be taken as a single dose after breakfast.
• A mild laxative should be administered to clean the bowel before initiation of niclosamide therapy in patients who are constipated.
• When treating dwarf tapeworms, urge patient to drink fruit juices. This helps to eliminate the accumulated intestinal mucus under which they lodge.
• Teach patient about the need for good personal hygiene, especially good handwashing technique. Advise patient to refrain from preparing food during infestation.
• Patient isn't considered cured until the stool has been negative for tapeworms for at least 3 months.

ethylnorepinephrine hydrochloride Bronkephrine

General

Classification: bronchodilator (adrenergic agonist). **Pregnancy risk category:** C.

Mechanism of action

Relaxes bronchial smooth muscle by acting on beta-adrenergic receptors.

Indications and dosage

• Relief of bronchospasm caused by asthma. **Adults:** 0.6 to 2 mg S.C. or I.M. **Children:** 0.2 to 1 mg S.C. or I.M.

Adverse reactions

CNS: *headache,* dizziness. **CV:** changes in blood pressure, *elevation in pulse rate,* palpitations. **GI:** nausea.

Interactions

Beta blockers: mutual inhibition of clinical effects. **CNS stimulants, xanthine derivatives:** enhanced CNS stimulation. **Digitalis glycosides, levodopa:** increased risk of cardiac arrhythmias. Monitor closely. **Nitrates, antihypertensives:** decreased effects of these agents. **Rauwolfia alkaloids, sympathomimetics:** enhanced effects. **Thyroid hormones:** increased risk of coronary insufficiency.

Nursing diagnoses

• Ineffective airway clearance related to patient's underlying respiratory condition.
• Knowledge deficit related to ethylnorepinephrine therapy.

Nursing interventions

• *Contraindicated* in patients with hypersensitivity to the drug; in patients with tachyarrhythmias, tachycardia caused by digitalis toxicity, narrow-angle glaucoma, or shock; and in those receiving general anesthesia with cyclopropane or halogenated inhalational anesthetics.
• *Use cautiously* in cardiovascular disease or history of stroke.
• Be aware that ethylnorepinephrine is safer than epinephrine for use in hypertensive or severely ill patients in whom significant pressor effects are undesirable.
• This drug is also valuable when used in children because of low incidence of adverse reactions; may be useful in diabetic asthmatics due to low glycogenolytic activity.
• Choose anatomic injection site carefully to avoid inadvertent intraneural or intravascular injection.

General

Classification: antianginal, antihypertensive (calcium channel blocker). **Pregnancy risk category:** C.

Mechanism of action

Inhibits calcium ion influx across cardiac and smooth muscle cells, thus decreasing myocardial contractility and oxygen demand, and dilates coronary arteries and arterioles.

Indications and dosage

• Chronic stable angina (used alone or in combination with beta blockers). **Adults:** initially, 20 mg P.O. t.i.d. (immediate-release only). Titrate dosage according to patient response. Usual dosage range is 20 to 40 mg t.i.d.

• Hypertension. **Adults:** initially, 20 to 40 mg P.O. t.i.d. (immediate-release) or 30 mg b.i.d. (sustained-release). Increase dosage according to patient response.

Adverse reactions

CNS: dizziness or light-headedness, headache, paresthesia, drowsiness, asthenia. **CV:** peripheral edema, palpitations, angina, tachycardia. **GI:** nausea, abdominal discomfort, dry mouth. **Skin:** rash, flushing.

Interactions

Antihypertensives: enhanced antihypertensive effect. **Beta-adrenergic blockers:** may increase cardiac depressant effects. Monitor patient closely. **Cimetidine:** may decrease metabolism of calcium channel blockers. Monitor for increased pharmacologic effect. **Cyclosporine:** nicardipine may increase plasma levels of cyclosporine. Monitor for toxicity. **Theophylline:** pharmacologic effects of theophylline may be enhanced. Monitor for toxicity.

Nursing diagnoses

• Pain related to ineffectiveness of nicardipine therapy.

• High risk for injury related to nicardipine-induced CNS reactions or orthostatic hypotension.

• Knowledge deficit related to nicardipine therapy.

Nursing interventions

• *Contraindicated* in patients with hypersensitivity to nicardipine and in advanced aortic stenosis.

• *Use cautiously* in cardiac conduction disturbances, hypotension, and CHF.

• Some patients may experience increased frequency, severity, or duration of chest pain at beginning of therapy or during dosage adjustments. The mechanism for this adverse reaction is not known. Advise patient to report chest pain immediately.

• Dosage of patients with renal impairment should be titrated slowly to achieve optimal response. Begin therapy with 20 mg P.O. t.i.d.

• Patients with hepatic impairment should receive lower initial doses (20 mg P.O. b.i.d.) and be carefully titrated to optimal response.

• Allow at least 3 days between dosage adjustments to achieve steady plasma levels.

• Measure blood pressure frequently during initial therapy. Maximum blood pressure response occurs about 1 hour after dosing with the immediate-release form and 2 to 4 hours after the sustained-release form. Check for potential orthostatic hypotension. Because large swings in blood pressure may occur based on blood level of drug, assess adequacy of antihypertensive effect 8 hours after dosing.

• When switching patients from the immediate-release form to the sustained-release preparation, the total daily dosage of the immediate-release form may be used as a guide; however, in many patients, it isn't a useful predictor of the total daily dosage of sustained-release drug. Individualize therapy and monitor closely.

etidronate disodium

Didronel

General

Classification: antihypercalcemic (pyrophosphate analogue). **Pregnancy risk category:** B.

Mechanism of action

Decreases osteoclastic activity by inhibiting osteocytic osteolysis. Also decreases mineral release and matrix or collagen breakdown in bone.

Indications and dosage

• Symptomatic Paget's disease. **Adults:** 5 mg/kg P.O. daily as a single dose 2 hours before a meal with water or juice. Patient should not eat for 2 hours after dose. May give up to 10 mg/kg daily in severe cases. Maximum dosage 20 mg/kg daily.
• Heterotopic ossification in spinal cord injuries. **Adults:** 20 mg/kg P.O. daily for 2 weeks, then 10 mg/kg daily for 10 weeks. Total treatment period is 12 weeks.
• Heterotopic ossification after total hip replacement. **Adults:** 20 mg/kg daily P.O. for 1 month before total hip replacement and for 3 months afterward.

Adverse reactions

Blood: *elevated serum phosphate.* **GI:** diarrhea, increased frequency of bowel movements, nausea (seen most frequently at 20 mg/kg daily). **Other:** increased or recurrent bone pain at pagetic sites, pain at previously asymptomatic sites, increased risk of fracture.

Interactions

None significant.

Nursing diagnoses

• High risk for injury related to the patient's underlying bone condition.
• Diarrhea related to etidronate-induced adverse GI reactions.
• Knowledge deficit related to etidronate therapy.

Nursing interventions

• *Use cautiously* in enterocolitis, impaired renal function.
• Etidronate has been used investigationally to prevent or treat osteoporosis.
• Therapy should not last more than 6 months. After 3 months, resume if needed. Don't give longer than 3 months at doses above 10 mg/kg daily.
• Don't give drug with food, milk, or antacids; may reduce absorption.
• Monitor renal function before and during therapy.
• Notify doctor if elevated serum phosphate occurs, especially in patients receiving higher doses. Be aware that serum phosphate usually returns to normal 2 to 4 weeks after drug is discontinued.
• Monitor effectiveness by regularly checking serum alkaline phosphatase and urinary hydroxyproline excretion (both lowered if therapy effective).
• Tell patient that improvement may not occur for up to 3 months but may continue for months after drug is stopped. Stress importance of good nutrition, especially diet high in calcium, and vitamin D.

General

Classification: nutritional agent (vitamin). **Pregnancy risk category:** A (C if greater than RDA).

Mechanism of action

Necessary for lipid metabolism, tissue respiration, and glycogenolysis. Also decreases synthesis of low-density lipoproteins and inhibits lipolysis in adipose tissue.

Indications and dosage

- Recommended daily allowance (RDA). **Neonates and infants to 6 months:** 5 mg. **Infants 6 months to 1 year:** 6 mg. **Children 1 to 3 years:** 9 mg. **Children 4 to 6 years:** 12 mg. **Children 7 to 10 years:** 13 mg. **Males 11 to 14 years:** 17 mg. **Males 15 to 18 years:** 20 mg. **Males 19 to 50 years:** 19 mg. **Males 51 years and over:** 15 mg. **Females 11 to 50 years:** 15 mg. **Females 51 years and over:** 13 mg. **Pregnant women:** 17 mg. **Lactating women:** 20 mg.
- Pellagra. **Adults:** 10 to 20 mg P.O., S.C., I.M., or I.V. daily, depending on severity of deficiency. Maximum daily dosage recommended is 500 mg; should be divided into 10 doses. **Children:** up to 300 mg P.O. or 100 mg I.V. daily, depending on severity of niacin deficiency.
- Peripheral vascular disease and circulatory disorders. **Adults:** 250 to 800 mg P.O. daily in divided doses.
- Adjunctive treatment of hyperlipidemias, especially with hypercholesterolemia. **Adults:** 1.5 to 3 g P.O. daily in three divided doses with or after meals, increased as needed and tolerated to a maximum of 6 g daily.

Adverse reactions

Most adverse reactions are dose-dependent. **CNS:** dizziness, transient headache. **CV:** *excessive peripheral vasodilation.* **GI:** *nausea, vomiting, diarrhea,* possible activation of peptic ulcer, epigastric or substernal pain. **Hepatic:** ***hepatic dysfunction.*** **Metabolic:** hyperglycemia, hyperuricemia. **Skin:** *flushing,* pruritus, dryness.

Interactions

Antihypertensives (sympathetic blocking type): may have an additive vasodilating effect and cause postural hypotension. Use together cautiously. Warn patient about postural hypotension.

Nursing diagnoses

- Altered peripheral tissue perfusion related to the patient's underlying condition.
- High risk for fluid volume deficit related to adverse drug reaction.
- Knowledge deficit related to niacin therapy.

Nursing interventions

- *Contraindicated* in hepatic dysfunction, active peptic ulcer disease, severe hypotension, or arterial hemorrhage.
- *Use cautiously* in gallbladder disease, diabetes mellitus, and gout.
- Monitor hepatic function and blood glucose early in therapy.
- Give with meals to minimize adverse GI effects.
- Aspirin (80 to 325 mg P.O. 30 minutes before niacin dose) may reduce the flushing response. Timed-release niacin may avoid excessive flushing effects with large doses. However, timed-release niacin has been associated with hepatic failure, even at low doses.
- **I.V. use:** Give I.V. no faster than 2 mg/minute. Explain harmlessness of flushing syndrome to ease anxiety.
- Stress that medication used to treat hyperlipoproteinemia or to dilate peripheral vessels is not "just a vitamin." Explain importance of adhering to therapeutic regimen.
- Also known as vitamin B_3 or nicotinic acid.

General

Classification: nonnarcotic analgesic (NSAID).
Pregnancy risk category: C.

Mechanism of action

Unknown, but believed to be associated with inhibition of prostaglandin biosynthesis.

Indications and dosage

• Acute and chronic management of osteoarthritis and pain. **Adults:** for acute pain, 200 to 400 mg P.O. q 6 to 8 hours p.r.n., not to exceed 1,200 mg daily. For patients weighing 132 lb (60 kg) or less, total daily dose should not exceed 20 mg/kg.

Adverse reactions

CNS: *asthenia, malaise,* dizziness, depression, nervousness. **CV:** anemia, hypertension, ***CHF,*** flushing, palpitations, edema. **EENT:** blurred vision, tinnitus, photophobia. **GI:** *dyspepsia, flatulence, abdominal pain, diarrhea, nausea,* constipation, gastritis, melena, vomiting, anorexia, peptic ulcer with or without bleeding or perforation, ulcerative stomatitis, thirst, dry mouth. **GU:** dysuria, urinary frequency. **Respiratory:** asthma. **Skin:** pruritus, rash. **Other:** chills, fever, hepatitis.

Interactions

Antacids: may decrease peak levels of the drug. Monitor for decreased effect of etodolac. **Aspirin:** reduces etodolac's protein-binding without altering its clearance. Clinical significance unknown. **Cyclosporine:** impaired elimination and increased risk of nephrotoxicity. Avoid concomitant use. **Digoxin, lithium, methotrexate:** etodolac may impair elimination of these drugs, resulting in increased levels and risk of toxicity. Monitor blood levels. **Warfarin:** etodolac decreases the protein-binding of warfarin but does not change its clearance. Although no dosage adjustment is necessary, monitor PT closely and watch for bleeding.

Nursing diagnoses

• Pain related to patient's underlying condition.
• High risk for injury related to etodolac-induced adverse CNS reactions.
• Knowledge deficit related to etodolac therapy.

Nursing interventions

• *Contraindicated* in patients with hypersensitivity to the drug and in patients with a history of NSAID-induced asthma, rhinitis, urticaria, or other allergic reactions.
• *Use cautiously* in patients with a history of GI bleeding, ulceration, and perforation and renal or hepatic impairment. Also use cautiously in patients with cardiac, renal, or hepatic failure who are using diuretics concomitantly.
• No apparent drug interaction occurs when etodolac is administered with diuretics, phenytoin, or glyburide.
• Watch closely for signs and symptoms of GI bleeding, especially if patient is receiving long-term therapy. Also note that peptic ulcer and GI bleeding and ulceration can sometimes occur without warning.
• Tell patient to take etodolac with milk or meals to minimize GI discomfort.
• When reviewing diagnostic tests, know that metabolites of etodolac may cause a false-positive test for urinary bilirubin. Decreased serum uric acid levels and borderline elevations of one or more liver tests may occur.

General

Classification: antibiotic (aminoglycoside). **Pregnancy risk category:** C.

Mechanism of action

Inhibits protein synthesis by binding directly to the 30S ribosomal subunit. Generally bactericidal.

Indications and dosage

• Serious infections caused by sensitive *Pseudomonas aeruginosa, Escherichia coli, Proteus, Klebsiella, Serratia, Enterobacter, Citrobacter, Staphylococcus.* **Adults and children over 12 years:** 3 to 6.5 mg/kg/day by I.M. injection or I.V. infusion. May be given q 12 hours to treat serious UTIs and q 8 to 12 hours to treat serious systemic infections. **Infants and children 6 weeks to 12 years:** 5.5 to 8 mg/kg/day by I.M. injection or I.V. infusion given either as 1.8 to 2.7 mg/kg q 8 hours or as 2.7 to 4 mg/kg q 12 hours. **Neonates under 6 weeks:** 4 to 6.5 mg/kg/day by I.M. injection or I.V. infusion given as 2 to 3.25 mg/kg q 12 hours. **Patients with impaired renal function:** Initial dose is the same as for patients with normal renal function. Subsequent doses and frequency determined by renal function and serum concentration of netilmicin.

Adverse reactions

CNS: headache, lethargy, ***neuromuscular blockade.***
EENT: *ototoxicity (tinnitus, vertigo, hearing loss).*
GU: *nephrotoxicity (oliguria; proteinuria; decreased creatinine clearance; increased BUN, nonprotein nitrogen, and serum creatinine levels).* **Other:** ***hypersensitivity reactions.***

Interactions

Cephalothin: increases nephrotoxicity. Use cautiously. **Dimenhydrinate:** may mask symptoms of ototoxicity. Use cautiously. **General anesthetics, neuromuscular blocking agents:** may potentiate neuromuscular blockade. **I.V. loop diuretics (such as furosemide):** increase ototoxicity. Use cautiously. **Other aminoglycosides, amphotericin B, cisplatin, methoxyflurane:** increases nephrotoxicity. Use cautiously. **Parenteral penicillins:** netilmicin inactivation. Don't mix together in I.V.

Nursing diagnoses

• Injury related to potential ineffectiveness of netilmicin to eradicate the infection.
• Altered urinary elimination related to netilmicin-induced nephrotoxicity.
• Knowledge deficit related to netilmicin therapy.

Nursing interventions

• *Use cautiously* in impaired renal function and in neonates, infants, and elderly patients.
• Obtain specimen for culture and sensitivity before first dose. Therapy may begin pending results.
• Weigh patient and obtain baseline renal function studies before therapy. Then monitor renal function (output, specific gravity, urinalysis, BUN and creatinine, and creatinine clearance). Notify doctor of signs of decreasing renal function.
• Patient should be well hydrated while taking drug to minimize irritation of the renal tubules.
• Watch for superinfection (continued fever and signs of new infections).
• **I.V. use:** After completing I.V. infusion, flush the line with 0.9% sodium chloride or D_5W.
• Draw blood for peak netilmicin level 1 hour after I.M. injection and 30 minutes to 1 hour after infusion ends; for trough levels, draw blood just before next dose. Don't draw blood in a heparinized tube. Peak blood levels above 16 mcg/ml and trough levels above 4 mcg/ml may be associated with toxicity.
• Evaluate patient's hearing before and during therapy. Notify doctor of complaints of tinnitus, vertigo, or hearing loss.

General

Classification: antineoplastic (podophyllotoxin derivative). **Pregnancy risk category:** D.

Mechanism of action

A semisynthetic derivative of podophyllotoxin that arrests cell mitosis.

Indications and dosage

- Testicular cancer. **Adults:** 50 to 100 mg/m^2 P.O. or I.V. on 5 consecutive days q 3 to 4 weeks; or 100 mg/m^2 on days 1, 3, and 5 q 3 to 4 weeks.
- Small-cell carcinoma of the lung, acute nonlymphocytic leukemia, Hodgkin's disease, malignant lymphoma, Ewing's sarcoma. **Adults:** 35 mg/m^2 I.V. or P.O. daily for 4 consecutive days or 50 mg/m^2 I.V. or P.O. daily for 5 consecutive days q 3 or 4 weeks.
- Kaposi's sarcoma. **Adults:** 150 mg/m^2 P.O. or I.V. daily for 3 consecutive days q 4 weeks.

Adverse reactions

Blood: *anemia, **myelosuppression** (dose-limiting), **leukopenia, thrombocytopenia.*** **CV:** hypotension from rapid infusion. **GI:** nausea and vomiting, anorexia, abdominal pain, *stomatitis.* **Local:** infrequent phlebitis. **Other:** occasional headache and fever, *reversible alopecia,* ***anaphylaxis*** (rare), peripheral neuropathy.

Interactions

Warfarin: etoposide may further increase PT.

Nursing diagnoses

- High risk for impaired skin integrity related to drug-induced adverse reactions.
- Altered protection related to etoposide-induced adverse hematologic reactions.
- Knowledge deficit related to etoposide therapy.

Nursing interventions

- *Contraindicated* for intrapleural and intrathecal administration.
- Know that etoposide has produced complete remissions in small-cell lung cancer and testicular cancer.
- Be aware that oral dosage is calculated according to body surface area; dose is rounded to the nearest 50 mg.
- Observe oral cavity for signs of ulceration.
- Store capsules in refrigerator.
- **I.V. use:** Exercise caution when preparing and administering this drug to avoid carcinogenic, mutagenic, and teratogenic risks. Follow institutional policy.
- Monitor blood pressure before infusion and at 30-minute intervals during infusion. If systolic blood pressure falls below 90 mm Hg, stop the infusion and notify the doctor.
- Have diphenhydramine, hydrocortisone, epinephrine, and airway available in case of an anaphylactic reaction.
- Dilute the drug for infusion in either D_5W or 0.9% sodium chloride solution to a concentration of 0.2 or 0.4 mg/ml. Higher concentrations may crystallize.
- Solutions diluted to 0.2 mg/ml are stable for 96 hours at room temperature in plastic or glass unprotected from light; solutions diluted to 0.4 mg/ml are stable for 48 hours under the same conditions.
- Do not administer through membrane-type inline filters because the diluent may dissolve the filter.
- Give drug by slow I.V. infusion (over at least 30 minutes) to prevent severe hypotension.
- Monitor CBC. Observe patient for signs of bone marrow suppression.

General

Classification: muscle stimulant (cholinesterase inhibitor). **Pregnancy risk category:** C.

Mechanism of action

Inhibits the destruction of acetylcholine released from the parasympathetic and somatic efferent nerves. Acetylcholine accumulates, promoting increased stimulation of the receptor.

Indications and dosage

- Antidote for nondepolarizing neuromuscular blockers. **Adults:** 0.5 to 2 mg I.V. (methylsulfate) slowly. Repeat p.r.n. to a total of 5 mg. (Give 0.6 to 1.2 mg atropine sulfate I.V. beforehand.)
- Postoperative abdominal distention and bladder atony. **Adults:** 0.5 to 1 mg I.M. or S.C. q 4 to 6 hours.
- Postoperative ileus. **Adults:** 0.25 to 1 mg I.M. or S.C. q 4 to 6 hours.
- Diagnosis of myasthenia gravis. **Adults:** 0.022 mg/kg I.M. 30 minutes after 0.4 to 0.6 mg of atropine sulfate. **Children:** 0.025 to 0.04 mg/kg. I.M. after 0.11 mg/kg atropine sulfate S.C.
- Treatment of myasthenia gravis. **Adults:** 15 to 30 mg P.O. (bromide) t.i.d. (range is 15 to 375 mg daily); or 0.5 to 2 mg S.C., I.M., or I.V. q 1 to 3 hours. Dosage must be individualized, depending on response and adverse reactions. Therapy may be required day and night. **Children:** 7.5 to 15 mg P.O. t.i.d. to q.i.d.

Note: 1:1,000 solution of injectable solution contains 1 mg/ml; 1:2,000 solution contains 0.5 mg/ml.

Adverse reactions

CNS: dizziness, weakness, confusion, jitters, sweating. **CV:** bradycardia, hypotension. **EENT:** blurred vision, lacrimation, miosis. **GI:** *vomiting, diarrhea, abdominal cramps,* excessive salivation. **GU:** urinary frequency. **Respiratory:** ***depression, bronchospasm, bronchoconstriction.*** **Skin:** rash. **Other:** *muscle cramps,* muscle fasciculations.

Interactions

Atropine, anticholinergic agents, procainamide, aminoglycosides, quinidine: may reverse cholinergic effect on muscle.

Nursing diagnoses

- Impaired physical mobility related to the patient's underlying condition.
- Diarrhea related to adverse reaction to neostigmine.
- Knowledge deficit related to neostigmine therapy.

Nursing interventions

- *Contraindicated* in hypersensitivity to cholinergics or to bromide, mechanical obstruction of the intestine or urinary tract, bradycardia, or hypotension.
- *Use with extreme caution* in bronchial asthma. *Use cautiously* in seizure disorders, recent coronary occlusion, peritonitis, vagotonia, hyperthyroidism, cardiac arrhythmias, and peptic ulcer.
- Stop all other cholinergics before giving this drug.
- Monitor vital signs frequently, especially respirations. Have atropine injection available and provide respiratory support as needed.
- Difficult to judge optimum dosage. Observe for improvement in strength, vision, and ptosis 45 to 60 minutes after each dose. Show patient how to observe and record variations in muscle strength.
- When using for myasthenia gravis, stress importance of taking drug exactly as ordered. Explain that drug may have to be taken for life. Schedule the dose before periods of fatigue (such as before meals if patient has dysphagia).
- Patient may develop resistance to neostigmine.
- Adverse GI reactions may be reduced by taking drug with milk or food.

General

Classification: antiulcer agent (histamine$_2$-receptor antagonist). **Pregnancy risk category:** B.

Mechanism of action

Competitively inhibits the action of histamine (H_2) at receptor sites of the parietal cells, decreasing gastric acid secretion.

Indications and dosage

- Duodenal ulcer. **Adults:** For acute therapy, 40 mg P.O. once daily h.s. For maintenance therapy, 20 mg once daily h.s.
- Pathologic hypersecretory conditions (such as Zollinger-Ellison syndrome). **Adults:** 20 mg P.O. q 6 hours. As much as 160 mg q 6 hours may be administered.
- Hospitalized patients with intractable ulcers or hypersecretory conditions, or patients who cannot take oral medication. **Adults:** 20 mg I.V. q 12 hours.
- Gastroesophageal reflux disease (GERD). **Adults:** 20 mg P.O. b.i.d. for up to 6 weeks. For esophagitis caused by GERD, give 20 to 40 mg b.i.d. for up to 12 weeks.

Adverse reactions

Blood: ***thrombocytopenia*** (rare). **CNS:** *headache,* dizziness, hallucinations. **GI:** diarrhea, constipation, nausea, flatulence. **GU:** increased BUN and creatinine. **Skin:** acne, pruritus, rash. **Local:** transient irritation at I.V. site.

Interactions

None significant.

Nursing diagnoses

- Pain related to the patient's underlying condition.
- High risk for injury related to famotidine-induced adverse CNS reactions.
- Knowledge deficit related to famotidine therapy.

Nursing interventions

- *Contraindicated* in patients with hypersensitivity to the drug.
- Be sure that gastric cancer has been ruled out before starting famotidine therapy.
- Advise patient not to take the drug for longer than 8 weeks unless doctor specifically orders it.
- Urge patient to avoid cigarette smoking as this may increase gastric acid secretion and worsen disease.
- Tell patient he may take antacids concomitantly with this drug to relieve pain, as long as he informs the doctor.
- Tell patient that he may take famotidine with a snack if he desires. Remind him that this drug is most effective if taken at bedtime. If drug is prescribed to be taken twice daily, tell patient to take at least one dose at bedtime.
- Store reconstituted oral suspension at a temperature below 86° F (30° C). Avoid freezing. Discard after 30 days.
- **I.V. use:** To prepare I.V. injection, dilute 2 ml (20 mg) famotidine with compatible I.V. solution to a total volume of either 5 or 10 ml, and inject slowly (over at least 2 minutes). Compatible solutions include sterile water for injection, 0.9% sodium chloride injection, 5% or 10% dextrose injection, 5% sodium bicarbonate injection, or lactated Ringer's injection.
- Alternatively, famotidine may be given by intermittent I.V. infusion. Dilute 20 mg (2 ml) famotidine in 100 ml of compatible solution, and infuse over 15 to 30 minutes. Solution is stable for 48 hours at room temperature after dilution.
- Store I.V. injection in the refrigerator at 35.6° to 46.4° F (2° to 8° C).

General
Classification: antibiotic (aminoglycoside). **Pregnancy risk category:** C.

Mechanism of action
Inhibits protein synthesis by binding directly to the 30S ribosomal subunit. Generally bactericidal.

Indications and dosage
• Infectious diarrhea caused by enteropathogenic *Escherichia coli*. **Adults:** 50 mg/kg daily P.O. in four divided doses for 2 to 3 days. **Children:** 50 to 100 mg/kg daily P.O. divided q 4 to 6 hours for 2 to 3 days.
• Suppression of intestinal bacteria preoperatively. **Adults:** 1 g P.O. q 1 hour for four doses, then 1 g q 4 hours for the balance of the 24 hours. A saline cathartic should precede therapy. **Children:** 40 to 100 mg/kg daily P.O. divided q 4 to 6 hours. First dose should follow saline cathartic.
• Adjunctive treatment in hepatic coma. **Adults:** 1 to 3 g P.O. q.i.d. for 5 to 6 days; or 200 ml of 1% or 100 ml of 2% solution as enema retained for 20 to 60 minutes q 6 hours.

Adverse reactions
CNS: headache, lethargy. **EENT:** *ototoxicity (tinnitus, vertigo, hearing loss).* **GI:** nausea, vomiting. **GU:** *nephrotoxicity (cells or casts in the urine, oliguria, proteinuria, decreased creatinine clearance, increased BUN and serum creatinine levels).* **Skin:** rash, urticaria. **Other:** ***hypersensitivity reactions.***

Interactions
Cephalothin: increases nephrotoxicity. Use together cautiously. **Dimenhydrinate:** may mask symptoms of ototoxicity. Use with caution. **I.V. loop diuretics (such as furosemide):** increase ototoxicity. Use cautiously. **Oral anticoagulants:** oral neomycin inhibits vitamin K-producing bacteria and may potentiate anticoagulant effect. **Other aminoglycosides, amphotericin B, cisplatin, methoxyflurane:** increases nephrotoxicity. Use together cautiously.

Nursing diagnoses
• High risk for injury related to ineffectiveness of neomycin to eradicate the infection.
• Altered urinary elimination related to neomycin-induced nephrotoxicity.
• Knowledge deficit related to neomycin therapy.

Nursing interventions
• *Contraindicated* in intestinal obstruction.
• *Use cautiously* in impaired renal function and ulcerative bowel lesions and in elderly patients. Never administer parenterally.
• Nonabsorbable at recommended dosage. However, more than 4 g/day may be systemically absorbed and lead to nephrotoxicity.
• Weigh patient and obtain baseline renal function studies before therapy begins.
• Obtain specimen for culture and sensitivity tests before first dose. Therapy may begin pending test results. Then watch for superinfection (fever or other signs of new infection).
• Monitor renal function (output, specific gravity, urinalysis, BUN and creatinine levels, and creatinine clearance). Notify doctor of signs of decreasing renal function. Make sure patient stays well hydrated while taking drug.
• Watch for respiratory depression in patients with renal disease, hypocalcemia, or neuromuscular diseases, such as myasthenia gravis.
• Evaluate hearing of patient with hepatic or renal disease before and during prolonged therapy. Notify doctor if patient complains of tinnitus, vertigo, or hearing loss. Onset of deafness may occur several weeks after drug is stopped.

General
Classification: anticonvulsant (dicarbamate derivative). **Pregnancy risk category:** C.

Mechanism of action
Unclear. Drug may act by elevating the seizure threshold or preventing the spread of seizure activity.

Indications and dosage
- Refractory partial seizures; Lennox-Gastaut syndrome. **Adults:** initially, 1,200 mg P.O. daily in two divided doses. Increase in increments of 1,200 mg daily to a maximum of 3,600 mg daily.

Adverse reactions
CNS: dizziness, insomnia, *somnolence*. **EENT:** blurred or double vision, rhinitis. **GI:** dyspepsia, *nausea, vomiting*. **Skin:** rash. **Other:** anorexia.

Interactions
Carbamazepine, phenytoin, valproate: potential increase in plasma levels when felbamate therapy added. Monitor plasma levels.

Nursing diagnoses
- High risk for injury related to underlying seizure disorder.
- Knowledge deficit related to felbamate therapy.

Nursing interventions
- *Use cautiously* in patients with hypersensitivity to carbamates.
- Also use cautiously with elderly patients and children. No studies of felbamate in geriatric patients have been conducted; and the safety and efficacy of felbamate in children other than those with Lennox-Gastaut syndrome is not known.
- Do not abruptly discontinue antiseizure drugs because of the possibility of increased seizures.

General

Classification: nonnarcotic analgesic, antipyretic, anti-inflammatory (NSAID). **Pregnancy risk category:** B (D in 3rd trimester).

Mechanism of action

Produces anti-inflammatory, analgesic, and antipyretic effects, possibly through inhibition of prostaglandin synthesis.

Indications and dosage

- Arthritis, primary dysmenorrhea (naproxen base). **Adults:** 250 to 500 mg P.O. b.i.d. (maximum dosage is 1,250 mg daily).
- Mild to moderate pain, primary dysmenorrhea (naproxen sodium). **Adults:** 2 tablets (275 mg each tablet) P.O. to start, followed by 275 mg q 6 to 8 hours p.r.n. (maximum daily dosage should not exceed 1,375 mg).

Adverse reactions

Blood: prolonged bleeding time, ***agranulocytosis,*** neutropenia. **CNS:** *headache,* drowsiness, *dizziness,* tinnitus. **CV:** peripheral edema, dyspnea. **EENT:** visual disturbances. **GI:** *epigastric distress, occult blood loss, nausea,* ***peptic ulceration.*** **GU:** nephrotoxicity. **Hepatic:** elevated enzymes. **Skin:** *pruritus, rash,* urticaria.

Interactions

Aspirin, alcohol, corticosteroids: may increase risk of adverse GI reactions. Advise taking drug with food or milk to minimize GI upset. **Methotrexate:** increased risk of toxicity. Monitor closely. **Oral anticoagulants, sulfonylureas, and drugs that are highly protein-bound:** increased risk of toxicity. Monitor closely. **Probenecid:** decreased elimination of naproxen. Monitor for toxicity.

Nursing diagnoses

- Pain related to the patient's underlying condition.
- High risk for trauma related to drowsiness or dizziness caused by CNS reaction to naproxen.
- Knowledge deficit related to naproxen therapy.

Nursing interventions

- *Contraindicated* in patients with hypersensitivity to the drug, aspirin, or other NSAIDs.
- *Use cautiously* in elderly patients and in patients with renal disease, CV disease, GI disorders, hepatic disease, a history of peptic ulcer disease, or angioedema.
- Serious GI toxicity can occur at any time in patients taking chronic NSAID therapy. Teach patient signs and symptoms of GI bleeding, and tell patient to report these to the doctor immediately.
- Monitor CBC and renal and hepatic function every 4 to 6 months or as indicated during long-term therapy. Advise patient to have periodic eye examinations.
- Tell patient taking naproxen that full therapeutic effect may be delayed 2 to 4 weeks.
- Warn patient against taking both naproxen and naproxen sodium at the same time.
- Naproxen sodium is more rapidly absorbed.
- Naproxen and naproxen sodium have also been used to manage pain of vascular headache, osteitis deformans (Paget's disease) of the bone, and Bartter's syndrome.
- Naproxen may interfere with certain urinary assays of 5-hydroxyindoleacetic acid and may cause false elevations of urinary 17-ketosteroid concentrations. Inform clinical laboratory personnel that patient is taking naproxen.
- Because of their antipyretic and anti-inflammatory actions, NSAIDs may mask the signs and symptoms of infection.

General

Classification: short-term adjunctive anorexigenic adent, indirect-acting sympathomimetic amine (amphetamine congener). **Pregnancy risk category:** C. **Controlled substance schedule**: IV.

Mechanism of action

Stimulates ventromedial nucleus of the hypothalamus. May also affect serotonin metabolism.

Indications and dosage

• Short-term adjunct in exogenous obesity. **Adults:** initially, 20 mg P.O. t.i.d. before meals. Maximum dosage is 40 mg t.i.d. Adjust dosage according to patient's response.

Adverse reactions

CNS: *drowsiness,* dizziness, incoordination, headache, euphoria or depression, anxiety, *insomnia,* weakness, fatigue, agitation. **CV:** *palpitations,* hypotension, hypertension, chest pain. **EENT:** eye irritation, blurred vision. **GI:** *diarrhea, dry mouth,* nausea, vomiting, abdominal pain, constipation. **GU:** dysuria, increased urinary frequency, impotence. **Skin:** rashes, urticaria, burning sensation. **Other:** sweating, chills, fever, increased libido.

Interactions

Alcohol, CNS depressants: enhanced CNS depression. **Centrally acting antihypertensives:** decreased antihypertensive effect. **MAO inhibitors:** severe hypertension; possible hypertensive crisis. Don't use together or within 14 days after an MAO inhibitor has been discontinued.

Nursing diagnoses

• Altered nutrition: More than body requirements, related to obesity.
• High risk for injury related to adverse CNS reactions to fenfluramine therapy.
• Knowledge deficit related to fenfluramine therapy.

Nursing interventions

• *Contraindicated* in glaucoma, hypersensitivity to sympathomimetic amines, symptomatic CV disease, alcoholism, or history of drug abuse.
• *Use cautiously* in hypertension, history of mental depression, and diabetes mellitus.
• Be aware that this drug has been proven effective for treating autistic children.
• Monitor blood and urine sugars. Because of possible hypoglycemia, patients with diabetes may have altered insulin or sulfonylurea requirements.
• Tell patient to report signs of excessive sedation, depression, or excessive stimulation. Be aware that fenfluramine differs pharmacologically from amphetamines in that it produces CNS depression more often than stimulation.
• Closely monitor blood pressure.
• Make sure patient is on a weight-reduction program.
• Avoid prolonged administration. Tolerance or dependence may occur.
• Do not discontinue fenfluramine abruptly; may precipitate an acute depressive reaction.

General

Classification: erythropoietic steroid (decanoate), anabolic steroid (decanoate), antineoplastic (phenproprionate) (anabolic steroid). **Pregnancy risk category:** X. **Controlled substance schedule:** III.

Mechanism of action

Promotes tissue-building processes and reverses catabolism. Also stimulates erythropoiesis.

Indications and dosage

- Severe debility or disease states, refractory anemias (decanoate). **Adults:** 100 to 200 mg I.M. weekly. Therapy should be intermittent.
- Tissue-building (decanoate). **Adults:** 50 to 100 mg I.M. q 3 to 4 weeks. **Children 2 to 13 years:** 25 to 50 mg I.M. q 3 to 4 weeks.
- Control of metastatic breast cancer (phenpropionate). **Adults:** 25 to 50 mg I.M. weekly. **Children 2 to 13 years:** 12.5 to 25 mg I.M. q 2 to 4 weeks.

Adverse reactions

Androgenic: in women—*acne, edema, oily skin, weight gain, hirsutism, hoarseness,* clitoral enlargement, decreased or increased libido. In men—prepubertal: premature epiphyseal closure, *acne,* priapism, *growth of body and facial hair,* phallic enlargement; postpubertal: testicular atrophy, oligospermia, decreased ejaculatory volume, impotence, gynecomastia, epididymitis. **CV:** edema. **GI:** gastroenteritis, nausea, vomiting, diarrhea, change in appetite. **GU:** bladder irritability. **Hepatic:** reversible jaundice, hepatotoxicity. **Hypoestrogenic:** in women—flushing; sweating; vaginitis with itching, drying, burning, or bleeding; menstrual irregularities with large doses. **Local:** pain at injection site, induration. **Other:** hypercalcemia, hypercalciuria.

Interactions

Antidiabetic agents: altered dosage requirements. **Hepatotoxic medications:** increased risk of hepatotoxicity. **Oral anticoagulants:** altered dosage requirements.

Nursing diagnoses

- High risk for injury related to the patient's underlying condition.
- Body image disturbance related to adverse androgenic reactions associated with nandrolone.
- Knowledge deficit related to nandrolone therapy.

Nursing interventions

- *Contraindicated* in prostatic hypertrophy with obstruction; male breast and prostatic cancer; cardiac, hepatic, or renal decompensation; nephrosis; in pregnancy; in breast-feeding women; and in premature infants.
- *Use cautiously* in prepubertal males; patients with diabetes or coronary disease; and patients taking corticotropin, corticosteroids, or anticoagulants.
- Avoid use in women of childbearing age until pregnancy is ruled out. Emphasize importance of using a nonhormonal contraceptive during therapy.
- Inject drug deep I.M.; rotate injection sites to prevent muscle atrophy.
- Hypercalcemia is most likely to occur in patients with mammary carcinoma; quantitative urine and serum calcium levels should be performed.
- Tell women to report menstrual irregularities.
- Watch for signs of virilization; they may be irreversible despite discontinuation of therapy.
- Observe boys under 7 years for precocious development of male sexual characteristics.
- Children should have wrist X-rays before therapy to establish level of bone maturation. Treatment may cause bone maturation to proceed more rapidly than linear growth; dosage should be intermittent and X-rays taken periodically.
- Watch for jaundice. If liver function tests are abnormal, therapy should be stopped.

General

Classification: nonnarcotic analgesic, antipyretic (NSAID). **Pregnancy risk category:** B (D in 3rd trimester).

Mechanism of action

Produces anti-inflammatory, analgesic, and antipyretic effects, possibly through inhibition of prostaglandin synthesis.

Indications and dosage

- Rheumatoid arthritis and osteoarthritis. **Adults:** 300 to 600 mg P.O. q.i.d. Maximum dosage is 3.2 g daily.
- Mild to moderate pain. **Adults:** 200 mg P.O. q 4 to 6 hours, p.r.n.

Adverse reactions

Blood: prolonged bleeding time, anemia. **CNS:** *headache, drowsiness, dizziness, somnolence.* **CV:** peripheral edema. **GI:** *epigastric distress, nausea,* ***GI bleeding,*** vomiting, occult blood loss, peptic ulceration, constipation, anorexia. **GU:** reversible renal failure. **Hepatic:** elevated enzymes. **Skin:** *pruritus,* rash, urticaria.

Interactions

Alcohol, corticosteroids: increased risk of adverse GI reactions. Avoid concomitant use. **Aspirin:** decreases fenoprofen half-life; may also increase GI toxicity. Avoid concomitant use. **Oral anticoagulants, sulfonylureas:** fenoprofen enhances pharmacologic effects of these drugs. Use together cautiously. **Phenobarbital:** enhanced metabolism of fenoprofen. Monitor for lack of effectiveness.

Nursing diagnoses

- Pain related to the patient's underlying condition.
- High risk for injury related to adverse CNS reactions to fenoprofen therapy.
- Knowledge deficit related to fenoprofen therapy.

Nursing interventions

- *Contraindicated* in patients with hypersensitivity to the drug, aspirin, or other NSAIDs.
- *Use cautiously* in elderly patients; in patients with GI disorders, angioedema, or CV disease; and in those with a history of peptic ulcer disease.
- Teach patient to recognize and report immediately signs and symptoms of GI bleeding. Serious GI toxicity can occur at any time in patients undergoing chronic NSAID therapy.
- Give dose 30 minutes before or 2 hours after meals. If adverse GI reactions occur, give with milk or meals.
- If patient is taking the drug for arthritis, inform him that full therapeutic effect may be delayed for 2 to 4 weeks.
- Check renal, hepatic, and auditory function periodically during prolonged therapy. Stop drug if abnormalities occur.
- Keep in mind that prothrombin time may be prolonged in patients receiving coumarin-type anticoagulants. Fenoprofen decreases platelet aggregation and may prolong bleeding time.
- Because fenoprofen may cause somnolence, warn the patient to avoid driving and other hazardous activities that require alertness until adverse CNS effects of the drug are known.
- Be aware that NSAIDs may mask the signs and symptoms of infection because of their antipyretic and anti-inflammatory actions.
- When interpreting laboratory test results, keep in mind that fenoprofen may cause false elevations in free and total serum triiodothyronine (T_3) levels as measured by the Amerlex-T assay. Fenoprofen or its metabolite may cross-react with the antibody used in the Amerlex-M assay. Limited data suggest that drug may alter free and total T_3 concentrations determined by the Corning method.

General

Classification: narcotic antagonist (opioid antagonist). **Pregnancy risk category:** B.

Mechanism of action

Displaces previously administered narcotic analgesics from their receptors (competitive antagonism). Has no pharmacologic activity of its own.

Indications and dosage

- Known or suspected narcotic-induced respiratory depression, including that caused by pentazocine and propoxyphene. **Adults:** 0.4 to 2 mg I.V., S.C., or I.M. May repeat q 2 to 3 minutes, p.r.n. If no response is observed after 10 mg has been administered, the diagnosis of narcotic-induced toxicity should be questioned.
- Postoperative narcotic depression. **Adults:** 0.1 to 0.2 mg I.V. q 2 to 3 minutes, p.r.n. Adult concentration is 0.4 mg/ml. **Children:** 0.01 mg/kg dose I.M., I.V., or S.C. May repeat q 2 to 3 minutes. (If initial dose of 0.01 mg/kg does not result in clinical improvement, up to 10 times this dose [0.1 mg/kg] may be necessary.) **Neonates** (asphyxia neonatorum): 0.01 mg/kg I.V. into umbilical vein. May repeat q 2 to 3 minutes for three doses.

Adverse reactions

With higher-than-recommended doses: **CV:** tachycardia, hypertension. **GI:** nausea, vomiting. **Other:** tremor, withdrawal symptoms (in narcotic-dependent patients).

Interactions

None significant.

Nursing diagnoses

- Ineffective breathing pattern related to known or suspected narcotic-induced respiratory depression.
- Decreased cardiac output related to naloxone-induced tachycardia.
- Knowledge deficit related to naloxone therapy.

Nursing interventions

- *Contraindicated* in patients with hypersensitivity to the drug.
- *Use cautiously* in cardiac irritability and opiate addiction. Abrupt reversal of opiate-induced CNS depression may result in nausea, vomiting, sweating, tachycardia, CNS excitement, and increased blood pressure.
- Naloxone is only effective in reversing respiratory depression caused by opiates. It's not effective against other drug-induced respiratory depression (such as from barbiturates and sedatives).
- Duration of action of a narcotic may exceed that of naloxone. Patient may relapse into respiratory depression.
- Monitor respiratory depth and rate. Be prepared to provide oxygen, ventilation, and other resuscitative measures.
- Respiratory rate increases within 1 to 2 minutes. Effect lasts 1 to 4 hours, but dosage may have to be repeated q 20 minutes.
- **I.V. use:** May be administered by continuous I.V. infusion, which is often necessary to control the adverse effects of epidurally administered morphine. May dilute adult concentration (0.4 mg) by mixing 0.5 ml with 9.5 ml sterile water or sodium chloride solution for injection to make neonatal concentration (0.02 mg/ml).
- Can see "overshoot" effect—respiratory rate exceeds the rate before respiratory depression.
- Naloxone has been used investigationally to treat the senile dementia of Alzheimer's disease.
- Also has been shown to improve circulation in refractory shock.
- Used by some researchers to relieve certain kinds of chronic constipation.

General

Classification: analgesic, anesthetic (opioid agonist). **Pregnancy risk category:** B (D for prolonged use or use of high doses at term). **Controlled substance schedule:** II.

Mechanism of action

Binds with opiate receptors at many sites in the CNS (brain, brain stem, and spinal cord), altering both perception of and emotional response to pain through an unknown mechanism.

Indications and dosage

- Adjunct to general anesthetic. **Adults:** 0.05 to 0.1 mg I.V. (citrate) repeated q 2 to 3 minutes, p.r.n. Dose should be reduced in elderly and high-risk patients.
- Postoperatively. **Adults:** 0.05 to 0.1 mg I.M. (citrate) q 1 to 2 hours p.r.n.
- Preoperatively. **Adults:** 0.05 to 0.1 mg I.M. 30 to 60 minutes before surgery. **Children 2 to 12 years:** 1.7 to 3.3 mcg/kg I.M.
- Management of chronic pain. **Adults:** apply one transdermal system patch to a portion of the upper torso on an area of skin that is not irritated and has not been irradiated. Initiate therapy with the 25-mcg/hour system; adjust dosage as needed and tolerated. Each system may be worn for 72 hours.

Adverse reactions

CNS: *sedation, somnolence, clouded sensorium, euphoria,* dizziness, seizures with large doses. **CV:** *hypotension,* bradycardia. **GI:** nausea, vomiting, *constipation,* ileus. **GU:** *urine retention.* **Local:** reaction at application site (erythema, papules, edema). **Other:** ***respiratory depression,*** muscle rigidity, physical dependence, *pruritus.*

Interactions

Alcohol, CNS depressants: additive effects. Use together cautiously.

Nursing diagnoses

- Pain related to patient's underlying condition.
- Ineffective breathing pattern related to fentanyl-induced respiratory depression.
- Knowledge deficit related to fentanyl therapy.

Nursing interventions

- *Contraindicated* in patients who have received MAO inhibitors within 14 days and in those with myasthenia gravis.
- *Use cautiously* in head injury, increased CSF pressure, asthma, COPD, respiratory depression, seizures, hepatic or renal disease, hypothyroidism, Addison's disease, alcoholism, increased intracranial pressure, CNS depression, and shock and in elderly or debilitated patients.
- Keep narcotic antagonist (naloxone) and resuscitative equipment available when giving drug I.V.
- **I.V. use:** Only staff trained in administration of I.V. anesthetics and managing their potential adverse reactions should administer I.V. fentanyl.
- **Epidural use:** Be aware that epidural injection or infusion has been used for postoperative analgesia, chronic pain management, or postpartum pain control. Drug may be administered with local anesthetics such as bupivacaine to enhance analgesic effects.
- **Transdermal use:** Remove transdermal system from package only immediately before applying. Hold in place for 10 to 20 seconds, and be sure the edges of the system are in contact with the patient's skin. Refer to dosage equivalent charts to calculate the fentanyl transdermal dose based on the daily morphine intake. An approximation: For every 90 mg of oral morphine or 15 mg of I.M. morphine per 24 hours, 25 mcg/hour of transdermal fentanyl is required. Make gradual dosage adjustments in patients using the transdermal system. Reaching steady-state levels of a new dose may take up to 6 days; patients should delay adjusting dose until after at least two applications. Some patients will require alternative means of opiate administration when the dose exceeds 300 mcg/hour.

General

Classification: antibiotic, urinary tract antiseptic (quinolone). **Pregnancy risk category:** B.

Mechanism of action

Inhibits microbial DNA synthesis.

Indications and dosage

• Acute and chronic UTIs caused by susceptible gram-negative organisms *(Proteus, Klebsiella, Enterobacter,* and *Escherichia coli).* **Adults:** 1 g P.O. q.i.d. for 7 to 14 days; 2 g daily for long-term use. **Children over 3 months:** 55 mg/kg P.O. daily divided q.i.d. for 7 to 14 days; 33 mg/kg daily for long-term use.

Adverse reactions

Blood: eosinophilia. **CNS:** drowsiness, weakness, headache, dizziness, vertigo, ***seizures,*** confusion, hallucinations. **EENT:** sensitivity to light, change in color perception, diplopia, blurred vision. **GI:** *abdominal pain, nausea, vomiting,* diarrhea. **Skin:** pruritus, photosensitivity, urticaria, rash. **Other:** angioedema, fever, chills, ***increased intracranial pressure and bulging fontanelles in infants and children.***

Interactions

Oral anticoagulants: increased anticoagulant effect.

Nursing diagnoses

• High risk for injury related to ineffectiveness of nalidixic acid to eradicate the infection.
• High risk for fluid volume deficit related to adverse GI reactions caused by nalidixic acid.
• Knowledge deficit related to nalidixic acid therapy.

Nursing interventions

• *Contraindicated* in seizure disorders.
• *Use with extreme caution* in prepubertal children; erosion of cartilage of immature animals has been reported.
• *Use cautiously* in patients with impaired hepatic or renal function or with severe cerebral arteriosclerosis.
• Not effective against *Pseudomonas* or infections outside of the urinary tract.
• Tell the patient to report visual disturbances; these usually disappear with reduced dose.
• Obtain specimen for culture and sensitivity tests before starting therapy and repeat p.r.n. Therapy may begin pending test results.
• Obtain CBC and renal and liver function studies during long-term therapy.
• Resistant bacteria may emerge within the first 48 hours of therapy.
• May cause a false-positive Clinitest reaction. Use Clinistix or Tes-Tape to monitor urine glucose. Also gives false elevations in urine vanillylmandelic acid and 17-ketosteroids. Repeat tests after therapy is completed.
• Avoid undue exposure to sunlight because of photosensitivity. Patient may continue to be photosensitive for as long as 3 months after drug is discontinued.

General

Classification: hematinic (iron supplement). **Pregnancy risk category:** A.

Mechanism of action

Provides elemental iron, an essential component in the formation of hemoglobin. Each 100 mg of ferrous fumarate provides 33 mg of elemental iron.

Indications and dosage

- Iron deficiency. **Adults:** 200 mg P.O. t.i.d. or q.i.d. **Children:** 3 mg/kg P.O. t.i.d., increased to 6 mg/kg t.i.d. as needed and tolerated.

Adverse reactions

GI: *nausea,* vomiting, *constipation, black stools.* **Other:** elixir may stain teeth.

Interactions

Antacids, levodopa, penicillamine, quinolones, tetracycline, vitamin E: decreased iron absorption. Separate doses by 2 to 4 hours. **Chloramphenicol:** watch for delayed response to iron therapy. **Vitamin C:** concurrent administration may increase iron absorption. Beneficial drug interaction.

Nursing diagnoses

- Activity intolerance related to patient's underlying condition.
- Constipation related to adverse GI reactions to ferrous fumarate.
- Knowledge deficit related to ferrous fumarate therapy.

Nursing interventions

- *Contraindicated* in hemosiderosis; also contraindicated in patients with hemochromatosis and hemolytic anemia unless iron deficiency anemia is also present.
- *Use cautiously* in peptic ulcer, regional enteritis, and ulcerative colitis. Also use cautiously on long-term basis.
- Teach parents to keep iron supplements out of children's reach and to administer to children carefully. Iron is toxic. As few as 3 or 4 tablets may cause poisoning in children.
- Tell patient to take iron supplements between meals and to take them with food if GI upset occurs, although absorption may be decreased. Enteric-coated products reduce GI upset but also reduce amount of iron absorbed. Warn patient not to crush or chew sustained-release iron preparations.
- Tell patient to take tablets with juice or water but not milk or antacids. Give with orange juice to promote iron absorption. To prevent staining teeth, use a straw to give iron elixir.
- Inform patient that certain foods may impair oral iron absorption, including yogurt, cheese, eggs, milk, whole-grain breads and cereals, tea, and coffee.
- If the patient misses a dose, tell him to take it as soon as he remembers, unless it's time for the next dose. Do not double-dose.
- Check for constipation; record color and amount of stool. Teach the patient dietary measures to avoid constipation. Inform him that the drug may turn his stools black but that this effect is harmless; however, it could mask the presence of melena.
- Monitor hemoglobin and reticulocyte counts during therapy.

General

Classification: analgesic, adjunct to anesthesia (opioid partial agonist; narcotic agonist-antagonist). **Pregnancy risk category:** B (D for prolonged use or use of high doses at term).

Mechanism of action

Binds with opiate receptors at many sites in the CNS (brain, brain stem, and spinal cord), altering both perception of and emotional response to pain through an unknown mechanism.

Indications and dosage

- Moderate to severe pain. **Adults:** 10 to 20 mg S.C., I.M., or I.V. q 3 to 6 hours, p.r.n. or around the clock. Maximum daily dosage is 160 mg.

Adverse reactions

CNS: *headache, sedation,* dizziness, nervousness, depression, restlessness, crying, euphoria, hostility, unusual dreams, confusion, hallucinations, delusions. **GI:** cramps, dyspepsia, bitter taste, *nausea, vomiting,* constipation. **GU:** urinary urgency. **Skin:** itching; burning; urticaria; *sweaty, clammy feeling.* **Other:** ***respiratory depression.***

Interactions

Alcohol, CNS depressants, general anesthetics, tranquilizers, sedatives, hypnotics, TCAs: respiratory depression, hypotension, profound sedation, coma. Use together with extreme caution. **Narcotic analgesics:** possible decreased analgesic effect. Avoid concomitant use.

Nursing diagnoses

- Pain related to patient's underlying condition.
- Ineffective breathing pattern related to nalbuphine-induced respiratory depression.
- Knowledge deficit related to nalbuphine therapy.

Nursing interventions

- *Contraindicated* in patients with hypersensitivity to the drug, emotional instability, history of drug abuse, head injury, or increased intracranial pressure.
- *Use cautiously* in hepatic and renal disease. These patients may overreact to customary doses.
- Causes respiratory depression, which at 10 mg is equal to the respiratory depression produced by 10 mg of morphine.
- Monitor respirations of neonates exposed to the drug during labor.
- **I.V. use:** Inject slowly (over at least 2 to 3 minutes) into a vein or into an I.V. line containing a compatible free-flowing I.V. solution, such as D_5W, 0.9% sodium chloride, or lactated Ringer's injection.
- Respiratory depression can be reversed with naloxone. Keep resuscitative equipment available, particularly when administering I.V.
- Psychological and physical dependence may occur.
- Monitor circulatory and respiratory status and bladder and bowel function. Hold dose and notify doctor if respirations are shallow or rate is below 12 breaths/minute.
- Constipation often severe with maintenance. Make sure stool softener or other laxative is ordered.
- Also acts as a narcotic antagonist; may precipitate abstinence syndrome. For patients who have chronically received opiates, administer 25% of the usual dose initially. Observe for signs of withdrawal.
- Warn patient to avoid hazardous activities that require alertness until CNS effects of the drug are known.

General

Classification: hematinic (iron supplement). **Pregnancy risk category:** A.

Mechanism of action

Provides elemental iron, an essential component in the formation of hemoglobin. Each 100 mg of ferrous gluconate provides 11.6 mg of elemental iron.

Indications and dosage

• Iron deficiency. **Adults:** 300 to 325 mg P.O. q.i.d., increased to 650 mg q.i.d. as needed and tolerated. **Children 2 years or older:** 8 mg/kg P.O. t.i.d., increased to 16 mg t.i.d. as needed and tolerated.

Adverse reactions

GI: *nausea*, vomiting, *constipation, black stools.*
Other: elixir may stain teeth.

Interactions

Antacids, levodopa, penicillamine, quinolones, tetracycline, vitamin E: decreased iron absorption. Separate doses if possible. **Chloramphenicol:** watch for delayed response to iron therapy. **Vitamin C:** may increase iron absorption. Beneficial drug interaction.

Nursing diagnoses

• Activity intolerance related to patient's underlying condition.
• Constipation related to adverse GI reactions to ferrous gluconate.
• Knowledge deficit related to ferrous gluconate therapy.

Nursing interventions

• *Contraindicated* in peptic ulcer, regional enteritis, ulcerative colitis, hemosiderosis, and hemochromatosis. Also contraindicated in patients with hemolytic anemia unless iron deficiency anemia is also present.
• *Use cautiously* on long-term basis.
• Teach parents to keep iron supplements out of children's reach and to administer to children carefully. Iron is toxic. As few as 3 or 4 tablets may cause poisoning in children.
• Tell patient to take iron supplements between meals and to take them with food if GI upset occurs, although absorption may be decreased. Enteric-coated products reduce GI upset but also reduce amount of iron absorbed. Warn patient not to crush or chew sustained-release iron preparations.
• Dilute liquid preparations in juice (preferably orange juice) or water, but not in milk or antacids. Give tablets with orange juice to promote absorption. To avoid staining teeth, give iron elixir through a straw; patient may take with water or fruit juice.
• Inform patient that certain foods may impair oral iron absorption, including yogurt, cheese, eggs, milk, whole-grain breads and cereals, tea, and coffee.
• If the patient misses a dose, tell him to take it as soon as he remembers, unless it's time for the next dose. Do not double-dose.
• Check for constipation; record color and amount of stool. Teach the patient dietary measures to avoid constipation. Inform him that the drug may turn his stools black but that this effect is harmless; however, it could mask the presence of melena.
• Monitor hemoglobin and reticulocyte counts during therapy.

General

Classification: antibiotic (penicillinase-resistant penicillin). **Pregnancy risk category:** B.

Mechanism of action

Bactericidal against microorganisms by inhibiting cell wall synthesis during active multiplication. Bacteria resist penicillins by producing penicillinases—enzymes that hydrolyze penicillin. Nafcillin resists these enzymes.

Indications and dosage

- Systemic infections caused by penicillinase-producing staphylococci. **Adults:** 2 to 4 g P.O. daily, divided into doses given q 6 hours; 2 to 12 g I.M. or I.V. daily, divided into doses given q 4 to 6 hours. **Children:** 50 to 100 mg/kg P.O. daily, divided into doses given q 4 to 6 hours; or 100 to 200 mg/kg I.M. or I.V. daily, divided into doses given q 4 to 6 hours.

Adverse reactions

Blood: transient leukopenia, neutropenia, granulocytopenia, ***thrombocytopenia*** with high doses. **GI:** *nausea*, vomiting, diarrhea. **Local:** *vein irritation, thrombophlebitis.* **Other:** hypersensitivity (chills, fever, *rash*, pruritus, urticaria, ***anaphylaxis***).

Interactions

None significant.

Nursing diagnoses

- High risk for injury related to ineffectiveness of nafcillin to eradicate the infection.
- High risk for fluid volume deficit related to nafcillin-induced adverse GI reactions.
- Knowledge deficit related to nafcillin therapy.

Nursing interventions

- *Use cautiously* in patients with other drug allergies, especially to cephalosporins (possible cross-allergenicity), and in GI distress.
- Obtain specimen for culture and sensitivity tests before first dose. Therapy may begin pending test results.
- Before giving nafcillin, ask patient if he's had any allergic reactions to penicillin. However, a negative history of penicillin allergy is no guarantee against a future allergic reaction.
- Tell patient to take medication exactly as prescribed, even if he feels better. Entire quantity prescribed should be taken.
- Tell patient to call the doctor if rash, fever, or chills develop. A rash is the most common allergic reaction.
- When given orally, drug may cause GI disturbances. Food may interfere with absorption; therefore, give 1 to 2 hours before or 2 to 3 hours after meals.
- **I.V. use:** When giving I.V., mix with D_5W or 0.9% sodium chloride solution.
- Give I.V. intermittently to prevent vein irritation. Change site every 48 hours.
- With large doses and prolonged therapy, bacterial and fungal superinfections may occur, especially in elderly, debilitated, or immunosuppressed patients. Close observation is essential.
- Give nafcillin at least 1 hour before bacteriostatic antibiotics.

General
Classification: hematinic (iron supplement). **Pregnancy risk category:** A.

Mechanism of action
Provides elemental iron, an essential component in the formation of hemoglobin.

Indications and dosage
• Iron deficiency. **Adults:** 325 mg P.O. t.i.d. or q.i.d. Alternatively, give 1 delayed-release capsule (160 or 525 mg) P.O. b.i.d. **Children:** 4 to 6 mg/kg daily in three divided doses.
• Prophylaxis for iron deficiency anemia. **Pregnant women:** 150 mg P.O. daily during the last two trimesters. **Premature or undernourished infants:** 1 to 2 mg/kg P.O. daily (as elemental iron) in divided doses.

Adverse reactions
GI: *nausea,* vomiting, *constipation, black stools.*
Other: elixir may stain teeth.

Interactions
Antacids, levodopa, penicillamine, quinolones, tetracycline, vitamin E: decreased iron absorption. Separate doses if possible. **Chloramphenicol:** watch for delayed response to iron therapy. **Vitamin C:** may increase iron absorption. Beneficial drug interaction.

Nursing diagnoses
• Activity intolerance related to patient's underlying condition.
• Constipation related to adverse GI reactions to ferrous sulfate.
• Knowledge deficit related to ferrous sulfate therapy.

Nursing interventions
• *Contraindicated* in hemosiderosis and hemochromatosis. Also contraindicated in patients with hemolytic anemia unless iron deficiency anemia is also present.
• *Use cautiously* in peptic ulcer, ulcerative colitis, and regional enteritis. Also use cautiously on long-term basis.
• Teach parents to keep iron supplements out of children's reach and to administer to children carefully. Iron is toxic. As few as 3 or 4 tablets may cause poisoning in children.
• Tell patient to take iron supplements between meals and to take them with food if GI upset occurs, although absorption may be decreased. Enteric-coated products reduce GI upset but also reduce amount of iron absorbed. Warn patient not to crush or chew sustained-release iron preparations.
• Dilute liquid preparations in juice (preferably orange juice) or water, but not in milk or antacids. Give tablets with orange juice to promote absorption. To avoid staining teeth, give iron elixir through a straw; patient may take with water or fruit juice.
• Inform patient that certain foods may impair oral iron absorption, including yogurt, cheese, eggs, milk, whole-grain breads and cereals, tea, and coffee.
• If the patient misses a dose, tell him to take it as soon as he remembers, unless it's time for the next dose. Do not double-dose.
• Check for constipation; record color and amount of stool. Teach the patient dietary measures to avoid constipation. Inform him that the drug may turn his stools black but that this effect is harmless; however, it could mask the presence of melena.
• Monitor hemoglobin and reticulocyte counts during therapy.

General

Classification: gonadotropin-releasing hormone (GnRH) analogue (synthetic decapeptide). **Pregnancy risk category:** X.

Mechanism of action

Acts on the pituitary to decrease the release of follicle-stimulating hormone and luteinizing hormone. The result is decreased ovarian stimulation, lowered circulating estrogens, and improvement of the symptoms associated with endometriosis.

Indications and dosage

• Management of endometriosis. **Women 18 years and older:** 1 spray in one nostril b.i.d. Maximum duration of therapy is 6 months.

Adverse reactions

CNS: *headaches, emotional lability, insomnia,* depression. **CV:** edema. **EENT:** *nasal irritation.* **GU:** *vaginal dryness.* **Skin:** *acne,* seborrhea, hirsutism. **Other:** *hot flashes, decreased libido, myalgia,* reduced breast size, weight gain or loss, increased libido, decreased bone density.

Interactions

None reported.

Nursing diagnoses

• Sexual dysfunction related to the patient's underlying condition.
• Impaired tissue integrity related to nafarelin-induced adverse reactions.
• Knowledge deficit related to nafarelin therapy.

Nursing interventions

• *Contraindicated* in patients with hypersensitivity to GnRH analogues or any components of the formulation (benzalkonium chloride, sorbitol, purified water, glacial acetic acid, hydrochloric acid, or sodium hydroxide). Also contraindicated in the presence of undiagnosed vaginal bleeding, in breast-feeding women, and during pregnancy (because it may harm the fetus).
• Studies have confirmed a small loss in bone density after 6 months of therapy, probably caused by the hypoestrogenic state induced by the drug. Patients with major risk factors for osteoporosis (chronic alcohol or tobacco users, strong family history of osteoporosis, or those who are using drugs that may reduce bone mass such as anticonvulsants or corticosteroids) should not receive additional courses of therapy and should strongly weigh the risks and benefits before an initial trial of the drug.
• Advise patient to contact her doctor if she develops a cold or rhinitis during therapy. If she requires a topical nasal decongestant, the manufacturer suggests that it be used at least 30 minutes after nafarelin treatment to reduce possible interference with nafarelin absorption.
• Advise patient to use nonhormonal form of contraception (such as barrier contraception). Although the drug will usually inhibit ovulation and stop menstruation, it is not a reliable contraceptive, particularly if the patient misses a few doses. She should stop the drug immediately and contact her doctor if she believes that she is pregnant.
• Teach patient that menstruation will stop with regular use of the drug. She should contact her doctor if menstruation persists or breakthrough bleeding occurs.
• Instruct patient to immediately report severe abdominal pain, bloating, swelling of the hands or feet, nausea, vomiting, diarrhea, substantial weight gain, or shortness of breath.

General

Classification: colony stimulating factor (biological response modifier). **Pregnancy risk category:** C.

Mechanism of action

A glycoprotein that stimulates proliferation and differentiation of hematopoietic cells. Filgrastim is specific for neutrophils.

Indications and dosage

- To decrease the incidence of infection in patients with nonmyeloid malignancies receiving myelosuppressive antineoplastics. **Adults and children:** 5 mcg/kg/day I.V. or S.C. as a single dose. Doses may be increased in increments of 5 mcg/kg for each chemotherapy cycle depending on the duration and severity of the nadir of the absolute neutrophil count (ANC).

Adverse reactions

Blood: ***thrombocytopenia.*** **GU:** hematuria, proteinuria. **Skin:** alopecia, exacerbation of preexisting conditions (such as psoriasis). **Other:** *skeletal pain,* fever, splenomegaly, osteoporosis.

Interactions

Chemotherapeutic agents: rapidly dividing myeloid cells are potentially sensitive to cytotoxic agents. Do not use filgrastim concomitantly with chemotherapy.

Nursing diagnoses

- High risk for infection related to myelosuppression induced by antineoplastics.
- Pain (skeletal) induced by filgrastim therapy.
- Knowledge deficit related to filgrastim therapy.

Nursing interventions

- *Contraindicated* in patients with hypersensitivity to proteins derived from *Escherichia coli.* Although the drug is a growth factor for neutrophils only, the potential exists for stimulation of myeloid tumor growth.
- Do not give the drug within 24 hours of cytotoxic chemotherapy.
- Be aware that a transiently increased neutrophil count is common 1 or 2 days after initiation of therapy. However, the drug should be given daily for up to 2 weeks or until the ANC has returned to 10,000/mm^3 after the expected chemotherapy-induced neutrophil nadir.
- Obtain a CBC and platelet count before therapy and monitor twice weekly during therapy. Note that patients who receive this drug have the potential for receiving higher doses of chemotherapy, which may increase the risk of chemotherapy-induced toxicities.
- Store in refrigerator at 36° to 46° F (2° to 8° C). Do not freeze; avoid shaking. The drug may be stored at room temperature for a maximum of 6 hours; discard any vial that has been at room temperature for more than 6 hours.
- The vials are intended for single use only and contain no preservatives. Once a dose is withdrawn, do not reenter the vial.
- If the patient is going to self-administer the drug, teach him how to administer it and dispose of used needles, syringes, and drug containers. Give him a copy of the "Information for patients" section of material included with the product information and ensure that he understands all information.
- Be aware that filgrastim is also known as granulocyte colony stimulating factor or G-CSF.

General

Classification: antihypertensive, antianginal (beta-adrenergic blocker). **Pregnancy risk category:** C.

Mechanism of action

Reduces cardiac oxygen demand by blocking catecholamine-induced increases in heart rate, blood pressure, and force of myocardial contraction. Depresses renin secretion.

Indications and dosage

• Management of angina pectoris. **Adults:** 40 mg P.O. once daily, initially. Dosage may be increased in 40- to 80-mg increments until optimum response occurs. Usual maintenance dosage range is 40 to 240 mg once daily.
• Hypertension. **Adults:** 40 mg P.O. once daily, initially. Dosage may be increased in 40- to 80-mg increments until optimum response occurs. Usual maintenance dosage range is 40 to 320 mg once daily. Doses of 640 mg may be necessary in rare cases.

Adverse reactions

CNS: fatigue, lethargy. **CV:** *bradycardia, hypotension, **CHF**,* peripheral vascular disease. **GI:** nausea, vomiting, diarrhea. **Metabolic:** hypoglycemia without tachycardia (in diabetic patients). **Skin:** rash. **Other:** *increased airway resistance,* fever.

Interactions

Antihypertensives: enhanced antihypertensive effect. **Digitalis glycosides:** excessive bradycardia and increased depressant effect on myocardium. Use together cautiously. **Epinephrine:** severe vasoconstriction and reflex bradycardia. Monitor blood pressure and observe patient carefully. **Indomethacin:** decreased antihypertensive effect. Monitor blood pressure and adjust dosage. **Insulin, oral antidiabetic agents:** can alter dosage requirements in previously stabilized diabetics. Observe patient carefully.

Nursing diagnoses

• Pain related to ineffectiveness of nadolol therapy.
• Fluid volume excess related to nadolol-induced CHF.
• Knowledge deficit related to nadolol therapy.

Nursing interventions

• *Contraindicated* in bronchial asthma, sinus bradycardia and greater than first-degree conduction block, and cardiogenic shock.
• *Use cautiously* in patients with heart failure, chronic bronchitis, renal or hepatic insufficiency, or emphysema. Elderly patients may experience enhanced adverse reactions. Dose may need to be adjusted.
• Always check patient's apical pulse before giving this drug. If slower than 60 beats/minute, withhold drug and call doctor.
• Monitor blood pressure frequently. If patient develops severe hypotension, administer a vasopressor, as ordered.
• Don't discontinue abruptly; can exacerbate angina and MI. Gradually reduce dosage over 1 to 2 weeks.
• Teach patient about his disease and therapy. Explain the importance of taking this drug as prescribed, even when he's feeling well. Tell outpatient not to discontinue drug suddenly, but to call doctor if unpleasant adverse reactions occur.
• Has been used in a limited number of patients with atrial flutter or fibrillation. Also has been used for a few patients in the treatment of migraine headaches.
• This drug masks common signs of shock, hyperthyroidism, and hypoglycemia.
• May be given without regard to meals.

General

Classification: androgen synthesis inhibitor (synthetic 4-azasteroid derivative steroid). **Pregnancy risk category:** X.

Mechanism of action

Competitively inhibits steroid 5α-reductase, an enzyme responsible for formation of the potent androgen 5α-dihydrotestosterone (DHT) from testosterone. Because DHT influences development of the prostate gland, decreasing levels of this hormone in adult males should relieve the symptoms associated with benign prostatic hyperplasia (BPH).

Indications and dosage

- Symptomatic BPH. **Adults:** 5 mg P.O. daily.

Adverse reactions

GU: impotence, decreased volume of ejaculate.
Other: decreased libido.

Interactions

Theophylline: small, clinically insignificant increases in theophylline clearance and decreases in theophylline half-life (10%) have been observed.

Nursing diagnoses

- Pain related to ineffectiveness of finasteride to relieve prostate enlargement.
- Urinary retention related to ineffectiveness of finasteride to relieve prostatic enlargement.
- Altered sexuality patterns related to adverse GU effects of finasteride therapy.
- Knowledge deficit related to finasteride.

Nursing interventions

- *Use cautiously* in patients with hepatic dysfunction because drug is metabolized extensively in the liver. No dosage adjustments are necessary in renal impairment; decreased urine excretion of metabolites is associated with increased excretion of metabolites in the feces.
- Before therapy, closely evaluate patient for conditions that might mimic BPH, including hypotonic bladder, prostate cancer, infection, stricture, or relevant neurologic conditions.
- Because it's impossible to identify prospectively which patients will respond to finasteride, a minimum of 6 months of therapy may be necessary.
- Crushed tablets shouldn't be handled by women who are or may become pregnant because of the risk of adverse effects on a male fetus.
- A patient whose partner is or may become pregnant should take precautions to avoid exposing her to his semen or should discontinue the drug.
- Although drug's elimination rate is decreased in elderly patients, dosage adjustments aren't necessary.
- Baseline and periodic digital rectal examinations are recommended. This drug will decrease serum prostate-specific antigen (PSA) levels, even in prostate cancer. However, in clinical trials, this drug didn't appear to decrease the rate of prostate cancer detection.
- Sustained increases in serum PSA levels should be carefully evaluated in patients receiving finasteride therapy. This could indicate noncompliance with therapy.
- Carefully monitor patients who have a large residual urine volume or severely diminished urine flow. Because not all patients respond to this drug, such patients may not be candidates for finasteride therapy.
- Long-term effects of this drug on the complications of BPH, including acute urinary obstruction, and the incidence of surgery are unknown.
- Patients should understand that finasteride may decrease the volume of ejaculate but doesn't appear to impair normal sexual function. However, impotence and decreased libido have occurred in less than 4% of patients treated with this drug.
- Investigators are currently determining the drug's effectiveness in preventing prostate cancer in certain high-risk individuals; as adjuvant treatment of prostate cancer; and as treatment of male pattern baldness, acne, and hirsutism.

General

Classification: nonnarcotic analgesic (NSAID).
Pregnancy risk category: C.

Mechanism of action

Produces analgesia by blocking generation of pain impulses, probably by inhibiting the synthesis of prostaglandins.

Indications and dosage

• Acute and chronic rheumatoid arthritis or osteoarthritis. **Adults:** initially, 1,000 mg P.O. daily as a single dose or in divided doses b.i.d. Maximum daily dose is 2,000 mg.

Adverse reactions

CNS: *dizziness, headache,* fatigue, increased sweating, insomnia, nervousness, somnolence. **CV:** vasculitis. **EENT:** *tinnitus.* **GI:** *diarrhea, dyspepsia, abdominal pain, constipation, flatulence, nausea,* dry mouth, gastritis, stomatitis, vomiting. **Skin:** *pruritus, rash.* **Other:** *edema.*

Interactions

Drugs that are highly bound to plasma proteins (such as warfarin): increased risk of adverse effects from displacement of drug by nabumetone. Use cautiously.

Nursing diagnoses

• Pain related to the patient's underlying condition.
• High risk for injury related to nabumetone-induced liver or kidney damage with toxic doses.
• Knowledge deficit related to nabumetone therapy.

Nursing interventions

• *Contraindicated* in patients with hypersensitivity to the drug and in patients with asthma, urticaria, or other allergic reactions to other NSAIDs or aspirin.
• *Use cautiously* in patients with renal or hepatic impairment; CHF, hypertension, or other conditions that may predispose the patient to fluid retention; and a history of peptic ulcer disease.
• Administer with food, milk, or antacids. Drug is absorbed more rapidly when administered with food or milk.
• Because NSAIDs impair the synthesis of renal prostaglandins, they can decrease renal blood flow and lead to reversible renal impairment, especially in patients with preexisting renal failure, liver dysfunction, or heart failure; in elderly patients; and in those taking diuretics. Monitor these patients closely during therapy.
• Serious GI toxicity, such as bleeding and ulceration, can occur in patients receiving chronic NSAID therapy. Such toxicity can occur at any time, sometimes without warning. Stress the importance of follow-up examinations to detect these adverse reactions. Teach patient signs and symptoms of GI bleeding, and tell him to notify the doctor immediately if these symptoms appear.
• During chronic therapy, periodically monitor renal and liver function, CBC, and hematocrit. Assess these patients for signs and symptoms of GI bleeding.
• Advise patient to limit alcohol intake because of the risk of additive GI toxicity.

flavoxate hydrochloride

Urispas

General

Classification: urinary tract spasmolytic (flavone derivative). **Pregnancy risk category:** C.

Mechanism of action

Has a direct spasmolytic effect on smooth muscles of the urinary tract. It also provides some local anesthesia and analgesia.

Indications and dosage

- Symptomatic relief of dysuria, frequency, urgency, nocturia, incontinence, and suprapubic pain associated with urologic disorders. **Adults and children over 12 years:** 100 to 200 mg P.O. t.i.d. to q.i.d.

Adverse reactions

CNS: *mental confusion* (especially in elderly patients), nervousness, dizziness, headache, drowsiness, difficulty with concentration. **CV:** tachycardia, palpitations. **EENT:** *dry throat, blurred vision,* disturbed eye accommodation. **GI:** *dry mouth,* abdominal pain, constipation (with high doses), nausea, vomiting. **Skin:** urticaria, dermatoses. **Other:** fever.

Interactions

None significant.

Nursing diagnoses

- Pain (bladder spasms) related to patient's underlying condition.
- High risk for injury related to flavoxate-induced blurred vision and drowsiness.
- Knowledge deficit related to flavoxate therapy.

Nursing interventions

- *Contraindicated* in pyloric or duodenal obstruction, obstructive intestinal lesions or ileus, achalasia, GI hemorrhage, or obstructive uropathies of lower urinary tract.
- *Use cautiously* in patients suspected of having glaucoma.
- Check patient's medical history for other drug use before giving drugs with anticholinergic adverse reactions.
- Warn patient to avoid driving and other hazardous activities that require alertness because of possible drowsiness, mental confusion, and blurred vision.
- Tell the patient to report adverse reactions or lack of response to drug.

General

Classification: immunosuppressant (monoclonal antibody). **Pregnancy risk category:** C.

Mechanism of action

Muromonab-CD3 is an IgG antibody that reacts in the T-lymphocyte membrane with a molecule (CD3) needed for antigen recognition. This drug depletes the blood of CD3-positive T cells, which leads to restoration of allograft function and reversal of rejection.

Indications and dosage

- Acute allograft rejection in renal transplant patients. **Adults:** 5 mg I.V. bolus once daily for 10 to 14 days. **Children:** 2.5 mg I.V. bolus once daily for 10 to 14 days.

Adverse reactions

CV: *chest pain.* **GI:** *nausea, vomiting,* diarrhea. **Other:** ***severe pulmonary edema,*** *fever, chills, tremor, dyspnea,* ***infection.***

Interactions

None reported.

Nursing diagnoses

- Altered protection related to organ rejection.
- Altered cardiopulmonary tissue perfusion related to muromonab-CD3 therapy.
- Knowledge deficit related to muromonab-CD3 therapy.

Nursing interventions

- *Contraindicated* in patients with fluid overload, as evidenced by chest X-ray or a weight gain greater than 3% within the week before treatment.
- Patients develop antibodies to this preparation that can lead to loss of effectiveness and more severe adverse reactions if a second course of therapy is attempted. Therefore, experts believe that this drug should be used for only a single course of treatment.
- Most adverse reactions develop within 30 minutes to 6 hours after the first dose.
- Treatment should begin in a facility where the patient can be monitored closely and that is equipped and staffed for CPR.
- Assess patient for signs of fluid overload before treatment.
- Chest X-ray must be taken within 24 hours before starting drug treatment.
- Inform patient of expected adverse reactions. Reassure him that they will be less severe as treatment progresses.
- Administering an antipyretic before giving the drug may help lower incidence of expected pyrexia and chills. Corticosteroids may also be administered before first injection to help decrease incidence of adverse reactions. Methylprednisolone sodium succinate (1 mg/kg) preinjection, followed by hydrocortisone sodium succinate (100 mg) 30 minutes postinjection, have been recommended to alleviate the severity of the first dose reaction.

General

Classification: ventricular antiarrhythmic (benzamide derivative). **Pregnancy risk category:** C.

Mechanism of action

A class Ic antiarrhythmic that depresses phase 0. Unlike class Ia and Ib agents, however, it does not prolong or shorten the action potential. All class I drugs have membrane stabilizing effects.

Indications and dosage

• Life-threatening ventricular arrhythmias, such as sustained ventricular tachycardia. **Adults:** 100 mg P.O. q 12 hours. May be increased in increments of 50 mg b.i.d. q 4 days until efficacy is achieved. Maximum dosage is 400 mg daily for most patients.

Initial dosage for patients with CHF is 50 mg q 12 hours.

Adverse reactions

CNS: *dizziness, headache,* fatigue, tremor. **CV:** ***new or worsened arrhythmias,*** chest pain, ***CHF, cardiac arrest.*** **EENT:** *blurred vision and other visual disturbances.* **GI:** nausea, constipation, abdominal pain. **Other:** *dyspnea,* edema, skin rash.

Interactions

Amiodarone, cimetidine, digoxin, propranolol: altered pharmacokinetics. Monitor for toxicity. **Digitalis glycosides:** flecainide may increase plasma digoxin levels by 15% to 25%. **Propranolol, beta-adrenergic blockers:** both flecainide and propranolol plasma levels increase by 20% to 30%. **Urine acidifying and alkalinizing agents:** extremes of urine pH may substantially alter excretion of flecainide.

Nursing diagnoses

• Decreased cardiac output related to ineffectiveness of flecainide therapy.
• Sensory/perceptual alterations (visual) related to flecainide-induced visual disturbances.
• Knowledge deficit related to flecainide therapy.

Nursing interventions

• *Contraindicated* in preexisting second- or third-degree AV block or right bundle branch block when associated with a left hemiblock, unless a pacemaker is present, and in cardiogenic shock.
• *Use cautiously* in preexisting CHF, cardiomyopathy, severe renal or hepatic disease, prolonged QT interval, sick sinus syndrome, or blood dyscrasias.
• Use only in patients with immediately life-threatening arrhythmias, such as sustained ventricular tachycardia. Findings from the Cardiac Arrhythmia Suppression Trial (CAST) include a greater-than-twofold increase in the number of deaths and nonfatal cardiac arrest in patients treated with flecainide.
• Flecainide can alter endocardial pacing thresholds. Determine pacing threshold 1 week before and after initiating therapy in patients with pacemakers.
• Correct hypokalemia or hyperkalemia before this drug is given becuase both may alter the effect of flecainide.
• Monitor blood levels, especially in patients with renal failure or CHF. Normal levels range from 0.2 to 1 mcg/ml. Adverse effects increase when trough blood levels exceed 1 mcg/ml.
• Expect to administer I.V. lidocaine while awaiting full therapeutic effect of flecainide.

General

Classification: viral vaccine. **Pregnancy risk category:** X.

Mechanism of action

Promotes active immunity to mumps.

Indications and dosage

• Immunization. **Adults and children over 1 year:** 1 vial (5,000 units) S.C.

Adverse reactions

Systemic: *slight fever,* rash, malaise, mild allergic reactions, febrile seizures (rare).

Interactions

Immune serum globulin, whole blood, plasma: antibodies in serum may interfere with immune response. Don't use vaccine within 3 months of transfusion. **Tuberculin skin test:** may temporarily decrease response to test. Defer skin testing.

Nursing diagnoses

• Altered protection related to lack of immunity to mumps virus.
• Hyperthermia related to vaccine-induced fever.
• Knowledge deficit related to live mumps virus vaccine.

Nursing interventions

• *Contraindicated* in immunosuppression; cancer; blood dyscrasias; corticosteroid or radiation therapy; gamma globulin disorders; active, untreated tuberculosis; or pregnancy.
• *Use cautiously* in patients with hypersensitivity to neomycin, chickens, ducks, eggs, or feathers. Defer in acute or febrile illness and for 3 months following transfusions or treatment with immune serum globulin.
• Keep epinephrine 1:1,000 available.
• Mumpsvax should not be given less than 1 month before or after immunization with other live virus vaccines, with the exception of Attenuvax, Meruvax, or monovalent or trivalent live, oral poliovirus vaccine, which may be administered simultaneously.
• Not recommended for infants under 12 months because retained maternal mumps antibodies may interfere with the immune response.
• Stress importance of avoiding pregnancy for 3 months after immunization. If necessary, provide contraceptive information.
• Treat fever with antipyretics.
• Do not give I.V.
• Store in refrigerator and protect from light. Solution may be used if red, pink, or yellow (but must be clear).
• Use only diluent supplied. Discard 8 hours after reconstituting.
• Obtain history of allergies, especially to antibiotics, and reaction to immunization.

General

Classification: antineoplastic (antimetabolite).
Pregnancy risk category: D.

Mechanism of action

Inhibits DNA synthesis.

Indications and dosage

- Brain, breast, head, neck, liver, gallbladder, and bile duct cancer. **Adults:** 0.1 to 0.6 mg/kg daily by intra-arterial infusion (use pump for continuous, uniform rate); or 0.4 to 0.6 mg/kg daily into hepatic artery.

Adverse reactions

Blood: ***leukopenia,*** anemia, ***thrombocytopenia.*** **CNS:** cerebellar ataxia, vertigo, nystagmus, seizures, depression, hemiplegia, hiccups, lethargy. **EENT:** blurred vision. **GI:** *anorexia, stomatitis, cramps, nausea, vomiting, diarrhea, bleeding, enteritis.* **Hepatic:** cholangitis, jaundice, elevated liver enzymes. **Skin:** *erythema,* dermatitis, pruritus, rash.

Interactions

None significant.

Nursing diagnoses

- Altered protection related to floxuridine-induced myelosuppression and immunosuppression.
- Altered oral mucous membrane related to floxuridine-induced stomatitis.
- Knowledge deficit related to floxuridine therapy.

Nursing interventions

- *Contraindicated* in patients with poor nutritional state, bone marrow suppression, or serious infection.
- *Use cautiously* after high-dose pelvic irradiation or use of alkylating agent and in impaired hepatic or renal function.
- Monitor for severe skin and GI adverse reactions; these require discontinuing drug. Use of antacid eases but probably won't prevent GI distress.
- Provide excellent mouth care to help prevent stomatitis.
- Monitor intake and output, CBC, and renal and hepatic function.
- Discontinue drug if WBC falls below 3,500/mm^3 or if platelet count falls below 100,000/mm^3.
- Make sure patient knows that therapeutic effect may be delayed from 1 to 6 weeks.
- Reconstitute drug with sterile water for injection. Dilute further in D_5W or 0.9% sodium chloride solution for actual infusion. Discard refrigerated solution after 2 weeks.
- To maintain continuous intra-arterial infusion, administer by infusion pump.
- Monitor arterial perfusion area. Check line for bleeding, blockage, displacement, or leakage.
- Follow institutional policy to reduce carcinogenic, mutagenic, and teratogenic risks.
- Avoid I.M. injections of any drugs in patients with thrombocytopenia to prevent bleeding.

General

Classification: narcotic analgesic (opioid). **Pregnancy risk category:** B (D for prolonged use or use of high doses at term). **Controlled substance schedule:** II.

Mechanism of action

Binds with opiate receptors at many sites in the CNS (brain, brain stem, and spinal cord), altering both perception of and emotional response to pain through an unknown mechanism.

Indications and dosage

- Severe pain. **Adults:** 4 to 15 mg S.C. or I.M.; or 30 to 60 mg P.O. or P.R. q 4 hours, p.r.n. or around the clock. May be injected I.V. over 4 to 5 minutes diluted in 4 to 5 ml water for injection. May also administer controlled-release tablets q 8 to 12 hours. As an epidural injection, 5 mg via an epidural catheter q 24 hours. **Children:** 0.1 to 0.2 mg/kg dose S.C. or I.M. q 4 hours. Maximum dosage is 15 mg.

In some situations, morphine may be administered by continuous I.V. infusion or by intraspinal and intrathecal injection.

Adverse reactions

CNS: *sedation, somnolence, clouded sensorium, euphoria,* seizures with large doses, dizziness, *nightmares* (with long-acting oral forms). **CV:** *hypotension,* bradycardia. **GI:** *nausea, vomiting, constipation,* ileus. **GU:** *urine retention.* **Other:** ***respiratory depression,*** *physical dependence, pruritus and skin flushing (with epidural administration).*

Interactions

Alcohol, CNS depressants: additional effects. Use together cautiously.

Nursing diagnoses

- Pain related to patient's underlying condition.
- Ineffective breathing pattern related to morphine-induced respiratory depression.
- Knowledge deficit related to morphine therapy.

Nursing interventions

- *Contraindicated* in patients with hypersensitivity to the drug or other opiate analgesics.
- *Use with extreme caution* in head injury, increased intracranial pressure, seizures, asthma, COPD, alcoholism, prostatic hypertrophy, severe hepatic or renal disease, acute abdominal conditions, hypothyroidism, Addison's disease, increased CSF pressure, urethral stricture, cardiac arrhythmias, reduced blood volume, and toxic psychosis and in elderly or debilitated patients.
- Monitor circulatory, respiratory, bladder, and bowel functions carefully. Drug may cause respiratory depression, hypotension, urine retention, nausea, vomiting, ileus, or altered level of consciousness. Hold dose and notify doctor if respirations are below 12 breaths/minute.
- Warn ambulatory patient to avoid hazardous activities that require mental alertness or physical coordination.
- Constipation often severe with maintenance. Make sure stool softener or other laxative is ordered.
- Drug of choice in relieving pain of MI. May cause transient decrease in blood pressure.
- Keep narcotic antagonist (naloxone) and resuscitative equipment available.
- Respiratory depression, hypotension, profound sedation, or coma may occur if used with general anesthetics, tranquilizers, sedatives, hypnotics, alcohol, TCAs, or MAO inhibitors. Reduce morphine dose. Use together with extreme caution. Monitor patient response.
- When used postoperatively, encourage turning, coughing, and deep breathing and use of the incentive spirometer to prevent atelectasis.
- When given epidurally, monitor for respiratory depression up to 24 hours after the injection. Check respiratory rate and depth every 30 to 60 minutes for 24 hours.

General

Classification: antifungal (bis-triazole derivative). **Pregnancy risk category:** C.

Mechanism of action

Inhibits fungal cytochrome P-450, an enzyme responsible for fungal sterol synthesis. This results in weakening of fungal cell walls.

Indications and dosage

- Oropharyngeal candidiasis. **Adults:** 200 mg P.O. or I.V. on the first day, followed by 100 mg once daily. Therapy should continue for 2 weeks.
- Esophageal candidiasis. **Adults:** 200 mg P.O. or I.V. on the first day, followed by 100 mg once daily. Higher doses (up to 400 mg daily) have been used, depending on patient's condition and tolerance of treatment. Patients should receive the drug for at least 3 weeks and for 2 weeks after symptoms resolve.
- Systemic candidiasis. **Adults:** 400 mg P.O. or I.V. on the first day, followed by 200 mg once daily. Treatment should continue for at least 4 weeks or for 2 weeks after symptoms resolve.
- Cryptococcal meningitis. **Adults:** 400 mg P.O. or I.V. on the first day, followed by 200 mg once daily. Higher doses (up to 400 mg daily) may be used. Treatment should continue for 10 to 12 weeks after cultures of CSF are negative.
- Suppression of relapse of cryptococcal meningitis in patients with AIDS. **Adults:** 200 mg P.O. or I.V. daily.

Adverse reactions

CNS: headache, dizziness. **GI:** *nausea,* vomiting, abdominal pain, diarrhea. **Skin:** rash, ***Stevens-Johnson syndrome (rare).*** **Other:** hepatotoxicity (rare), elevated liver enzymes.

Interactions

Cyclosporine, phenytoin: may cause increased plasma concentrations of these drugs. Monitor serum cyclosporine or phenytoin levels. **Isoniazid, phenytoin, rifampin, valproic acid, oral sulfonylureas:** increased incidence of abnormally elevated hepatic transaminases. Monitor closely. **Oral antidiabetic agents (tolbutamide, glyburide, glipizide):** may cause increased plasma concentrations of these drugs. Monitor for enhanced hypoglycemic effect. **Rifampin:** enhanced metabolism of fluconazole. Monitor for lack of response. **Warfarin:** increased risk of bleeding. Monitor prothrombin time.

Nursing diagnoses

- High risk for injury related to ineffectiveness of fluconazole to eradicate the infection.
- High risk for fluid volume deficit related to fluconazole-induced nausea.
- Knowledge deficit related to fluconazole therapy.

Nursing interventions

- *Contraindicated* in patients with hypersensitivity to the drug.
- *Use cautiously* in patients with hypersensitivity to other antifungal azole compounds because there is no information regarding cross-sensitivity.
- Because the drug is excreted unchanged by the kidneys, adjust dosage in patients with renal failure. Reduce dosage by 50% if creatinine clearance is 21 to 50 ml/minute and by 75% if creatinine clearance is 11 to 20 ml/minute. Give patients receiving regular hemodialysis treatment the usual dose after each dialysis session.
- **I.V. use:** May be administered by continuous infusion at a rate not to exceed 200 mg/hour. Use an infusion pump. Do not connect in series with other infusions to prevent air embolism. Do not add any other drugs to the solution.
- Remove protective wrapping of I.V. fluconazole just before use to help ensure sterility. The plastic container may show some opacity from moisture absorbed during sterilization. This is normal, will not affect the drug, and will diminish over time.

General

Classification: antiarrhythmic (sodium channel blocker). **Pregnancy risk category:** B.

Mechanism of action

A class I antiarrhythmic that reduces the fast inward current carried by sodium ions.

Indications and dosage

• Life-threatening ventricular arrhythmias. **Adults:** individualized dosage is based on clinical response and patient tolerance. Therapy should begin in the hospital. Most patients respond to 600 to 900 mg P.O. daily, given in divided doses q 8 hours. Increase daily dosage q 3 days by 150 mg until the desired clinical effect is seen.
• Hepatic or renal function impairment. **Adults:** start therapy at 600 mg P.O. daily or less. Monitor closely and adjust dosage carefully.

Adverse reactions

CNS: *dizziness, headache, fatigue,* anxiety, hypoesthesia, asthenia, nervousness, paresthesia, sleep disorders. **CV:** ***proarrhythmic events,*** *ECG abnormalities (including conduction defects, sinus pause, junctional rhythm, or AV block),* ***CHF,*** *palpitations,* ***sustained ventricular tachycardia,*** *chest pain, sinus bradycardia,* ***sinus arrest.*** **EENT:** blurred vision. **GI:** *nausea, vomiting, abdominal pain, dyspepsia, diarrhea, dry mouth.* **GU:** urine retention. **Skin:** rash. **Other:** dyspnea, drug fever, sweating, musculoskeletal pain.

Interactions

Cimetidine: increased plasma levels of and decreased clearance of moricizine. Begin moricizine therapy at low dosage (not more than 600 mg daily) and monitor plasma levels and therapeutic effect closely. **Propranolol, digoxin:** additive prolongation of the PR interval. Monitor closely. **Theophylline:** increased theophylline clearance and reduced plasma levels. Monitor plasma levels and therapeutic response; adjust theophylline dosage as needed.

Nursing diagnoses

• Decreased cardiac output related to ineffectiveness of moricizine to correct arrhythmia.
• Altered protection related to moricizine-induced proarrhythmias.
• Knowledge deficit related to moricizine therapy.

Nursing interventions

• *Contraindicated* in patients with preexisting second- or third-degree AV block, right bundle-branch block when associated with left hemiblock (bifascicular block) unless a pacemaker is present, in patients with severe hepatic insufficiency, and in patients in cardiogenic shock and those with hypersensitivity to the drug.
• *Use with extreme caution* in patients with sick sinus syndrome. The drug may cause sinus bradycardia or sinus arrest.
• The drug should be used only for patients with life-threatening ventricular arrhythmias.
• When substituting another antiarrhythmic, withdraw previous antiarrhythmic therapy for one to two half-lives of the drug before starting moricizine at recommended dosage. Patients who have shown a tendency to develop life-threatening arrhythmias after withdrawal of drug therapy should be hospitalized during withdrawal and adjustment to moricizine. Start moricizine 8 to 12 hours after the last dose of mexilitine, 3 to 6 hours after the last dose of procainamide, 8 to 12 hours after the last dose of propafenone, 6 to 12 hours after the last dose of quinidine, or 8 to 12 hours after the last dose of tocainide.
• Hypokalemia, hyperkalemia, and hypomagnesemia may alter the effects of the drug. Determine electrolyte status and correct imbalances before therapy.
• Patients with hepatic or renal dysfunction will exhibit decreased moricizine clearance.

General

Classification: antifungal (fluorinated pyrimidine). **Pregnancy risk category:** C.

Mechanism of action

Appears to penetrate fungal cells, where it is converted to fluorouracil, a known metabolic antagonist. Causes defective protein synthesis.

Indications and dosage

- Severe fungal infections caused by susceptible strains of *Candida* (including septicemia, endocarditis, urinary tract and pulmonary infections) and *Cryptococcus* (meningitis, pulmonary infection, and possibly UTIs). **Adults and children over 50 kg:** 50 to 150 mg/kg P.O. daily q 6 hours. **Adults and children under 50 kg:** 1.5 to 4.5 g/m^2 P.O. daily in four divided doses.

  Severe infections, such as meningitis, may require doses up to 250 mg/kg.

Adverse reactions

Blood: anemia, ***leukopenia, bone marrow suppression, thrombocytopenia.*** **CNS:** dizziness, drowsiness, confusion, headache, vertigo. **GI:** *nausea, vomiting, diarrhea,* abdominal bloating. **Hepatic:** elevated AST, ALT. **Metabolic:** elevated serum alkaline phosphatase, BUN, serum creatinine. **Skin:** occasional rash.

Interactions

None significant.

Nursing diagnoses

- High risk for injury related to ineffectiveness of flucytosine in eradicating the fungal infection.
- Altered protection related to flucytosine-induced hematologic adverse reactions.
- Knowledge deficit related to flucytosine therapy.

Nursing interventions

- *Use with extreme caution* in patients with impaired hepatic or renal function or bone marrow depression. Patients with renal dysfunction should have dosage based on plasma flucytosine levels.
- Check to be sure appropriate tests have been done before administering first dose. Hematologic tests and renal and liver function studies should precede therapy and should be repeated at frequent intervals. Before treatment, susceptibility tests should establish that the organism is flucytosine-sensitive. Monitor repeat susceptibility tests weekly to detect drug resistance.
- Monitor intake and output; report any marked change.
- If possible, monitor blood level assays of drug regularly to maintain flucytosine at therapeutic level (25 to 120 mcg/ml). Higher blood levels may be toxic.
- Expect to administer drug concurrently with amphotericin B for synergistic effects.
- To help reduce adverse GI reactions, give capsules over a 15-minute period.
- Inform patient that adequate therapeutic response may take weeks or months.
- Be aware that flucytosine is also known as 5-FC.

molindone hydrochloride

Moban

General

Classification: antipsychotic (dihydroindolone).
Pregnancy risk category: C.

Mechanism of action

Blocks postsynaptic dopamine receptors in the brain.

Indications and dosage

- Psychotic disorders. **Adults:** 50 to 75 mg P.O. daily, increasing to maximum of 225 mg daily. Doses up to 400 mg may be required.

Adverse reactions

Blood: transient leukopenia. **CNS:** *extrapyramidal reactions (moderate incidence), tardive dyskinesia, sedation (moderate incidence),* pseudoparkinsonism, EEG changes, dizziness. **CV:** *orthostatic hypotension,* tachycardia, ECG changes. **EENT:** *blurred vision.* **GI:** *dry mouth, constipation.* **GU:** *urine retention,* dark urine, menstrual irregularities, gynecomastia, inhibited ejaculation. **Hepatic:** cholestatic jaundice, abnormal liver function tests. **Metabolic:** hyperprolactinemia. **Skin:** *mild photosensitivity,* dermal allergic reactions. **Other:** rarely, ***neuroleptic malignant syndrome*** (fever, tachycardia, tachypnea, profuse diaphoresis).

Interactions

Alcohol, other CNS depressants: increased CNS depression. Avoid concomitant use.

Nursing diagnoses

- Altered thought processes related to the patient's underlying condition.
- Constipation related to adverse reactions to molindone.
- Knowledge deficit related to molindone therapy.

Nursing interventions

- *Contraindicated* in coma or severe CNS depression.
- *Use cautiously* when increased physical activity would be harmful, as this agent increases activity; in seizures (may lower seizure threshold), suicide risk, suspected brain tumor, or intestinal obstruction.
- Tardive dyskinesia may occur after prolonged use. It may not appear until months or years later and may disappear spontaneously or persist for life despite discontinuation of drug.
- Neuroleptic malignant syndrome is rare, but frequently fatal. It is not necessarily related to length of drug use or type of neuroleptic, but over 60% of affected patients are men. Watch for symptoms.
- Acute dystonic reactions may be treated with I.V. diphenhydramine.
- Warn against activities that require alertness or good psychomotor coordination until CNS effects of the drug are known. Drowsiness and dizziness usually subside after first few weeks.
- Dry mouth may be relieved with sugarless gum, sour hard candy, or rinsing with mouthwash.
- Drug is the only dihydroindolone derivative.
- Dose of 10 mg is therapeutic equivalent of 100 mg chlorpromazine.
- May be administered in a single daily dose.

General

Classification: mineralocorticoid replacement (mineralocorticoid, glucocorticoid). **Pregnancy risk category:** C.

Mechanism of action

Increases sodium reabsorption and potassium and hydrogen secretion at the nephron's distal convoluted tubule.

Indications and dosage

• Adrenal insufficiency (partial replacement), adrenogenital syndrome. **Adults:** 0.1 to 0.2 mg P.O. daily.

Adverse reactions

CV: *sodium and water retention,* hypertension, cardiac hypertrophy, edema. **Metabolic:** hypokalemia.

Interactions

Potassium-depleting drugs such as thiazide diuretics: enhanced potassium-wasting effects of fludrocortisone. Monitor serum potassium levels.

Nursing diagnoses

• Fluid volume deficit related to the patient's underlying condition.
• Fluid volume excess related to high risk of sodium and water retention.
• Knowledge deficit related to fludrocortisone therapy.

Nursing interventions

• *Contraindicated* in hypertension, CHF, or cardiac disease.
• *Use cautiously* in patients with Addison's disease.
• Be aware that fludrocortisone is also prescribed to treat chronic severe orthostatic hypotension caused by levodopa therapy or diabetes mellitus.
• Know that fludrocortisone has potent mineralocorticoid effects. Usual doses, however, produce little glucocorticoid effect.
• Expect to use fludrocortisone with cortisone or hydrocortisone in adrenal insufficiency.
• Monitor patient's blood pressure and serum electrolyte levels regularly. Weigh patient daily; report sudden weight gain to doctor.
• Inform patient that mild peripheral edema is common. Tell him to report worsening symptoms, such as hypotension, weakness, cramping, and palpitations, to the doctor.
• Unless contraindicated, give low-sodium diet high in potassium and protein. Potassium supplement may be needed.
• Be alert for additional potassium depletion from diuretics and amphotericin B.

General

Classification: antineoplastic (antibiotic). **Pregnancy risk category:** D.

Mechanism of action

Not fully understood; probably cell cycle-nonspecific. Reacts with DNA, producing cytotoxic effect.

Indications and dosage

- Combination initial therapy for acute nonlymphocytic leukemia (ANL). **Adults:** induction begins with 12 mg/m² I.V. daily on days 1 through 3, in combination with cytosine arabinoside 100 mg/m² daily on days 1 through 7. A second induction may be given if response is not adequate. Maintenance therapy: 12 mg/m² on days 1 and 2 with cytosine arabinoside administered on days 1 through 5.

Adverse reactions

Blood: ***myelosuppression.*** **CNS:** ***seizures,*** headache. **CV:** ***CHF, arrhythmias,*** tachycardia. **EENT:** conjunctivitis. **GI:** *bleeding, abdominal pain, diarrhea, nausea, mucositis, stomatitis, vomiting.* **Respiratory:** dyspnea, cough. **Skin:** petechiae, ecchymoses. **Other:** alopecia, jaundice, fever, hyperuricemia, renal failure.

Interactions

Heparin: incompatible when mixed together.

Nursing diagnoses

- High risk for fluid volume deficit related to adverse drug reactions.
- Altered protection related to drug-induced myelosuppression.
- Knowledge deficit related to mitoxantrone therapy.

Nursing interventions

- *Contraindicated* in patients with hypersensitivity to mitoxantrone.
- *Use cautiously* in patients with prior exposure to anthracyclines or other cardiotoxic drugs.
- Uric acid nephropathy can be avoided by adequately hydrating the patient before and during therapy. Administer allopurinol as ordered.
- Patients with significant myelosuppression should not receive mitoxantrone unless the benefits outweigh the risks.
- Hematologic and chemistry laboratory parameters should be monitored closely.
- **I.V. use:** Available as an aqueous solution of 2 mg/ml in volumes of 10, 12.5, and 15 ml. Dilute in at least 50 ml of 0.9% sodium chloride injection or D_5W injection. Administer by direct injection into a free-flowing I.V. of 0.9% sodium chloride or D_5W injection over at least 3 minutes. Mixing with other drugs is not recommended.
- Store undiluted solution at room temperature. Once diluted, the mixture is stable for 48 hours at room temperature.
- Exercise extreme caution when preparing or administering mitoxantrone to avoid mutagenic, teratogenic, and carcinogenic risks. Use a biological containment cabinet, wear gloves and mask, and use syringes with luer-lock fittings. Clean spills with a calcium hypochlorite solution (6 parts calcium hypochlorite to 13 parts of water for each 1 part of mitoxantrone). Correctly dispose of needles, vials, and unused drug, and avoid contaminating work surfaces. Avoid inhalation of dust or vapors and contact with skin or mucous membranes. If eye contact occurs, irrigate with water or sodium chloride solution and consult an ophthalmologist. If skin contact occurs, irrigate the area with water.
- Treat infections with antibiotics, as ordered. If severe nonhematologic toxicity occurs during the first course of therapy, delay the second course until patient recovers.
- Inform patients that urine may appear blue-green within 24 hours after administration and some bluish discoloration of the sclera may occur, but that these effects are not harmful.

General

Classification: antidote (benzodiazepine antagonist). **Pregnancy risk category:** C.

Mechanism of action

Competitively inhibits the actions of benzodiazepines on the gamma-aminobutyric acid-benzodiazepine receptor complex.

Indications and dosage

- Complete or partial reversal of the sedative effects of benzodiazepines after anesthesia or short diagnostic procedures (conscious sedation). **Adults:** initially, 0.2 mg I.V. over 15 seconds. If patient does not reach the desired level of consciousness after 45 seconds, repeat dose. Repeat at 1-minute intervals until a cumulative dose of 1 mg has been given (initial dose plus four additional doses). Most patients respond after 0.6 to 1 mg of drug. In case of resedation, dosage may be repeated after 20 minutes; however, no more than 1 mg should be given at any one time, and no more than 3 mg/hour.
- Management of suspected benzodiazepine overdose. **Adults:** initially, 0.2 mg I.V. over 15 seconds. If patient does not reach the desired level of consciousness after 30 seconds, administer 0.3 mg over 30 seconds. If patient still does not respond adequately, give 0.5 mg over 30 seconds; repeat 0.5-mg doses at 1-minute intervals until a cumulative dose of 3 mg has been given. Most patients with benzodiazepine overdose respond to cumulative doses between 1 and 3 mg; rarely, patients who respond partially after 3 mg may require additional doses. Do not give more than 5 mg over 5 minutes initially. Sedation that persists after this dosage is unlikely to be caused by benzodiazepines. In case of resedation, dosage may be repeated after 20 minutes; however, no more than 1 mg should be given at any one time, and no more than 3 mg/hour.

Adverse reactions

CNS: *dizziness, abnormal or blurred vision, headache,* ***seizures,*** fatigue, agitation, emotional lability. **CV:** ***arrhythmias,*** cutaneous vasodilation. **GI:** nausea, vomiting. **Local:** *pain at injection site.* **Other:** *increased sweating.*

Interactions

Antidepressants; any drug that can cause seizures or arrhythmias: seizures or arrhythmias can develop after the effects of the benzodiazepine overdose is removed. Use flumazenil with caution in cases of mixed overdose.

Nursing diagnoses

- High risk for injury related to flumazenil-induced seizure activity.
- Decreased cardiac output related to flumazenil-induced arrhythmias.
- Knowledge deficit related to flumazenil therapy.

Nursing interventions

- *Contraindicated* in patients with hypersensitivity to flumazenil or benzodiazepines; patients who show evidence of serious tricyclic or tetracyclic antidepressant overdose; those who received the benzodiazepine to treat a potentially life-threatening condition (such as status epilepticus); and in benzodiazepine-dependent patients because the drug may precipitate seizures.
- *Use cautiously* in patients at high risk for developing seizures (including patients undergoing concurrent sedative-hypnotic drug withdrawal; patients who have recently received multiple doses of a parenteral benzodiazepine; patients displaying some signs of seizure activity (such as myoclonus); patients who may be at risk for unrecognized benzodiazepine dependence (such as intensive-care-unit patients); patients with head injury (because of the risk of precipitating seizures); those who have received neuromuscular blockers; and psychiatric patients because the drug has precipitated panic attacks in those with panic disorder.
- **I.V. use:** Administer drug into an I.V. line in a large vein with a free-flowing I.V. solution to minimize pain at the injection site. Compatible solutions include D_5W, lactated Ringer's injection, or 0.9% sodium chloride.

General

Classification: antineoplastic, antiadrenal agent (chlorophenothane [DDT] analogue). **Pregnancy risk category:** C.

Mechanism of action

Selectively destroys adrenocortical tissue and hinders extra-adrenal metabolism of cortisol.

Indications and dosage

- Inoperable adrenocortical cancer. **Adults:** initially, 1 to 6 g P.O. daily divided t.i.d. or q.i.d.; increased to 9 to 10 g P.O. daily, divided t.i.d. or q.i.d. Dosage is adjusted until maximum tolerated dosage is achieved (varies from 2 to 16 g daily but is usually 8 to 10 g daily). **Children:** initially, 0.1 to 0.5 mg/kg P.O. (1 to 2 g daily) in divided doses. Increase dosage based upon patient tolerance and response. Usual dose is 5 to 7 g daily in divided doses.

Adverse reactions

CNS: *depression, somnolence, lethargy, vertigo;* brain damage and dysfunction in long-term, high-dose therapy. **GI:** *severe nausea, vomiting,* diarrhea, anorexia. **Metabolic:** adrenal insufficiency. **Skin:** dermatitis, maculopapular rash.

Interactions

None significant.

Nursing diagnoses

- High risk for fluid volume deficit related to drug-induced adverse reactions.
- High risk for impaired skin integrity related to drug-induced adverse reactions.
- Knowledge deficit related to mitotane therapy.

Nursing interventions

- *Contraindicated* in patients with hypersensitivity to the drug.
- *Use cautiously* in patients with hepatic disease; however, dosage need not be routinely reduced in such patients.
- Drug should not be used in a patient with shock or trauma. Use of corticosteroids may avoid acute adrenocorticoid insufficiency and is usually required. Glucocorticoid dosage should be increased in periods of physiologic stress such as infection or trauma.
- Assess and record behavioral and neurologic signs daily throughout therapy. Prolonged therapy has been associated with significant neurologic impairment.
- Give antiemetic before administering to reduce nausea.
- Dosage may be reduced if GI or skin adverse reactions are severe.
- Obese patients may need higher dosage and may have longer-lasting adverse reactions, since drug distributes mostly to body fat.
- Warn ambulatory patient of CNS adverse reactions; advise him to avoid hazardous tasks requiring mental alertness or physical coordination.
- Monitor effectiveness by reduction in pain, weakness, anorexia.
- Adequate trial is at least 3 months, but therapy can continue if clinical benefits are observed.

General

Classification: anti-inflammatory agent (glucocorticoid). **Pregnancy risk category:** C.

Mechanism of action

Decreases inflammation, mainly by stabilizing leukocyte lysosomal membranes. Also suppresses the immune response, stimulates bone marrow, and influences protein, fat, and carbohydrate metabolism.

Indications and dosage

• Steroid-dependent asthma. **Adults and children over 6 years:** 2 oral inhalations (500 mcg) b.i.d. Don't exceed 4 inhalations b.i.d.

Adverse reactions

CNS: headache. **EENT:** watery eyes, throat irritation, hoarseness. **GI:** nausea, vomiting, dry mouth. **Other:** development of nasopharyngeal fungal infections.

Interactions

None significant.

Nursing diagnoses

• Ineffective airway clearance related to the patient's underlying condition.

• Altered oral mucous membrane related to drug-induced fungal infections.
• Knowledge deficit related to flunisolide therapy.

Nursing interventions

• *Contraindicated* in patients with hypersensitivity to the drug and in those with status asthmaticus or respiratory infections. Not recommended for use in asthma controlled by bronchodilators or other noncorticosteroids alone or for nonasthmatic bronchial diseases.
• If patient is a child receiving long-term therapy, tell parents that periodic growth measurements will be performed to check for evidence of hypothalamic-pituitary-adrenal axis suppression.
• Teach patient how to use a spacer device to ensure proper dosage administration.
• Teach patient to keep inhaler clean and unobstructed. Tell him to wash it with warm water and dry thoroughly after use.
• If patient is also using a bronchodilator, tell him to use it several minutes before flunisolide.
• Tell patient to allow 1 minute to elapse before repeating inhalations and to hold breath for a few seconds to enhance action of drug.
• Warn patient never to use flunisolide to relieve an emergency asthma attack because drug takes too long to work.
• Check mucous membranes frequently for signs of fungal infection. To prevent such infection, tell patient to gargle or rinse his mouth with water after using the inhaler. Caution him not to swallow the water.
• Store medication between 36° and 86° F (2° and 30° C). Tell patient to warm cannister to room temperature before use by keeping it in his pocket. If the canister is cold, the proper dose of medication may not be delivered.
• If patient has received long-term oral corticosteroid therapy, withdraw medication slowly.

General

Classification: antiulcer agent, gastric mucosal protectant (prostaglandin E_1 analogue). **Pregnancy risk category:** X.

Mechanism of action

Replaces gastric prostaglandins that are depleted by NSAID therapy. It also decreases basal and stimulated gastric acid secretion and may increase gastric mucus and bicarbonate production.

Indications and dosage

• Prevention of NSAID-induced gastric ulcers in elderly or debilitated patients at high risk of complications from gastric ulcer, and patients with a history of NSAID-induced ulcers. **Adults:** 200 mcg P.O. q.i.d. with food. If this dosage isn't tolerated, it may be decreased to 100 mcg P.O. q.i.d.

Adverse reactions

CNS: headache. **GI:** diarrhea, abdominal pain, nausea, flatulence, dyspepsia, vomiting, constipation. **GU:** hypermenorrhea, dysmenorrhea, spotting, cramps, menstrual disorders.

Interactions

Antacids: reduced plasma levels when administered concomitantly. Not considered significant.

Nursing diagnoses

• Pain related to the patient's underlying condition.
• Diarrhea related to adverse GI reactions to misoprostol.
• Knowledge deficit related to misoprostol therapy.

Nursing interventions

• *Contraindicated* for use in pregnant women and in patients who have a history of an allergic response to prostaglandins.
• Misoprostol should not be routinely administered to women of childbearing age unless they are at high risk of developing ulcers or complications from NSAID-induced ulcers.
• Special precautions must be taken to prevent the use of this drug during pregnancy. The patient must be fully aware of the dangers of misoprostol to a fetus, and must receive both oral and written warnings regarding these dangers. She must be capable of complying with effective contraceptive means, and must have a negative serum pregnancy test within 2 weeks of initiating therapy.
• Misoprostol therapy must not begin until the second or third day of the next normal menstrual period.
• Instruct *ALL* patients not to share misoprostol with anyone else. They should be aware that when taken by a pregnant patient this drug may cause miscarriage, often with potentially life-threatening bleeding. Concomitant ingestion of food or antacids seems to reduce maximal plasma concentrations of misoprostol, but this doesn't appear to impair the drug's effectiveness.
• Used investigationally for the prophylaxis and treatment of gastric ulcers, reflux esophagitis, alcohol-induced gastritis, hemorrhagic gastritis, and fat malabsorptions in patients with cystic fibrosis.

General

Classification: antineoplastic (antimetabolite).
Pregnancy risk category: D.

Mechanism of action

Inhibits DNA synthesis.

Indications and dosage

• Colon, rectal, breast, ovarian, cervical, bladder, liver, and pancreatic cancer. **Adults:** 12.5 mg/kg I.V. daily for 3 to 5 days q 4 weeks; or 15 mg/kg weekly for 6 weeks. (Dosages recommended based on lean body weight.) Maximum single recommended dose is 800 mg, although higher single doses (up to 1.5 g) have been used. The injectable form has been given orally but is not recommended.
• Multiple actinic (solar) keratoses; superficial basal cell carcinoma. **Adults:** apply cream or topical solution b.i.d.

Adverse reactions

Blood: ***leukopenia,*** thrombocytopenia, anemia; WBC nadir 9 to 14 days after first dose; platelet nadir in 7 to 14 days. **CNS:** acute cerebellar syndrome, ataxia, confusion, disorientation, euphoria, headache, nystagmus. **GI:** *stomatitis, GI ulcer, nausea, vomiting, diarrhea, anorexia.* **Skin:** (I.V. use) *dermatitis,* hyperpigmentation, nail changes, pigmented palmar creases. **Local:** *erythema, pain, burning, pruritus;* (topical use) contact dermatitis, *hyperpigmentation,* soreness, suppuration, swelling. **Other:** *reversible alopecia, weakness, malaise.*

Interactions

Leucovorin calcium, prior treatment with alkylating agents: increased toxicity of fluorouracil. Use with extreme caution.

Nursing diagnoses

• Altered protection related to fluorouracil-induced myelosuppression and immunosuppression.
• Altered oral mucous membrane related to fluorouracil-induced stomatitis.
• Knowledge deficit related to fluorouracil therapy.

Nursing interventions

• *Contraindicated* in poor nutritional states and bone marrow suppression (leukocyte counts less than or equal to 5,000/mm^3 or platelet counts less than or equal to 100,000/mm^3) and in those who have had major surgery within the previous month.
• *Use cautiously* after high-dose pelvic irradiation or use of alkylating agents or in patients with impaired hepatic or renal function or widespread neoplastic infiltration of bone marrow.
• Give antiemetic before administering drug to reduce nausea. Watch for stomatitis or diarrhea. Use topical oral anesthetic to soothe lesions. Discontinue drug if diarrhea occurs.
• Monitor WBC and platelet counts daily. Consider protective isolation if WBC count is below 2,000/mm^3. Watch for ecchymoses, petechiae, easy bruising, and anemia.
• Encourage good and frequent oral hygiene to prevent superinfection of denuded mucosa.
• Warn patient to avoid exposure to strong sunlight or ultraviolet light. Encourage use of sunscreens. If erythematous, desquamative rash of the hands and feet develops, treat with pyridoxine (50 to 150 mg P.O. daily) for 5 to 7 days.
• **I.V. use:** Slowing infusion rate from 2 to 8 hours lessens toxicity. Don't refrigerate drug or use cloudy solution. If crystals form, redissolve by warming. Use plastic I.V. containers for administering continuous infusions to keep solution stable.
• Follow institutional policy to reduce carcinogenic, mutagenic, and teratogenic risks.
• **Topical use:** Apply with caution near eyes, nose, and mouth; avoid occlusive dressings.
• Know that application to large ulcerated areas may cause systemic toxicity. Ingestion and systemic absorption may cause leukopenia, thrombocytopenia, stomatitis, diarrhea, or GI ulceration, bleeding, and hemorrhage.
• Sometimes ordered as 5-fluorouracil or 5-FU. The numeral 5 is part of drug name and should not be confused with dosage units.

General

Classification: antihypertensive (peripheral vasodilator). **Pregnancy risk category:** C.

Mechanism of action

Produces direct arteriolar vasodilation.

Indications and dosage

- Severe hypertension. **Adults:** 5 mg P.O. initially as a single dose. Effective dosage range is usually 10 to 40 mg daily. Maximum dosage is 100 mg daily. **Children under 12 years:** 0.2 mg/kg as a single daily dose. Effective dosage range usually is 0.25 to 1 mg/kg daily. Maximum dosage is 50 mg.

Adverse reactions

CV: *edema, tachycardia, pericardial effusion and tamponade,* ***CHF,*** ECG changes. **Skin:** rash, ***Stevens-Johnson syndrome.*** **Other:** *hypertrichosis* (elongation, thickening, and enhanced pigmentation of fine body hair), breast tenderness.

Interactions

Guanethidine: severe orthostatic hypotension. Advise patient to stand up slowly.

Nursing diagnoses

- Altered tissue perfusion (renal, cerebral, cardiopulmonary, and peripheral) related to the patient's underlying condition.
- Fluid volume excess related to minoxidil-induced adverse reactions.
- Knowledge deficit related to minoxidil therapy.

Nursing interventions

- *Contraindicated* in pheochromocytoma. Patients with malignant hypertension should be hospitalized during initial therapy.
- A potent vasodilator; use only when other antihypertensives have failed.
- Instruct patient to take his own pulse. Patient should report an increase greater than 20 beats/minute to the doctor.
- Closely monitor blood pressure and pulse at beginning of therapy.
- Monitor intake and output and check for weight gain and edema. Tell outpatients to weigh themselves at least weekly and report substantial weight gain (more than 5 lb [2.27 kg] per week).
- Elderly patients may be more sensitive to hypotensive effects.
- About 8 out of 10 patients will experience hypertrichosis within 3 to 6 weeks of beginning treatment. Unwanted hair can be controlled with a depilatory or shaving. Assure patient that extra hair will disappear within 1 to 6 months of stopping minoxidil. Advise patient, however, not to discontinue drug without doctor's approval.
- Drug is usually prescribed with a beta-blocking drug to control tachycardia and a diuretic to counteract fluid retention. Make sure patient complies with total treatment regimen.
- Teach patient about his disease and therapy. Explain the importance of taking this drug as prescribed, even when he's feeling well. Tell outpatient not to discontinue drug suddenly, but to call the doctor if unpleasant adverse reactions occur.
- A patient package insert has been prepared by the manufacturer of minoxidil, describing in layman's terms the drug and its adverse reactions. Be sure your patient receives this insert and reads it thoroughly. Provide an oral explanation also.
- Instruct patient to check with doctor or pharmacist before taking OTC medications.
- Available as a topical solution (Rogaine) for the treatment of androgenetic alopecia in both males and females.
- Minoxidil is removed by hemodialysis. Be sure to administer dose after dialysis.

General

Classification: antidepressant (serotonin uptake inhibitor). **Pregnancy risk category:** B.

Mechanism of action

Inhibits the CNS neuronal uptake of serotonin. Not a tricyclic derivative; considered an atypical antidepressant.

Indications and dosage

- Short-term management of depressive illness. **Adults:** initially, 20 mg P.O. in morning; increase dosage according to patient response. May be given b.i.d. in morning and at noon. Maximum dosage is 80 mg/day.

Adverse reactions

CNS: *nervousness, anxiety, insomnia, headache, drowsiness, tremor, dizziness,* abnormal dreams. **CV:** palpitations, flushing, bradycardia, ***arrhythmias.*** **EENT:** flulike syndrome, nasal congestion, upper respiratory infection, pharyngitis, cough, sinusitis, visual disturbances, tinnitus, respiratory distress. **GI:** *nausea, diarrhea, dry mouth, anorexia, dyspepsia,* constipation, abdominal pain, vomiting, taste change, flatulence, increased appetite. **GU:** sexual dysfunction, urine retention. **Other:** muscle pain, *weight loss, rash, pruritus, urticaria, asthenia,* edema, lymphadenopathy.

Interactions

Diazepam: half-life may be prolonged. Drugs highly bound to plasma proteins (warfarin, digitoxin) can displace drug and cause toxic effects. **Insulin, oral antidiabetic agents:** fluoxetine alters blood glucose levels and may alter requirements for antidiabetic medication. Adjust dosage as ordered. **TCAs:** risk of increased adverse CNS effects. Avoid concomitant use. **Tryptophan:** agitation, GI distress, and restlessness.

Nursing diagnoses

- Ineffective individual coping related to the patient's underlying condition.
- Sleep pattern disturbance related to fluoxetine-induced insomnia and drowsiness.
- Knowledge deficit related to fluoxetine therapy.

Nursing interventions

- *Contraindicated* in patients with hypersensitivity to the drug and in patients taking MAO inhibitors within 14 days of starting therapy.
- *Use cautiously* in patients at high risk for suicide and in patients with a history of hepatic, renal, or CV disease; diabetes mellitus; or a history of seizures.
- Because fluoxetine commonly causes nervousness and insomnia, tell patient to avoid taking it in the afternoon.
- Warn patient to avoid driving or other hazardous activities that require alertness until CNS effects of the drug are known. Although fluoxetine is less sedating than other antidepressants, it may cause dizziness or drowsiness in some patients.
- Expect lower dosages or less frequent dosing for elderly or debilitated patients and patients with renal or hepatic dysfunction.
- Tell patient that clinical effects of dosage changes may not be evident for weeks and that full antidepressant effects may not appear for 4 or more weeks of treatment.
- Advise patient not to take any other drugs without consulting the doctor.
- If skin rash or pruritus occur (usually early in therapy), treat with antihistamines or topical corticosteroids.

General

Classification: antibiotic (tetracycline). **Pregnancy risk category:** D.

Mechanism of action

Exerts bacteriostatic effect by binding to the 30S ribosomal subunit of microorganisms, thus inhibiting protein synthesis.

Indications and dosage

- Infections caused by sensitive gram-negative and gram-positive organisms, trachoma, amebiasis. **Adults:** 200 mg I.V., then 100 mg I.V. q 12 hours (don't exceed 400 mg/day); or 200 mg P.O. initially, then 100 mg P.O. q 12 hours. **Children over 8 years:** initially, 4 mg/kg P.O. or I.V., followed by 2 mg/kg q 12 hours. (Give I.V. in 500- to 1,000-ml solution without calcium over 6 hours.)
- Gonorrhea in patients sensitive to penicillin. **Adults:** initially, 200 mg P.O., then 100 mg q 12 hours for at least 4 days.
- Syphilis in patients sensitive to penicillin. **Adults:** initially, 200 mg P.O., then 100 mg q 12 hours for 10 to 15 days.
- Meningococcal carrier state. 100 mg P.O. q 12 hours for 5 days.
- Uncomplicated urethral, endocervical, or rectal infection caused by *Chlamydia trachomatis* or *Ureaplasma urealyticam.* **Adults:** 100 mg P.O. b.i.d. for at least 7 days.
- Uncomplicated gonoccocal urethritis in men. **Adults:** 100 mg P.O. b.i.d. for 5 days.

Adverse reactions

Blood: neutropenia, eosinophilia. **CNS:** *light-headedness, dizziness from vestibular toxicity.* **CV:** pericarditis. **EENT:** dysphagia, glossitis. **GI:** *anorexia,* epigastric distress, *nausea,* vomiting, *diarrhea,* enterocolitis, inflammatory lesions in anogenital region. **Metabolic:** increased BUN. **Skin:** *maculopapular and erythematous rashes, photosensitivity, increased pigmentation, urticaria.* **Local:** *thrombophlebitis.* **Other:** ***hypersensitivity, teeth discoloration.***

Interactions

Antacids and laxatives containing aluminum, magnesium, or calcium: decrease minocycline absorption. Give minocycline 1 hour before or 2 hours after any of the above. **Ferrous sulfate and other iron products, zinc:** decrease minocycline absorption. Give tetracyclines 3 hours after or 2 hours before iron. **Methoxyflurane:** may cause severe nephrotoxicity with minocycline. **Oral contraceptives:** decreased contraceptive effectiveness and increased risk of breakthrough bleeding.

Nursing diagnoses

- High risk for infection related to ineffectiveness of minocycline to eradicate the infection.
- High risk for fluid volume deficit related to adverse GI reactions to minocycline therapy.
- Knowledge deficit related to minocycline.

Nursing interactions

- *Use with extreme caution* in patients with impaired renal or hepatic function. Use during last half of pregnancy and in children under 8 years may cause permanent discoloration of teeth, enamel defects, and retardation of bone growth. If used in young adults, observe for brown pigmentation of teeth.
- With large doses or prolonged therapy, monitor for superinfection. Check patient's tongue for signs of monilia infection.
- Parenteral form may cause false-positive reading of Clinitest. All forms may cause false-negative reading of Clinistix or Tes-Tape.
- Check expiration date. Outdated or deteriorated tetracyclines have been associated with reversible nephrotoxicity.

General

Classification: androgen replacement, antineoplastic (androgen). **Pregnancy risk category:** X. **Controlled substance schedule:** III.

Mechanism of action

Stimulates target tissues to develop normally in androgen-deficient men.

Indications and dosage

• Hypogonadism and impotence caused by testicular deficiency. **Adults:** 2 to 10 mg P.O. daily.
• Palliation of breast cancer in women. **Adults:** 15 to 30 mg P.O. daily in divided doses. (Individualize dosages and reduce to minimum when effect is noted.)
• Postpartum breast engorgement. **Adults:** 2.5 mg P.O. followed by 5 to 10 mg daily for 5 days.

Adverse reactions

Androgenic: in women—*acne, edema, oily skin, weight gain, hirsutism, hoarseness,* clitoral enlargement, change in libido. In men—prepubertal: premature epiphyseal closure, *acne,* priapism, *growth of body and facial hair,* phallic enlargement; postpubertal: testicular atrophy, oligospermia, decreased ejaculatory volume, impotence, gynecomastia, epididymitis. **CV:** edema. **GI:** gastroenteritis, nausea, vomiting, constipation, change in appetite, diarrhea. **GU:** bladder irritability. **Hepatic:** reversible jaundice. **Hypoestrogenic:** in women—flushing; sweating; vaginitis with itching, drying, burning, or bleeding; menstrual irregularities; emotional lability. **Other:** hypercalcemia.

Interactions

Antidiabetic agents: altered dosage requirements. Monitor blood glucose levels in diabetics. **Hepatotoxic medications:** increased risk of hepatotoxicity. Monitor closely. **Oral anticoagulants:** altered dosage requirements. Monitor PT.

Nursing diagnoses

• Sexual dysfunction related to hormonal dysfunction.
• Body image disturbance related to adverse androgenic reactions associated with fluoxymesterone.
• Knowledge deficit related to fluoxymesterone therapy.

Nursing interventions

• *Contraindicated* in prostatic hypertrophy with obstruction; carcinoma of male breast; prostatic cancer; cardiac, hepatic, or renal decompensation; nephrosis; hypercalcemia; in premature infants; during pregnancy; and in breast-feeding women.
• *Use cautiously* in prepubertal males; diabetes or coronary disease; and patients taking corticotropin, corticosteroids, or anticoagulants.
• Avoid use in women of childbearing age until pregnancy is ruled out. Stress importance of using a nonhormonal contraceptive during therapy.
• Be aware that when used in breast cancer, subjective effects may not be seen for about 1 month and objective effects not for 3 months.
• To decrease risk of vaginitis, advise washing after intercourse and wearing cotton underwear.
• Inform women taking drug for breast cancer palliation that virilization may occur because of dosage required. Tell patient to report such effects immediately, as they may be irreversible.
• Tell women to report menstrual irregularities; discontinue therapy pending etiologic determination.
• Watch for signs of jaundice, which may be reversed by dosage adjustment. If liver function tests are abnormal, therapy should be stopped.
• Observe patient on concomitant anticoagulant therapy for ecchymotic areas, petechiae, or abnormal bleeding. Monitor PT.
• Watch for signs of hypoglycemia in patients with diabetes. Check blood glucose levels. Dosage of antidiabetic drug may need adjustment.
• Tell patient to eat a diet high in calories and protein unless contraindicated; to eat small, frequent meals; and to take drug with food if GI upset occurs.

General

Classification: laxative (lubricant oil). **Pregnancy risk category:** C.

Mechanism of action

Increases water retention in the stool by creating a barrier between colon wall and feces that prevents colonic reabsorption of fecal water.

Indications and dosage

• Constipation; preparation for bowel studies or surgery. **Adults:** 5 to 45 ml P.O. h.s.; or 120 ml enema. **Children:** 5 to 20 ml P.O. h.s.; or 30 to 60 ml enema.

Adverse reactions

GI: *nausea;* vomiting; diarrhea in excessive use; *abdominal cramps,* especially in severe constipation; decreased absorption of nutrients and fat-soluble vitamins, resulting in deficiency; and slowed healing after hemorrhoidectomy. **Skin:** pruritus. **Other:** laxative dependence in long-term or excessive use, ***lipid pneumonitis.***

Interactions

Docusate salts: may increase mineral oil absorption and cause lipid pneumonia. Don't administer together. **Fat-soluble vitamins (A,D,E,K):** absorption may be decreased after prolonged administration.

Nursing diagnoses

• Constipation related to interruption of normal pattern of elimination characterized by infrequent or absent stools.
• Pain related to mineral oil-induced abdominal cramping.
• Knowledge deficit related to mineral oil therapy.

Nursing interventions

• *Contraindicated* in abdominal pain, nausea, vomiting, or other symptoms of appendicitis or acute surgical abdomen; and in fecal impaction, or intestinal obstruction or perforation. Enema contraindicated in children under 2 years.
• *Use cautiously* in young children; in elderly or debilitated patients because of susceptibility to lipid pneumonitis through aspiration, absorption, and transport from intestinal mucosa; and in rectal bleeding.
• Don't give drug with meals or immediately after, as it delays passage of food from stomach. More active on an empty stomach.
• To be taken only at bedtime. Warn patient not to take for more than 1 week.
• Give with fruit juices or carbonated drinks to disguise taste.
• Use when patient needs to ease the strain of evacuation.
• Warn patient of possible rectal leakage from excessive dosages so he can avoid soiling clothing.
• Before giving for constipation, determine if patient has adequate fluid intake, exercise, and diet. Tell him that dietary sources of bulk include bran and other cereals, fresh fruit, and vegetables.
• Onset of action is 6 to 8 hours.

General

Classification: antipsychotic (piperazine phenothiazine). **Pregnancy risk category:** C.

Mechanism of action

Blocks postsynaptic dopamine receptors in the brain.

Indications and dosage

• Psychotic disorders. **Adults:** initially, 0.5 to 10 mg (hydrochloride) P.O. daily in divided doses q 6 to 8 hours; may increase cautiously to 20 mg. Higher doses (50 to 100 mg) have been given. Maintenance dosage is 1 to 5 mg daily. I.M. doses are ⅓ to ½ oral doses. Lower dosages for geriatric patients (1 to 2.5 mg daily). **Children:** 0.25 to 3.5 mg (hydrochloride) P.O. daily in divided doses q 4 to 6 hours; or ⅓ to ½ of oral dose I.M.; maximum dosage is 10 mg daily. **Adults and children over 12 years:** 12.5 to 25 mg of long-acting esters (decanoate, enanthate) I.M. or S.C. q 1 to 6 weeks. Maintenance dosage is 25 to 100 mg p.r.n.

Adverse reactions

Blood: transient leukopenia, ***agranulocytosis.*** **CNS:** *extrapyramidal reactions (high incidence), tardive dyskinesia,* sedation (low incidence), pseudoparkinsonism, EEG changes, dizziness. **CV:** *orthostatic hypotension,* tachycardia, ECG changes. **EENT:** ocular changes, *blurred vision.* **GI:** *dry mouth, constipation.* **GU:** *urine retention,* dark urine, menstrual irregularities, gynecomastia, inhibited ejaculation. **Hepatic:** cholestatic jaundice, abnormal liver function tests. **Metabolic:** hyperprolactinemia. **Skin:** *photosensitivity,* allergic reactions. **Other:** weight gain; appetite increase; rarely, ***neuroleptic malignant syndrome*** (fever, tachycardia, tachypnea, diaphoresis). **With abrupt withdrawal of long-term therapy:** gastritis, nausea, vomiting, dizziness, tremor, feeling of warmth or cold, sweating, tachycardia, headache, insomnia.

Interactions

Alcohol, other CNS depressants: increased CNS depression. Avoid concomitant use. **Antacids:** inhibits absorption of oral phenothiazines. Separate antacid and phenothiazine doses by at least 2 hours. **Anticholinergics:** additive effects. Avoid concomitant use. **Barbiturates, lithium:** may decrease phenothiazine effect. Observe patient. **Centrally acting antihypertensives:** decreased antihypertensive effect.

Nursing diagnoses

• Impaired thought processes related to the patient's underlying condition.
• Sensory/perceptual alterations (visual) related to adverse drug reactions.
• Knowledge deficit related to fluphenazine therapy.

Nursing interventions

• *Contraindicated* in coma, CNS depression, bone marrow suppression, blood dyscrasias, subcortical or hepatic damage, and renal insufficiency and with use of spinal or epidural anesthetic or adrenergic blockers.
• *Use cautiously* in elderly or debilitated patients; in acutely ill or dehydrated children; and in hepatic disease; pheochromocytoma; arteriosclerotic, cerebrovascular, or CV disease; peptic ulcer; exposure to extreme heat or cold; respiratory disorders, hypocalcemia; seizure disorders; severe reactions to insulin or electroshock therapy; suspected brain tumor; intestinal obstruction; glaucoma; or prostatic hypertrophy. Use parenteral form cautiously in asthmatic patients and patients allergic to sulfites.

General

Classification: inotropic agent, vasodilator (bipyridine derivative). **Pregnancy risk category:** C.

Mechanism of action

Produces inotropic action by increasing cellular levels of cyclic adenosine monophosphate. Produces vasodilation by directly relaxing vascular smooth muscle.

Indications and dosage

• Short-term treatment of CHF. **Adults:** initial loading dose of 50 mcg/kg I.V., slowly administered over 10 minutes, followed by continuous I.V. infusion of 0.375 to 0.75 mcg/kg/minute. Adjust infusion dose according to clinical and hemodynamic responses. Typically given with digoxin and diuretics.

Adverse reactions

CNS: headache. **CV:** ***ventricular arrhythmias,*** *ventricular ectopic activity,* nonsustained ventricular tachycardia, ***sustained ventricular tachycardia.***

Interactions

Furosemide: immediate precipitation when mixed with I.V. milrinone. Don't administer through same I.V. line.

Nursing diagnoses

• Fluid volume excess related to ineffectiveness of milrinone to relieve CHF.
• Decreased cardiac output related to milrinone-induced arrhythmias.
• Knowledge deficit related to milrinone therapy.

Nursing interventions

• *Contraindicated* in patients with hypersensitivity to the drug and in patients with severe obstructive pulmonic or aortic valvular disease in lieu of surgery; also avoid use during acute phase of MI because safety and efficacy have not been established.
• *Use cautiously* in patients with atrial flutter or fibrillation because drug slightly shortens AV node conduction time and may increase ventricular response rate. If patient is to receive a digitalis glycoside, such therapy should begin before milrinone.
• Monitor patient concurrently receiving diuretics, especially if such therapy has decreased cardiac filling pressure.
• Be aware that inotropic agents may aggravate outflow tract obstruction in patients with hypertrophic subaortic stenosis.
• Patients treated with milrinone have exhibited supraventricular and ventricular arrhythmias. Studies have shown that milrinone isn't arrhythmogenic; however, patients receiving drug may be taking several other medications concurrently, which may increase potential for arrhythmias. Monitor patients who are at increased risk for arrhythmias.
• Monitor fluid and electrolyte status, blood pressure, heart rate, and renal function during therapy. Excessive decrease in blood pressure requires discontinuation or slower rate of infusion.
• Improvement of cardiac output may result in enhanced urine output. Expect dosage reduction in patient's diuretic therapy as CHF improves. Remember that potassium loss produced by excessive diuresis may predispose patient to digitalis toxicity.
• **I.V. use:** Prepare I.V. infusion solution using 0.45% or 0.9% sodium chloride injection or D_5W. Prepare 100 mcg/ml solution by adding 180 ml diluent per 20-mg (20-ml) vial. Prepare 150 mcg/ml solution by adding 113 ml diluent per 20-mg (20-ml) vial. Prepare 200 mcg/ml solution by adding 80 ml diluent per 20-mg (20-ml) vial.
• Dosage adjustments are necessary in patients with renal failure. If creatinine clearance is 50 ml/minute/1.73 m^2 or less, dosage should be carefully titrated to maximum clinical effect and shouldn't exceed 1.13 mg/kg/day. Consult manufacturer's literature for specific infusion rate information.

General

Classification: sedative-hypnotic (benzodiazepine). **Pregnancy risk category:** D. **Controlled substance schedule:** IV.

Mechanism of action

Acts on the limbic system, thalamus, and hypothalamus of the CNS to produce hypnotic effects.

Indications and dosage

- Insomnia. **Adults:** 15 to 30 mg P.O. h.s. May repeat dose once. **Adults over 65 years:** 15 mg P.O. h.s.

Adverse reactions

Blood: leukopenia, granulocytopenia. **CNS:** *daytime sedation, dizziness, drowsiness, disturbed coordination,* lethargy, confusion, *headache.* **GI:** nausea, vomiting, heartburn. **Metabolic:** elevated liver enzymes.

Interactions

Alcohol or other CNS depressants, including narcotic analgesics: excessive CNS depression. Use together cautiously. **Cimetidine:** increased sedation. Monitor carefully.

Nursing diagnoses

- Sleep pattern disturbance related to underlying patient problem.
- High risk for trauma related to adverse CNS reactions caused by flurazepam.
- Knowledge deficit related to flurazepam therapy.

Nursing interventions

- *Contraindicated* in patients with hypersensitivity to benzodiazepines.
- *Use cautiously* in patients with impaired hepatic or renal function, mental depression, suicidal tendencies, or history of drug abuse.
- Check hepatic and renal function and CBC before and periodically during long-term therapy. Drug may cause elevations in certain liver function tests (AST, ALT, total and direct bilirubin, and alkaline phosphatase).
- Assess an elderly patient's mental status before initiating therapy; such patients are more sensitive to the drug's adverse CNS reactions.
- Prevent hoarding or overdosing by patients who are depressed, suicidal, or drug-dependent or who have a history of drug abuse. Know that dependence is possible with long-term use.
- Warn patients to avoid hazardous activities requiring mental alertness or physical coordination. Supervise walking; raise bed rails, especially for elderly patients.
- Encourage patient to continue drug if it doesn't relieve insomnia the first night. Explain that effectiveness increases on second, third, and fourth nights of use because active metabolite accumulates.
- If flurazepam overdose occurs, be prepared to administer flumazenil (a specific benzodiazepine antagonist). Know that the duration of action of flumazenil is shorter than that of flurazepam, so resedation is possible.

General

Classification: sedative-hypnotic (benzodiazepine). **Pregnancy risk category:** D. **Controlled substance schedule:** IV.

Mechanism of action

Depresses the CNS at the limbic and subcortical levels of the brain.

Indications and dosage

- Preoperative sedation (to induce sleepiness or drowsiness and relieve apprehension). **Adults:** 0.07 mg to 0.08 mg/kg I.M. approximately 1 hour before surgery. May be administered with atropine or scopolamine and reduced doses of narcotics.
- Conscious sedation before short diagnostic or endoscopic procedures. **Adults:** initially, 0.035 mg/kg slowly I.V.(not to exceed 2.5 mg). Dose is then titrated in small amounts to a total dosage of 0.1 mg/kg.
- Induction of general anesthesia. **Adults:** 0.3 to 0.35 mg/kg I.V. over 20 to 30 seconds. Additional increments of 25% of the initial dose may be needed to complete induction. Up to 0.6 mg/kg total dosage may be given.

Adverse reactions

CNS: headache, oversedation, involuntary movements, combativeness. **CV:** variations in blood pressure and pulse rate. **GI:** nausea, vomiting, hiccups. **Local:** pain and tenderness at injection site. **Other:** decreased respiratory rate, apnea.

Interactions

CNS depressants: may increase the risk of apnea. Prepare to adjust drug dosage.

Nursing diagnoses

- Anxiety related to upcoming surgery or diagnostic procedure.
- Ineffective breathing pattern related to midazolam-induced respiratory depression.
- Knowledge deficit related to midazolam therapy.

Nursing interventions

- *Contraindicated* in acute narrow-angle glaucoma, shock, coma, or acute alcohol intoxication.
- *Use cautiously* in CHF, COPD, or renal disease and in elderly or debilitated patients.
- **I.V. use:** Before administering, have oxygen and resuscitation equipment available in case of severe respiratory depression. Excessive dosage or rapid infusion has been associated with respiratory arrest, particularly in elderly or debilitated patients. Administer slowly over at least 2 minutes, and wait at least 2 minutes when titrating doses to effect.
- When administering I.V., take care to avoid extravasation.
- Monitor blood pressure, heart rate and rhythm, respirations, airway integrity, and arterial oxygen saturation during procedure, especially in patients who have also been premedicated with narcotics.
- Midazolam has a beneficial amnestic effect, which diminishes patient's recall of perioperative events. This effect requires extra caution when teaching patients; written information, instruction of family members, and follow-up contact may be required.
- Advise caution with hazardous activities requiring mental alertness or physical coordination.
- When injecting I.M., give deep into a large muscle mass. May be mixed in the same syringe with morphine sulfate, meperidine, atropine sulfate, or scopolamine.
- If midazolam overdose occurs, flumazenil (a specific benzodiazepine antagonist) may be useful. The duration of action of flumazenil is shorter than that of midazolam, and resedation is possible.

General

Classification: antiarthritic agent (NSAID). **Pregnancy risk category:** B.

Mechanism of action

Interferes with prostaglandin synthesis.

Indications and dosage

- Rheumatoid arthritis and osteoarthritis. **Adults:** 200 to 300 mg P.O. daily, divided b.i.d. to q.i.d.

Adverse reactions

CNS: *headache,* anxiety, insomnia, increased reflexes, tremor, amnesia, asthenia, drowsiness, malaise, depression, dizziness. **CV:** *edema.* **EENT:** rhinitis, tinnitus, visual changes. **GI:** *dyspepsia, diarrhea, abdominal pain, nausea,* constipation, ***GI bleeding,*** flatulence, vomiting. **GU:** *symptoms suggesting urinary tract infection.* **Hepatic:** elevated liver enzymes. **Skin:** rash. **Other:** weight changes.

Interactions

Aspirin: decreased flurbiprofen levels. Concomitant use is not recommended. **Diuretics:** possible decreased diuretic effect. Monitor patient closely. **Oral anticoagulants:** increased bleeding tendencies. Monitor patient closely.

Nursing diagnoses

- Pain related to the patient's underlying condition.
- Diarrhea related to adverse GI reactions to flurbiprofen therapy.
- Knowledge deficit related to flurbiprofen therapy.

Nursing interventions

- *Contraindicated* in patients with hypersensitivity, including asthma or urticaria, to aspirin or NSAIDs.
- Teach patient the signs and symptoms of GI bleeding, and tell him to discontinue the drug and call the doctor if these symptoms appear. Serious GI toxicity can occur at any time with patients on long-term NSAID therapy.
- Closely monitor elderly or debilitated patients and patients with impaired hepatic or renal function. Such patients may be at risk for renal toxicity and should receive lower doses. Periodically monitor renal function.
- Monitor liver function studies, hematocrit determinations, and results of eye examinations if the patient is receiving long-term therapy.
- Tell patient to take drug with food, milk, or antacid if GI upset occurs.
- Advise patient to avoid hazardous activities that require mental alertness until the CNS effects of the drug are known.
- Tell patient to call doctor immediately if edema, substantial weight gain, black stools, skin rash, itching, or visual disturbances occur.

General

Classification: antifungal (imidazole derivative).
Pregnancy risk category: C.

Mechanism of action

Inhibits purine transport and DNA, RNA, and protein synthesis; increases cell wall permeability, making the fungus more susceptible to osmotic pressure.

Indications and dosage

- Systemic fungal infections (coccidioidomycosis, candidiasis, cryptococcosis, paracoccidioidomycosis), chronic mucocutaneous candidiasis. **Adults:** 200 to 3,600 mg/day by I.V. infusion. Dosages may vary with diagnosis and with infective agent. May divide daily dosage over 3 infusions, 200 to 1,200 mg per infusion. Dilute in at least 200 ml of 0.9% sodium chloride. Repeated courses may be needed because of relapse or reinfection. **Children 1 year and over:** 20 to 40 mg/kg/day by I.V. infusion. Do not exceed 15 mg/kg per infusion.
- Fungal meningitis. **Adults:** 20 mg intrathecally as an adjunct to I.V. administration, q 3 to 7 days.

Adverse reactions

Blood: transient decreases in hematocrit, thrombocytopenia. **CNS:** dizziness, drowsiness. **CV:** ***cardiorespiratory arrest.*** **GI:** *nausea, vomiting,* diarrhea. **Metabolic:** *transient decrease in serum sodium.* **Skin:** *pruritic rash.* **Local:** *phlebitis at injection site.* **Other:** fever, chills.

Interactions

Oral anticoagulants: enhanced anticoagulant effect. Monitor closely.

Nursing diagnoses

- High risk for infection related to ineffectiveness of miconazole to eradicate the fungal infection.
- Impaired tissue integrity related to miconazole-induced pruritic rash.
- Knowledge deficit related to miconazole therapy.

Nursing interventions

- *Use cautiously.* Acute cardiorespiratory arrest has occurred with the first dose. The first dose should be given under continuous medical supervision with emergency resuscitative equipment immediately available.
- **I.V. use:** Use of I.V. miconazole has been replaced largely by newer drugs that are better tolerated.
- Rapid injection of undiluted miconazole may produce arrhythmias. Dilute infusion with at least 200 ml of 0.9% sodium chloride solution and infuse over 30 to 60 minutes.
- Premedication with antiemetic may lessen nausea and vomiting.
- Avoid administration at mealtime in order to lessen GI adverse reactions.
- Pruritic rash may persist for weeks after drug is discontinued. Pruritus may be controlled with oral or I.V. diphenhydramine.
- In treatment of fungal meningitis and urinary bladder infections, must be supplemented with intrathecal administration and bladder irrigation, respectively.
- Inform patient that adequate therapeutic response may take weeks or months.
- Monitor levels of hemoglobin, hematocrit, electrolytes, and lipids regularly. Transient elevations in serum cholesterol and triglycerides may be due to castor oil vehicle.

General

Classification: antineoplastic (nonsteroidal antiandrogen). **Pregnancy risk category:** D.

Mechanism of action

Inhibits androgen uptake or prevents binding of androgens in nucleus of cells within target tissues.

Indications and dosage

- Treatment of metastatic prostatic carcinoma (stage D_2) in combination with luteinizing hormone-releasing hormone analogs such as leuprolide acetate. **Adults:** 250 mg P.O. q. 8 hours.

Adverse reactions

CNS: *loss of libido.* **CV:** edema, hypertension. **GI:** *diarrhea, nausea, vomiting.* **GU:** *impotence.* **Metabolic:** elevated hepatic enzymes, hepatitis. **Skin:** rash, photosensitivity. **Other:** *hot flashes, gynecomastia.*

Interactions

None reported.

Nursing diagnoses

- High risk for fluid volume deficit related to adverse drug reactions.
- Sexual dysfunction related to drug-induced impotence.
- Knowledge deficit related to flutamide therapy.

Nursing interventions

- *Contraindicated* in patients with hypersensitivity to flutamide.
- Monitor liver function studies if patient is receiving prolonged therapy with flutamide.
- Inform patient that flutamide must be taken continuously with agent used for medical castration (such as leuprolide) to allow the full benefits of therapy. Leuprolide suppresses testosterone production, whereas flutamide inhibits testosterone action at the cellular level. Together they impair the growth of androgen-responsive tumors. Tell patient not to discontinue either drug without consulting the doctor.

General

Classification: antibiotic (extended-spectrum penicillin). **Pregnancy risk category:** B.

Mechanism of action

Bactericidal against microorganisms by inhibiting cell wall synthesis during active multiplication. Bacteria resist mezlocillin by producing penicillinases—enzymes that hydrolyze mezlocillin.

Indications and dosage

• Systemic infections caused by susceptible strains of gram-positive and especially gram-negative organisms (including *Proteus, Pseudomonas aeruginosa). **Adults:** 200 to 300 mg/kg daily I.V. or I.M. given in 4 to 6 divided doses. Usual dose is 3 g q 4 hours or 4 g q 6 hours. For very serious infections, up to 24 g daily may be administered. **Children up to 12 years:** 50 mg/kg q 4 hours by I.V. infusion or direct I.V. injection.

Adverse reactions

Blood: ***bleeding with high doses,*** neutropenia, eosinophilia, leukopenia, ***thrombocytopenia.*** **CNS:** neuromuscular irritability. **GI:** nausea, diarrhea. **Metabolic:** *hypokalemia.* **Local:** pain at injection site, vein irritation, phlebitis. **Other:** hypersensitivity (edema, fever, chills, rash, pruritus, urticaria, ***anaphylaxis****), overgrowth of nonsusceptible organisms.*

Interactions

Aminoglycoside antibiotics (such as gentamicin and tobramycin): chemically incompatible. Don't mix together in I.V. solution. Give 1 hour apart, especially in patients with renal insufficiency. **Probenecid:** increases blood levels of mezlocillin. Probenecid may be used for this purpose.

Nursing diagnoses

• High risk for injury related to ineffectiveness of mezlocillin to eradicate the infection.
• Impaired tissue integrity related to mezlocillin-induced thrombophlebitis at the injection site.
• Knowledge deficit related to mezlocillin therapy.

Nursing interventions

• *Use cautiously* in patients with hypersensitivity to cephalosporins (possible cross-hypersensitivity) and in bleeding tendencies, uremia, and hypokalemia.
• Before giving mezlocillin, ask patient if he's had any allergic reactions to penicillin. A negative history of penicillin allergy, however, is no guarantee against future allergic reaction.
• Obtain specimen for culture and sensitivity before first dose. Therapy may begin pending test results.
• Dosage should be altered in patients with impaired renal function.
• Check CBC and platelets frequently. Drug may cause thrombocytopenia.
• Monitor serum potassium level.
• Patient with high serum level of this drug may have seizures. Institute seizure precautions.
• **I.V. use:** When giving I.V., mix with D_5W or other suitable I.V. fluids. Give I.V. intermittently to prevent vein irritation. Change site every 48 hours.
• With large doses and prolonged therapy, bacterial and fungal superinfections may occur, especially in elderly, debilitated, or immunosuppressed patients. Monitor patient closely.
• Compared with similar antibiotics, such as carbenicillin and ticarcillin, mezlocillin is less likely to cause hypokalemia.
• Give mezlocillin at least 1 hour before bacteriostatic antibiotics.

General

Classification: antihypertensive (ACE inhibitor).
Pregnancy risk category: D.

Mechanism of action

Inhibits ACE, preventing conversion of angiotensin I to angiotensin II. This decreases peripheral arterial resistance, resulting in decreased aldosterone secretion, which reduces sodium and water retention and lowers blood pressure. Fosinopril also has antihypertensive activity in patients with low-renin hypertension.

Indications and dosage

- Hypertension. **Adults:** initially, 10 mg P.O. daily; adjust dose based on blood pressure response at peak and trough levels. Usual dose is 20 to 40 mg, up to 80 mg. Dose may be divided.

Adverse reactions

CNS: headache, dizziness, fatigue, light-headedness, syncope, memory disturbances, mood change, paresthesia, sleep disturbance, drowsiness, weakness, ***CVA.*** **CV:** chest pain, angina, ***MI, hypertensive crisis,*** rhythm disturbances, palpitations, hypotension, flushing, claudications, orthostatic hypotension. **EENT:** tinnitus, vision disturbances, eye irritation, epistaxis. **GI:** nausea, vomiting, diarrhea, pancreatitis, hepatitis, dysphagia, abdominal distention, abdominal pain, flatulence, constipation, heartburn, appetite change, weight change, dry mouth. **GU:** sexual dysfunction, decreased libido, urinary frequency, renal insufficiency, acute renal failure. **Respiratory:** cough, ***bronchospasm,*** pharyngitis, sinusitis, rhinitis, laryngitis, hoarseness. **Skin:** urticaria, rash, photosensitivity, pruritus. **Other:** ***angioedema,*** fever, arthralgia, musculoskeletal pain, myalgia, jaundice, gout.

Interactions

Antacids: may impair absorption. Separate administration times by at least 2 hours. **Diuretics, other antihypertensives:** risk of excessive hypotension. Discontinue diuretic or lower dose of fosinopril as needed. **Lithium:** increased serum lithium levels and lithium toxicity. Avoid concomitant use. **Potassium-sparing diuretics, potassium supplements, sodium substitutes containing potassium:** risk of hyperkalemia. Avoid concomitant use.

Nursing diagnoses

- High risk for injury related to patient's underlying condition.
- Knowledge deficit related to fosinopril therapy.

Nursing interventions

- *Contraindicated* in patients with hypersensitivity to ACE inhibitors or with a history of angioedema.
- *Use cautiously* in impaired renal or hepatic function; in renal insufficiency or diabetes mellitus; and with use of potassium-sparing diuretics, potassium supplements, and sodium substitutes containing potassium. Avoid use in pregnant or breast-feeding women.
- If possible, discontinue diuretic therapy 2 to 3 days before starting fosinopril to reduce potential for excessive hypotensive response. If fosinopril does not adequately control blood pressure, diuretic may be reinstituted with care.
- Assess renal and hepatic function before and periodically throughout therapy. Monitor CBC with differential counts before and every 2 weeks for the first 3 months of therapy, and periodically thereafter. Monitor potassium levels.
- Tell patient to take drug on an empty stomach, 1 hour before or 2 hours after meals, or 2 hours after taking antacids. Warn him to take drug with caution in hot weather and during exercise and to avoid sodium substitutes.
- Tell patient to report any signs of infection; easy bruising or bleeding; swelling of tongue, lips, face, mucous membranes, eyes, lips, or extremities; difficulty swallowing or breathing; and hoarseness.

General

Classification: ventricular antiarrhythmic (lidocaine analogue). **Pregnancy risk category:** C.

Mechanism of action

A class Ib antiarrhythmic that depresses phase 0. It shortens the action potential. All class I drugs have membrane-stabilizing effects.

Indications and dosage

• Treatment of refractory ventricular arrhythmias, including ventricular tachycardia and premature ventricular contractions. **Adults:** 200 to 400 mg P.O. followed by 200 mg q 8 hours. May increase dose to 400 mg q 8 hours if satisfactory control is not obtained. (Some patients may respond well to an every-12-hour schedule. May give up to 450 mg q 12 hours.)

• Where available, mexiletine may be given I.V. **Adults:** following a loading dose of 200 to 250 mg I.V. at a rate of 25 mg/minute, prepare an infusion solution of 250 mg mexiletine/500 ml D_5W. Administer the first 120 ml (60 mg) over 1 hour. If clinical response is inadequate, give another bolus of 200 mg over 10 to 20 minutes. Maintenance dose is 0.5 mg/minute (1 ml/minute of prepared solution).

Adverse reactions

CNS: *tremor, dizziness,* blurred vision, ataxia, diplopia, confusion, nystagmus, nervousness, headache. **CV:** hypotension, bradycardia, widened QRS complex, ***new or worsened arrhythmias.*** **GI:** nausea, vomiting. **Skin:** rash.

Interactions

Cimetidine: increased mexiletine blood levels. Monitor carefully. **Phenytoin, rifampin, phenobarbital:** decreased mexiletine blood levels. Monitor carefully.

Nursing diagnoses

• Decreased cardiac output related to ineffectiveness of mexiletine.

• High risk for injury related to mexiletine-induced CNS reactions.

• Knowledge deficit related to mexiletine therapy.

Nursing interventions

• *Contraindicated* in cardiogenic shock or preexisting second- or third-degree AV block (if pacemaker is not present).

• Early sign of mexiletine toxicity is tremor, usually a fine tremor of the hands. This progresses to dizziness and later to ataxia and nystagmus as the drug's blood level increases. Question your patient about these symptoms.

• When changing from lidocaine to mexiletine, stop the infusion when the first mexiletine dose is given. Keep the infusion line open, however, until the arrhythmia appears to be satisfactorily controlled.

• May administer oral dose with meals to lessen GI distress.

• Therapeutic levels range from 0.75 to 2 mcg/ml.

• Monitor blood pressure and heart rate and rhythm frequently. Notify doctor of any significant change.

• Patients who respond well to mexiletine can often be maintained on a q 12 hour schedule. Notify doctor if you feel the patient is a good candidate for q 12 hour therapy. Twice-daily dosage eases compliance.

• **I.V. use:** Mexiletine injection is compatible with 0.9% sodium chloride, D_5W, 5% sodium bicarbonate, 1/6 M sodium lactate, and 10% fructose (levulose).

General
Classification: diuretic, antihypertensive (loop diuretic). **Pregnancy risk category:** C.

Mechanism of action
Inhibits reabsorption of sodium and chloride at the proximal portion of the ascending loop of Henle.

Indications and dosage
- Edema, acute pulmonary edema. **Adults:** 20 to 80 mg P.O. daily in a.m.; second dose can be given in 6 to 8 hours; carefully titrated up to 600 mg daily if needed. Or 20 to 40 mg I.M. or I.V., increased by 20 mg q 2 hours until desired response is achieved. I.V. dose should be given slowly over 1 to 2 minutes. For acute edema, 40 mg I.V. slowly, then 40 mg I.V. in 1½ hours if needed.
- Hypertension. **Adults:** 40 mg P.O. b.i.d. Adjust dose according to response. **Infants and children:** 2 mg/kg P.O. daily; dose increased by 1 to 2 mg/kg in 6 to 8 hours if needed; carefully titrated up to 6 mg/kg daily if needed.

Adverse reactions
Blood: ***agranulocytosis,*** leukopenia, thrombocytopenia. **CV:** volume depletion and dehydration, orthostatic hypotension. **EENT:** transient deafness with too-rapid I.V. injection. **GI:** abdominal discomfort and pain, diarrhea (with oral solution). **Metabolic:** hypokalemia; hypochloremic alkalosis; asymptomatic hyperuricemia; dilutional hyponatremia, hypocalcemia, or hypomagnesemia; hyperglycemia and impaired glucose tolerance. **Skin:** dermatitis.

Interactions
Aminoglycoside antibiotics: potentiated ototoxicity. **Antihypertensives:** increased risk of hypotension. **Chloral hydrate:** sweating, flushing with I.V. furosemide. **Clofibrate:** enhanced furosemide effects. **NSAIDs:** inhibited diuretic response.

Nursing diagnoses
- Fluid volume excess related to the patient's underlying condition as evidenced by edema.
- Altered urinary elimination related to diuretic therapy.
- Knowledge deficit related to furosemide therapy.

Nursing interventions
- *Contraindicated* in patients with anuria.
- *Use cautiously* in cardiogenic shock complicated by pulmonary edema, anuria, hepatic coma, or electrolyte imbalances. Drug is not routinely administered to women of childbearing age because its safety in pregnancy hasn't been established.
- Monitor blood pressure and pulse rate during rapid diuresis and routinely with chronic use; can lead to profound water and electrolyte depletion.
- Sulfonamide-sensitive patients may have allergic reactions to furosemide.
- If oliguria or azotemia develops or worsens, doctor may stop drug.
- Monitor serum electrolyte, BUN, and carbon dioxide frequently. Also monitor serum potassium level. Watch for signs of hypokalemia. Patients also on a digitalis glycoside have an increased risk of digitalis toxicity from the potassium-depleting effect.
- Monitor blood glucose levels in patients with diabetes. May treat severe hyperglycemia with oral antidiabetic agents.
- Monitor blood uric acid, especially in patients with a history of gout.
- **I.V. use:** Promotes calcium excretion. I.V. furosemide often used to treat hypercalcemia.
- To prepare parenteral furosemide for I.V. infusion, mix drug with D_5W, 0.9% sodium chloride solution, or lactated Ringer's solution. Use prepared infusion solution within 24 hours.
- Don't use parenteral route in infants and children unless oral dosage form is not practical.
- Give P.O. and I.M. preparations in a.m. to prevent nocturia. Give second doses in early afternoon.
- Elderly patients are especially susceptible to excessive diuresis, with potential for circulatory collapse and thromboembolic complications.
- Advise patients to report immediately ringing in ears, severe abdominal pain, or sore throat and fever; may indicate furosemide toxicity.

General

Classification: amebicide and trichomonacide (nitroimidazole). **Pregnancy risk category:** B.

Mechanism of action

A direct-acting trichomonacide and amebicide that works at intestinal and extraintestinal sites.

Indications and dosage

- Amebic hepatic abscess. **Adults:** 500 to 750 mg P.O. t.i.d. for 5 to 10 days. **Children:** 35 to 50 mg/kg daily (in three doses) for 10 days.
- Intestinal amebiasis. **Adults:** 750 mg P.O. t.i.d. for 5 to 10 days. **Children:** 35 to 50 mg/kg daily (oral iodoquinal in three doses) for 10 days.
- Trichomoniasis. **Adults** (both male and female): 250 mg P.O. t.i.d. for 7 days or 2 g P.O. in single dose; 4 to 6 weeks should elapse between courses of therapy.
- Treatment of bacterial infections caused by anaerobic microorganisms. **Adults:** Loading dose is 15 mg/kg I.V. (hydrochloride) over 1 hour. Maintenance dose is 7.5 mg/kg I.V. or P.O. q 6 hours. Administer first maintenance dose 6 hours following loading dose. Maximum dosage not to exceed 4 g daily.
- Giardiasis. **Adults:** 250 mg P.O. t.i.d. for 5 days. **Children:** 5 mg/kg P.O. t.i.d. for 5 days.

Adverse reactions

Blood: transient leukopenia, neutropenia. **CNS:** vertigo, headache, ataxia, incoordination, confusion, irritability, depression, restlessness, weakness, fatigue, drowsiness, insomnia, sensory neuropathy, paresthesia of extremities, psychic stimulation, seizures, neuromyopathy. **CV:** ECG change (flattened T wave), edema (with I.V. preparation). **GI:** abdominal cramping, stomatitis, *vomiting, anorexia,* diarrhea, constipation, proctitis, dry mouth. **GU:** darkened urine, polyuria, dysuria, pyuria, incontinence, cystitis, decreased libido, dyspareunia, dryness of vagina and vulva, sense of pelvic pressure. **Skin:** pruritus, flushing, rash. **Local:** *thrombophlebitis after I.V. infusion.* **Other:** overgrowth of nonsusceptible organisms, especially *Candida,* metallic taste, fever, gynecomastia.

Interactions

Alcohol: Disulfiram-like reaction (nausea, vomiting, headache, cramps, flushing). Don't use together. **Cimetidine:** increased risk of metronidazole toxicity. **Disulfiram:** acute psychoses and confusional states. Don't use together. **Oral anticoagulants:** increased anticoagulant effects. **Phenytoin, phenobarbital:** decreased metronidazole effectiveness.

Nursing diagnoses

- High risk for injury related to dosage regimen inadequate to alleviate infection.
- Altered nutrition: Less than body requirements, related to anorexia, nausea, and vomiting.
- Knowledge deficit related to metronidazole.

Nursing interventions

- *Use cautiously* in patients with a history of blood dyscrasia or CNS disorder, retinal or visual field changes, hepatic disease, alcoholism, or in conjunction with hepatotoxic drugs.
- If indicated during pregnancy for trichomoniasis, the 7-day regimen is preferred.
- Tell patient to avoid alcohol or alcohol-containing medications during therapy and for at least 48 hours after therapy is completed.
- Asymptomatic sexual partners of patients being treated for *Trichomonas vaginalis* infection should be treated simultaneously to avoid reinfection.
- **I.V. use:** Administer by slow infusion. Don't give I.V. push.

General

Classification: skeletal muscle relaxant (nondepolarizing neuromuscular blocker). **Pregnancy risk category:** C.

Mechanism of action

Precise mechanism unknown; the drug has no cytotoxic effects in animals. It appears to reduce hypercalcemia by inhibiting the resorption of bone and reducing bone turnover in patients with increased bone turnover.

Indications and dosage

- Treatment of symptomatic, unresponsive hypercalcemia caused by cancer. **Adults:** 200 mg/m^2 I.V. daily for 5 consecutive days or until serum calcium is normal. Administer as a constant infusion over 24 hours. Lower doses (100 mg/m^2) may be given to patients with mild hypercalcemia.

Adverse reactions

Blood: anemia, leukopenia. **CNS:** lethargy, confusion. **CV:** tachycardia, lower extremity edema, decreased mean systolic and diastolic blood pressures. **EENT:** visual or hearing impairment, acute optic neuritis. **GI:** nausea and vomiting, diarrhea, constipation. **GU:** ***acute renal failure,*** *increased BUN and creatinine levels.* **Respiratory:** dyspnea, crackles and rhonchi, pulmonary infiltrates, pleural effusion. **Metabolic:** *hypophosphatemia, hypocalcemia, decreased serum bicarbonate.*

Interactions

Nephrotoxic drugs, such as aminoglycosides or amphotericin B: increased risk of nephrotoxicity. Avoid concomitant use.

Nursing diagnoses

- Pain related to the underlying disease.
- Diarrhea related to adverse effects of the drug.
- Knowledge deficit related to gallium nitrate therapy.

Nursing interventions

- *Contraindicated* in patients with severe renal impairment. Keep in mind the association of hypercalcemia with decreased renal function in cancer patients. This drug should *not* be used in patients with asymptomatic hypercalcemia (generally, serum calcium levels of less than 12 mg/dl).
- Be sure the patient is adequately hydrated, either with oral fluids or I.V. sodium chloride solution, before using the drug and during the infusion. It is important to establish an adequate urine flow (2 liters per day) before treatment. Diuretic therapy is not recommended before the correction of hypovolemia. Avoid overhydration, especially in patients with decreased CV function.
- **I.V. use:** Dilute the daily dose in 1 liter of 0.9% sodium chloride injection or D_5W. Because the drug contains no preservatives, discard the unused portion.
- Rapid I.V. infusion or dosage over 200 mg/m^2 may increase the risk of nephrotoxicity or cause nausea and vomiting.
- If patient requires treatment with a potentially nephrotoxic drug such as an aminoglycoside, discontinue gallium nitrate therapy and continue hydration for several days after administration of the nephrotoxic drug. Monitor renal function closely.
- Monitor renal function, including intake and output and BUN and serum creatinine levels, during therapy. Discontinue the drug if serum creatinine rises above 2.5 mg/dl.
- Monitor serum calcium levels, and assess patient for signs of hypocalcemia (including a positive Chvostek's sign). If hypocalcemia occurs, discontinue the drug. Treatment of hypocalcemia may be required.
- Overdosage is usually treated with vigorous hydration, sometimes with diuretics, for 2 to 3 days. Carefully monitor the patient's intake and output and renal function. Short-term therapy with I.V. calcium may be needed.
- Transient hypophosphatemia is common. Patients may require oral phosphorus supplements.
- Advise patient to report hearing or vision problems.

General

Classification: antihypertensive (beta-adrenergic blocking agent). **Pregnancy risk category:** B.

Mechanism of action

Blocks cardiac beta receptors and depresses renin secretion.

Indications and dosage

- Hypertension; may be used alone or in combination with other antihypertensives. **Adults:** 50 mg b.i.d. or 100 mg once daily P.O. initially. Up to 200 to 400 mg daily in two to three divided doses. (No dosage recommendations for children.)
- Early intervention in acute MI. **Adults:** Three injections of 5-mg I.V. boluses q 2 minutes; 15 minutes after last dose, administer 50 mg P.O. q 6 hours for 48 hours. Maintenance dosage is 100 mg P.O. b.i.d.
- Angina pectoris. **Adults:** initially, 100 mg P.O. daily as a single dose. Increase dosage weekly until an adequate response or a pronounced decrease in heart rate is seen. Daily dosage beyond 400 mg has not been studied.

Adverse reactions

CNS: fatigue, lethargy, dizziness. **CV:** *bradycardia, hypotension, **CHF**,* peripheral vascular disease. **GI:** nausea, vomiting, diarrhea. **Skin:** rash. **Respiratory:** dyspnea, ***bronchospasm.*** **Other:** fever, arthralgia.

Interactions

Barbiturates, rifampin: increased metabolism of metoprolol. Monitor for decreased effect. **Chlorpromazine, cimetidine, verapamil:** decreased hepatic clearance. Monitor for greater beta-blocking effect. **Digitalis glycosides:** excessive bradycardia and increased depressant effect on myocardium. Use together cautiously. **Indomethacin:** decrease in antihypertensive effect. Monitor blood pressure and adjust dosage. **Insulin, oral antidiabetic agents:** can alter dosage requirements in previously stabilized diabetics. Observe patient carefully.

Nursing diagnoses

- Altered tissue perfusion (renal, cerebral, cardiopulmonary, and peripheral) related to the patient's underlying condition.
- High risk for injury related to adverse reactions to metoprolol.
- Knowledge deficit related to metoprolol therapy.

Nursing interventions

- *Contraindicated* in patients with hypersensitivity to the drug or other beta blockers and in patients with sinus bradycardia, heart block greater than first degree, cardiogenic shock, or overt cardiac failure.
- *Use cautiously* in heart failure, diabetes, respiratory or hepatic disease, or in patients taking other antihypertensives. Always check patient's apical pulse rate before giving this drug. If it's slower than 60 beats/minute, hold drug and call doctor.
- Although most patients with asthma and bronchitis can take this drug without worsening their condition, use doses over 100 mg daily cautiously.
- Monitor blood pressure frequently.
- Teach patient the importance of taking this drug as prescribed, even when he's feeling well. Tell outpatient not to discontinue this drug suddenly because this can exacerbate angina and MI. Drug must be withdrawn gradually over 1 to 2 weeks. Instruct patient to call doctor if unpleasant adverse reactions occur.
- Instruct patient to check with doctor or pharmacist before taking OTC medications.
- This drug masks common signs of shock and hypoglycemia.
- Food may increase absorption of metoprolol. Give consistently with meals.

General

Classification: antiviral (synthetic nucleoside). **Pregnancy risk category:** C.

Mechanism of action

Inhibits viral DNA synthesis of CMV.

Indications and dosage

- CMV retinitis treatment in immunocompromised individuals, including patients with AIDS. **Adults:** induction treatment – initially, 5 mg/kg I.V. q 12 hours for 14 to 21 days (normal renal function); maintenance treatment – 5 mg/kg I.V. daily for 7 days each week, or 6 mg/kg daily for 5 days each week.

Adverse reactions

Blood: *granulocytopenia,* ***thrombocytopenia.*** **CNS:** altered dreams, confusion, ataxia, dizziness, headache. **CV:** arrhythmias, hypotension, hypertension. **EENT:** retinal detachment in CMV retinitis patients. **GI:** nausea, vomiting, diarrhea, anorexia. **GU:** hematuria. **Local:** injection site inflammation, pain, phlebitis.

Interactions

Cytotoxic agents: additive toxic effects, especially hematologic effects and stomatitis. **Imipenem/cilastatin:** reports of seizure activity with concomitant use. **Probenecid:** increased ganciclovir blood levels. **Zidovudine:** increased incidence of granulocytopenia with concurrent use.

Nursing diagnoses

- High risk for injury related to ineffectiveness of ganciclovir to eradicate the infection.
- Altered protection related to ganciclovir-induced blood disorders.
- Knowledge deficit related to ganciclovir therapy.

Nursing interventions

- *Contraindicated* in patients with an absolute neutrophil count below 500/mm^3 or a platelet count below 25,000/mm^3.
- Dosage of ganciclovir should be reduced in patients with renal dysfunction.
- **I.V. use:** Do not administer S.C. or I.M.
- Infusion must take place over at least 1 hour. Use an infusion pump. Infusions faster than 60 minutes will result in increased toxicity. Do not administer as an I.V. bolus.
- Ganciclovir infusion therapy should be accompanied by adequate hydration.
- Because of the frequency of granulocytopenia and thrombocytopenia, neutrophil and platelet counts should be obtained every 2 days during twice-daily ganciclovir dosing and at least weekly thereafter.
- Use caution when preparing ganciclovir solution, which is alkaline.

General

Classification: diuretic, antihypertensive (quinazoline [thiazide-like]). **Pregnancy risk category:** D.

Mechanism of action

Although not a thiazide diuretic, metolazone acts in a similar fashion. It increases urine excretion of sodium and water by inhibiting sodium reabsorption in the cortical diluting site of the ascending loop of Henle.

Indications and dosage

- Edema in congestive heart failure. **Adults:** 5 to 10 mg P.O. daily.
- Edema in renal disease. **Adults:** 5 to 20 mg P.O. daily.
- Hypertension. **Adults:** 2.5 to 5 mg (Diulo or Zaroxolyn) P.O. daily. (Maintenance dosage determined by blood pressure.) Or 0.5 mg (Mykrox) once daily in the morning. Increase to 1 mg P.O. daily as needed.

Adverse reactions

Blood: ***aplastic anemia, agranulocytosis,*** leukopenia, thrombocytopenia. **CV:** volume depletion and dehydration, orthostatic hypotension. **GI:** anorexia, nausea, pancreatitis. **Hepatic:** hepatic encephalopathy. **Metabolic:** asymptomatic hyperuricemia, hyperglycemia and impairment of glucose tolerance, fluid and electrolyte imbalances (including dilutional hyponatremia and hypochloremia, hypokalemia, and hypercalcemia), metabolic alkalosis, gout. **Skin:** dermatitis, photosensitivity, rash. **Other:** hypersensitivity reactions, such as pneumonitis and vasculitis.

Interactions

Cholestyramine, colestipol: intestinal absorption of thiazides decreased. Keep doses as separate as possible. **Diazoxide:** increased antihypertensive, hyperglycemic, and hyperuricemic effects. Use together cautiously. **NSAIDs:** decreased diuretic effect. Avoid concomitant use.

Nursing diagnoses

- Fluid volume excess related to sodium and water retention.
- Altered urinary elimination related to metolazone therapy.
- Knowledge deficit related to metolazone therapy.

Nursing interventions

- *Contraindicated* in anuria, hepatic coma or precoma, or hypersensitivity to thiazides or other sulfonamide-derived drugs.
- *Use cautiously* in hyperuricemia or gout and impaired renal or hepatic function.
- Mykrox tablets are more rapidly and completely absorbed than other brands; because dosage is different, don't interchange Mykrox with Diulo or Zaroxolyn.
- Monitor intake and output, weight, blood pressure, and serum electrolytes.
- Consult with doctor and dietitian to provide high-potassium diet. Watch for hypokalemia. Patients also on digitalis glycosides may have an increased risk of digitalis toxicity from the potassium-depleting effect of this diuretic.
- Check insulin requirements in patients with diabetes. Also monitor blood uric acid, especially in patients with a history of gout.
- In hypertension, therapeutic response may be delayed several days.
- Elderly patients are especially susceptible to excessive diuresis.
- A thiazide-related diuretic. However, unlike thiazide diuretics, metolazone is effective in patients with decreased renal function.
- Discontinue before tests for parathyroid function are performed.
- Advise patient to avoid sudden posture changes and rise slowly to avoid orthostatic hypotension.
- Advise patient to use a sunscreen.

General

Classification: antilipemic (fibric acid deviative).
Pregnancy risk category: B.

Mechanism of action

Inhibits peripheral lipolysis and also reduces triglyceride synthesis in the liver. Lowers serum triglyceride levels and increases high-density-lipoprotein cholesterol levels.

Indications and dosage

• Treatment of type IV hyperlipidemia (hypertriglyceridemia) and severe hypercholesterolemia unresponsive to diet and other drugs; to reduce the risk of coronary heart disease in patients intolerant of or refractory to treatment with bile acid sequestrants or niacin. **Adults:** 1,200 mg P.O. administered in two divided doses. Usual dosage range is 900 to 1,500 mg daily. If no beneficial effect is seen after 3 months of therapy, drug should be discontinued.

Adverse reactions

Blood: anemia, leukopenia. **CNS:** blurred vision, headache, dizziness. **GI:** *abdominal and epigastric pain, diarrhea, nausea,* vomiting, flatulence. **Hepatic:** bile duct obstruction, elevated enzymes. **Skin:** rash, dermatitis, pruritus. **Other:** painful extremities.

Interactions

Oral anticoagulants: gemfibrozil may enhance the clinical effects of oral anticoagulants. Monitor patient closely.

Nursing diagnoses

• High risk for injury related to elevated blood lipids and cholesterol levels.
• Sensory/perceptual alterations (visual) related to adverse drug reactions.
• Knowledge deficit related to gemfibrozil therapy.

Nursing interventions

• *Contraindicated* in hepatic or severe renal dysfunction—including primary biliary cirrhosis—and preexisting gallbladder disease.
• CBC and liver function tests should be done periodically during the first 12 months of therapy.
• Gemfibrozil is very closely related to clofibrate both chemically and pharmacologically.
• Instruct patient to take drug 30 minutes before breakfast and dinner.
• Should not be used indiscriminately. May pose risk of gallstones, heart disease, and cancer.
• Observe bowel movements for evidence of steatorrhea or other signs of bile duct obstruction.
• Because of possible dizziness and blurred vision, patient should avoid driving or other hazardous activities until CNS effects of the drug are known.
• Teach patient about proper dietary management (restricting total fat and cholesterol intake), weight control, and exercise. Explain their importance in controlling elevated serum lipids.

General
Classification: antiemetic, GI stimulant (para-aminobenzoic acid derivative). **Pregnancy risk category:** B.

Mechanism of action
Stimulates motility of the upper GI tract by increasing lower esophageal sphincter tone. Also blocks dopamine receptors at the chemoreceptor trigger zone.

Indications and dosage
- Prevention or reduction of nausea and vomiting induced by cisplatin and other chemotherapeutic agents. **Adults:** 2 mg/kg I.V. q 2 hours for 5 doses, beginning 30 minutes before cisplatin administration.
- To facilitate small-bowel intubation and to aid in radiologic examinations. **Adults:** 10 mg (2 ml) I.V. as a single dose over 1 to 2 minutes. **Children 6 to 14 years:** 2.5 to 5 mg I.V. (0.5 to 1 ml). **Children under 6 years:** 0.1 mg/kg I.V.
- Delayed gastric emptying secondary to diabetic gastroparesis. **Adults:** 10 mg P.O. 30 minutes before meals and h.s. for 2 to 8 weeks.
- Gastroesophageal reflux. **Adults:** 10 to 15 mg P.O. q.i.d., p.r.n. Take 30 minutes before meals.

Adverse reactions
CNS: *restlessness, anxiety, drowsiness,* fatigue, *lassitude,* insomnia, headache, dizziness, *extrapyramidal symptoms, tardive dyskinesia, dystonic reactions,* sedation. **CV:** transient hypertension. **GI:** nausea, bowel disturbances. **Skin:** rash. **Other:** fever, prolactin secretion, loss of libido.

Interactions
Alcohol, CNS depressants: additive CNS depression. Avoid concomitant use. **Anticholinergics, narcotic analgesics:** antagonize GI motility effects of metoclopramide. Use together cautiously. **Phenothiazines, butyrophenones:** increased risk of extrapyramidal effects. Monitor closely.

Nursing diagnoses
- High risk for fluid volume deficit related to nausea and vomiting induced by chemotherapy.
- Altered thought processes related to adverse CNS reactions to metoclopramide.
- Knowledge deficit related to metoclopramide therapy.

Nursing interventions
- *Contraindicated* whenever stimulation of GI motility might be dangerous (hemorrhage, obstruction, or perforation) and in pheochromocytoma or seizure disorder.
- Elderly patients are more likely to experience extrapyramidal symptoms and tardive dyskinesia.
- Safety and effectiveness have not been established for therapy that continues longer than 12 weeks.
- Monitor blood pressure frequently in patients receiving I.V. dosage.
- **I.V. use:** I.V. infusions should be given slowly over at least 15 minutes. Protection from light is unnecessary if the infusion mixture is administered within 24 hours.
- Diphenhydramine 25 mg I.V. may be prescribed to counteract the extrapyramidal adverse effects associated with high metoclopramide doses.
- Warn patient to avoid activities requiring alertness for 2 hours after taking each dose.
- Oral form is being used investigationally to treat nausea and vomiting.

General

Classification: antibiotic (aminoglycoside). **Pregnancy risk category:** C.

Mechanism of action

Inhibits protein synthesis by binding directly to the 30S ribosomal subunit. Generally bactericidal.

Indications and dosage

• Serious infections caused by sensitive *Pseudomonas aeruginosa, Escherichia coli, Proteus, Klebsiella, Serratia, Enterobacter, Citrobacter, or Staphylococcus*. **Adults with normal renal function:** 3 mg/kg daily in divided doses q 8 hours I.M. or I.V. infusion (in 50 to 200 ml of 0.9% sodium chloride solution or D_5W infused over 2 hours). May be given by direct I.V. push. For life-threatening infections, up to 5 mg/kg daily in 3 to 4 divided doses. **Children with normal renal function:** 2 to 2.5 mg/kg I.M. or I.V. infusion q 8 hours. **Infants and neonates over 1 week with normal renal function:** 2.5 mg/kg q 8 hours I.M. or I.V. infusion. **Neonates under 1 week:** 2.5 mg/kg I.V. q 12 hours. For I.V. infusion, dilute in 0.9% sodium chloride solution or D_5W and infuse over 30 minutes to 2 hours.

• Meningitis. **Adults:** systemic therapy as above; or 4 to 8 mg intrathecally daily. **Children:** systemic therapy as above; or 1 to 2 mg intrathecally daily.

• Endocarditis prophylaxis for GI or GU procedure or surgery. **Adults:** 1.5 mg/kg I.M. or I.V. 30 minutes beforehand. Maximum dose: 80 mg. Give with ampicillin (vancomycin in penicillin-allergic patients). Repeat in 8 hours. **Children:** 2.5 mg/kg I.M. or I.V. 30 minutes before procedure or surgery. Maximum dose should not exceed 80 mg. Give with ampicillin (vancomycin in penicillin-allergic patients). After 8 hours, give half initial dose. **Patients with impaired renal function:** initial dose is same as for normal renal function. Subsequent doses and frequency determined by renal function studies and serum concentrations of gentamicin.

Adverse reactions

CNS: headache, lethargy, ***neuromuscular blockade.***
EENT: *ototoxicity (tinnitus, vertigo, hearing loss).*
GU: *nephrotoxicity (cells or casts in the urine; oliguria; proteinuria; decreased creatinine clearance; increased BUN, nonprotein nitrogen, and serum creatinine levels).* **Other:** ***hypersensitivity reactions, hepatic necrosis.***

Interactions

Cephalothin: increases nephrotoxicity. **Dimenhydrinate:** may mask symptoms of ototoxicity. **General anesthetics, neuromuscular blockers:** may potentiate neuromuscular blockade. **I.V. loop diuretics:** increase ototoxicity. **Other aminoglycosides, methoxyflurane:** increase ototoxicity and nephrotoxicity. **Parenteral penicillins:** gentamicin inactivation in vitro. Don't combine I.V.

Nursing diagnoses

• High risk for injury related to dosage regimen inadequate to alleviate infection.
• Sensory/perceptual alterations (auditory) related to ototoxicity induced by drug therapy.
• Knowledge deficit related to gentamicin.

Nursing interventions

• Obtain specimen for culture and sensitivity tests; therapy may begin pending test results.
• Monitor renal function and notify doctor of signs of decreasing renal function.
• Patient should be well hydrated to minimize chemical irritation of the renal tubules.
• Notify doctor of complaints of tinnitus, vertigo, or hearing loss.
• Monitor for superinfection.
• Usual duration of therapy is 7 to 10 days. If no response in 3 to 5 days, therapy may be stopped and new specimens obtained.
• Peak blood levels above 12 mcg/ml and trough levels (those drawn just before next dose) above 2 mcg/ml may indicate higher incidence of toxicity.
• Draw blood for peak gentamicin level 1 hour after I.M. injection and 30 minutes to 1 hour after infusion ends; for trough levels, draw blood just before next dose.
• Hemodialysis (8 hours) removes up to 50% of drug.

General

Classification: vasoconstrictor (ergot alkaloid). **Pregnancy risk category:** C.

Mechanism of action

Specifically blocks serotonin (a neurotransmitter) in the peripheral nervous system. In the CNS, the drug acts as a serotonin agonist.

Indications and dosage

- Prevention of frequent, severe, uncontrollable, or disabling migraine or vascular headache. **Adults:** 4 to 8 mg P.O. daily with meals.
- Control of diarrhea caused by carcinoid disease. **Adults:** initially, 2 mg P.O. t.i.d., increased p.r.n. to 4 to 16 mg t.i.d.

Adverse reactions

Blood: neutropenia, eosinophilia. **CNS:** insomnia, drowsiness, *euphoria, vertigo,* ataxia, *light-headedness,* hyperesthesia, weakness, hallucinations or feelings of dissociation. **CV:** ***fibrotic thickening of cardiac valves and aorta, inferior vena cava, and common iliac branches (retroperitoneal fibrosis);*** vasoconstriction, causing chest pain, abdominal pain, vascular insufficiency of lower limbs; cold, numb, painful extremities with or without paresthesias and diminished or absent pulses; postural hypotension; tachycardia; peripheral edema; murmurs; bruits. **EENT:** nasal stuffiness. **GI:** nausea, vomiting, diarrhea, constipation, epigastric pain. **Skin:** hair loss, dermatitis, sweating, flushing, rash. **Other:** ***pulmonary fibrosis,*** causing dyspnea, tightness and pain in chest, pleural friction rubs and effusion, arthralgia, myalgia.

Interactions

None significant.

Nursing diagnoses

- Pain related to the patient's underlying condition.
- High risk for injury related to adverse drug reactions.
- Knowledge deficit related to methysergide therapy.

Nursing interventions

- *Contraindicated* in severe hypertension, arteriosclerosis, peripheral vascular insufficiency, renal or hepatic disease, severe coronary artery diseases, thromboembolic disorders, phlebitis or cellulitis of lower limbs, fibrotic processes, valvular heart disease; and in debilitated patients.
- *Use cautiously* in peptic ulcers or suspected coronary artery disease. ECG and cardiac status evaluation advisable before giving to patients over 40 years.
- GI effects may be prevented by gradual introduction of medication and by administering with meals.
- Obtain laboratory studies of cardiac and renal function, blood count, and sedimentation rate before and during therapy.
- Drug may be gradually withdrawn every 6 months; then restart after at least 3 or 4 weeks.
- Stop gradually over 2 to 3 weeks; stopping abruptly may cause rebound headaches.
- Patient should keep daily weight record and report rapid weight gain. Teach him to check for peripheral edema.
- Give drug for 3 weeks before evaluating effectiveness.
- Tell patient to report to doctor promptly if he experiences cold, numb, or painful hands and feet; leg cramps when walking; pelvic, chest, or flank pain.
- Not for treatment of migraine or vascular headache in progress or for tension headaches.
- Indicated only for patients who are unresponsive to other drugs and who can be kept under close medical supervision.

General

Classification: antidiabetic (sulfonylurea). **Pregnancy risk category:** C.

Mechanism of action

Stimulates insulin release from pancreatic beta cells and reduces glucose output. Extrapancreatic effect increases peripheral sensitivity to insulin.

Indications and dosage

- Adjunct to diet for lowering blood glucose in patients with non-insulin-dependent diabetes mellitus (type II). **Adults:** initially, 5 mg P.O. daily before breakfast. Elderly patients or those with liver disease may be started on 2.5 mg. Usual maintenance dosage is 10 to 15 mg. Maximum recommended daily dosage is 40 mg.
- Insulin therapy replacement. **Adults:** if insulin dosage is more than 20 units daily, give as above in addition to 50% of the insulin. If insulin dosage is less than 20 units, insulin may be discontinued.

Adverse reactions

CNS: dizziness. **GI:** nausea, vomiting, constipation. **Hepatic:** cholestatic jaundice. **Metabolic:** ***hypoglycemia.*** **Skin:** rash, pruritus, facial flushing.

Interactions

Anabolic steroids, chloramphenicol, clofibrate, guanethidine, MAO inhibitors, phenylbutazone, probenecid, salicylates, sulfonamides: increased hypoglycemic activity. Monitor blood glucose level. **Beta blockers, clonidine:** prolonged hypoglycemic effect and masked symptoms of hypoglycemia. **Corticosteroids, glucagon, rifampin, thiazide diuretics:** decreased hypoglycemic response. Monitor blood glucose level. **Hydantoins:** increased blood levels of hydantoins. **Oral anticoagulants:** increased hypoglycemic activity or enhanced anticoagulant effect. Monitor blood glucose and PT.

Nursing diagnoses

- Altered nutrition: More than body requirements, related to the patient's inability to produce sufficient insulin to maintain normal blood glucose levels.
- High risk for injury related to glipizide-induced hypoglycemia.
- Knowledge deficit related to glipizide therapy.

Nursing interventions

- *Contraindicated* in diabetic ketoacidosis, with or without coma. This drug also should not be used during pregnancy or breast-feeding.
- *Use cautiously* in renal and hepatic disease and sulfonamide hypersensitivity.
- Elderly patients may be more sensitive to this drug's adverse reactions.
- Patient transferring from insulin therapy to an oral antidiabetic agent requires blood glucose monitoring at least t.i.d. before meals. May require hospitalization during transition.
- During periods of increased stress, such as infection, fever, surgery, or trauma, patient may require insulin therapy. Monitor patient closely for hyperglycemia in these situations.
- Instruct patient about nature of disease; importance of following therapeutic regimen, adhering to specific diet, losing weight, exercising, following personal hygiene program, and avoiding infection; how and when to perform self-monitoring of blood glucose level; and recognition of hypoglycemia and hyperglycemia.
- Some patients taking glipizide may be effectively controlled on a once-daily regimen, while others show better response with divided dosing.
- Give approximately 30 minutes before meals.
- Glipizide is a second-generation sulfonylurea. Frequency of adverse reactions seems lower than with first-generation drugs.
- Glipizide has a mild diuretic effect. May be useful in patients who have CHF or cirrhosis.
- Teach patient not to change drug dosage without the doctor's orders. Report abnormal blood or urine glucose tests.
- Be sure patient understands that he should not take any other medication, including OTC drugs, without first checking with the doctor.

General

Classification: sedative-hypnotic (piperidinedione derivative). **Pregnancy risk category:** B. **Controlled substance schedule:** III.

Mechanism of action

Raises threshold of arousal centers in the brain stem.

Indications and dosage

• Insomnia. **Adults:** 200 to 400 mg P.O. 15 minutes before bedtime. **Children over 3 months:** 50 mg P.O. at bedtime, increased to 200 mg, if necessary. Maximum dosage is 400 mg daily.

Adverse reactions

Blood: thrombocytopenic purpura, neutropenia, ***aplastic anemia***. **CNS:** *morning drowsiness, dizziness,* headache, paradoxical excitation. **CV:** hypotension. **GI:** nausea, vomiting, diarrhea, esophagitis. **Skin:** rash, pruritus.

Interactions

Alcohol or other CNS depressants, including narcotic analgesics: excessive CNS and respiratory depression. Use together cautiously.

Nursing diagnoses

• Sleep pattern disturbance related to underlying patient problem.
• High risk for trauma related to adverse CNS reactions caused by methyprylon.
• Knowledge deficit related to methyprylon therapy.

Nursing interventions

• *Contraindicated* in patients with hypersensitivity to the drug and in patients with intermittent porphyria.
• *Use cautiously* in renal or hepatic impairment.
• Periodic blood counts are advisable during repeated or long-term use.
• May cause drug dependence after long-term use. Withdrawal should be gradual and closely monitored.
• Take precautions to prevent hoarding or self-overdosing by patients who are depressed, suicidal, or drug-dependent or who have a history of drug abuse.
• Advise caution with hazardous activities requiring mental alertness or physical coordination, including driving. Supervise walking; raise bed rails, especially for elderly patients.
• Value of this drug as a sedative has not been established.
• Symptoms of overdosage include somnolence, confusion, constricted pupils, respiratory depression, hypotension, and coma. Hemodialysis is useful in severe intoxication.
• Suppresses REM sleep, as do barbiturates. Patient may experience increased dreaming after drug is discontinued.

General

Classification: antihypoglycemic, diagnostic agent. **Pregnancy risk category:** B.

Mechanism of action

Raises blood glucose level by promoting catalytic depolymerization of hepatic glycogen to glucose.

Indications and dosage

- Coma of insulin-shock therapy. **Adults:** 0.5 to 1 mg S.C., I.M., or I.V. 1 hour after coma develops; may repeat within 25 minutes, if necessary. In very deep coma, also give glucose 10% to 50% I.V. for faster response. When patient responds, give additional carbohydrate immediately.
- Severe insulin-induced hypoglycemia during diabetic therapy. **Adults and children:** 0.5 to 1 mg S.C., I.M., or I.V.; may repeat q 20 minutes for 2 doses, if necessary. If coma persists, give glucose 10% to 50% I.V.
- Diagnostic aid for radiologic examination. **Adults:** 0.25 to 2 mg I.V. or I.M. before initiation of radiologic procedure.

Adverse reactions

GI: nausea, vomiting. **Other:** ***hypersensitivity.***

Interactions

Phenytoin: inhibited glucagon-induced insulin release. Use cautiously.

Nursing diagnoses

- High risk for injury related to the patient's severe hypoglycemia.
- High risk for fluid volume deficit related to glucagon-induced vomiting.
- Knowledge deficit related to glucagon therapy.

Nursing interventions

- *Use cautiously* in patients with insulinoma pheochromocytoma.
- Unstable hypoglycemic diabetics may not respond to glucagon. Give dextrose I.V. instead.
- It is vital to arouse the patient from coma as quickly as possible and to give additional carbohydrates orally to prevent secondary hypoglycemic reactions.
- **I.V. use:** Reconstitute 1-unit vial with 1 ml of diluent; reconstitute 10-unit vial with 10 ml of diluent. Use only the diluent supplied by the manufacturer when preparing doses of 2 mg or less. For larger doses, dilute with sterile water for injection.
- For I.V. drip infusion, use dextrose solution, which is compatible with glucagon; drug forms a precipitate in chloride solutions. Give directly into vein or into I.V. tubing of a free-flowing compatible solution over 2 to 5 minutes. Interrupt primary infusion during glucagon injection if you're using the same I.V. line.
- Instruct patient and family in proper glucagon administration, recognition of hypoglycemia, and urgency of calling a doctor immediately in emergencies.
- May be used as diagnostic aid in radiologic examination of the stomach, duodenum, small bowel, and colon when a hypotonic state is advantageous.
- Has a positive inotropic and chronotropic action on the heart. May be used to treat overdosage of beta-adrenergic blockers.

General

Classification: androgen replacement (androgen). **Pregnancy risk category:** X. **Controlled substance schedule:** III.

Mechanism of action

Stimulates target tissues to develop normally in androgen-deficient males.

Indications and dosage

• Breast engorgement of nonnursing mothers. **Adults:** 80 mg P.O. daily, or 40 mg buccal daily for 3 to 5 days.
• Breast cancer in women 1 to 5 years postmenopausal. **Adults:** 200 mg P.O. daily; or 100 mg buccal daily.
• Eunuchoidism and eunuchism, male climacteric symptoms. **Adults:** 10 to 40 mg P.O. daily; or 5 to 20 mg buccal daily.
• Postpubertal cryptorchidism. **Adults:** 30 mg P.O. daily; or 15 mg buccal daily.

Adverse reactions

Androgenic: in women—*acne, edema, oily skin, weight gain, hirsutism, hoarseness,* clitoral enlargement, changes in libido. In men—prepubertal: premature epiphyseal closure, *acne,* priapism, *growth of body and facial hair,* phallic enlargement; postpubertal: testicular atrophy, oligospermia, decreased ejaculatory volume, impotence, gynecomastia, epididymitis. **CV:** edema. **GI:** gastroenteritis, constipation, nausea, vomiting, diarrhea, change in appetite. **GU:** bladder irritability. **Hepatic:** reversible jaundice. **Hypoestrogenic:** in women—flushing, sweating, vaginitis, menstrual irregularities. **Local:** irritation of oral mucosa with buccal administration. **Other:** hypercalcemia.

Interactions

Hepatotoxic medications: increased risk of hepatotoxicity. **Oral anticoagulants:** altered dosage requirements. **Oral antidiabetic agents:** altered dosage requirements.

Nursing diagnoses

• Sexual dysfunction related to hormonal dysfunction.
• Body image disturbance related to adverse androgenic reactions associated with methyltestosterone therapy.
• Knowledge deficit related to methyltestosterone therapy.

Nursing interventions

• *Contraindicated* in pregnancy and in breast-feeding women; in elderly, asthenic men who may react adversely to androgen overstimulation; in hypercalcemia; cardiac, hepatic, or renal decompensation; prostatic or breast cancer in men; benign prostatic hypertrophy with obstruction; conditions aggravated by fluid retention; hypertension; and in premature infants.
• *Use cautiously* in MI or coronary artery disease.
• In children, X-ray of wrist bones should establish level of bone maturation before therapy. During treatment, bone maturation may proceed more rapidly than linear growth. Dosage should be intermittent and X-rays should be taken periodically to monitor bone maturation.
• In metastatic breast cancer, hypercalcemia may indicate progression of bone metastasis.
• Therapeutic response in breast cancer is usually apparent within 3 months. Therapy should be stopped if signs of disease progression appear.
• Watch for ecchymoses, petechiae, and abnormal bleeding in patients receiving anticoagulants.
• Report signs of virilization in women.
• Use with diet high in calories and protein. Give small, frequent feedings.
• Buccal tablets twice as potent as oral tablets. Tell patient to avoid eating, drinking, chewing, or smoking while buccal tablet is in place, and that tablet is not to be swallowed. Place in upper or lower buccal pouch between cheek and gum. Tablet dissolves in 30 to 60 minutes. Instruct patient to change tablet absorption site with each dose to minimize risk of irritation.

General

Classification: sedative-hypnotic (piperidinedione). **Pregnancy risk category:** C. **Controlled substance schedule:** III.

Mechanism of action

Unknown.

Indications and dosage

• Insomnia. **Adults:** 250 to 500 mg P.O. h.s. May be repeated, but not less than 4 hours before intended awakening. Total daily dosage should not exceed 1 g.

Adverse reactions

CNS: *residual sedation, dizziness, ataxia,* paradoxical excitation, headache, vertigo. **EENT:** blurred vision. **GI:** dry mouth, irritation, nausea. **GU:** bladder atony. **Skin:** rash, urticaria.

Interactions

Alcohol or other CNS depressants, including narcotic analgesics: excessive CNS depression. Use together cautiously. **Oral anticoagulants:** glutethimide enhances the metabolism of coumarin derivatives. Monitor for decreased effect.

Nursing diagnoses

• Sleep pattern disturbance related to underlying patient problem.
• High risk for trauma related to adverse CNS reactions caused by glutethimide.
• Knowledge deficit related to glutethimide therapy.

Nursing interventions

• *Contraindicated* in patients with hypersensitivity to the drug and in patients with uncontrolled pain, severe renal impairment, or porphyria.
• *Use cautiously* in patients with mental depression, suicidal tendencies, history of drug abuse, and conditions that may be worsened by the drug's anticholinergic activity (prostatic hypertrophy, stenosing peptic ulcer, pyloroduodenal or bladder-neck obstruction, narrow-angle glaucoma, and cardiac arrhythmias).
• Drug is effective for short-term use only.
• Advise caution with activities requiring mental alertness or physical coordination. Supervise walking; raise bed rails, especially for elderly patients.
• Take precautions to prevent hoarding or self-overdosing by patients who are depressed, suicidal, or drug-dependent or who have a history of drug abuse.
• Abrupt withdrawal after long-term use may produce nausea, vomiting, nervousness, tremor, chills, fever, nightmares, insomnia, tachycardia, delirium, numbness of extremities, hallucinations, dysphagia, and seizures. Withdraw drug gradually.
• Assess patient for anticholinergic symptoms, including mydriasis, dry mouth, tachycardia, or urine retention.
• Monitor PT carefully when patient on glutethimide starts or ends anticoagulant therapy. Anticoagulant dose may need to be adjusted.
• Suppresses REM sleep, as do barbiturates. Patient may experience increased dreaming after drug is discontinued.

General

Classification: anti-inflammatory, immunosuppressant (glucocorticoid). **Pregnancy risk category:** C.

Mechanism of action

Decreases inflammation, mainly by stabilizing leukocyte lysosomal membranes. Also suppresses the immune response, stimulates bone marrow, and influences protein, fat, and carbohydrate metabolism.

Indications and dosage

- Severe inflammation or immunosuppression. **Adults:** 2 to 60 mg P.O. in four divided doses; or 40 to 80 mg (acetate) I.M. daily, or 10 to 250 mg (succinate) I.M. or I.V. q 4 hours; or 4 to 30 mg (acetate) into joints and soft tissue, p.r.n. **Children:** 117 mcg to 1.66 mg/kg (succinate) I.V. in three or four divided doses.
- Shock. **Adults:** 100 to 250 mg (succinate) I.V. at 2- to 6-hour intervals.
- To decrease damage following spinal cord trauma. **Adults:** 30 mg/kg (succinate) I.V. as bolus injection within 8 hours of injury; then continuous infusion of 5.4 mg/kg/hour for next 23 hours.

Adverse reactions

CNS: *euphoria, insomnia,* psychotic behavior, pseudotumor cerebri. **CV:** ***CHF,*** hypertension, edema. **EENT:** cataracts, glaucoma. **GI:** *peptic ulcer,* GI irritation, increased appetite. **Metabolic:** possible hypokalemia, hyperglycemia and carbohydrate intolerance, growth suppression in children. **Skin:** delayed wound healing, acne, skin eruptions. **Other:** muscle weakness, osteoporosis, pancreatitis, hirsutism, susceptibility to infections. Acute adrenal insufficiency may occur with increased stress or abrupt withdrawal after long-term therapy. **Withdrawal symptoms:** rebound inflammation, fatigue, weakness, arthralgia, fever, dizziness, lethargy, depression, orthostatic hypotension, dyspnea, anorexia, hypoglycemia. ***Sudden withdrawal may be fatal.***

Interactions

Barbiturates, phenytoin, rifampin: decreased corticosteroid effect. **NSAIDs, indomethacin, aspirin:** risk of GI distress and bleeding. **Oral anticoagulants:** altered dosage requirements. **Potassium-depleting drugs such as thiazide diuretics:** enhanced potassium-wasting effects. **Skin-test antigens:** decreased response. **Vaccines and toxoids:** decreased antibody response and increased risk of neurologic complications.

Nursing diagnoses

- Impaired tissue integrity related to the patient's underlying condition.
- High risk for injury related to adverse reactions to methylprednisolone.
- Knowledge deficit related to methylprednisolone therapy.

Nursing interventions

- *Contraindicated* in systemic fungal infections and in patients allergic to any component of the formulation.
- *Use cautiously* in patients with GI ulceration or renal disease, hypertension, osteoporosis, varicella, vaccinia, exanthema, diabetes mellitus, Cushing's syndrome, thromboembolic disorders, seizures, myasthenia gravis, metastatic cancer, CHF, tuberculosis, ocular herpes simplex, hypoalbuminemia, emotional instability, and psychotic tendencies.
- Gradually reduce dosage after long-term therapy. Tell patient not to discontinue drug abruptly or without doctor's consent.
- Inject diluted drug into vein or free-flowing compatible I.V. solution over 1 minute. For shock, give over 10 minutes to prevent arrhythmias and circulatory collapse. Give I.M. injection deep into gluteal muscle. Avoid S.C. injection. Give P.O. dose with food when possible.

General

Classification: antidiabetic (sulfonylurea). **Pregnancy risk category:** B.

Mechanism of action

Stimulates insulin release from the pancreatic beta cells and reduces glucose output by the liver. An extrapancreatic effect increases peripheral sensitivity to insulin and causes a mild diuretic effect.

Indications and dosage

• Adjunct to diet in lowering blood glucose in patients with non-insulin-dependent diabetes mellitus (type II). **Adults:** initially, 2.5 to 5 mg P.O. (regular tablets) daily administered with breakfast. Patients who are more sensitive to antidiabetic drugs should be started at 1.25 mg daily. Usual maintenance dosage is 1.25 to 20 mg daily, given either as a single dose or in divided doses.

Alternatively, use micronized formulation. Initial dose is 1.5 to 3 mg daily. Patients who are more sensitive to antidiabetic agents should be started at 0.75 mg daily.

• Insulin therapy replacement. **Adults:** if insulin dosage is more than 40 units daily, patient may be started on 5 mg glyburide (regular tablets) or 3 mg glyburide (micronized formulation) daily in addition to 50% of the insulin dosage.

Adverse reactions

GI: nausea, epigastric fullness, heartburn. **Hepatic:** cholestatic jaundice. **Metabolic:** ***hypoglycemia.*** **Skin:** rash, pruritus, facial flushing.

Interactions

Anabolic steroids, chloramphenicol, clofibrate, guanethidine, MAO inhibitors, phenylbutazone, salicylates, sulfonamides: increased hypoglycemic activity. Monitor blood glucose level. **Beta blockers, clonidine:** prolonged hypoglycemic effect and masked symptoms of hypoglycemia. Use together cautiously. **Corticosteroids, glucagon, rifampin, thiazide diuretics:** decreased hypoglycemic response. Monitor blood glucose level. **Hydantoins:** increased blood levels of hydantoins. Monitor blood levels closely. **Oral anticoagulants:** increased hypoglycemic activity or enhanced anticoagulant effect. Monitor blood glucose and PT.

Nursing diagnoses

• Altered nutrition: More than body requirements, related to the patient's inability to produce sufficient insulin to maintain normal blood glucose levels.

• High risk for injury related to glyburide-induced hypoglycemia.

• Knowledge deficit related to glyburide therapy.

Nursing interventions

• *Contraindicated* in diabetic ketoacidosis, with or without coma. This drug also should not be used during pregnancy or breast-feeding.

• *Use cautiously* in sulfonamide hypersensitivity and severe renal impairment.

• Micronized glyburide contains the drug in a smaller particle size and is not bioequivalent to regular glyburide tablets. Patients who have been taking Micronase or DiaBeta should be retitrated.

• Patient transferring from insulin therapy to an oral antidiabetic agent requires blood glucose monitoring at least t.i.d. before meals. Patient may require hospitalization during transition.

• During periods of increased stress, patient may require insulin therapy. Monitor patient closely for hyperglycemia.

• A maintenance dosage of 5 mg glyburide (regular tablets) provides approximately the same degree of blood glucose control as 250 to 375 mg chlorpropamide, 250 to 375 mg tolazamide, 500 to 750 mg acetohexamide, or 1,000 to 1,500 mg tolbutamide.

• Patients taking more than 10 mg daily may achieve better results with twice-daily dosage.

• Glyburide exerts a mild diuretic effect. May be useful in patients who have CHF or cirrhosis.

• Teach patient not to change drug dosage without the doctor's orders. Report abnormal blood or urine glucose tests.

General

Classification: CNS stimulant, analeptic (piperidine). **Pregnancy risk category:** C. **Controlled substance schedule:** II.

Mechanism of action

Main site of activity appears to be the cerebral cortex and the reticular activating system. Promotes nerve impulse transmission by releasing stored norepinephrine from nerve terminals in the brain. In children with attention deficit disorder with hyperactivity (ADDH), amphetamines have a paradoxical calming effect.

Indications and dosage

• ADDH. **Children 6 years and older:** initial dose 5 to 10 mg of tablets P.O. daily before breakfast and lunch, with 5- to 10-mg increments weekly as needed, up to 60 mg daily.
• Narcolepsy. **Adults:** 10 mg P.O. b.i.d. or t.i.d. half hour before meals. (Dosage varies with patient needs; range is 5 to 50 mg daily.)

Adverse reactions

Blood: thrombocytopenia. **CNS:** *nervousness, insomnia,* dizziness, headache, akathisia, dyskinesia, *Tourette's disorder.* **CV:** *palpitations,* angina, *tachycardia,* changes in blood pressure and pulse rate. **EENT:** difficulty with accommodation and blurring of vision. **GI:** nausea, dry throat, abdominal pain, anorexia, weight loss. **Skin:** rash, urticaria, ***exfoliative dermatitis, erythema multiforme,*** thrombocytopenic purpura. **Other:** growth suppression.

Interactions

Anticonvulsants, tricyclic antidepressants, oral anticoagulants: methylphenidate may increase plasma levels of these drugs and enhance their pharmacologic effects. **Centrally acting antihypertensives:** decreased antihypertensive effect. **MAO inhibitors:** severe hypertension; possible hypertensive crisis. Don't use together or within 14 days after an MAO inhibitor has been discontinued.

Nursing diagnoses

• High risk for injury related to patient's underlying disorder.
• Sleep pattern disturbance related to methylphenidate-induced insomnia.
• Knowledge deficit related to methylphenidate therapy.

Nursing interventions

• *Contraindicated* in symptomatic cardiac disease; hyperthyroidism; moderate to severe hypertension; angina pectoris; advanced arteriosclerosis; severe endogenous or exogenous depression; glaucoma; parkinsonism; history of drug abuse or dependency; or history of marked anxiety, tension, or agitation.
• *Use cautiously* in elderly, debilitated, or hyperexcitable patients, and those with CV disease, diabetes, or seizures.
• May precipitate Tourette syndrome in children. Monitor especially at start of therapy.
• Monitor blood pressure. Observe for excessive stimulation. Don't use to prevent fatigue.
• May alter daily insulin needs in patients with diabetes. May decrease seizure threshold in patients with seizure disorders.
• Drug of choice for ADDH.
• Tolerance or psychic dependence may develop. After long-term use, lower dosage gradually to prevent acute rebound depression.
• Fatigue may result as drug effects wear off.
• Tell patient to avoid drinks containing caffeine. Also warn patient to avoid activities that require alertness or good psychomotor coordination until CNS effects of drug are known.
• Monitor height and weight in children on prolonged therapy; drug may suppress growth.
• Give at least 6 hours before bedtime to prevent insomnia. Administer after meals to reduce appetite-suppressive effects.

General

Classification: osmotic laxative (trihydric alcohol). **Pregnancy risk category:** C.

Mechanism of action

Draws water from the tissues into the feces and thus stimulates evacuation.

Indications and dosage

- Constipation. **Adults and children over 6 years:** 3 g as a rectal suppository; or 5 to 15 ml as an enema. **Children under 6 years:** 1 to 1.5 g as a rectal suppository; or 2 to 5 ml as an enema.

Adverse reactions

GI: *cramping pain,* rectal discomfort, hyperemia of rectal mucosa.

Interactions

None significant.

Nursing diagnoses

- Constipation related to interruption of normal pattern of elimination characterized by infrequent or absent stools.
- Pain related to glycerin-induced abdominal cramping.
- Knowledge deficit related to glycerin therapy.

Nursing interventions

- *Contraindicated* in patients with hypersensitivity to the drug and in those with intestinal obstruction, undiagnosed abdominal pain, vomiting or other signs of appendicitis, fecal impaction, or acute surgical abdomen.
- A hyperosmolar laxative used mainly to reestablish proper toilet habits in laxative-dependent patients.
- Must be retained for at least 15 minutes; usually acts within 1 hour. Entire suppository need not melt to be effective.

General

Classification: oxytocic (ergot alkaloid). **Pregnancy risk category:** not applicable.

Mechanism of action

Increases motor activity of the uterus by direct stimulation.

Indications and dosage

• Prevention and treatment of postpartum hemorrhage caused by uterine atony or subinvolution. **Adults:** 0.2 mg I.M. q 2 to 5 hours for maximum of five doses; or I.V. (excessive uterine bleeding or other emergencies) over 1 minute while blood pressure and uterine contractions are monitored. (I.V. dose may be diluted to 5 ml with 0.9% sodium chloride solution. Following initial I.M. or I.V. dose, may give 0.2 to 0.4 mg P.O. q 6 to 12 hours for 2 to 7 days. Decrease dosage if severe cramping occurs.)

Adverse reactions

CNS: dizziness, headache, ***seizures.*** **CV:** ***hypertension, MI,*** transient chest pain, dyspnea, palpitations, peripheral vasoconstriction, gangrene. **EENT:** tinnitus. **GI:** *nausea, vomiting.* **Other:** sweating, ***hypersensitivity, uterine tetany.***

Interactions

Regional anesthetics, vasoconstrictors, dopamine, I.V. oxytocin: excessive vasoconstriction.

Nursing diagnoses

• Fluid volume deficit related to postpartum hemorrhage.
• Pain related to methylergonovine-induced uterine cramping.
• Knowledge deficit related to methylergonovine therapy.

Nursing interventions

• *Contraindicated* for induction of labor; before delivery of placenta; in patients with hypertension, toxemia, or sensitivity to ergot preparations; and in threatened spontaneous abortion.
• *Use cautiously* in sepsis; obliterative vascular disease; and hepatic, renal, or cardiac disease.
• Monitor and record blood pressure, pulse rate, and uterine response; report any sudden change in vital signs, frequent periods of uterine relaxation, and character and amount of vaginal bleeding.
• Contractions begin 5 to 15 minutes after P.O. administration; 2 to 5 minutes after I.M. injection. May continue 3 hours or more after P.O. or I.M. administration.
• Store in tightly closed, light-resistant containers. Discard if discolored.
• **I.V. use:** Drug should not be routinely administered I.V. because of the risk of severe hypertension and CVA. If it must be given by this route, administer slowly over 1 minute with careful blood pressure monitoring. Contractions begin immediately after I.V. use and continue for up to 45 minutes.
• Store I.V. solutions below 8° C (46.4° F). Avoid freezing. Daily stock may be kept at room temperature for 60 to 90 days.

General
Classification: antimuscarinic, GI antispasmodic (anticholinergic). **Pregnancy risk category:** B.

Mechanism of action
Inhibits cholinergic (muscarinic) actions of acetylcholine on autonomic effectors innervated by postganglionic cholinergic nerves.

Indications and dosage
• Neuromuscular blockade reversal. **Adults:** 0.2 mg I.V. for each 1 mg neostigmine or 5 mg of pyridostigmine. May be given I.V. without dilution or may be added to dextrose injection and given by infusion.
• Preoperatively to diminish secretions and block cardiac vagal reflexes. **Adults and children 2 years and older:** 0.0044 mg/kg I.V. or I.M. 30 to 60 minutes before anesthesia. **Children under 2 years:** 0.0088 mg/kg I.M. 30 minutes before anesthesia.
• Adjunctive therapy in peptic ulcers and other GI disorders. **Adults:** 1 to 2 mg P.O. t.i.d. or 0.1 mg I.M. t.i.d. or q.i.d. Dosage must be individualized. Maximum P.O. dose is 8 mg/day.

Adverse reactions
CNS: disorientation, irritability, incoherence, weakness, nervousness, drowsiness, dizziness, headache. **CV:** palpitations, tachycardia, paradoxical bradycardia. **EENT:** *dilated pupils, blurred vision,* photophobia, increased intraocular pressure, difficulty swallowing. **GI:** *constipation, dry mouth,* nausea, vomiting, epigastric distress. **GU:** *urinary hesitancy, urine retention,* impotence. **Skin:** urticaria, decreased sweating or anhidrosis, other dermal manifestations. **Local:** burning at injection site. **Other:** bronchial plugging, fever.

Interactions
Amantadine, antihistamines, antiparkinsonian agents, disopyramide, glutethimide, meperidine, phenothiazines, procainamide, quinidine: additive adverse effects. Avoid concomitant use. **Ketoconazole:** anticholinergics may interfere with ketoconazole absorption. Avoid concomitant use. **Methotrimeprazine:** anticholinergics may enhance risk of extrapyramidal reactions. Avoid concomitant use.

Nursing diagnoses
• Altered health maintenance related to the patient's underlying condition.
• Sensory/perceptual alterations (visual) related to adverse drug reaction.
• Knowledge deficit related to glycopyrrolate therapy.

Nursing interventions
• *Contraindicated* in narrow-angle glaucoma, obstructive uropathy, obstructive GI disease, myasthenia gravis, paralytic ileus, intestinal atony, unstable cardiovascular status, or toxic megacolon.
• *Use cautiously* in patients with autonomic neuropathy, hyperthyroidism, coronary artery disease, cardiac arrhythmias, CHF, hypertension, hiatal hernia associated with reflux esophagitis, hepatic or renal disease, and ulcerative colitis and in patients over 40 years. Use with caution in hot or humid environments.
• **I.V. use:** Don't mix with I.V. solution containing sodum bicarbonate or alkaline solutions with a pH of more than 6.
• Monitor vital signs and watch for adverse reactions. Call doctor promptly.
• Advise patient to report signs of urinary hesitancy or urine retention and to avoid activities that require alertness until CNS effects of the drug are known.
• Administer 30 minutes to 1 hour before meals.

General

Classification: antihypertensive (centrally acting antiadrenergic agent). **Pregnancy risk category:** B.

Mechanism of action

Inhibits the central vasomotor centers, thereby decreasing sympathetic outflow.

Indications and dosage

• Sustained mild to severe hypertension; should not be used for acute treatment of hypertensive emergencies. **Adults:** initially, 250 mg of tablets or suspension P.O. b.i.d. to t.i.d. in first 48 hours. Then increase as needed q 2 days (maintenance dosage is 500 mg to 2 g daily in two to four divided doses, with a maximum dosage of 3 g). I.V. dosage, 250 to 500 mg q 6 hours, diluted in D_5W and administered over 30 to 60 minutes. (Maximum dosage is 1 g q 6 hours; switch to oral antihypertensives as soon as possible.) **Children:** initially, 10 mg/kg P.O. daily in two to three divided doses; or 20 to 40 mg/kg I.V. daily in four divided doses. (Increase dose daily until desired response occurs; maximum daily dose is 65 mg/kg, 2 g/m^2, or 3 g/day, whichever is least.)

Adverse reactions

Blood: ***hemolytic anemia,*** reversible granulocytopenia, thrombocytopenia. **CNS:** *sedation,* headache, asthenia, weakness, dizziness, *decreased mental acuity,* involuntary choreoathetotic movements, psychic disturbances, depression, nightmares. **CV:** bradycardia, *orthostatic hypotension,* aggravated angina, myocarditis, *edema, and weight gain.* **EENT:** *nasal stuffiness.* **GI:** dry mouth, diarrhea, pancreatitis. **Hepatic:** ***hepatic necrosis.*** **Skin:** rash. **Other:** gynecomastia, lactation, ***drug-induced fever,*** impotence.

Interactions

Levodopa: additive hypotensive effects; possible increased CNS adverse reactions. **Norepinephrine, phenothiazines, TCAs, amphetamines:** possible hypertensive effects. Monitor carefully.

Nursing diagnoses

• Altered tissue perfusion (renal, cerebral, cardiopulmonary, peripheral) related to the patient's underlying condition.
• High risk for injury related to methyldopa-induced adverse reactions.
• Knowledge deficit related to methyldopa therapy.

Nursing interventions

• *Use cautiously* in patients receiving other antihypertensives or MAO inhibitors and in patients with impaired hepatic function. Monitor blood pressure and pulse rate.
• Methyldopa is used to treat hypertension in pregnant women, apparently without ill effects to the fetus if the patient is closely monitored.
• **I.V. use:** Observe for involuntary choreoathetoid movements. Report to doctor.
• Watch for adverse reactions, particularly unexplained fever. Report to doctor.
• After dialysis, monitor for hypertension. Patient may need extra dose of methyldopa.
• If patient has received this drug for several months, positive direct Coombs' test indicates hemolytic anemia.
• If patient requires blood transfusion, make sure he gets direct and indirect Coombs' tests to avoid cross-matching problems.
• Monitor CBC before and during therapy. Monitor hepatic function periodically.
• Weigh patient daily. Notify doctor of weight increase.
• Explain the importance of taking this drug as prescribed, even when feeling well. Tell the outpatient not to stop this drug suddenly.
• Warn patient that drug may impair mental alertness. Once-daily dosage at bedtime will minimize daytime drowsiness.
• Instruct patient to check with doctor or pharmacist before taking OTC medications.

General

Classification: antirheumatic (gold derivative).
Pregnancy risk category: C.

Mechanism of action

Anti-inflammatory effects in rheumatoid arthritis are probably caused by inhibition of sulfhydryl systems, which alter cellular metabolism. Gold salts may also alter enzyme function and immune response and suppress phagocytic activity.

Indications and dosage

• Rheumatoid arthritis. **Adults:** initially, 10 mg I.M., followed by 25 mg in 1 week. Then, 25 to 50 mg weekly until 14 to 20 doses have been given. If improvement occurs without toxicity, continue 25 to 50 mg q 2 weeks for 4 doses; then, 25 to 50 mg q 3 weeks for 4 doses; then, 25 to 50 mg q month indefinitely as maintenance therapy. If relapse occurs during maintenance therapy, resume injections at weekly intervals. **Children:** initially, 10 mg I.M. After 1 week, begin weekly injections of 1 mg/kg I.M., not to excced 50 mg weekly. After 14 to 20 doses, reduce frequency to every other week or once every 3 weeks.

Adverse reactions

Adverse reactions to gold are considered severe and potentially life-threatening. Report any reactions to the doctor immediately.
Blood: ***thrombocytopenia*** (with or without purpura), ***aplastic anemia, agranulocytosis,*** leukopenia, eosinophilia. **CNS:** *dizziness,* syncope, sweating. **CV:** bradycardia, hypotension. **EENT:** corneal gold deposition, corneal ulcers. **GI:** *metallic taste, stomatitis,* difficulty swallowing, nausea, vomiting. **GU:** albuminuria, proteinuria, ***nephrotic syndrome,*** nephritis, acute tubular necrosis. **Hepatic:** hepatitis, jaundice. **Skin:** *rash and dermatitis in 20% of patients. (If drug is not stopped, may lead to fatal* ***exfoliative dermatitis.****)* **Other:** ***anaphylaxis, angioneurotic edema.***

Interactions

Phenytoin: may increase phenytoin blood levels.

Nursing diagnoses

• Pain related to patient's underlying condition.
• Altered oral mucous membrane related to gold sodium thiomalate-related reaction.
• Knowledge deficit related to gold sodium thiomalate therapy.

Nursing interventions

• *Contraindicated* in severe uncontrollable diabetes, renal disease, hepatic dysfunction, hypertension, heart failure, systemic lupus erythematosus, Sjögren's syndrome, skin rash, and drug allergies or hypersensitivities.
• *Use cautiously* with other drugs that cause blood dyscrasias.
• Most adverse reactions are readily reversible if drug is stopped immediately.
• Color of drug is pale yellow; don't use if it darkens.
• Observe patient for 15 minutes after injection for possible anaphylactoid reaction.
• Inform patient that benefits of therapy may not appear for 3 to 4 months or longer.
• Increased joint pain may occur for 1 to 2 days after injection. This usually subsides after a few injections.
• Advise patient to lie down and to remain recumbent for 10 minutes after injection.
• CBC, including platelet count, should be performed before every second injection during therapy.
• Advise patient to report any skin rashes or problems immediately. Pruritus often precedes dermatitis.
• Advise patient that stomatitis is often preceded by a metallic taste, which should be reported to the doctor at once. Teach careful oral hygiene.
• Stress importance of medical follow-ups.
• Serious toxicity is usually treated with high-dose corticosteroids such as prednisone, 40 to 100 mg daily in divided doses.

methylcellulose

Citrucel◇, Cologel◇

General

Classification: bulk-forming laxative (absorbent).
Pregnancy risk category: C.

Mechanism of action

Absorbs water and expands to increase bulk and moisture content of the stool. The increased bulk encourages peristalsis and bowel movement.

Indications and dosage

• Chronic constipation. **Adults:** 1 heaping tablespoon in 8 ounces cold water daily to t.i.d. **Children 6 to 12 years:** 1 level tablespoon in 4 ounces cold water daily to t.i.d.

Adverse reactions

GI: *nausea,* vomiting, diarrhea (all after excessive use); esophageal, gastric, small intestinal, or colonic strictures when drug is chewed or taken in dry form; *abdominal cramps,* especially in severe constipation. **Other:** laxative dependence in long-term or excessive use.

Interactions

None significant.

Nursing diagnoses

• Constipation related to interruption of normal pattern of elimination characterized by infrequent or absent stools.
• Pain related to methylcellulose-induced abdominal cramping.
• Knowledge deficit related to methylcellulose therapy.

Nursing interventions

• *Contraindicated* in abdominal pain, nausea, vomiting, or other symptoms of appendicitis or acute surgical abdomen; and in intestinal obstruction or ulceration, disabling adhesion, or difficulty swallowing.
• Laxative effect usually takes 12 to 24 hours, but may be delayed 3 days.
• Tell patient to take drug with at least 8 oz (240 ml) of pleasant-tasting liquid to mask grittiness.
• Especially useful in postpartum constipation, debilitated patients, chronic laxative abuse, irritable bowel syndrome, diverticular disease, colostomies, and to empty colon before barium enema examinations.
• Before giving for constipation, determine if patient has adequate fluid intake, exercise, and diet. Tell him that dietary sources of bulk include bran and other cereals, fresh fruit, and vegetables.
• Not absorbed systemically; nontoxic.

General

Classification: fertility agent (gonadotropin releasing hormone). **Pregnancy risk category:** B.

Mechanism of action

Mimics the action of gonadotropin releasing hormone, which results in the synthesis and release of luteinizing hormone (LH) from the anterior pituitary. LH subsequently acts upon the reproductive organs to regulate hormone synthesis.

Indications and dosage

- Induction of ovulation in women with primary hypothalamic amenorrhea. **Women:** 5 mcg I.V. q 90 minutes for 21 days. If no response follows three treatment intervals, dosage may be increased.

Adverse reactions

GU: ovarian hyperstimulation. **Local:** hematoma, infection, inflammation, mild phlebitis. **Other:** multiple pregnancy.

Interactions

None reported.

Nursing diagnoses

- Sexual dysfunction related to the patient's underlying condition.
- High risk for infection related to need for maintaining an I.V. site for extended period.
- Knowledge deficit related to therapy with gonadorelin.

Nursing interventions

- *Contraindicated* in women with ovarian cysts or conditions that could be complicated by pregnancy; and in patients who are anovulatory from any cause other than a hypothalamic disorder.
- Anaphylaxis has been reported with similar drugs. Teach the patient how to recognize the signs and symptoms of hypersensitivity reactions and encourage her to report these promptly.
- Patient should understand that a multiple pregnancy is possible.
- Close monitoring of dosage as well as ultrasonography of the ovaries to monitor drug response is necessary.
- Patients usually require pelvic ultrasound on days 7 and 14 after establishment of a baseline scan.
- Encourage patients to adhere to the close monitoring schedule required by the therapy. Inspect the I.V. site at each visit.
- **I.V. use:** To mimic the naturally occurring hormone, gonadorelin acetate must be administered in a pulsatile fashion with the ambulatory infusion pump. The pulse period is set at 1 minute (drug is infused over 1 minute) and pulse interval is set at 90 minutes.
- To administer 2.5 mcg/pulse, reconstitute the 0.8-mg vial with 8 ml of supplied diluent, and set the pump to deliver 25 microliters/pulse. To administer 5 mcg/pulse, use the same dosage strength and dilution but set the pump to deliver 50 microliters/pulse.
- Some patients may require higher I.V. doses. To administer 10 mcg/pulse, reconstitute the 3.2-mg vial with 8 ml of supplied diluent, and set the pump to deliver 25 microliters/pulse. To administer 20 mcg/pulse, use the same dosage strength and dilution but set the pump to deliver 50 microliters/pulse.
- Instruct the patient about proper aseptic technique and care of the I.V. site. Cannula and I.V. site should be changed every 48 hours.
- Advise patient to report signs of infection, hematoma, inflammation, or phlebitis at the injection site. Patient should also immediately report severe abdominal pain, bloating, swelling of the hands or feet, nausea, vomiting, diarrhea, substantial weight gain, or shortness of breath.

methyclothiazide

Aquatensen, Duretic†, Enduron

General

Classification: diuretic, antihypertensive (thiazide). **Pregnancy risk category:** D

Mechanism of action

A thiazide diuretic that increases urine excretion of sodium and water by inhibiting sodium reabsorption in the cortical diluting site of the nephron.

Indications and dosage

- Edema, hypertension. **Adults:** 2.5 to 10 mg of tablets P.O. daily. **Children:** 0.05 to 2 mg/kg or 1.5 to 6 mg/m^2 P.O. as a single daily dose.

Adverse reactions

Blood: ***aplastic anemia, agranulocytosis,*** leukopenia, thrombocytopenia. **CV:** volume depletion and dehydration, orthostatic hypotension. **GI:** anorexia, nausea, pancreatitis. **Hepatic:** hepatic encephalopathy. **Metabolic:** asymptomatic hyperuricemia, gout, hyperglycemia and impairment of glucose tolerance, fluid and electrolyte imbalances (including dilutional hyponatremia and hypochloremia, hypokalemia, and hypercalcemia), metabolic alkalosis. **Skin:** dermatitis, photosensitivity, rash. **Other:** hypersensitivity reactions, such as pneumonitis and vasculitis.

Interactions

Cholestyramine, colestipol: intestinal absorption of thiazides decreased. Keep doses as separate as possible. **Diazoxide:** increased antihypertensive, hyperglycemic, and hyperuricemic effects. Use together cautiously.

Nursing diagnoses

- Fluid volume excess related to ineffectiveness of methyclothiazide to relieve edema.
- Altered urinary elimination related to methyclothiazide therapy.
- Knowledge deficit related to methyclothiazide therapy.

Nursing interventions

- *Contraindicated* in renal decompensation, anuria, or hypersensitivity to other thiazides or other sulfonamide-derived drugs.
- *Use cautiously* in potassium depletion, renal disease or dysfunction, impaired hepatic function, and progressive hepatic disease.
- Monitor intake and output, weight, blood pressure, and serum electrolytes.
- Consult with doctor and dietitian to provide high-potassium diet. Foods rich in potassium include citrus fruits, tomatoes, bananas, dates, and apricots. Watch for hypokalemia (for example, muscle weakness and cramps). Patients also on digitalis glycosides have an increased risk of digitalis toxicity from the potassium-depleting effect of this diuretic. May use with potassium-sparing diuretic to prevent potassium loss.
- Check insulin requirements in patients with diabetes. May treat severe hyperglycemia with oral antidiabetic agents.
- Monitor serum creatinine and BUN regularly. Not as effective if these levels are more than twice normal.
- Monitor blood uric acid, especially in patients with a history of gout.
- In hypertension, therapeutic response may be delayed several days.
- Give in the morning to prevent nocturia.
- Elderly patients are especially susceptible to excessive diuresis.
- Thiazides and thiazide-like diuretics should be stopped before tests for parathyroid function are performed.
- Advise patient to avoid sudden posture changes and rise slowly to avoid orthostatic hypotension.
- Advise patient to use a sunscreen.

gonadorelin hydrochloride

Factrel

General

Classification: diagnostic agent (luteinizing hormone-releasing hormone [LHRH]). **Pregnancy risk category:** B.

Mechanism of action

A synthetic luteinizing hormone that releases LHRH.

Indications and dosage

- Evaluation of the functional capacity and response of gonadotropic hormones. **Adults:** 100 mcg S.C. or I.V. In women for whom the phase of the menstrual cycle can be established, perform the test between day 1 and day 7.

Adverse reactions

CNS: headache, flushing, light-headedness. **GI:** nausea, abdominal discomfort. **Local:** swelling (occasionally with pain and pruritus) when administered S.C.; rash after long-term S.C. administration.

Interactions

Digoxin, oral contraceptives: may depress gonadotropin levels. Monitor results carefully. **Levodopa, spironolactone:** may elevate gonadotropin levels. Monitor results carefully.

Nursing diagnoses

- Sexual dysfunction related to the patient's underlying condition.
- Pain related to gonadorelin-induced headache and abdominal discomfort.
- Knowledge deficit related to the gonadorelin hydrochloride test.

Nursing interventions

- *Use cautiously* in patients who are allergic to other drugs, although hypersensitivity reactions have not yet been reported. Keep epinephrine readily available.
- As a single injection, gonadorelin can evaluate the functional capacity and response of the gonadotropins of the anterior pituitary. Prolonged or repeated administration may be necessary to measure pituitary gonadotropic reserve.
- The gonadorelin test can be performed concomitantly with other post-treatment evaluations.
- For specific test methodology and interpretation of test results, refer to the manufacturer's full product information. Ask pharmacist for a copy.
- **I.V. use:** Reconstitute vial with 1 to 2 ml of accompanying sterile diluent. Inject drug directly into vein over 3 to 5 minutes. Alternatively, inject into an I.V. line containing a free-flowing compatible solution. Prepare solution immediately before use. After reconstitution, store at room temperature and use within 1 day. Discard unused reconstituted solution and diluent.

General

Classification: anticonvulsant (succinimide derivative). **Pregnancy risk category:** C.

Mechanism of action

Increases seizure threshold. Reduces the paroxysmal spike-and-wave pattern of absence seizures by depressing nerve transmission in the motor cortex.

Indications and dosage

- Refractory absence seizures. **Adults and children:** initially, 300 mg P.O. daily. May increase by 300 mg weekly. Maximum daily dosage is 1.2 g in divided doses.

Adverse reactions

Blood: eosinophilia, ***leukopenia,*** monocytosis, ***pancytopenia.*** **CNS:** *drowsiness, ataxia, dizziness,* irritability, nervousness, headache, insomnia, confusion, depression, aggressiveness. **EENT:** blurred vision, photophobia, periorbital edema. **GI:** *nausea, vomiting, anorexia,* diarrhea, weight loss, abdominal or epigastric pain. **Skin:** urticaria, pruritic and erythematous rashes.

Interactions

None significant.

Nursing diagnoses

- Altered thought processes related to patient's underlying absence seizure disorder.
- Altered protection related to methsuximide-induced blood disorders.
- Knowledge deficit related to methsuximide therapy.

Nursing interventions

- *Contraindicated* in hypersensitivity to succinimide derivatives.
- *Use cautiously* in hepatic or renal dysfunction.
- Never change or withdraw drug suddenly. Abrupt withdrawal may precipitate absence seizures. Call doctor immediately if adverse reactions develop.
- Warn patient to avoid activities that require alertness and good psychomotor coordination until CNS effects of the drug are known.
- Obtain CBC, urinalysis, and liver function tests periodically.
- Tell patient to call doctor promptly if lupus-like syndrome develops.
- May color urine pink or brown.
- Not as popular an anticonvulsant as ethosuximide.

General

Classification: gonadotropin (ovulation stimulant; spermatogenesis stimulant). **Pregnancy risk category:** C.

Mechanism of action

Serves as a substitute for luteinizing hormone to stimulate ovulation of a human menopausal gonadotropin-prepared follicle. Also promotes secretion of gonadal steroid hormones by stimulating the interstitial cells of the testes (Leydig's cells) to produce androgen.

Indications and dosage

- Anovulation and infertility. **Women:** 10,000 units I.M. 1 day after last dose of menotropins.
- Hypogonadism. **Men:** 500 to 1,000 units I.M. three times weekly for 3 weeks, then twice weekly for 3 weeks; or 4,000 units I.M. three times weekly for 6 to 9 months, then 2,000 units three times weekly for 3 more months.
- Nonobstructive cryptorchidism. **Boys 4 to 9 years:** 5,000 units I.M. every other day for four doses.

Adverse reactions

CNS: headache, fatigue, irritability, restlessness, depression. **GU:** early puberty (growth of testes, penis, pubic and axillary hair; voice change; down on upper lip; growth of body hair). **Local:** *pain at injection site.* **Other:** gynecomastia, edema.

Interactions

None significant.

Nursing diagnoses

- Sexual dysfunction related to the patient's underlying condition.
- Pain related to gonadotropin administration.
- Knowledge deficit related to gonadotropin therapy.

Nursing interventions

- *Contraindicated* in patients with pituitary hypertrophy or tumor, prostate cancer, and early puberty (usual onset between ages 10 and 13), undiagnosed vaginal bleeding, uterine fibroids, ovarian cyst, and a history of thrombophlebitis.
- *Use cautiously* in epilepsy, migraine, asthma, and cardiac or renal disease.
- When used with menotropins to induce ovulation, multiple births are possible.
- Usually used only after failure of clomiphene in anovulatory patients.
- In infertility, encourage daily intercourse from day before chorionic gonadotropin is given until ovulation occurs.
- Inspect genitalia of boys for signs of early puberty.
- Be alert to symptoms of ectopic pregnancy. Usually evident between week 8 to 12 of gestation.
- Reconstitute with 1 to 2 ml of supplied diluent just before use. Use reconstituted solutions within 24 hours.
- For I.M. use only. Don't inject I.V. Rotate injection sites to prevent muscle atrophy.
- Instruct the patient to immediately report severe abdominal pain, bloating, swelling of the hands or feet, nausea, vomiting, diarrhea, substantial weight gain, or shortness of breath.
- Also known as HCG.

General

Classification: repigmenting agent, antipsoriatic agent (psoralen derivative). **Pregnancy risk category:** C.

Mechanism of action

May enhance melanogenesis, either directly or secondarily, to an inflammatory process.

Indications and dosage

• To induce repigmentation in vitiligo; psoriasis. **Adults and children over 12 years:** 0.6 mg/kg P.O. 1.5 to 2 hours before measured periods of high-intensity long-wave ultraviolet exposure, 2 to 3 times weekly at least 48 hours apart.

Topical solution: Apply to small, well-defined vitiliginous lesions and allow to dry (1 to 2 minutes); reapply 2 to 2.5 hours before measured periods of long-wave ultraviolet exposure. After exposure, wash lesions with soap and water. Protect area with opaque sunscreen. Although manufacturer recommends treatment weekly, some clinicians may treat q 3 to 5 days.

Adverse reactions

CNS: nervousness, insomnia, depression, vertigo, headache. **GI:** *discomfort, nausea, diarrhea.* **Skin:** edema, erythema, painful blistering, burning, peeling, pruritus.

Interactions

Photosensitizing agents: do not use together. May increase toxicity.

Nursing diagnoses

• Impaired skin integrity related to underlying condition.
• Pain related to headache from adverse reactions to drug.
• Knowledge deficit related to methoxsalen therapy.

Nursing interventions

• *Contraindicated* in hepatic insufficiency, porphyria, acute lupus erythematosus, or hydromorphic and polymorphic light eruptions.
• *Use cautiously* in patients with familial history of sunlight allergy, GI diseases, and chronic infection.
• Regulate therapy carefully. Overdosage or overexposure to light can cause serious burning or blistering. Patients should avoid excessive sunlight during therapy.
• Drug should be taken with meals or milk. Patient should avoid the following foods: limes, figs, parsley, parsnips, mustard, carrots, and celery.
• During light exposure treatments, protect eyes and lips.
• Monthly liver function tests should be done on patients with vitiligo (especially at beginning of therapy).

goserelin acetate

Zoladex

General

Classification: luteinizing hormone-releasing hormone (synthetic decapeptide). **Pregnancy risk category:** X.

Mechanism of action

A luteinizing hormone-releasing hormone (LHRH) analogue that acts on the pituitary to decrease the release of follicle-stimulating hormone and luteinizing hormone. In males, the result is dramatically lowered serum levels of testosterone.

Indications and dosage

• Palliative treatment of advanced carcinoma of the prostate. **Adults:** 1 implant S.C. q 28 days into the upper abdominal wall.

Adverse reactions

Blood: anemia. **CNS:** lethargy, pain (worsened in the first 30 days), dizziness, insomnia, anxiety, depression, headache, chills, fever. **CV:** edema, ***CHF, arrhythmias, CVA,*** hypertension, ***MI,*** peripheral vascular disorder, chest pain. **EENT:** upper respiratory infection. **GI:** nausea, vomiting, diarrhea, constipation, ulcer. **GU:** *impotence,* renal insufficiency, urinary obstruction, urinary tract infection. **Respiratory:** COPD. **Skin:** rash, sweating. **Other:** *hot flashes, sexual dysfunction,* gout, hyperglycemia, weight increase, breast swelling and tenderness.

Interactions

None reported.

Nursing diagnoses

• Anxiety related to goserelin-induced adverse reactions.
• Sexual dysfunction related to goserelin-induced impotence.
• Knowledge deficit related to goserelin therapy.

Nursing interventions

• *Contraindicated* during pregnancy.
• At the beginning of therapy, LHRH analogs such as goserelin may cause a worsening of the symptoms of prostatic cancer because the drug initially causes an increase in testosterone serum levels. A few patients may experience increased bone pain. Rarely, disease exacerbation (either spinal cord compression or ureteral obstruction) has occurred.
• Advise the patient to report every 28 days for a new implant. A delay of a couple of days is permissible, however.
• The implant comes in a preloaded syringe. If the package is damaged, do not use the syringe. Make sure that the drug is visible in the translucent chamber of the syringe.
• The drug is administered into the upper abdominal wall using aspetic technique. After cleaning the area with an alcohol swab (and injecting a local anesthetic), stretch the patient's skin with one hand while grasping the barrel of the syringe with the other. Insert the needle into the S.C. fat, then change direction of the needle so that it parallels the abdominal wall. The needle should then be pushed in until the hub touches the patient's skin, then withdrawn about 1 cm (this creates a gap for the drug to be injected) before depressing the plunger completely.
• To avoid the need for a new syringe and injection site, do not aspirate after inserting the needle.

General

Classification: sedative, analgesic, antipruritic (phenothiazine). **Pregnancy risk category:** C.

Mechanism of action

Acts on the limbic system, thalamus, and hypothalamus to produce hypnotic effects.

Indications and dosage

- Postoperative analgesia. **Adults and children over 12 years:** initially, 2.5 to 7.5 mg I.M. q 4 to 6 hours, then adjust dose.
- Preanesthetic medication. **Adults and children over 12 years:** 2 to 20 mg I.M. 45 minutes to 3 hours before surgery.
- Sedation, analgesia. **Adults and children over 12 years:** 10 to 20 mg deep I.M. q 4 to 6 hours as required; or 6 to 25 mg P.O. daily in three divided doses with meals. For severe pain, dosage may be increased to 50 to 75 mg daily in two or three divided doses with meals. **Adults over 65 years:** 5 to 10 mg I.M. q 4 to 6 hours.
- Psychosis. **Adults:** 6 to 25 mg P.O. daily in three divided doses with meals. Dosage may be gradually increased as needed and tolerated to 50 to 75 mg daily in two or three divided doses.
- Sedation and analgesia during labor. **Adults:** 15 to 20 mg I.M.

Adverse reactions

Blood: ***agranulocytosis*** and other dyscrasias after long-term high dosage. **CNS:** *fainting, weakness, dizziness,* drowsiness, excessive sedation, amnesia, disorientation, euphoria, headache, slurred speech. **CV:** *orthostatic hypotension,* palpitations. **EENT:** nasal congestion. **GI:** dry mouth, nausea, vomiting, abdominal discomfort. **GU:** difficulty urinating. **Local:** *pain, inflammation, swelling at injection site.*

Interactions

All antihypertensive agents: increased orthostatic hypotension. Don't use together. **Epinephrine:** methotrimeprazine reverses the effect of epinephrine on blood pressure, worsening hypotension. Don't use together.

Nursing diagnoses

- Pain related to the patient's underlying condition.
- High risk for injury related to methotrimeprazine-induced drowsiness.
- Knowledge deficit related to methotrimeprazine therapy.

Nursing interventions

- *Contraindicated* in patients receiving concurrent antihypertensive drug therapy, including MAO inhibitors; in patients with a history of seizure disorders; in hypersensitivity to phenothiazines; in severe cardiac, hepatic, or renal disease; in previous overdose of CNS depressant; and in coma.
- *Use with extreme caution* in elderly or debilitated patients with cardiac disease or in those who may be affected by drop in blood pressure.
- *Use injectable form cautiously* in asthmatic patients or in patients with sulfite sensitivity.
- Check pulse rate, blood pressure, and circulation often in debilitated patients while giving dose.
- Expect drop in blood pressure 10 to 20 minutes after I.M. injection. May last 4 to 12 hours.
- Keep patient in bed or closely supervised for 6 to 12 hours after each of the first several injections because orthostatic hypotension may occur. Combat severe hypotension with phenylephrine, methoxamine, or levarterenol. Don't use epinephrine because it may worsen hypotension.
- Inject I.M. into large muscle masses. Rotate sites. Do not administer subcutaneously.
- Warn patient to avoid hazardous activities that require mental alertness or physical coordination.
- Assess patient for anticholinergic symptoms, including mydriasis, dry mouth, or urine retention.
- In prolonged use, monitor liver function and blood studies periodically.
- Monitor for neuroleptic malignant syndrome.
- Methotrimeprazine interferes with provocative and blocking tests for pheochromocytoma.

General
Classification: antifungal (penicillin antibiotic). **Pregnancy risk category:** C.

Mechanism of action
Arrests fungal cell activity by disrupting its mitotic spindle structure.

Indications and dosage
• Ringworm infections of skin, hair, nails (tinea corporis, tinea pedis, tinea capitis) when caused by *Trichophyton, Microsporum*, or *Epidermophyton*. **Adults:** 500 mg (microsize) P.O. daily in single or divided doses. Severe infections may require up to 1 g daily. Alternatively, may give 330 to 375 mg (ultramicrosize) in single or divided doses.
• Tinea pedis and tinea unguium. **Adults:** 0.75 to 1 g (microsize) P.O. daily; or 660 to 750 mg (ultramicrosize) P.O. daily. **Children:** 11 mg/kg (microsize) P.O. daily or 7.3 mg/kg P.O. (ultramicrosize) daily.

Adverse reactions
Blood: leukopenia, ***granulocytopenia.*** **CNS:** headaches, transient decrease in hearing, fatigue with large doses, occasional mental confusion, impaired performance of routine activities, psychotic symptoms, dizziness, insomnia. **GI:** nausea, vomiting, excessive thirst, flatulence, diarrhea. **Metabolic:** porphyria. **Skin:** rash, urticaria, photosensitivity. **Other:** estrogen-like effects in children, oral thrush.

Interactions
Alcohol: may cause tachycardia, diaphoresis, and flushing. Avoid alcohol. **Barbiturates:** decreased griseofulvin blood levels due to decreased absorption or increased metabolism. Avoid using together or administer griseofulvin t.i.d. **Coumarin anticoagulants:** decreased effectiveness. Monitor prothrombin times when used concurrently. **Oral contraceptives:** decreased effectiveness. Suggest alternate methods of contraception.

Nursing diagnoses
• High risk for injury related to ineffectiveness of griseofulvin to eradicate the fungus infection.
• Altered protection related to griseofulvin-induced granulocytopenia.
• Knowledge deficit related to griseofulvin therapy.

Nursing interventions
• *Contraindicated* in porphyria or hepatocellular failure. Because griseofulvin is a penicillin derivative, use cautiously in penicillin-sensitive patients. Use only when topical treatment fails to arrest mycotic disease.
• CBC should be repeated regularly.
• Advise patient that prolonged treatment may be needed to control infection and prevent relapse, even if symptoms abate in first few days of therapy. Tell patient to keep skin clean and dry and to maintain good hygiene. Caution him to avoid intense sunlight.
• Most effectively absorbed and causes least GI distress when given after high-fat meal.
• Effective treatment of tinea pedis may require concomitant use of topical agent.
• Diagnosis of infecting organism should be verified in laboratory. Continue drug until clinical and laboratory examinations confirm complete eradication.
• Because griseofulvin ultramicrosize is dispersed in polyethylene glycol, it is absorbed more rapidly and completely than microsize preparations and is effective at one-half to two-thirds the usual griseofulvin dose.
• Advise patient to avoid alcoholic beverages.

General

Classification: antineoplastic (antimetabolite).
Pregnancy risk category: D.

Mechanism of action

Prevents reduction of folic acid to tetrahydrofolate by binding to dihydrofolate reductase.

Indications and dosage

- Trophoblastic tumors (choriocarcinoma, hydatidiform mole). **Adults:** 15 to 30 mg P.O. or I.M. (sodium) daily for 5 days. Repeat after 1 or more weeks, according to response or toxicity.
- Acute lymphoblastic and lymphatic leukemia. **Adults and children:** 3.3 mg/m² P.O., I.M., or I.V. daily for 4 to 6 weeks or until remission occurs; then 20 to 30 mg/m² P.O. or I.M. twice weekly.
- Meningeal leukemia. **Adults and children:** 10 to 15 mg/m² intrathecally q 2 to 5 days until CSF is normal. Use only 20-, 50-, or 100-mg vials of powder with no preservatives; dilute using 0.9% sodium chloride injection *without* preservatives or Elliot's B solution. Use only new vials of drug and diluent. Use immediately.
- Burkitt's lymphoma (Stage I or Stage II). **Adults:** 10 to 25 mg P.O. daily for 4 to 8 days with 1-week rest intervals.
- Lymphosarcoma (Stage III). **Adults:** 0.625 to 2.5 mg/kg daily P.O., I.M., or I.V.

- Mycosis fungoides. **Adults:** 2.5 to 10 mg P.O. daily or 50 mg I.M. weekly; or 25 mg I.M. twice weekly.
- Psoriasis. **Adults:** 10 to 25 mg P.O., I.M., or I.V. as single weekly dose.
- Rheumatoid arthritis. **Adults:** Initially 7.5 mg P.O. weekly, either in a single dose or divided as 2.5 mg q 12 hours for three doses weekly. Maximum dosage is 20 mg weekly.

Adverse reactions

Blood: WBC and platelet nadir on day 7; ***anemia, leukopenia, thrombocytopenia*** (all dose-related). **CNS:** ***arachnoiditis*** *within hours of intrathecal use;* subacute neurotoxicity (weeks later); ***necrotizing demyelinating leukoencephalopathy*** (years later). **EENT:** pharyngitis. **GI:** gingivitis, *stomatitis; diarrhea leading to* ***hemorrhagic enteritis and intestinal perforation;*** *nausea; vomiting.* **GU:** nephropathy, *tubular necrosis.* **Hepatic:** acute toxicity (elevated transaminases), *chronic toxicity* (cirrhosis, ***hepatic fibrosis***). **Metabolic:** hyperuricemia. **Respiratory:** ***pulmonary fibrosis,*** pneumonitis. **Skin:** *urticaria;* pruritus; hyperpigmentation; exposure to sun may aggravate psoriatic lesions, rash, photosensitivity. **Other:** alopecia; ***pulmonary interstitial infiltrates;*** osteoporosis in children (long-term use).

Interactions

Digoxin: may decrease serum digoxin levels. Monitor closely. **Folic acid derivatives:** antagonized methotrexate effect. **Phenytoin:** may decrease serum phenytoin levels. Monitor closely. **Probenecid, phenylbutazone, NSAIDs, salicylates, sulfonamides:** increased methotrexate toxicity; don't use together. **Vaccines:** ineffective; risk of disseminated infection with live virus vaccines.

Nursing diagnoses

- Altered protection related to methotrexate-induced myelosuppression and immunosuppression.
- Altered oral mucous membrane related to methotrexate-induced stomatitis.
- Knowledge deficit related to methotrexate therapy.

Nursing interventions

- *Use cautiously* and with modified dosage in impaired hepatic or renal function, bone marrow suppression, aplasia, leukopenia, thrombocytopenia, or anemia. Also use cautiously in infection, peptic ulcer, and ulcerative colitis and in very young, elderly, or debilitated patients.
- Perform baseline pulmonary function tests. Watch for increases in AST (SGOT), ALT (SGPT), and alkaline phosphatase. Monitor serum uric acid. Monitor intake and output daily. Encourage fluid intake.
- Take temperature daily, and monitor for cough, dyspnea, cyanosis, bleeding, and infection.
- Follow institutional policy in preparing drug.

General

Classification: expectorant (propanediol derivative). **Pregnancy risk category:** C.

Mechanism of action

Increases production of respiratory tract fluids to help liquefy and reduce the viscosity of tenacious secretions.

Indications and dosage

- As expectorant. **Adults:** 100 to 400 mg P.O. q 4 hours. Maximum 2,400 mg daily. **Children 6 to 12 years:** 100 to 200 mg P.O. q 4 hours. Maximum 600 mg daily. **Children 2 to 5 years:** 50 to 100 mg P.O. q 4 hours. Maximum 300 mg daily.

Adverse reactions

CNS: drowsiness. **GI:** stomach pain, diarrhea, vomiting and nausea occur with large doses.

Interactions

Heparin: increased risk of bleeding. Use together cautiously.

Nursing diagnoses

- Ineffective airway clearance related to the patient's underlying condition.
- Fluid volume deficit related to guaifenesin-induced nausea and vomiting.
- Knowledge deficit related to guaifenesin therapy.

Nursing interventions

- *Contraindicated* in patients with hypersensitivity to the drug.
- May interfere with certain laboratory tests for 5-hydroxyindoleacetic acid and vanillylmandelic acid.
- Drug is used to liquefy thick, tenacious sputum, but efficacy has not been established. Simply increasing fluid intake may prove beneficial. Tell patient to take each dose with a glass of water.
- Monitor cough type and frequency. Be sure patient understands that persistent cough may indicate a serious condition and that he should call the doctor if cough lasts longer than 1 week, recurs frequently, or is associated with high fever, rash, or severe headache.
- Encourage deep-breathing exercises.

General

Classification: skeletal muscle relaxant (carbonate derivative of guaifenesin). **Pregnancy risk category:** C.

Mechanism of action

Reduces transmission of impulses from the spinal cord to skeletal muscle.

Indications and dosage

- As an adjunct in acute, painful musculoskeletal conditions. **Adults:** 1.5 g P.O. q.i.d. for 2 to 3 days, then 1 g q.i.d., or not more than 500 mg (5 ml) I.M. into each gluteal region. May repeat q 8 hours. Or 1 to 3 g daily (10 to 30 ml) I.V. directly into vein at 3 ml/minute, or 10 ml may be added to no more than 250 ml of D_5W or 0.9% sodium chloride solution. Maximum dosage is 3 g daily.
- Supportive therapy in tetanus management. **Adults:** 1 to 2 g into tubing of running I.V. or 1 to 3 g in infusion bottle q 6 hours. **Children:** 15 mg/kg I.V. q 6 hours.

Adverse reactions

Blood: hemolysis, decreased hemoglobin (I.V. only). **CNS:** drowsiness, dizziness, light-headedness, headache, syncope, mild muscular incoordination (I.M. or I.V. only), ***seizures*** (I.V. only). **CV:** hypotension, bradycardia (I.M. or I.V. only). **GI:** nausea, anorexia, GI upset, metallic taste. **GU:** hematuria (I.V. only), discoloration of urine. **Skin:** urticaria, pruritus, rash. **Local:** thrombophlebitis, extravasation (I.V. only). **Other:** fever, flushing, ***anaphylactic reactions*** (I.M. or I.V. only).

Interactions

Alcohol and CNS depressants: increased CNS depression. Avoid concomitant use.

Nursing diagnoses

- Pain related to the patient's underlying condition.
- High risk for injury related to drug-induced drowsiness.
- Knowledge deficit related to methocarbamol therapy.

Nursing interventions

- *Contraindicated* in impaired renal function (injectable form), myasthenia gravis, seizure disorder (injectable form); in children under 12 years (except in tetanus); and in patients receiving anticholinesterase agents.
- **I.V. use:** Infuse slowly, not to exceed 300 mg/minute (3 ml/minute). Drug irritates veins and may aggravate seizures and cause phlebitis and fainting if injected rapidly. Keep patient supine during infusion. Avoid extravasation.
- Give I.M. deeply, only into upper outer quadrant of buttocks with maximum of 5 ml in each buttock.
- Do not give subcutaneously.
- In tetanus management, use methocarbamol with tetanus antitoxin, penicillin, tracheotomy, and aggressive supportive care.
- Watch for orthostatic hypotension, especially with parenteral administration. Keep patient supine for 15 minutes afterward, and supervise ambulation. Advise patient to get up slowly.
- Watch for sensitivity reactions, such as fever and skin eruptions. Have epinephrine, antihistamines, and corticosteroids available.
- Warn patient to avoid activities that require alertness until CNS effects of the drug are known.
- Avoid combining with alcohol or other depressants.
- Advise patient to follow doctor's orders regarding physical activity.
- Tell patient urine may turn green, black, or brown.
- Give tablets with meals or milk to prevent GI distress.
- Prepare liquid by crushing tablets into water or saline solution. Give through nasogastric tube.
- Obtain CBC periodically during prolonged therapy.
- May interfere with urine tests for 5-hydroxyindoleacetic acid and vanillylmandelic acid.

General

Classification: antihypertensive (antiadrenergic agent). **Pregnancy risk category:** C.

Mechanism of action

Inhibits the central vasomotor centers, thereby decreasing sympathetic outflow.

Indications and dosage

- Treatment of hypertension. **Adults:** initially, 4 mg P.O. b.i.d. Dosage may be increased in increments of 4 to 8 mg/day q 1 to 2 weeks (maximum dosage is 32 mg b.i.d). To ensure adequate overnight blood pressure control, give last dose h.s.

Adverse reactions

CNS: *drowsiness, sedation, dizziness, weakness,* headache, ataxia, depression. **CV:** ***severe rebound hypertension.*** **GI:** *dry mouth.* **GU:** sexual dysfunction.

Interactions

CNS depressants: may cause increased sedation. Use together cautiously. **TCAs, MAO inhibitors:** may decrease antihypertensive effect.

Nursing diagnoses

- Altered tissue perfusion (renal, cerebral, cardiopulmonary, peripheral) related to the patient's underlying condition.
- High risk for injury related to guanabenz-induced adverse reactions.
- Knowledge deficit related to guanabenz therapy.

Nursing interventions

- *Use cautiously* in vascular insufficiency, coronary insufficiency, recent MI, cerebrovascular disease, or severe hepatic or renal failure.
- Don't stop guanabenz therapy abruptly. Rebound hypertension may occur.
- Advise patient to avoid driving and other hazardous tasks that require alertness until the CNS effects of the drug are known.
- Elderly patients may be more sensitive to hypotensive effects.
- Warn patient that his tolerance to alcohol or other CNS depressants may be diminished.
- Guanabenz can be used alone or in combination with a thiazide diuretic.
- Teach patient about his disease and therapy. Explain the importance of taking this drug as prescribed, even when he's feeling well. Tell outpatient not to discontinue drug suddenly, but to call the doctor if unpleasant adverse reactions occur.
- Instruct patient to check with doctor or pharmacist before taking OTC medications.
- To relieve dry mouth, tell patient to chew sugarless gum or dissolve ice chips in the mouth.
- Has been used investigationally as an adjunct in the treatment of opiate withdrawal (4 mg P.O. b.i.d.).

General

Classification: antihyperthyroid (thyroid hormone antagonist). **Pregnancy risk category:** D.

Mechanism of action

Inhibits oxidation of iodine in the thyroid gland, blocking iodine's ability to combine with tyrosine to form thyroxine. May also prevent the coupling of monoiodotyrosine and diiodotyrosine to form thyroxine and triiodothyronine.

Indications and dosage

• Hyperthyroidism. **Adults:** 5 mg P.O. t.i.d. if mild; 10 to 15 mg P.O. t.i.d. if moderately severe; and 20 mg P.O. t.i.d. if severe. Continue until patient is euthyroid, then start maintenance dosage of 5 mg daily to t.i.d. Maximum dosage 150 mg daily. **Children:** 0.4 mg/kg P.O. daily divided q 8 hours. Continue until patient is euthyroid, then start maintenance dosage of 0.2 mg/kg daily divided q 8 hours.
• Preparation for thyroidectomy. **Adults and children:** same doses as for hyperthyroidism until patient is euthyroid; then iodine may be added for 10 days before surgery.
• Thyrotoxic crisis. **Adults and children:** same doses as for hyperthyroidism, with concomitant iodine therapy and propranolol.

Adverse reactions

Blood: ***agranulocytosis,*** leukopenia, granulopenia, thrombocytopenia (appear to be dose-related). **CNS:** headache, drowsiness, vertigo. **GI:** diarrhea, nausea, vomiting (may be dose-related). **Hepatic:** jaundice. **Skin:** rash, urticaria, skin discoloration. **Other:** arthralgia, myalgia, salivary gland enlargement, loss of taste, drug fever, lymphadenopathy.

Interactions

None significant.

Nursing diagnoses

• Activity intolerance related to increased metabolic rate.
• High risk for infection related to methimazole-induced blood reaction.
• Knowledge deficit related to methimazole therapy.

Nursing interventions

• *Use cautiously* in pregnancy. Pregnant women may require less drug as pregnancy progresses. Monitor thyroid function studies closely. Thyroid may be added to regimen. Drugs may be stopped during last few weeks of pregnancy.
• Also use cautiously in breast-feeding women. Although drug is excreted in breast milk, small doses given to the mother (15 mg/day or less) do not pose a major risk to the infant if infant's thyroid function is monitored frequently (at biweekly or weekly intervals).
• Watch for signs of hypothyroidism (mental depression; cold intolerance; hard, nonpitting edema). Dosage may need to be adjusted.
• Monitor CBC periodically to detect impending leukopenia, thrombocytopenia, and agranulocytosis. Also monitor hepatic function.
• Doses of over 30 mg/day increase the risk of agranulocytosis.
• Warn patient to report immediately: fever, sore throat, or mouth sores (possible signs of developing agranulocytosis). Agranulocytosis can develop too rapidly to be detected by periodic blood cell counts. Tell patient also to immediately report skin eruptions (sign of hypersensitivity).
• Drug should be stopped if severe rash or enlarged cervical lymph nodes develop.
• Tell patient to ask doctor about using iodized salt and eating shellfish during treatment.
• Warn patient against OTC cough medicines; many contain iodine.
• Give with meals to reduce adverse GI reactions.
• Store in light-resistant container.

General

Classification: antihypertensive (adrenergic neuron blocker). **Pregnancy risk category:** B.

Mechanism of action

Acts peripherally, inhibiting norepinephrine release and depleting norepinephrine stores in adrenergic nerve endings.

Indications and dosage

• Treatment of hypertension. **Adults:** initially, 5 mg P.O. b.i.d. Dosage can be adjusted until blood pressure is controlled. Most patients require doses of 20 to 75 mg/day, usually given b.i.d.; however, tolerance to hypotensive effect may require titration of dosage to 100 to 400 mg daily, given in three to four divided doses.

Adverse reactions

CNS: *fatigue, dizziness,* drowsiness, faintness. **CV:** *orthostatic hypotension,* edema. **GI:** diarrhea. **Other:** impotence, ejaculation disturbances.

Interactions

MAO inhibitors, ephedrine, norepinephrine, methylphenidate, TCAs, amphetamines, phenothiazines: may inhibit the antihypertensive effect of guanadrel. Adjust dose accordingly.

Nursing diagnoses

• Altered tissue perfusion (renal, cerebral, cardiopulmonary, peripheral) related to the patient's underlying condition.
• High risk for injury related to guanadrel-induced hypotension and CNS adverse reactions.
• Knowledge deficit related to guanadrel therapy.

Nursing interventions

• *Contraindicated* in known or suspected pheochromocytoma or frank CHF.
• *Use cautiously* in known peripheral vascular disease, asthma, and history of peptic ulcer disease.
• Guanadrel should be discontinued 48 to 72 hours before surgery to minimize the risk of vascular collapse during anesthesia.
• Don't give concurrently or within 1 week of therapy with an MAO inhibitor.
• Patient response varies widely with this drug and dosage must be individualized. Monitor both supine and standing blood pressure, especially during the period of dosage adjustment.
• Teach patient about his disease and therapy. Explain the importance of taking this drug as prescribed, even when he's feeling well. Tell patient not to discontinue this drug suddenly, but to call the doctor if unpleasant adverse reactions occur.
• Instruct patient to check with doctor or pharmacist before taking OTC medications.
• Tell outpatient to avoid strenuous exercise, and warn that hot showers may cause hypotensive reaction.
• Inform patient that orthostatic hypotension can be minimized by rising slowly from a supine position and by avoiding sudden position changes.
• Elderly patients may be more sensitive to hypotensive effects.

General

Classification: antibiotic (penicillinase-resistant penicillin). **Pregnancy risk category:** B.

Mechanism of action

Inhibits cell wall synthesis during active multiplication (bactericidal). Bacteria resist penicillins by producing penicillinases—enzymes that convert penicillins to inactive penicilloic acid. Methicillin resists these enzymes.

Indications and dosage

• Systemic infections caused by penicillinase-producing staphylococci. **Adults:** 4 to 12 g I.M. or I.V. daily, divided into doses given q 4 to 6 hours. **Children:** 100 to 300 mg/kg I.M. or I.V. daily, divided into doses given q 4 to 6 hours.

Adverse reactions

Blood: ***agranulocytosis,*** *eosinophilia,* hemolytic anemia, transient neutropenia. **CNS:** neuropathy, ***seizures with high doses.*** **GI:** glossitis, stomatitis. **GU:** interstitial nephritis. **Local:** *vein irritation, thrombophlebitis.* **Other:** *hypersensitivity (chills, fever, edema, rash, urticaria,* ***anaphylaxis***), overgrowth of nonsusceptible organisms.

Interactions

Probenecid: increases blood levels of methicillin and other penicillins. Probenecid may be used for this purpose.

Nursing diagnoses

• High risk for injury related to ineffectiveness of methicillin to eradicate the infection.
• Impaired tissue integrity related to methicillin-induced thrombophlebitis at the injection site.
• Knowledge deficit related to methicillin therapy.

Nursing interventions

• *Use cautiously* in patients with other drug allergies, especially to cephalosporins (possible cross-allergenicity), and in infants.
• Obtain specimen for culture and sensitivity tests before first dose. Therapy may begin pending test results.
• Methicillin-resistant strains of staphylococci should be treated with vancomycin.
• Before giving methicillin, ask patient if he's had any allergic reactions to penicillin. However, a negative history of penicillin allergy is no guarantee against a future allergic reaction.
• Closely monitor renal function. Urinalysis should be done frequently to detect interstitial nephritis.
• If patient has high blood level of this drug, he may have seizures. Institute seizure precautions.
• **I.V. use:** When giving I.V., mix with 0.9% sodium chloride solution. Don't mix with others because methicillin may be inactivated. Initial dilution must be made with sterile water for injection.
• Give I.V. intermittently to prevent vein irritation. Change site every 48 hours.
• With large doses and prolonged therapy, bacterial and fungal superinfections may occur, especially in elderly, debilitated, or immunosuppressed patients. Close observation is essential.
• Periodic assessment of hepatic, renal, and hematopoietic function is required during prolonged therapy.
• Give methicillin at least 1 hour before bacteriostatic antibiotics.

General

Classification: antihypertensive (adrenergic neuron blocking agent). **Pregnancy risk category:** C.

Mechanism of action

Acts peripherally, inhibiting norepinephrine release and depleting norepinephrine stores in adrenergic nerve endings.

Indications and dosage

• For moderate to severe hypertension; usually used in combination with other antihypertensives. **Adults:** initially, 10 mg P.O. daily. Increase by 10 mg at weekly to monthly intervals, p.r.n. Usual dose is 25 to 50 mg of tablets daily, but some patients may require up to 300 mg. **Children:** initially, 200 mcg/kg P.O. daily. Increase gradually q 1 to 3 weeks to maximum of 8 times initial dose.

Adverse reactions

CNS: *dizziness, weakness, syncope.* **CV:** *orthostatic hypotension, bradycardia,* ***CHF, arrhythmias.*** **EENT:** *nasal stuffiness.* **GI:** *diarrhea.* **Other:** *edema, weight gain, inhibition of ejaculation.*

Interactions

Levodopa, alcohol: may increase hypotensive effect of guanethidine. Use together cautiously. **MAO inhibitors, ephedrine, norepinephrine, methylphenidate, TCAs, amphetamines, phenothiazines:** may inhibit the antihypertensive effect of guanethidine. Adjust dose accordingly.

Nursing diagnoses

• Altered tissue perfusion (renal, cerebral, cardiopulmonary, and peripheral) related to the patient's underlying condition.
• High risk for injury related to orthostatic hypotension and adverse CNS effects of guanethidine.
• Knowledge deficit related to guanethidine therapy.

Nursing interventions

• *Contraindicated* in pheochromocytoma.
• *Use cautiously* in severe cardiac disease, recent MI, cerebrovascular disease, peptic ulcer, impaired renal function, or bronchial asthma, or in patients taking other antihypertensives.
• Full antihypertensive effect may not appear for 1 to 3 weeks.
• Discontinue drug 2 to 3 weeks before elective surgery to reduce the possibility of vascular collapse and cardiac arrest during anesthesia.
• Teach patient about his disease and therapy. Explain the importance of taking this drug as prescribed. Tell patient not to discontinue this drug suddenly, but to call the doctor if unpleasant adverse reactions occur.
• Instruct patient to check with doctor or pharmacist before taking OTC medications.
• Tell outpatient to avoid strenuous exercise, and warn that hot showers may cause hypotensive reaction. Explain that a hot environment may also potentiate the hypotensive effects of guanethidine.
• Instruct patient on low-sodium diet. Monitor for possible weight gain and edema.
• Inform patient that orthostatic hypotension can be minimized by rising slowly and avoiding sudden position changes. Dry mouth can be relieved with sugarless chewing gum, sour hard candy, or ice chips.
• Elderly patients may be more sensitive to hypotensive effects.
• If patient develops diarrhea, doctor may prescribe atropine or paregoric.

General

Classification: urinary tract antiseptic (formaldehyde pro-drug). **Pregnancy risk category:** C.

Mechanism of action

In acid urine, methenamines are hydrolyzed to ammonia and to formaldehyde, which is responsible for antibacterial action against gram-positive and gram-negative organisms. Mandelic and hippuric acids, with which methenamines are combined, are also antibacterial by unknown mechanisms.

Indications and dosage

- Long-term prophylaxis or suppression of chronic urinary tract infections. **Adults and children over 12 years:** 1 g (hippurate) P.O. q 12 hours. **Children 6 to 12 years:** 500 mg to 1 g (hippurate) P.O. q 12 hours.
- UTIs, infected residual urine in patients with neurogenic bladder. **Adults:** 1 g (mandelate) P.O. q.i.d. after meals. **Children 6 to 12 years:** 500 mg (mandelate) P.O. q.i.d. after meals. **Children under 6 years:** 50 mg/kg (mandelate) P.O. divided in four doses after meals.

Adverse reactions

GI: nausea, vomiting, diarrhea. **GU:** with high doses, urinary tract irritation, dysuria, frequency, albuminuria, hematuria. **Hepatic:** elevated liver enzymes. **Skin:** rashes.

Interactions

Acetazolamide: antagonizes methenamine effect. Use together cautiously. **Urine alkalinizing agents:** inhibit methenamine action. Don't use together.

Nursing diagnoses

- High risk for injury related to ineffectiveness of methenamine to eradicate the infection.
- High risk for fluid volume deficit related to methenamine-induced adverse GI reactions.
- Knowledge deficit related to methenamine therapy.

Nursing interventions

- *Contraindicated* in renal insufficiency, severe hepatic disease, or severe dehydration.
- Ineffective against *Candida* infection.
- Oral suspension contains vegetable oil. Administer cautiously to elderly or debilitated patients because aspiration could cause lipid pneumonia.
- Monitor intake and output. Intake should be at least 1,500 to 2,000 ml daily.
- Obtain a clean-catch urine specimen for culture and sensitivity tests before starting therapy, and repeat p.r.n. Therapy may begin pending test results.
- Limit intake of alkaline foods, such as vegetables, milk, and peanuts. May drink cranberry, plum, and prune juices. These juices or ascorbic acid may be used to acidify urine.
- Warn patient not to take antacids, including Alka-Seltzer and sodium bicarbonate.
- For best results, maintain urine pH at 5.5 or below. Use Nitrazine paper to check pH. Large doses of ascorbic acid (12 g/day) may be necessary to effectively acidify urine.
- *Proteus* and *Pseudomonas* tend to raise urine pH; urine acidifiers are usually necessary when treating these infections.
- Obtain liver function studies periodically during long-term therapy.
- Administer after meals to minimize GI upset.
- If rash appears, withhold dose and contact doctor.

guanfacine hydrochloride

Tenex

General

Classification: antihypertensive (centrally acting antiadrenergic). **Pregnancy risk category:** B.

Mechanism of action

Inhibits the central vasomotor center, thereby decreasing sympathetic outflow.

Indications and dosage

- Treatment of mild to moderate hypertension. **Adults:** initially, 0.5 to 1 mg P.O. daily, h.s. Average dose is 1 to 3 mg daily.

Adverse reactions

CNS: *drowsiness, dizziness,* fatigue, headache, insomnia. **CV:** bradycardia, orthostatic hypotension, rebound hypertension. **GI:** *constipation,* diarrhea, dry mouth, nausea. **Skin:** dermatitis, pruritus.

Interactions

None significant.

Nursing diagnoses

- Altered tissue perfusion (renal, cerebral, cardiopulmonary, and peripheral) related to the patient's underlying condition.
- High risk for injury related to guanfacine-induced adverse reactions.
- Knowledge deficit related to guanfacine therapy.

Nursing interventions

- *Use cautiously* in severe coronary insufficiency, recent MI, cerebrovascular disease, or chronic renal or hepatic insufficiency.
- Warn patients not to discontinue therapy abruptly. Rebound hypertension is less common than with similar drugs, such as clonidine, but may occur.
- Guanfacine reportedly has no adverse effect on blood lipids.
- May be used alone or with a diuretic.
- Note incidence and severity of adverse reactions increase with higher dosages.
- Teach patient about his disease and therapy. Explain the importance of taking this drug as prescribed, even when he's feeling well. Tell outpatient not to discontinue drug suddenly, but to call the doctor if unpleasant adverse reactions occur.
- Instruct patient to check with doctor or pharmacist before taking OTC medications.
- Because guanfacine causes drowsiness, advise patient to avoid activities that require alertness until response to the drug is established.
- Guanfacine appears to be as effective as methyldopa and clonidine; long half-life permits once-daily dosing.

General

Classification: antihistamine (H_1-receptor antagonist), antipruritic (phenothiazine). **Pregnancy risk category:** C.

Mechanism of action

Competes with histamine for H_1-receptor sites on effector cells. Prevents but does not reverse histamine-mediated responses.

Indications and dosage

- Allergic rhinitis; pruritus. **Adults:** 8 mg P.O. b.i.d. to q.i.d. or (chewable tablets) 7.2 mg b.i.d. to q.i.d. **Children over 3 years:** 4 mg P.O. b.i.d. to q.i.d. or (chewable tablets) 3.6 mg b.i.d. to q.i.d.

Adverse reactions

CNS: (especially in elderly patients) *drowsiness,* dizziness, headache. **GI:** nausea, *dry mouth and throat.* **GU:** urine retention. **Hepatic:** cholestatic jaundice. **Skin:** rash.

Interactions

CNS depressants: increased sedation. Use together cautiously. **MAO inhibitors:** increased anticholinergic effects. Don't use together. **Phenothiazines:** increased effects. Don't use together.

M

Nursing diagnoses

- Ineffective airway clearance related to the patient's underlying condition.
- High risk for injury related to methdilazine-induced drowsiness.
- Knowledge deficit related to methdilazine therapy.

Nursing interventions

- *Contraindicated* in acute asthmatic attacks.
- *Use cautiously* in elderly or debilitated patients; acutely ill or dehydrated children; in patients with a history of seizures; in pulmonary, hepatic, or CV disease; and in asthma, hypertension, prostatic hypertrophy, bladder-neck obstruction, CNS depression, and stenosing peptic ulcers.
- Warn patient against drinking alcoholic beverages during therapy and against driving or other activities that require alertness until CNS response to drug is determined.
- Reduce GI distress by giving with food or milk.
- Coffee or tea may reduce drowsiness. Sugarless gum or sour hard candy, or ice chips may relieve dry mouth.
- If tolerance develops, another antihistamine may be substituted.
- Available as chewable tablet for children. Instruct child to chew completely and swallow promptly; may cause local anesthetic effect in mouth, which increases the risk of choking.
- Warn patient to stop taking drug 4 days before allergy skin tests to preserve accuracy of tests.
- Antihistamines are not recommended for use by women who are breast-feeding because small amounts of drug are excreted in breast milk.

General

Classification: bacterial vaccine. **Pregnancy risk category:** C.

Mechanism of action

Promotes active immunity to *Haemophilus influenzae* type B (Hib) infection. Conjugate vaccines covalently link Haemophilus antigen to other highly antigenic substances such as diptheria toxoid fragments. This process enhances the antigenicity of the vaccine and ensures an immune response from undeveloped immune systems found in infants.

Indications and dosage

• Immunization against Hib infection.
—***Conjugate vaccine, diphtheria CRM$_{197}$ protein conjugate.*** **Infants:** 0.5 ml I.M. HibTITER at age 2 months. Repeat at ages 4 months and 6 months. A booster dose is required at age 15 months. **Previously unvaccinated infants 2 to 6 months:** 0.5 ml I.M. HibTITER. Repeat in 2 months and again in 4 months for a total of three doses. Give a booster dose at age 15 months. **Previously unvaccinated infants 7 to 11 months:** 0.5 ml I.M. Repeat in 2 months for a total of two doses. Give a booster dose at age 15 months (but no sooner than 2 months after the last vaccination). **Previously unvaccinated infants 12 to 14 months:** 0.5 ml I.M. Give a booster dose at age 15 months (but no sooner than 2 months after the first vaccination). **Previously unvaccinated children 15 months to 5 years:** 0.5 ml I.M. A booster dose is not required.
—***Conjugate vaccine, diphtheria toxoid conjugate.*** **Previously unvaccinated children 15 months to 5 years:** 0.5 ml I.M. ProHIBiT. A booster dose is not required. Not recommended for use in children under age 15 months.
—***Conjugate vaccine, meningococcal protein conjugate.*** **Infants:** 0.5 ml I.M. PedvaxHIB at age 2 months. Repeat at age 4 months. A booster dose is required at age 12 months. **Previously unvaccinated infants 2 to 6 months:** 0.5 ml I.M. PedvaxHIB. Repeat in 2 months. Give a booster dose at age 12 months. **Previously unvaccinated infants 7 to 11 months:** 0.5 ml I.M. Repeat in 2 months. Give a booster dose at age 15 months (but no sooner than 2 months after the last vaccination). **Previously unvaccinated infants 12 to 14 months:** 0.5 ml I.M. Give a booster dose at age 15 months (but no sooner than 2 months after the first vaccination). **Previously unvaccinated children 15 months to 5 years:** 0.5 ml I.M. A booster dose is not required.

Adverse reactions

Systemic: fever, ***anaphylaxis.*** **Local:** *erythema and pain at injection site.*

Interactions

Immunosuppressive agents: may suppress antibody response to Hib vaccine.

Nursing diagnoses

• Altered protection related to lack of immunity to Hib infection.
• Ineffective breathing pattern related to vaccine-induced anaphylaxis.
• Knowledge deficit related to the vaccine.

Nursing interventions

• *Contraindicated* in immunosuppression and febrile illness. Defer immunization in acute illness.
• Don't administer intradermally or I.V. Administer into anterolateral aspect of upper thigh in small children. May be injected into deltoid muscle of larger children if sufficient muscle mass is present.
• Keep in mind that diphtheria toxoid conjugate vaccine (ProHIBiT) is not recommended for children under age 15 months.
• This vaccine will *not* protect children against any other microorganisms that cause meningitis. Will protect against Hib only.
• This vaccine and DPT can be given simultaneously. A combination product is commercially available.
• Not routinely given to children over 5 years or adults unless they're at high risk for infection.

methazolamide Neptazane

General
Classification: antiglaucoma agent (carbonic anhydrase inhibitor). **Pregnancy risk category:** C.

Mechanism of action
Decreases secretion of aqueous humor in the eye, thereby lowering intraocular pressure.

Indications and dosage
- Glaucoma (open-angle, or preoperatively in obstructive or narrow-angle). **Adults:** 50 to 100 mg b.i.d. or t.i.d.

Adverse reactions
Blood: ***aplastic anemia,*** hemolytic anemia, leukopenia. **CNS:** drowsiness, paresthesia. **EENT:** transient myopia. **GI:** nausea, vomiting, anorexia. **GU:** crystalluria, renal calculi. **Metabolic:** hyperchloremic acidosis, hypokalemia, asymptomatic hyperuricemia. **Skin:** rash.

Interactions
NSAIDs: decreased diuretic effectiveness. Avoid concomitant use.

Nursing diagnoses
- High risk for injury related to intraocular pressure above normal.
- Altered protection related to methazolamide-induced blood disorders.
- Knowledge deficit related to methazolamide therapy.

Nursing interventions
- *Contraindicated* in severe or absolute glaucoma; for long-term use in chronic noncongestive narrow-angle glaucoma; in patients with depressed serum sodium or potassium levels, renal or hepatic disease or dysfunction, adrenal gland dysfunction, or hyperchloremic acidosis.
- *Use cautiously* in respiratory acidosis, emphysema, and chronic pulmonary disease.
- Monitor intake and output, weight, and serum electrolytes.
- May cause false-positive urine protein tests by alkalinizing urine.
- Elderly patients are especially susceptible to excessive diuresis.
- Diuretic effect decreases in acidosis.
- Anticipate that drug will be given every day for glaucoma but intermittently for edema. Caution patient to comply with prescribed dosage to lessen risk of metabolic acidosis.
- Evaluate the patient with glaucoma for eye pain to make sure drug is effective in decreasing intraocular pressure.

General

Classification: anxiolytic (benzodiazepine). **Pregnancy risk category:** D. **Controlled substance schedule:** IV.

Mechanism of action

Depresses the CNS at the limbic and subcortical levels of the brain.

Indications and dosage

- Relief of anxiety and tension. **Adults:** Usual dose is 20 to 40 mg P.O. t.i.d. or q.i.d. Optimal daily dosage is generally 80 to 160 mg. Daily dosages up to 600 mg have been given. In elderly or debilitated patients, initial dosage is 20 mg once or twice daily.

Adverse reactions

CNS: *drowsiness, lethargy, hangover,* fainting. **CV:** transient hypotension. **GI:** dry mouth, nausea and vomiting, discomfort.

Interactions

Alcohol, other CNS depressants: increased CNS depression. Avoid concomitant use. **Cigarette smoking:** increased clearance of benzodiazepines. Monitor for lack of effect. **Cimetidine:** possible increased sedation. Monitor carefully. **Digoxin:** benzodiazepines may increase serum levels of digoxin, increasing risk of toxicity. Monitor closely.

Nursing diagnoses

- Anxiety related to the patient's underlying condition.
- High risk for injury related to halazepam-induced CNS reactions.
- Knowledge deficit related to halazepam therapy.

Nursing interventions

- *Contraindicated* in patients with hypersensitivity to the drug and in patients with acute narrow-angle glaucoma, psychoses, or anxiety-free psychiatric disorders.
- *Use cautiously* in hepatic or renal impairment.
- Reduce dosage in elderly or debilitated patients.
- Possibility of abuse and addiction exists. Do not withdraw drug abruptly after long-term use; withdrawal symptoms may occur.
- Warn patient not to combine drug with alcohol or other depressants and to avoid hazardous activities that require alertness and psychomotor coordination until CNS effects are known.
- Caution patient against giving medication to others.
- Periodic hepatic, renal, and hematopoietic function studies should be performed in patients receiving repeated or prolonged therapy.
- Drug should not be prescribed for everyday stress or for long-term use (more than 4 months).
- If halazepam overdose occurs, flumazenil (a specific benzodiazepine antagonist) may be useful. Know that the duration of action of halazepam is longer than that of flumazenil, and resedation is possible.

General

Classification: antimuscarinic, GI antispasmodic (anticholinergic). **Pregnancy risk category:** C.

Mechanism of action

Competitively blocks acetylcholine, which decreases GI motility and inhibits gastric acid secretion.

Indications and dosage

- Adjunctive therapy in peptic ulcer, pylorospasm, spastic colon, biliary dyskinesia, pancreatitis, and certain forms of gastritis. **Adults:** 50 to 100 mg P.O. q 6 hours. **Children over 1 year:** 12.5 to 50 mg P.O. q.i.d. **Children under 1 year:** 12.5 to 25 mg P.O. q.i.d. **Neonates:** 12.5 mg P.O. b.i.d. to t.i.d.

Adverse reactions

CNS: headache, insomnia, drowsiness, dizziness, *confusion or excitement in elderly patients,* nervousness, weakness. **CV:** *palpitations,* tachycardia. **EENT:** *blurred vision,* mydriasis, increased ocular tension, cycloplegia, photophobia. **GI:** *dry mouth,* dysphagia, *constipation,* heartburn, loss of taste, nausea, vomiting, *paralytic ileus.* **GU:** *urinary hesitancy, urine retention,* impotence. **Skin:** urticaria, decreased sweating or possible anhidrosis, other dermal manifestations. **Other:** fever, allergic reactions.

M

Overdosage may cause curare-like symptoms.

Interactions

Amantadine, antihistamines, antiparkinsonian agents, disopyramide, glutethimide, meperidine, phenothiazines, procainamide, quinidine: additive adverse effects. Avoid concomitant use. **Ketoconazole:** anticholinergics may interfere with ketoconazole absorption. Avoid concomitant use. **Methotrimeprazine:** anticholinergics may enhance risk of extrapyramidal reactions. Avoid concomitant use.

Nursing diagnoses

- Pain related to the patient's underlying condition.
- Urinary retention related to adverse drug reaction.
- Knowledge deficit related to methantheline therapy.

Nursing interventions

- *Contraindicated* in narrow-angle glaucoma, obstructive uropathy, obstructive disease of GI tract, severe ulcerative colitis, myasthenia gravis, hypersensitivity to anticholinergics, paralytic ileus, intestinal atony, unstable CV status in acute hemorrhage, or toxic megacolon.
- *Use cautiously* in autonomic neuropathy, hyperthyroidism, coronary artery disease, cardiac arrhythmias, CHF, hypertension, hiatal hernia associated with reflux esophagitis, hepatic or renal disease, and ulcerative colitis or in patients over 40 years because of the increased incidence of glaucoma. Also use cautiously in hot or humid environments. Drug-induced heatstroke can develop.
- Give 30 minutes to 1 hour before meals and at bedtime. Bedtime dose can be larger and should be given at least 2 hours after last meal of day.
- If patient is also taking antihistamines, he may experience increased dryness of mouth.
- Monitor patient's vital signs and urine output carefully.
- Instruct patient to avoid driving and other hazardous activities if he is drowsy, dizzy, or has blurred vision; to drink plenty of fluids to help prevent constipation; and to report any rash or skin eruption.
- Gum or sugarless hard candy may relieve dry mouth.
- Therapeutic effects appear in 30 to 45 minutes; persist for 4 to 6 hours after oral administration.

haloperidol

Apo-Haloperidol†, Haldol**; Haldol Decanoate; Haldol

General

Classification: antipsychotic (butyrophenone).
Pregnancy risk category: C.

Mechanism of action

Blocks postsynaptic dopamine receptors in the brain.

Indications and dosage

- Psychotic disorders. **Adults:** Dosage varies for each patient. Initial range is 0.5 to 5 mg P.O. b.i.d. or t.i.d.; or 2 to 5 mg I.M. q 4 to 8 hours, increasing rapidly if necessary for prompt control. Maximum dosage is 100 mg P.O. daily. Doses over 100 mg have been used for patients with severely resistant conditions.
- Chronic psychotic patients who require prolonged therapy. **Adults:** 50 to 100 mg (decanoate) I.M. q 4 weeks.
- Control of tics, vocal utterances in Gilles de la Tourette's syndrome. **Adults:** 0.5 to 5 mg P.O. b.i.d. or t.i.d., increasing p.r.n.

Adverse reactions

Blood: transient leukopenia and leukocytosis. **CNS:** *high incidence of severe extrapyramidal reactions, tardive dyskinesia,* low incidence of sedation. **CV:** low incidence of CV effects with therapeutic dosages. **EENT:** *blurred vision.* **GI:** *dry mouth.* **GU:** urine retention, menstrual irregularities, gynecomastia. **Skin:** rash. **Other:** rarely, ***neuroleptic malignant syndrome*** (fever, tachycardia, tachypnea, profuse diaphoresis).

Interactions

Alcohol, other CNS depressants: increased CNS depression. Avoid concomitant use. **Lithium:** lethargy and confusion with high doses. Observe patient. **Methyldopa:** possible symptoms of dementia. Observe patient.

Nursing diagnoses

- Impaired thought processes related to the patient's underlying condition.
- Impaired physical mobility related to high risk for extrapyramidal effects.
- Knowledge deficit related to haloperidol therapy.

Nursing interventions

- *Contraindicated* in parkinsonism, coma, or CNS depression.
- *Use cautiously* in elderly and debilitated patients; in severe CV disorders, allergies, glaucoma, and urine retention; and in conjunction with anticonvulsant, anticoagulant, antiparkinsonian, or lithium medications.
- Tardive dyskinesia may occur after prolonged use. It may not appear until months or years later and may disappear spontaneously or persist for life despite discontinuation of drug.
- Neuroleptic malignant syndrome is rare, but frequently fatal. It is not necessarily related to length of drug use or type of neuroleptic, but over 60% of affected patients are men. Watch for symptoms.
- Acute dystonic reactions may be treated with I.V. diphenhydramine.
- Elderly patients usually require lower initial doses and a more gradual dosage titration.
- Haloperidol is the least sedating of the antipsychotic agents. However, warn patient against activities that require alertness and good psychomotor coordination until CNS effects of the drug are known. Drowsiness and dizziness usually subside after a few weeks.
- Protect medication from light. Slight yellowing of injection or concentrate is common; does not affect potency. Discard markedly discolored solutions.
- Do not withdraw drug abruptly unless required by severe adverse reactions.
- Dry mouth may be relieved by sugarless gum, sour hard candy, and rinsing with mouthwash.
- Dose of 2 mg is therapeutic equivalent of 100 mg chlorpromazine.
- Especially useful for agitation associated with senile dementia.
- When changing from tablets to decanoate injection, patient should receive 10 to 15 times the oral dose once a month (maximum 100 mg).
- Don't administer the decanoate form I.V.

General

Classification: analgesic, opiate detoxification adjunct (opioid). **Pregnancy risk category:** B (D with prolonged use or high doses at term). **Controlled substance schedule:** II.

Mechanism of action

Binds with opiate receptors at many sites in the CNS (brain, brain stem, and spinal cord), altering both perception of and emotional response to pain.

Indications and dosage

• Severe pain. **Adults:** 2.5 to 10 mg P.O., I.M., or S.C. q 6 to 8 hours, p.r.n. or around the clock.
• Narcotic abstinence syndrome. **Adults:** 15 to 40 mg P.O. daily (highly individualized). Maintenance dosage is 20 to 120 mg P.O. daily. Adjust dose as needed. Daily dosages greater than 120 mg require special state and federal approval.

Adverse reactions

CNS: *sedation, somnolence, clouded sensorium, euphoria,* dizziness, seizures with large doses. **CV:** *hypotension,* bradycardia. **GI:** *nausea, vomiting, constipation,* ileus. **GU:** *urine retention.* **Local:** pain at injection site, tissue irritation, induration following S.C. injection. **Other:** ***respiratory depression,*** decreased libido, sweating, physical dependence.

Interactions

Alcohol, CNS depressants: additive effects. Use together cautiously. **Ammonium chloride and other urine acidifiers, phenytoin:** may reduce methadone effect. Monitor for decreased pain control. **Rifampin:** withdrawal symptoms; reduced blood levels of methadone. Use together cautiously.

Nursing diagnoses

• Pain related to the patient's underlying condition.
• Ineffective breathing pattern related to methadone-induced respiratory depression.
• Knowledge deficit related to methadone therapy.

Nursing interventions

• Contraindicated in patients with hypersensitivity to the drug or other opiate analgesics.
• *Use with extreme caution* in elderly or debilitated patients or in patients with acute abdominal conditions, severe hepatic or renal impairment, hypothyroidism, Addison's disease, prostatic hypertrophy, urethral stricture, head injury, increased intracranial pressure, asthma, COPD, respiratory depression, and CNS depression.
• When used as an adjunct in the treatment of narcotic addiction ("maintenance"), withdrawal will usually be delayed and mild. Safe use as maintenance drug in adolescent addicts not established.
• Oral liquid form legally required in maintenance programs. Completely dissolve tablets in 120 ml of orange juice or powdered citrus drink.
• Oral dose is half as potent as injected dose.
• Rotate injection sites.
• Has cumulative effect; marked sedation can occur after repeated doses.
• Monitor circulatory and respiratory status and bladder and bowel function. Patient may need a laxative.
• Warn ambulatory patient to avoid activities that require mental alertness or physical coordination.
• When used for severe, chronic pain, tolerance may develop with long-term use, requiring a higher dose to achieve the same degree of analgesia. This is *not* a sign of addiction.
• Patient treated for narcotic abstinence syndrome will usually require an additional analgesic if pain control is necessary.
• Use with general anesthetics, tranquilizers, sedatives, hypnotics, alcohol, tricyclic antidepressants, or MAO inhibitors may cause respiratory depression, hypotension, profound sedation, or coma. Use together with extreme caution. Monitor patient response.

General

Classification: anticoagulant (blood derivative.)
Pregnancy risk category: C.

Mechanism of action

Accelerates formation of an antithrombin III-thrombin complex and inactivates thrombin and prevents conversion of fibrinogen to fibrin.

Indications and dosage

Heparin dosing is highly individualized, depending upon disease state, age, and renal and hepatic status.

• Treatment of deep vein thrombosis, MI, pulmonary embolism. **Adults:** initially, 5,000 to 10,000 units I.V. push, then adjust according to partial thromboplastin time (PTT) and give I.V. q 4 hours (usually 4,000 to 5,000 units); or 5,000 to 7,500 units I.V. bolus, then 1,000 units/hour by I.V. infusion pump. Wait 8 hours following bolus dose; adjust hourly rate according to PTT.

• Prophylaxis of embolism, venous thrombosis, pulmonary embolism, atrial fibrillation with embolism; prophylaxis of postoperative deep vein thrombosis. **Adults:** 5,000 units S.C. q 12 hours. In surgical patients, give first dose 2 hours before procedure; follow with 5,000 units S.C. q 8 to 12 hours for 5 to 7 days or until patient is ambulatory.

Adverse reactions

Blood: ***hemorrhage with excessive dosage,*** *overly prolonged clotting time,* ***thrombocytopenia.*** **Local:** irritation, mild pain, hematoma, ulceration, cutaneous or subcutaneous necrosis. **Other:** ***"white clot" syndrome,*** hypersensitivity reactions.

Interactions

Oral anticoagulants: additive anticoagulation. Monitor PT and PTT. **Salicylates:** increased anticoagulant effect. **Thrombolytics:** increased risk of hemorrhage. Monitor closely.

Nursing diagnoses

• Altered tissue perfusion (renal, cerebral, cardiopulmonary, GI, peripheral) related to the patient's underlying condition.
• High risk for fluid volume deficit related to adverse effects of heparin therapy.
• Knowledge deficit related to heparin therapy.

Nursing interventions

• Conditionally *contraindicated* in active bleeding; blood dyscrasia; or bleeding tendencies such as hemophilia, thrombocytopenia, or hepatic disease with hypoprothrombinemia; suspected intracranial hemorrhage; suppurative thrombophlebitis; inaccessible ulcerative lesions (especially of GI tract); open ulcerative wounds; extensive denudation of skin; ascorbic acid deficiency and other conditions causing increased capillary permeability; during or after brain, eye, or spinal cord surgery; during spinal tap or spinal anesthesia; during continuous tube drainage of stomach or small intestine; in subacute bacterial endocarditis; shock; advanced renal disease; threatened abortion.
• *Use cautiously* during menses; in mild hepatic or renal disease or alcoholism; in patients with high-risk occupations; immediately postpartum; in patients with history of allergies, asthma, GI ulcers.
• Monitor platelet counts regularly; thrombocytopenia caused by heparin associated with an arterial thrombosis is called "white clot" syndrome.
• Measure PTT carefully and regularly. Anticoagulation is present when PTT values are 1.5 to 2 times control values.
• Low-dose injections given sequentially between iliac crests in lower abdomen deep into subcutaneous fat. Inject drug slowly S.C. into fat pad. Leave needle in place for 10 seconds after injection; then withdraw needle. Alternate site every 12 hours—right for a.m., left for p.m.
• **I.V. use:** I.V. administration preferred because of long-term effect and irregular absorption when given S.C. Whenever possible, administer I.V. heparin using infusion pump to provide maximum safety. Never piggyback other drugs into an infusion line while heparin infusion is running.
• Avoid excessive I.M. injections of other drugs to prevent or minimize hematomas.
• Abrupt withdrawal may cause increased coagulability.

General

Classification: vasopressor (adrenergic). **Pregnancy risk category:** D.

Mechanism of action

Predominantly stimulates alpha-adrenergic receptors within the sympathetic nervous system.

Indications and dosage

- Prevention of hypotension. **Adults:** 2 to 10 mg I.M. or S.C.
- Severe shock. **Adults:** 0.5 to 5 mg direct I.V. followed by I.V. infusion.
- Treatment of hypotension caused by shock. **Adults:** 15 to 100 mg in 500 ml 0.9% sodium chloride solution or D_5W I.V. infusion. Adjust rate to maintain blood pressure.
- **Children** (all indications): 0.01 mg/kg as single I.V. injection; 1 mg/25 ml D_5W as I.V. infusion. Adjust rate to maintain blood pressure. Or 0.1 mg/kg I.M. as single dose, p.r.n. Allow 10 minutes to elapse before increasing dose because maximum effect is not immediately apparent.

Adverse reactions

CNS: apprehension, restlessness, dizziness, headache, tremor, weakness; with excessive use, ***seizures.*** **CV:** hypertension; hypotension; precordial pain; palpitations; ***arrhythmias,*** including sinus or ***ventricular tachycardia;*** bradycardia; premature supraventricular contractions; AV dissociation. **GI:** nausea, vomiting. **GU:** decreased urine output. **Metabolic:** hyperglycemia. **Skin:** flushing, pallor, sweating. **Local:** abscess, necrosis, and sloughing upon extravasation. **Other:** ***metabolic acidosis in hypovolemia,*** *increased body temperature,* ***respiratory distress.***

Interactions

General anesthetics: increased risk of adverse cardiac effects. Monitor closely. **MAO inhibitors:** may cause hypertensive crisis. Don't use together.

Nursing diagnoses

- Ineffective breathing pattern related to metaraminol-induced adverse effects.
- Altered cardiopulmonary tissue perfusion related to metaraminol-induced adverse effects.
- Knowledge deficit related to metaraminol therapy.

Nursing interventions

- *Contraindicated* in peripheral or mesenteric thrombosis, pulmonary edema, hypercarbia, or acidosis and during anesthesia with cyclopropane and halogenated hydrocarbon anesthetics.
- *Use cautiously* in hypertension, thyroid disease, diabetes, cirrhosis, malaria, or sulfite sensitivity and in patients taking digitalis glycosides.
- Replace volume deficit before giving this drug.
- **I.V. use:** Use a central venous catheter or large veins to minimize risk of extravasation. If it occurs, stop infusion immediately and call doctor. Use a continuous infusion pump to regulate infusion flow rate and a piggyback setup so I.V. can continue if this drug is stopped. Watch site for signs of extravasation.
- During infusion, check blood pressure every 5 minutes until stabilized; then every 15 minutes. Monitor ECG, blood pressure, cardiac output, central venous pressure, pulmonary artery wedge pressure, pulse rate, urine output, and color and temperature of extremities.
- When discontinuing this drug, slow infusion rate gradually. Continue monitoring vital signs, watching for possible severe hypotension. Keep equipment nearby to start drug again, if necessary.
- Blood pressure should be raised to slightly less than the patient's normal level. Rapidly induced hypertensive response can cause acute pulmonary edema, arrhythmias, and cardiac arrest.
- With an excessive vasopressor response, elevated blood pressure may persist after stopping the drug.
- Report persistent decreased urine output.
- Keep atropine, phentolamine, and propranolol on hand to reverse effects of metaraminol.
- Closely monitor patients with diabetes. Adjustment in insulin dose may be needed.
- Metaraminol shouldn't be mixed with other drugs.

General
Classification: hepatitis B prophylaxis (immune serum). **Pregnancy risk category:** C.

Mechanism of action
Provides passive immunity to hepatitis B.

Indications and dosage
• Hepatitis B exposure in high-risk patients. **Adults and children:** 0.06 ml/kg I.M. within 7 days after exposure. Repeat 28 days after exposure. **Neonates born to women who test positive for hepatitis B surface antigen (HBsAg):** 0.5 ml within 12 hours of birth. Repeat dose at ages 3 months and 6 months.

Adverse reactions
Systemic: ***anaphylaxis.***

Interactions
Other vaccines: Hepatitis B immune globulin may interfere with response to live virus vaccines. Defer administration for 3 months.

Nursing diagnoses
• Altered protection related to lack of immunity to hepatitis B.
• Ineffective breathing pattern related to immunization-induced anaphylaxis.
• Knowledge deficit related to hepatitis B immune globulin.

Nursing interventions
• *Contraindicated* in patients with a history of anaphylactic reactions to immune serum.
• Anterolateral aspect of thigh or deltoid areas are the preferred injection sites in adults; anterolateral aspect of thigh is preferred for neonates and children under 3 years.
• Health care personnel should receive immunization if exposed to hepatitis B (for example, by needle stick or direct contact).
• Obtain history of allergies and reaction to immunizations.

General

Classification: bronchodilator (adrenergic). **Pregnancy risk category:** C.

Mechanism of action

Relaxes bronchial smooth muscle by acting on beta$_2$-adrenergic receptors.

Indications and dosage

- Acute episodes of bronchial asthma. **Adults and children:** 2 to 3 inhalations. Should not repeat inhalations more often than q 3 to 4 hours. Should not exceed 12 inhalations daily.
- Bronchial asthma and reversible bronchospasm. **Adults:** 20 mg P.O. q 6 to 8 hours. **Children over 9 years or over 27 kg:** 20 mg P.O. q 6 to 8 hours (0.4 mg to 0.9 mg/kg/dose t.i.d.). **Children 6 to 9 years or less than 27 kg:** 10 mg P.O. q 6 to 8 hours (0.4 mg to 0.9 mg/kg/dose t.i.d.).

Not recommended for children under 6 years.

Adverse reactions

CNS: nervousness, weakness, drowsiness, tremor. **CV:** tachycardia, hypertension, palpitations; *with excessive use, **cardiac arrest.*** **GI:** vomiting, nausea, bad taste in mouth. **Other:** paradoxical bronchiolar constriction with excessive use.

Interactions

Levodopa: risk of cardiac arrhythmias. Avoid concomitant use. **Propranolol and other beta blockers:** blocked bronchodilating effect of metaproterenol. Monitor patient carefully if used together.

Nursing diagnoses

- Ineffective airway clearance related to patient's underlying condition.
- Noncompliance related to medication regimen.
- Knowledge deficit related to metaproterenol therapy.

Nursing interventions

- *Contraindicated* in tachycardia and arrhythmias associated with tachycardia. *Use cautiously* in hypertension, coronary artery disease, hyperthyroidism, and diabetes.
- Safe use of inhalant in children under 12 years not established.
- Teach patient how to administer metered dose correctly. Instructions: shake container; exhale through nose; administer aerosol while inhaling deeply on mouthpiece of inhaler; and hold breath for a few seconds, then exhale slowly. Allow 2 minutes between inhalations. Store drug in light-resistant container.
- Metaproterenol inhalations should precede steroid inhalations (when prescribed) by 10 to 15 minutes to maximize therapy.
- Warn patient about the possibility of paradoxical bronchospasm. If this occurs, the drug should be discontinued immediately.
- Patients may use tablets and aerosol concomitantly. Monitor closely for toxicity.
- Metaproterenol reportedly produces less cardiac stimulation than other sympathomimetics, especially isoproterenol.
- Inhalant solution diluted in sodium chloride solution is administered by IPPB. When used full strength it's given via hand nebulizer.
- Tell patient to notify doctor if no response is derived from dosage. Warn against changing dose without calling doctor.
- If more than one inhalation is ordered, the patient should wait at least 2 minutes before repeating the procedure for a second dose.
- Tell patient who is also using a steroid inhaler to use the bronchodilator first, then wait about 5 minutes before using the steroid. This allows the bronchodilator to open air passages for maximum effectiveness.

General
Classification: hepatitis B prophylaxis (vaccine).
Pregnancy risk category: C.

Mechanism of action
Promotes active immunity to hepatitis B.

Indications and dosage
• Immunization against hepatitis B infection; primary preexposure prophylaxis against hepatitis B; or postexposure prophylaxis (with hepatitis B immune globulin).

Engerix-B—**Adults and children over 10 years:** initially, 20 mcg (1-ml adult formulation) I.M., followed by second dose of 20 mcg 30 days later. Give third dose of 20 mcg 6 months after initial dose. **Neonates, children to 10 years:** initially, 10 mcg (0.5-ml pediatric formulation) I.M., followed by second dose of 10 mcg 30 days later. Give third dose of 10 mcg 6 months after initial dose. **Adults undergoing dialysis or receiving immunosuppressant therapy:** initially, 40 mcg I.M. (divided into two 20-mcg doses and administered at different sites). Follow with second dose of 40 mcg in 30 days and final dose of 40 mcg 6 months after initial dose.

Note: Certain populations (neonates born to infected mothers, persons recently exposed to the virus, and travelers to high-risk areas) may receive vaccine on an abbreviated schedule, with initial dose followed by second dose in 1 month, and third dose after 2 months. For prolonged maintenance of protective antibody titers, a booster dose is recommended 12 months after initial dose.

Recombivax HB—**Adults:** initially, 10 mcg (1-ml adult formulation) I.M., followed by second dose of 10 mcg 30 days later. Give third dose of 10 mcg 6 months after initial dose. **Children 11 to 19 years:** initially, 5 mcg (0.5-ml pediatric formulation) I.M., followed by second dose of 5 mcg 30 days later. Give third dose of 5 mcg 6 months after initial dose. **Neonates and children to 11 years:** initially, 2.5 mcg (0.25-ml pediatric formulation) I.M., followed by second dose of 2.5 mcg 30 days later. Give third dose of 2.5 mcg 6 months after initial dose. **Adults undergoing dialysis or receiving immunosuppressant therapy:** initially, 40 mcg I.M. (use dialysis formulation, which contains 40 mcg/ml). Follow with second dose of 40 mcg in 30 days and final dose of 40 mcg 6 months after the initial dose.

Adverse reactions
Systemic: slight fever, transient malaise, headache, dizziness, nausea, vomiting, flulike symptoms, myalgia. **Local:** discomfort at injection site, local inflammation.

Interactions
None reported.

Nursing diagnoses
• Altered protection related to lack of immunity to hepatitis.
• Hyperthermia related to vaccine-induced fever.
• Knowledge deficit related to hepatitis B vaccine.

Nursing interventions
• *Contraindicated* in patients with a history of severe hypersensitivity reaction to yeast. Recombinant vaccines are derived from yeast cultures.
• *Use cautiously* in any serious, active infections; in compromised cardiac or pulmonary status; and in those for whom a febrile or systemic reaction could pose a serious risk.
• Recombinant hepatitis B vaccine is not made with any human plasma products.
• The CDC reports that response to hepatitis B vaccine is significantly better when administered in the arm rather than the buttock. Adults should receive the vaccine in the deltoid muscle; infants and young children, in the anterolateral aspect of the thigh. Never administer I.V.
• May be administered S.C., but may lead to an increased incidence or severity of local reactions. Use only in persons at risk for hemorrhage, such as hemophiliacs.
• Although anaphylaxis has not been reported, epinephrine should be available when administering this drug to counteract possible reactions.
• The recommended dosage regimen provides immunity for at least 5 years.

General

Classification: antipsychotic (phenothiazine). **Pregnancy risk category:** C.

Mechanism of action

Blocks postsynaptic dopamine receptors in the brain.

Indications and dosage

- Alcoholism. **Adults and children over 12 years:** 25 mg P.O. b.i.d. up to maximum of 200 mg daily.
- Behavioral problems associated with chronic brain syndrome. **Adults and children over 12 years:** 25 mg P.O. t.i.d. up to 300 mg daily.
- Psychoneurotic manifestations (anxiety). **Adults and children over 12 years:** 10 mg P.O. t.i.d. up to maximum of 150 mg daily.
- Schizophrenia. **Adults and children over 12 years:** initially, 50 mg P.O. t.i.d. or 25 mg I.M. repeated in 30 to 60 minutes, p.r.n.

Adverse reactions

Blood: transient leukopenia, ***agranulocytosis.*** **CNS:** extrapyramidal reactions (low incidence), *tardive dyskinesia, sedation (high incidence),* EEG changes, dizziness. **CV:** *orthostatic hypotension,* tachycardia, ECG changes. **EENT:** *ocular changes, blurred vision,* pigmentary retinopathy. **GI:** *dry mouth, constipation.* **GU:** *urine retention,* dark urine, menstrual irregularities, gynecomastia, inhibited ejaculation. **Hepatic:** cholestatic jaundice, abnormal liver function tests. **Metabolic:** hyperprolactinemia. **Skin:** *mild photosensitivity,* dermal allergic reactions. **Local:** pain at I.M. injection site, sterile abscess. **Other:** weight gain; increased appetite; rarely, ***neuroleptic malignant syndrome.*** **After abrupt withdrawal of long-term therapy:** gastritis, nausea, vomiting, dizziness, tremor, feeling of warmth or cold, sweating, tachycardia, headache, insomnia.

Interactions

Alcohol, other CNS depressants: increased CNS depression. Avoid concomitant use. **Antacids:** inhibit absorption of oral phenothiazines. Separate doses by at least 2 hours. **Barbiturates:** may decrease phenothiazine effect. Observe patient.

Nursing diagnoses

- Altered health maintenance related to the patient's underlying condition.
- Sensory/perceptual alterations (visual) related to adverse drug reactions.
- Knowledge deficit related to mesoridazine therapy.

Nursing interventions

- *Contraindicated* in coma, CNS depression, bone marrow suppression, subcortical damage, and with spinal or epidural anesthetics or adrenergic blockers.
- *Use cautiously* in elderly or debilitated patients; in acutely ill or dehydrated children; and in hepatic disease, arteriosclerosis or CV disease, exposure to extreme heat or cold, respiratory disorders, hypocalcemia, seizure disorders, reactions to insulin or electroshock therapy, suspected brain tumor or intestinal obstruction, glaucoma, and prostatic hypertrophy.
- Tardive dyskinesia may occur after prolonged use.
- Neuroleptic malignant syndrome is rare, but frequently fatal. Watch for symptoms.
- Hold dose and notify doctor if patient develops jaundice, symptoms of blood dyscrasias, persistent extrapyramidal reactions, or any such reactions in pregnancy or in children.
- Monitor therapy with bilirubins, CBC and liver function, and ophthalmic tests.
- Have patient report urine retention or constipation. Tell him drug may discolor urine.
- Tell patient to protect himself from sunlight.
- Warn against activities requiring alertness until CNS effects of the drug are known.
- Obtain baseline measures of blood pressure before starting therapy and monitor regularly. Watch for orthostatic hypotension.
- Give deep I.M., only in upper outer quadrant of buttocks. Massage slowly afterward.
- Prevent contact of drug with skin and clothing.
- Don't withdraw drug abruptly.

General

Classification: antihypertensive (peripheral vasodilator). **Pregnancy risk category:** C.

Mechanism of action

Directly relaxes arteriolar smooth muscle.

Indications and dosage

• Essential hypertension (oral, alone or in combination with other antihypertensives); reduction of afterload in severe CHF (with nitrates); severe essential hypertension (parenteral to lower blood pressure quickly). **Adults:** initially, 10 mg P.O. q.i.d.; gradually increased to 50 mg q.i.d. Maximum recommended dosage is 200 mg daily, but some patients may require 300 to 400 mg daily. Can be given b.i.d. for CHF. *I.V.*—10 to 20 mg given slowly and repeated as necessary, generally q 4 to 6 hours. Switch to oral antihypertensives as soon as possible. *I.M.*—20 to 40 mg repeated as necessary, generally q 4 to 6 hours. Switch to oral antihypertensives as soon as possible. **Children:** initially, 0.75 mg/kg P.O. daily in four divided doses (25 mg/m² daily). May increase gradually to 10 times this dosage, if necessary. *I.V.*—give slowly 1.7 to 3.5 mg/kg daily or 50 to 100 mg/m² daily in four to six divided doses. *I.M.*—1.7 to 3.5 mg/kg daily or 50 to 100 mg/m² daily in four to six divided doses.

Adverse reactions

Blood: neutropenia, leukopenia. **CNS:** peripheral neuritis, *headache,* dizziness. **CV:** orthostatic hypotension, *tachycardia,* arrhythmias, *angina, palpitations, sodium retention.* **GI:** *nausea, vomiting, diarrhea, anorexia.* **Skin:** rash. **Other:** *lupus erythematosus-like syndrome (especially with high doses), weight gain.*

Interactions

Diazoxide, MAO inhibitors: may cause severe hypotension. Use together cautiously.

Nursing diagnoses

• Altered tissue perfusion (renal, cerebral, cardiopulmonary, and peripheral) related to the patient's underlying condition.
• Pain related to hydralazine-induced headache.
• Knowledge deficit related to hydralazine therapy.

Nursing interventions

• *Use cautiously* in cardiac disease, CVA, or severe renal impairment and in those taking other antihypertensives.
• Monitor patient's blood pressure, pulse rate, and body weight frequently. Some clinicians combine hydralazine therapy with diuretics and beta-adrenergic blockers to decrease sodium retention and tachycardia and to prevent anginal attacks.
• Watch patient closely for signs of lupus erythematosus-like syndrome (sore throat, fever, muscle and joint aches, skin rash). Call doctor immediately if any of these develop.
• Teach patient about his disease and therapy. Explain the importance of taking this drug as prescribed, even when he's feeling well. Tell outpatient not to discontinue this drug suddenly, but to call the doctor if unpleasant adverse reactions occur.
• Instruct patient to check with doctor or pharmacist before taking OTC medications.
• Inform patient that orthostatic hypotension can be minimized by rising slowly and avoiding sudden position changes.
• Elderly patients may be more sensitive to hypotensive effects.
• Give this drug with meals to increase absorption
• Compliance may be improved by administering this drug b.i.d. Check with doctor.
• CBC, lupus erythematosus cell preparation, and antinuclear antibody titer determinations should be done before therapy and periodically during long-term therapy.
• Has been prescribed during pregnancy for treatment of eclampsia. Administered I.V.
• **I.V. use:** Give slowly and repeat as necessary, generally q 4 to 6 hours. Switch to oral antihypertensives as soon as possible.

General

Classification: anti-inflammatory (salicylate).
Pregnancy risk category: B.

Mechanism of action

Exact mechanism unknown; mesalamine is one of the active metabolites of sulfasalazine. Probably acts topically by inhibiting prostaglandin production in the colon.

Indications and dosage

• Treatment of active mild to moderate distal ulcerative colitis, proctitis, or proctosigmoiditis.
Adults: 500 mg P.R. (suppository) b.i.d., or 1 rectal unit as a retention enema once daily (preferably h.s.). Drug should be retained overnight (for about 8 hours). Usual course of therapy is 3 to 6 weeks.

Adverse reactions

CNS: headache, dizziness, fatigue, malaise. **GI:** abdominal pain, cramps, discomfort, flatulence, diarrhea, rectal pain, bloating, nausea, *pancolitis*. **Skin:** itching, rash, urticaria, hair loss. **Other:** wheezing, ***anaphylaxis*** (rare), fever.

Interactions

None significant.

Nursing diagnoses

• Pain related to the underlying condition.
• Diarrhea related to adverse effects of the medication.
• Knowledge deficit related to mesalamine therapy.

Nursing interventions

• *Contraindicated* in patients sensitive to the drug or its components.
• *Use cautiously* in renal impairment. Problems have not been documented, but the nephrotoxic potential from absorbed mesalamine exists. Patients on long-term mesalamine therapy should have periodic renal function studies.
• Mesalamine may rarely cause allergic reactions in patients sensitive to sulfites because it contains potassium metabisulfite.
• Instruct patient to carefully follow instructions supplied with medication.
• Patients intolerant of sulfasalazine may also be hypersensitive to mesalamine. Instruct these patients to discontinue drug if they have a fever or rash.

General

Classification: diuretic, antihypertensive (thiazide diuretic). **Pregnancy risk category:** D.

Mechanism of action

Increases urine excretion of sodium and water by inhibiting sodium reabsorption in the cortical diluting site of the nephron.

Indications and dosage

• Edema. **Adults:** initially, 25 to 100 mg P.O. daily or intermittently for maintenance dosage. **Children over 6 months:** 2.2 mg/kg P.O. daily divided b.i.d. **Children under 6 months:** up to 3.3 mg/kg P.O. daily divided b.i.d.

• Hypertension. **Adults:** 25 to 150 mg P.O. daily as single dose or two divided doses. Dosages above 50 mg daily are associated with reduction in serum potassium.

Adverse reactions

Blood: ***aplastic anemia, agranulocytosis,*** leukopenia, thrombocytopenia. **CV:** volume depletion and dehydration, orthostatic hypotension. **GI:** anorexia, nausea, pancreatitis. **Hepatic:** hepatic encephalopathy. **Metabolic:** hypokalemia, asymptomatic hyperuricemia, hyperglycemia and impairment of glucose tolerance, fluid and electrolyte imbalances including dilutional hyponatremia and hypochloremia, metabolic alkalosis, hypercalcemia, gout. **Skin:** dermatitis, photosensitivity, rash. **Other:** hypersensitivity reactions, such as pneumonitis and vasculitis.

Interactions

Antidiabetic agents: dosage adjustments may be necessary. Monitor blood glucose levels. **Cholestyramine, colestipol:** intestinal absorption of thiazides decreased. Keep doses as separate as possible. **Diazoxide:** increased antihypertensive, hyperglycemic, and hyperuricemic effects. Use together cautiously. **NSAIDs:** decreased diuretic effectiveness. Avoid concomitant use.

Nursing diagnoses

• Fluid volume excess related to ineffectiveness of hydrochlorothiazide to relieve edema.

• Altered urinary elimination related to hydrochlorothiazide therapy.

• Knowledge deficit related to hydrochlorothiazide therapy.

Nursing interventions

• *Contraindicated* in anuria or hypersensitivity to other thiazides or other sulfonamide derivatives.

• *Use cautiously* in severe renal disease, impaired hepatic function, and progressive hepatic disease.

• Monitor intake and output, weight, blood pressure, and serum electrolytes.

• Consult with doctor and dietitian to provide high-potassium diet. Watch for hypokalemia (for example, muscle weakness and cramps). Patients also on a digitalis glycoside have an increased risk of digitalis toxicity from the potassium-depleting effect of this diuretic. May use with potassium-sparing diuretic to prevent potassium loss.

• Foods rich in potassium include citrus fruits, tomatoes, bananas, dates, and apricots.

• Monitor serum creatinine and BUN regularly. Not as effective if these levels are more than twice normal.

• Monitor blood uric acid, especially in patients with a history of gout.

• Check insulin requirements in patients with diabetes. May treat severe hyperglycemia with oral antidiabetic agents.

• In hypertension, therapeutic response may be delayed several days.

• Give in the morning to prevent nocturia. Studies have shown that the drug is as effective when administered once daily as it is when given more frequently.

• Elderly patients are especially susceptible to excessive diuresis.

• Thiazides and thiazide-like diuretics should be stopped before tests for parathyroid function are performed.

• Advise patient to avoid sudden posture changes and rise slowly to avoid orthostatic hypotension.

• Advise patient to use a sunscreen.

General

Classification: antineoplastic (antimetabolite).
Pregnancy risk category: D.

Mechanism of action

Inhibits RNA and DNA synthesis.

Indications and dosage

• Acute lymphoblastic leukemia (in children), acute myeloblastic leukemia, chronic myelocytic leukemia. **Adults:** 80 to 100 mg/m² (rounded to the nearest 25 mg) P.O. daily as a single dose up to 5 mg/kg daily. **Children:** 75 mg/m² (rounded to the nearest 25 mg) P.O. daily.

Usual maintenance for adults and children: 1.5 to 2.5 mg/kg daily.

Adverse reactions

Blood: ***leukopenia,*** *thrombocytopenia, and anemia; all may persist several days after drug is stopped.* **GI:** *nausea, vomiting, and anorexia in 25% of patients;* painful oral ulcers. **Hepatic:** biliary stasis, *jaundice,* ***hepatic necrosis.*** **Metabolic:** hyperuricemia. **Skin:** rash, hyperpigmentation.

Interactions

Allopurinol: slowed inactivation of mercaptopurine. Decrease mercaptopurine to ¼ or ⅓ normal dose. **Hepatotoxic drugs:** may enhance liver toxicity of mercaptopurine. **Nondepolarizing neuromuscular blockers:** antagonized muscle relaxant effect. Notify anesthesiologist that patient is receiving mercaptopurine. **Warfarin:** enhanced anticoagulant effect.

Nursing diagnoses

• Altered protection related to mercaptopurine-induced myelosuppression and immunosuppression.
• Altered oral mucous membrane related to mercaptopurine-induced stomatitis.
• Knowledge deficit related to mercaptopurine therapy.

Nursing interventions

• *Contraindicated* in patients whose disease has exhibited resistance to the drug.
• *Use cautiously.* Dosage modifications may be required after chemotherapy or radiation therapy, in depressed neutrophil or platelet count, and in impaired hepatic or renal function.
• Observe for signs of bleeding and infection.
• Hepatic dysfunction is reversible when drug is stopped. Watch for jaundice, clay-colored stools, and frothy dark urine. Drug should be stopped if hepatic tenderness occurs.
• Monitor blood counts, serum transaminase, alkaline phosphatase, and bilirubin weekly during induction and monthly during maintenance.
• Warn patient to watch for signs of infection (fever, sore throat, fatigue) and bleeding (easy bruising, nosebleeds, bleeding gums, melena). Take temperature daily.
• Monitor intake and output. Encourage fluid intake (3 liters daily).
• Sometimes ordered as 6-mercaptopurine or 6-MP. The numeral 6 is part of drug name and does not signify number of dosage units.
• Warn patient that improvement may take 2 to 4 weeks or longer.
• Adverse GI reactions less common in children than in adults.
• Avoid all I.M. injections when platelets are below 100,000/mm³.
• Monitor serum uric acid. If allopurinol is necessary, use cautiously.

General

Classification: adrenocorticoid replacement (glucocorticoid, mineralocorticoid). **Pregnancy risk category:** C.

Mechanism of action

Decreases inflammation, mainly by stabilizing leukocyte lysosomal membranes. Also suppresses the immune response, stimulates bone marrow, and influences metabolism.

Indications and dosage

- Severe inflammation, adrenal insufficiency. **Adults:** 5 to 30 mg P.O. b.i.d., t.i.d., or q.i.d. (as much as 80 mg q.i.d. may be given in acute situations); or initially, 100 to 250 mg (succinate) I.M. or I.V., then 50 to 100 mg I.M., as indicated; or 15 to 240 mg (phosphate) I.M. or I.V. q 12 hours; or 5 to 75 mg (acetate) into joints and soft tissue.
- Shock. **Adults:** 500 mg to 2 g (succinate) q 2 to 6 hours. **Children:** 0.16 to 1 mg/kg (phosphate or succinate) I.M. or I.V., b.i.d. or t.i.d.

Adverse reactions

CNS: *euphoria, insomnia,* psychotic behavior, pseudotumor cerebri. **CV:** ***CHF,*** hypertension, edema. **EENT:** cataracts, glaucoma. **GI:** *peptic ulcer,* GI irritation, increased appetite. **Metabolic:** possible hypokalemia, hyperglycemia and carbohydrate intolerance, growth suppression in children. **Skin:** delayed wound healing, acne, various skin eruptions. **Other:** muscle weakness, osteoporosis, pancreatitis, hirsutism, susceptibility to infections. ***Sudden withdrawal may be fatal.***

Interactions

Aspirin, NSAIDs: increased risk of GI bleeding. Give together cautiously. **Barbiturates, phenytoin, rifampin:** decreased corticosteroid effect. May need increased corticosteroid dose. **Live attenuated virus vaccines, other vaccines and toxoids:** decreased antibody response and increased risk of neurologic complications. Avoid concomitant use. **Oral anticoagulants:** altered dosage requirements. Monitor PT. **Potassium-depleting drugs:** enhanced potassium-wasting effects of hydrocortisone. Monitor serum potassium levels.

Nursing diagnoses

- Fluid volume deficit related to volume depletion from adrenal insufficiency.
- High risk for injury related to hydrocortisone-induced adverse reactions.
- Knowledge deficit related to hydrocortisone therapy.

Nursing interventions

- *Contraindicated* in systemic fungal infections. Certain injectable forms contain sulfites, which can cause allergic reactions.
- *Use cautiously* in patients with GI ulceration or renal disease, hypertension, osteoporosis, varicella, vaccinia, exanthema, diabetes mellitus, Cushing's syndrome, thromboembolic disorders, seizures, myasthenia gravis, metastatic cancer, CHF, tuberculosis, ocular herpes simplex, hypoalbuminemia, emotional instability, and psychotic tendencies and in children.
- Gradually reduce drug dosage after long-term therapy. Don't discontinue drug abruptly.
- Always titrate to lowest effective dose.
- Monitor patient's weight, blood pressure, and serum electrolytes.
- May mask or exacerbate infections.
- Instruct patient to carry a card stating need for supplemental glucocorticoids during stress.
- Warn patients on long-term therapy about cushingoid symptoms.

General

Classification: anxiolytic (carbamate). **Pregnancy risk category:** D. **Controlled substance schedule:** IV.

Mechanism of action

Depresses the CNS at the limbic and subcortical levels of the brain.

Indications and dosage

• Anxiety and tension. **Adults:** 1.2 to 1.6 g P.O. in three or four equally divided doses. Maximum dosage is 2.4 g daily. **Children 6 to 12 years:** 100 to 200 mg P.O. b.i.d. or t.i.d. Not recommended for children under 6 years.

Adverse reactions

Blood: ***thrombocytopenia, leukopenia,*** eosinophilia. **CNS:** *drowsiness,* ataxia, dizziness, slurred speech, headache, vertigo. **CV:** palpitation, tachycardia, hypotension. **GI:** anorexia, nausea, vomiting, diarrhea, stomatitis. **Skin:** pruritus, urticaria, erythematous maculopapular rash.

Interactions

Alcohol, other CNS depressants: increased CNS depression. Avoid concomitant use.

Nursing diagnoses

• Anxiety related to the patient's underlying condition.
• Altered peripheral tissue perfusion related to adverse reactions to meprobamate.
• Knowledge deficit related to meprobamate therapy.

Nursing interventions

• *Contraindicated* in patients with hypersensitivity to meprobamate, carisoprodol, mebutamate, tybamate, and carbromal and in renal insufficiency or porphyria.
• *Use cautiously* in patients with impaired hepatic or renal function, seizure disorders, or suicidal tendencies and in patients with a history of aspirin hypersensitivity.
• Dosage should be reduced in elderly or debilitated patients.
• Possibility of abuse and addiction exists with long-term use. Meprobamate should not be used for everyday stress. Withdraw drug gradually (over 2 weeks) or withdrawal symptoms may occur, including severe generalized tonic-clonic seizures.
• Warn patient to avoid hazardous activities that require alertness or good psychomotor coordination until CNS effects of the drug are known.
• Warn patient not to combine drug with alcohol or other depressants.
• Give drug with meals to reduce GI distress.
• Therapeutic blood levels 0.5 to 2 mg/100 ml; levels above 20 mg/100 ml may cause coma and death.
• Periodic evaluation of CBC and renal and hepatic function tests are indicated in patients receiving high doses.
• Tell patient to report any unusual bruising or bleeding, fever, or sore throat. These symptoms may indicate serious hematologic toxicity.
• Meprobamate may interfere with certain laboratory tests for urinary 17-ketogenic steroids and 17-hydroxycorticosteroids.

General
Classification: diuretic, antihypertensive (thiazide diuretic). **Pregnancy risk category:** B.

Mechanism of action
Increases urine excretion of sodium and water by inhibiting sodium reabsorption in the cortical diluting site of the ascending loop of Henle.

Indications and dosage
- Edema. **Adults:** 25 to 200 mg P.O. daily in divided doses (maintenance dosages may be on intermittent or alternate-day schedule). **Children:** 1 mg/kg P.O. daily.
- Hypertension. **Adults:** 50 to 100 mg P.O. daily or b.i.d.

Adverse reactions
Blood: ***aplastic anemia, agranulocytosis,*** leukopenia, thrombocytopenia. **CV:** volume depletion and dehydration, orthostatic hypotension. **GI:** anorexia, nausea, pancreatitis. **Hepatic:** hepatic encephalopathy. **Metabolic:** hypokalemia, asymptomatic hyperuricemia, hyperglycemia and impairment of glucose tolerance, fluid and electrolyte imbalances including dilutional hyponatremia and hypochloremia, metabolic alkalosis, hypercalcemia, gout. **Skin:** dermatitis, photosensitivity, rash. **Other:** hypersensitivity reactions, such as pneumonitis and vasculitis.

Interactions
Cholestyramine, colestipol: intestinal absorption of thiazides decreased. Keep doses as separate as possible. **Diazoxide:** increased antihypertensive, hyperglycemic, and hyperuricemic effects. Use together cautiously. **NSAIDs:** decreased diuretic effectiveness.

Nursing diagnoses
- Fluid volume excess related to the patient's underlying condition, as evidenced by edema.
- Altered urinary elimination related to diuretic therapy.
- Knowledge deficit related to hydroflumethiazide therapy.

Nursing interventions
- *Contraindicated* in anuria or hypersensitivity to other thiazides or other sulfonamide-derived drugs.
- *Use cautiously* in severe renal disease, impaired hepatic function, and progressive hepatic disease.
- Monitor intake and output, weight, blood pressure, and serum electrolytes.
- Consult with doctor and dietitian to provide high-potassium diet. Watch for hypokalemia. May use with potassium-sparing diuretic to prevent potassium loss. Patients also on a digitalis glycoside have an increased risk of digitalis toxicity from the potassium-depleting effects of this diuretic.
- Monitor serum creatinine and BUN regularly. Not as effective if these levels are more than twice normal.
- Monitor blood uric acid, especially in patients with a history of gout.
- Check insulin requirements in patients with diabetes. May treat severe hyperglycemia with oral antidiabetic agents.
- Give in the morning to prevent nocturia.
- In hypertension, therapeutic response may be delayed several days.
- Elderly patients are especially susceptible to excessive diuresis.
- Thiazides and thiazide-like diuretics should be stopped before tests for parathyroid function are performed.
- Advise patient to avoid sudden posture changes and rise slowly to avoid orthostatic hypotension.
- Advise patient to use a sunscreen because of possible photosensitivity reactions.

General

Classification: anticonvulsant, nonspecific CNS depressant (barbiturate). **Pregnancy risk category:** D. **Controlled substance schedule:** IV.

Mechanism of action

Depresses monosynaptic and polysynaptic transmission in the CNS and increases the threshold for seizure activity in the motor cortex.

Indications and dosage

• Generalized tonic-clonic or absence seizures. **Adults:** 400 to 600 mg P.O. daily or in divided doses. **Children:** 6 to 12 mg/kg P.O. daily, divided q 6 to 8 hours (smaller doses are given initially and increased over 4 to 5 days p.r.n.).

Adverse reactions

Blood: megaloblastic anemia, ***agranulocytosis,*** thrombocytopenia. **CNS:** *dizziness,* headache, *hangover,* confusion, paradoxical excitation, exacerbation of existing pain, drowsiness. **CV:** hypotension, bradycardia. **GI:** nausea, vomiting, epigastric pain. **Skin:** urticaria, morbilliform rash, blisters, purpura, ***erythema multiforme.*** **Other:** allergic reactions (facial edema).

Interactions

Alcohol and other CNS depressants, including narcotic analgesics: excessive CNS depression. Use cautiously. **Griseofulvin:** decreased absorption of griseofulvin. **MAO inhibitors:** potentiated barbiturate effect. Monitor patient for increased CNS and respiratory depression. **Oral anticoagulants, estrogens and oral contraceptives, doxycycline, corticosteroids:** mephobarbital may enhance the metabolism of these drugs. Monitor for decreased effect. **Rifampin:** may decrease barbiturate levels. Monitor for decreased effect.

Nursing diagnoses

• High risk for injury related to patient's underlying seizure disorder.
• Impaired skin integrity related to mephobarbital-induced dermal adverse reaction.
• Knowledge deficit related to mephobarbital therapy.

Nursing interventions

• *Contraindicated* in barbiturate hypersensitivity, porphyria, or respiratory disease with dyspnea or obstruction.
• *Use cautiously* in hepatic, renal, cardiac, or respiratory function impairment; myasthenia gravis; and myxedema.
• Never withdraw drug suddenly. Call doctor at once if adverse reactions develop.
• Warn patient to avoid activities that require alertness and good psychomotor coordination until CNS effects of drug are known.
• Store in light-resistant container.
• In adults, give total or largest dose at night if seizures occur then.
• Three-quarters of drug is metabolized to phenobarbital; therapeutic blood levels as phenobarbital are 15 to 40 mcg/ml.
• Periodically monitor CBC, BUN, and creatinine levels.
• Women who use oral contraceptives should consider alternative birth control methods when receiving this drug because it may enhance contraceptive hormone metabolism and decrease its effectiveness.
• Like other barbiturates, suppresses REM sleep. When drug is discontinued, patient may experience increased dreaming.

General

Classification: analgesic, antitussive (opioid). **Pregnancy risk category:** B (D for prolonged use or use of high doses at term). **Controlled substance schedule:** II.

Mechanism of action

Binds with opiate receptors at many sites in the CNS, altering both perception of and emotional response to pain through an unknown mechanism. Also suppresses the cough reflex by direct action on the cough center in the medulla.

Indications and dosage

- Moderate to severe pain. **Adults:** 1 to 6 mg P.O. q 4 to 6 hours, p.r.n. or around the clock; or 2 to 4 mg I.M., S.C., or I.V. q 4 to 6 hours, p.r.n., or q 6 to 8 hours around the clock. Give I.V. dose over 3 to 5 minutes. Or 3 mg P.R. h.s., p.r.n., or q 6 to 8 hours around the clock.
- Cough. **Adults:** 1 mg P.O. q 3 to 4 hours p.r.n. **Children 6 to 12 years:** 0.5 mg P.O. q 3 to 4 hours p.r.n.

Adverse reactions

CNS: *sedation, somnolence, clouded sensorium,* dizziness, *euphoria,* seizures with large doses. **CV:** *hypotension,* bradycardia. **GI:** *nausea, vomiting, constipation, ileus.* **GU:** *urine retention.* **Local:** induration with repeated S.C. injections. **Other:** ***respiratory depression,*** physical dependence.

Interactions

General anesthetics, other narcotic analgesics, tranquilizers, sedatives, hypnotics, alcohol, TCAs, MAO inhibitors: increased CNS depression. Use together with extreme caution.

Nursing diagnoses

- Pain related to patient's underlying condition.
- Ineffective breathing pattern related to hydromorphone-induced respiratory depression.
- Knowledge deficit related to hydromorphone therapy.

Nursing interventions

- *Contraindicated* in patients with status asthmaticus.
- *Use with extreme caution* in patients with increased CSF pressure, respiratory depression, hepatic or renal disease, hypothyroidism, shock, Addison's disease, acute alcoholism, seizures, head injury, severe CNS depression, brain tumor, bronchial asthma, and COPD and in elderly or debilitated patients.
- Monitor respiratory and circulatory status and bowel function.
- Keep narcotic antagonist (naloxone) available.
- **I.V. use:** Respiratory depression and hypotension can occur with I.V. administration. Give very slowly and monitor constantly. Keep resuscitative equipment available.
- Rotate injection sites to avoid induration with S.C. injection.
- Commonly abused narcotic.
- Warn ambulatory patient to avoid hazardous activities that require mental alertness and physical coordination.
- For better analgesic effect, give before patient has intense pain.
- When used postoperatively, encourage turning, coughing, and deep breathing to avoid atelectasis.
- May worsen or mask gallbladder pain.

General

Classification: anticonvulsant (hydantoin derivative). **Pregnancy risk category:** C.

Mechanism of action

Stabilizes neuronal membranes and limits seizure activity by either increasing efflux or decreasing influx of sodium ions across cell membranes in the motor cortex during generation of nerve impulses.

Indications and dosage

• Generalized tonic-clonic or complex-partial seizures. **Adults:** 50 to 100 mg P.O. daily. May increase by 50 to 100 mg at weekly intervals up to 200 mg t.i.d. **Children:** initially, 50 to 100 mg P.O. daily or 100 to 450 mg/m^2 daily in three divided doses. May increase slowly by 50 to 100 mg at weekly intervals up to 200 mg t.i.d., divided q 8 hours. Dosage must be adjusted individually.

Adverse reactions

Blood: ***leukopenia, neutropenia, agranulocytosis, thrombocytopenia, pancytopenia,*** eosinophilia. **CNS:** ataxia, *drowsiness,* fatigue, irritability, choreiform movements, depression, tremor, sleeplessness, dizziness (usually transient). **EENT:** conjunctivitis, diplopia, nystagmus. **GI:** gingival hyperplasia, nausea and vomiting (with prolonged use). **Skin:** *rash,* ***exfoliative dermatitis,*** photosensitivity. **Other:** hypertrichosis, edema, dysarthria, lymphadenopathy, polyarthropathy, ***pulmonary fibrosis.***

Interactions

Alcohol, folic acid: monitor for decreased mephenytoin activity. **Oral anticoagulants, antihistamines, chloramphenicol, cimetidine, diazepam, diazoxide, disulfiram, isoniazid, phenylbutazone, salicylates, sulfamethizole, valproate:** monitor for increased mephenytoin activity and toxicity.

Nursing diagnoses

• High risk for injury related to patient's underlying seizure activity.
• Altered protection related to myelosuppression and immunosuppression secondary to blood dyscrasias.
• Knowledge deficit related to mephenytoin therapy.

Nursing interventions

• *Contraindicated* in hydantoin hypersensitivity.
• *Use cautiously* in patients receiving other hydantoin derivatives.
• Periodically monitor liver function studies with long-term use. Check baseline CBC and platelet count and periodically thereafter. Discontinue drug if neutrophil count becomes less than 1,600/mm^3.
• Never withdraw drug suddenly. Call doctor if adverse reactions develop.
• Therapeutic blood level of mephenytoin and its active metabolite is 25 to 40 mcg/ml.
• Heavy use of alcohol may diminish benefit of drug.
• Potentially life-threatening blood dyscrasias limit this drug's usefulness.
• Tell patient to notify doctor if fever, sore throat, bleeding, or rash occurs.
• Warn patient to avoid activities that require alertness and good psychomotor coordination until CNS effects of the drug are known.

General

Classification: antimalarial, anti-inflammatory agent (4-aminoquinoline). **Pregnancy risk category:** C.

Mechanism of action

May bind to and alter the properties of DNA.

Indications and dosage

• Suppressive prophylaxis of malarial attacks. **Adults and children:** 5 mg (base)/kg body weight P.O. (not to exceed 310 mg) weekly on same day of the week (begin 2 weeks before entering and continue for 8 weeks after leaving endemic area). If not started before exposure, double initial dose (620 mg for adults, 10 mg/kg for children) in two divided doses P.O. 6 hours apart.

• Treatment of acute malarial attacks. **Adults and children over 15 years:** initially, 800 mg (sulfate) P.O., then 400 mg after 6 to 8 hours, then 400 mg daily for 2 days (total 2 g sulfate salt). **Children 11 to 15 years:** 600 mg (sulfate) P.O. stat, then 200 mg 8 hours later, then 200 mg 24 hours later (total 1 g sulfate salt). **Children 6 to 10 years:** 400 mg (sulfate) P.O. stat, then two doses of 200 mg at 8-hour intervals (total 800 mg sulfate salt). **Children 2 to 5 years:** 400 mg (sulfate) P.O. stat, then 200 mg 8 hours later (total 600 mg sulfate salt). **Children under 1 year:** 100 mg (sulfate) P.O. stat; then three doses of 100 mg 6 to 9 hours apart (total 400 mg sulfate salt).

• Lupus erythematosus. **Adults:** 400 mg P.O. daily or b.i.d., continued for several weeks or months, depending on response. Prolonged maintenance dosage – 200 to 400 mg P.O. daily.

• Rheumatoid arthritis. **Adults:** initially, 400 to 600 mg P.O. daily. When good response occurs (usually in 4 to 12 weeks), cut dosage in half.

Adverse reactions

Blood: ***agranulocytosis, leukopenia,*** thrombocytopenia, ***hemolysis in patients with G6PD deficiency, aplastic anemia.*** **CNS:** irritability, nightmares, ataxia, seizures, psychic stimulation, toxic psychosis, vertigo, tinnitus, nystagmus, lassitude, fatigue, dizziness, hypoactive deep tendon reflexes, skeletal muscle weakness. **EENT:** visual disturbances, ototoxicity. **GI:** anorexia, abdominal cramps, diarrhea, nausea, vomiting. **Skin:** pruritus, lichen planus-like eruptions, skin and mucosal pigmentary changes, pleomorphic skin eruptions. **Other:** weight loss, alopecia, bleaching of hair.

Interactions

Cimetidine: decreased hepatic metabolism of hydroxychloroquine. Monitor for toxicity. **Magnesium and aluminum salts, kaolin:** Decreased GI absorption. Separate administration times.

Nursing diagnoses

• High risk for injury related to ineffectiveness of hydroxychloroquine.
• Sensory/perceptual alterations (visual and auditory) related to adverse drug reactions.
• Knowledge deficit related to hydroxychloroquine.

Nursing interventions

• *Contraindicated* in patients with retinal or visual field changes, or porphyria.
• *Use with extreme caution* in presence of severe GI, neurologic, or blood disorders.
• *Use cautiously* in patients with hepatic disease, alcoholism, G6PD deficiency, or psoriasis.
• Monitor CBC and liver function during prolonged therapy.
• Watch for signs of overdosage: headache, drowsiness, visual disturbances, CV collapse, and seizures.
• Tell patient to report blurred vision, increased photosensitivity, or muscle weakness.
• Tell patient to take drug right before or after meals on same day of each week.

General

Classification: analgesic, adjunct to anesthesia (opioid). **Pregnancy risk category:** B (D with prolonged use or high doses at term). **Controlled substance schedule:** II.

Mechanism of action

Binds with opiate receptors in the CNS, altering both perception of and emotional response to pain.

Indications and dosage

• Moderate to severe pain. **Adults:** 50 to 150 mg P.O., I.M., or S.C. q 3 to 4 hours, p.r.n. or around the clock; or 15 to 35 mg/hour by continuous I.V. infusion. **Children:** 1 to 1.8 mg/kg P.O., I.M., or S.C. q 4 to 6 hours. Maximum dosage is 100 mg q 4 hours, p.r.n. or around the clock.
• Preoperatively. **Adults:** 50 to 100 mg I.M. or S.C. 30 to 90 minutes before surgery. **Children:** 1 to 2.2 mg/kg I.M. or S.C. 30 to 90 minutes before surgery.

Adverse reactions

CNS: *sedation, somnolence, clouded sensorium, euphoria,* paradoxical excitement, tremor, dizziness, seizures with large doses. **CV:** *hypotension,* bradycardia, tachycardia. **GI:** *nausea, vomiting, constipation,* ileus. **GU:** *urine retention.* **Local:** pain at injection site, local tissue irritation and induration after S.C. injection; phlebitis after I.V. use. **Other:** ***respiratory depression,*** physical dependence, muscle twitching.

M

Interactions

Alcohol, CNS depressants: additive effects. Use together cautiously. **MAO inhibitors, barbiturates, isoniazid:** increased CNS excitation or depression can be severe or fatal. Don't use together. **Phenytoin:** decreased blood levels of meperidine. Monitor for decreased analgesia.

Nursing diagnoses

• Pain related to patient's underlying condition.
• Ineffective breathing pattern related to meperidine-induced respiratory depression.
• Knowledge deficit related to meperidine therapy.

Nursing interventions

• *Contraindicated* in hypersensitivity to the drug or other opiate analgesics and in patients who have received MAO inhibitors within 14 days.
• *Use with extreme caution* in increased intracranial pressure, increased CSF pressure, shock, CNS depression, head injury, asthma, COPD, respiratory depression, supraventricular tachycardias, seizures, acute abdominal conditions, hepatic or renal disease, hypothyroidism, Addison's disease, urethral stricture, prostatic hypertrophy, and alcoholism; in children under 12 years; and in elderly or debilitated patients.
• Monitor for increased toxic effect (drug and its metabolite accumulate).
• Give slow I.V., preferably as a diluted solution; keep narcotic antagonist (naloxone) available.
• Warn patient to avoid activities requiring mental alertness or physical coordination.
• Monitor respirations of neonates exposed to drug during labor. Have resuscitation equipment and naloxone available.
• P.O. dose less than half as effective as parenteral dose. When changing from parenteral to P.O. route, dose should be increased. Give before patient has intense pain (better analgesic effect).
• Monitor respiratory and CV status carefully. Don't give if respirations are below 12 breaths/minute, if respiratory rate or depth is decreased, or if change in pupils is noted.
• Monitor bowel and bladder function in postoperative patients.
• Don't withdraw abruptly after long-term use.
• Use with other narcotic analgesics, general anesthetics, phenothiazines, sedatives, hypnotics, tricyclic antidepressants, or alcohol may cause respiratory depression, hypotension, profound sedation, or coma. Reduce meperidine dose. Use together with extreme caution.
• Encourage turning, coughing, and deep breathing postoperatively to prevent atelectasis.

General
Classification: progestin, antineoplastic (progestin). **Pregnancy risk category:** X.

Mechanism of action
Suppresses ovulation, possibly by inhibiting pituitary gonadotropin secretion. Forms a thick cervical mucus.

Indications and dosage
• Menstrual disorders. **Women:** 125 to 375 mg I.M. q 4 weeks. Stop after 4 cycles.
• Uterine cancer. **Women:** 1 to 5 g I.M. weekly.

Adverse reactions
CNS: dizziness, migraine headache, lethargy, depression. **CV:** hypertension, thrombophlebitis, ***pulmonary embolism,*** edema. **GI:** nausea, vomiting, abdominal cramps. **GU:** breakthrough bleeding, dysmenorrhea, amenorrhea, cervical erosion, abnormal secretions, uterine fibromas, vaginal candidiasis. **Hepatic:** cholestatic jaundice. **Metabolic:** hyperglycemia. **Skin:** melasma, rash. **Local:** irritation and pain at injection site. **Other:** breast tenderness, enlargement, or secretion; decreased libido.

Interactions
Barbiturates, carbamazepine, rifampin: decreased progestogen effects. Monitor for diminished therapeutic response. **Bromocriptine:** may cause amenorrhea, interfering with the effects of bromocriptine. Avoid concomitant use. **Corticosteroids:** possible enhanced effects. Monitor closely. **Dantrolene, other hepatotoxic medications:** increased risk of hepatotoxicity. Monitor closely. **Oral anticoagulants:** dosage adjustments may be necessary. Monitor PT.

Nursing diagnoses
• Sexual dysfunction related to the patient's underlying condition.
• Fluid volume excess related to hydroxyprogesterone-induced edema.
• Knowledge deficit related to hydroxyprogesterone therapy.

Nursing interventions
• *Contraindicated* in thromboembolic disorders, breast cancer, undiagnosed abnormal vaginal bleeding, severe hepatic disease, or missed abortion or in pregnant women.
• *Use cautiously* in diabetes mellitus, seizure disorder, migraine, cardiac or renal disease, asthma, and mental illness.
• FDA regulations require that, before receiving first dose, patients read package insert explaining possible adverse effects of drug. Provide verbal explanation also. Patient should report any unusual symptoms immediately and should stop drug and call doctor if visual disturbances or migraine occurs.
• Hydroxyprogesterone should not be used to induce withdrawal bleeding or as a test for pregnancy; drug may cause birth defects and masculinization of female fetus.
• Warn patient that edema and weight gain are likely. Monitor weight routinely and recommend sodium-restricted diet as needed.
• Instruct patient to report breast pain or tenderness, vaginal discharge or bleeding, and swelling of the hands or feet.
• Give sesame oil- and castor oil-based solutions deep I.M. in gluteal muscle. Rotate injection sites to prevent muscle atrophy.
• Effect lasts 7 to 14 days.
• Teach patient how to perform a monthly breast self-examination.
• Instruct patient that normal menstrual cycles may not resume for 2 to 3 months after drug is stopped.

General

Classification: ovulation stimulant, spermatogenesis stimulant (gonadotropin). **Pregnancy risk category:** C.

Mechanism of action

Menotropins, when administered to women who have not had primary ovarian failure, mimics follicle-stimulating hormone (FSH) in inducing follicular growth and luteinizing hormone (LH) in aiding follicular maturation.

Indications and dosage

- Anovulation. **Women:** 75 IU each of FSH and LH I.M. daily for 9 to 12 days, followed by 10,000 units of human chorionic gonadotropin (HCG) I.M. 1 day after last dose of menotropins. Repeat for one to three menstrual cycles until ovulation occurs.
- Infertility with ovulation. **Women:** 75 IU each of FSH and LH I.M. daily for 9 to 12 days, followed by 10,000 units HCG I.M. 1 day after last dose of menotropins. Repeat for two menstrual cycles and then increase to 150 IU each of FSH and LH I.M. daily for 9 to 12 days, followed by 10,000 units HCG I.M. 1 day after last dose of menotropins. Repeat for two menstrual cycles.
- Infertility. **Men:** 1 ampule I.M. three times weekly (given concomitantly with 2,000 units HCG twice weekly) for at least 4 months.

Adverse reactions

Blood: hemoconcentration with fluid loss into abdomen. **GI:** nausea, vomiting, diarrhea. **GU:** in women—*ovarian enlargement with pain and abdominal distention,* multiple births, ovarian hyperstimulation syndrome (sudden ovarian enlargement, ascites with or without pain, or pleural effusion); in men—*gynecomastia.* **Other:** fever.

Interactions

None significant.

Nursing diagnoses

- Sexual dysfunction related to the patient's underlying condition.
- Pain related to ovarian enlargement induced by menotropins.
- Knowledge deficit related to menotropins therapy.

Nursing interventions

- *Contraindicated* in patients with hypersensitivity to the drug; in those with ovarian failure, high urinary gonadotropin levels, thyroid or adrenal dysfunction, pituitary tumor, abnormal uterine bleeding, uterine fibroids, or ovarian cysts or enlargement; and in pregnant patients.
- *Use cautiously* in patients with cardiac, renal, or pulmonary disease; seizure disorder; migraine headache; history of thrombophlebitis; or polycystic ovary syndrome.
- Close monitoring of patient response is critical to ensure adequate ovarian stimulation without hyperstimulation.
- Tell patient that there is a possibility of multiple births.
- In infertility, encourage daily intercourse from day before HCG is given until ovulation occurs.
- Pregnancy usually occurs 4 to 6 weeks after therapy.
- Reconstitute with 1 to 2 ml sterile sodium chloride injection. Use immediately.
- Rotate injection sites to prevent muscle atrophy.
- Instruct patient to immediately report severe abdominal pain, bloating, swelling of the hands or feet, nausea, vomiting, diarrhea, substantial weight gain, or shortness of breath.

General

Classification: antineoplastic (antimetabolite).
Pregnancy risk category: D.

Mechanism of action

Inhibits DNA synthesis.

Indications and dosage

• Melanoma; resistant chronic myelocytic leukemia; recurrent, metastatic, or inoperable ovarian cancer; head and neck cancers. **Adults:** 80 mg/kg P.O. as single dose q 3 days; or 20 to 30 mg/kg P.O. as a single daily dose.

Adverse reactions

Blood: ***leukopenia,*** thrombocytopenia, anemia, *megaloblastosis; dose-limiting and dose-related* ***bone marrow suppression,*** *with rapid recovery.* **CNS:** drowsiness, hallucinations. **GI:** *anorexia, nausea, vomiting, diarrhea,* stomatitis. **GU:** increased BUN and serum creatinine levels. **Metabolic:** hyperuricemia. **Skin:** rash, pruritus.

Interactions

Cytotoxic drugs, radiation therapy: enhanced toxicity of hydroxyurea. Use together cautiously.

Nursing diagnoses

• Altered protection related to hydroxyurea-induced myelosuppression and immunosuppression.
• Altered oral mucous membrane related to hydroxyurea-induced stomatitis.
• Knowledge deficit related to hydroxyurea therapy.

Nursing interventions

• *Contraindicated* in patients with hypersensitivity to the drug.
• *Use cautiously* in renal dysfunction. Discontinue if WBC count is below 2,500/mm^3 or if platelet count is below 100,000/mm^3.
• Dosage modification may be required after chemotherapy or radiation therapy.
• Warn patient to watch for signs of infection (fever, sore throat, fatigue) and bleeding (easy bruising, nosebleeds, bleeding gums, melena). Take temperature daily.
• If patient can't swallow capsule, he may empty contents into water and take immediately.
• Monitor intake and output; keep patient hydrated.
• Routinely measure BUN, uric acid, and serum creatinine levels.
• Drug crosses blood-brain barrier.
• Auditory and visual hallucinations and blood toxicity increase when decreased renal function exists.
• Patients who receive concomitant radiation therapy may experience an increased incidence or severity of GI distress or stomatitis.
• Avoid all I.M. injections when platelet counts are below 100,000/mm^3.
• Has been used investigationally to relieve symptoms of sickle cell anemia. Dosage is highly variable; in early trials, the median dose was 20 mg/kg daily.

General

Classification: antineoplastic (alkylating agent).
Pregnancy risk category: D.

Mechanism of action

Cross-links strands of cellular DNA and interferes with RNA transcription, causing an imbalance of growth that leads to cell death. Cell cycle-non-specific.

Indications and dosage

• Multiple myeloma. **Adults:** initially, 6 mg P.O. daily for 2 to 3 weeks, then stop drug for up to 4 weeks or until WBC and platelet counts stop dropping and begin to rise again; resume with maintenance dosage of 2 mg daily. Stop drug if WBC count is below 3,000/mm^3 or platelet count is below 100,000/mm^3. Alternative therapy: give 0.15 mg/kg P.O. daily for 7 days, or 0.25 mg/kg for 4 days; repeat q 4 to 6 weeks.

For patients who can't tolerate oral therapy, give 16 mg/m^2 by I.V. infusion over 15 to 20 minutes. Give at 2-week intervals for four doses. After patient has recovered from toxicity, drug is given at 4-week intervals.

• Nonresectable advanced ovarian cancer. **Adults:** 0.2 mg/kg P.O. daily for 5 days. Repeat q 4 to 5 weeks, depending on bone marrow recovery.

Adverse reactions

Blood: ***thrombocytopenia, leukopenia, agranulocytosis.*** **Skin:** dermatitis, pruritus, rash, alopecia. **Other:** ***pneumonitis and pulmonary fibrosis, anaphylaxis.***

Interactions

Anticoagulants, aspirin: may increase GI bleeding. Use together cautiously. **Carmustine:** I.V. melphalan may lower the threshold for carmustine lung toxicity. Monitor closely. **Cisplatin:** may alter renal clearance of melphalan by causing nephrotoxicity. Monitor renal function; adjust dosage as ordered. **Cyclosporine:** severe renal failure has been reported in patients who followed a single I.V. dose of melphalan with standard doses of cyclosporine. Avoid use. **Nalidixic acid:** increased incidence of severe hemorrhagic necrotic enterocolitis in pediatric patients. Avoid use.

Nursing diagnoses

• High risk for injury related to hemorrhage secondary to thrombocytopenia and myelosuppression.
• High risk for infection related to the immunosuppressant effects of drug therapy.
• Knowledge deficit related to melphalan therapy.

Nursing interventions

• *Contraindicated* in hypersensitivity to the drug and in diseases known to be resistant to the drug. Patients with hypersensitivity to chlorambucil may exhibit cross-sensitivity to melphalan.
• Not recommended in severe leukopenia, thrombocytopenia, or anemia or in chronic lymphocytic leukemia.
• Monitor serum uric acid and CBC.
• Avoid all I.M. injections when platelet count is below 100,000/mm^3.
• Therapeutic effects are often accompanied by toxicity. Reduce dosage in renal impairment.
• Administer on empty stomach.
• Warn patient to watch for signs of infection and bleeding. Take temperature daily. Tell patient to avoid OTC products containing aspirin.
• **I.V. use:** Reconstitute immediately before administering with the 10 ml of sterile diluent supplied by the manufacturer. Shake vigorously until clear. Solution will contain 5 mg melphalan/ml. Immediately dilute the required dose in 0.9% sodium chloride injection. Final concentration shouldn't exceed 0.45 mg/ml.
• Dilute and administer promptly. Within 30 minutes, the reconstituted product begins to degrade. After final dilution, nearly 1% of the drug degrades every 10 minutes. Don't refrigerate; a precipitate will form.
• Follow institutional guidelines for the safe handling, preparation, administration, and disposal of chemotherapeutic drugs.

General

Classification: anxiolytic, sedative, antipruritic, antiemetic, antispasmodic (antihistamine). **Pregnancy risk category:** C.

Mechanism of action

Depresses the CNS at the limbic and subcortical levels of the brain.

Indications and dosage

- Anxiety and tension. **Adults:** 25 to 100 mg P.O. t.i.d. or q.i.d.
- Hyperkinesia. **Children 6 years and over:** 50 to 100 mg P.O. daily in divided doses. **Children under 6 years:** 50 mg P.O. daily in divided doses.
- Preoperative and postoperative adjunctive therapy. **Adults:** 25 to 100 mg I.M. q 4 to 6 hours. **Children:** 1.1 mg/kg I.M. q 4 to 6 hours.
- Rashes, pruritus. **Adults:** 25 mg P.O. t.i.d. or q.i.d. **Children 6 years and over:** 50 to 100 mg P.O. daily in divided doses. **Children under 6 years:** 50 mg P.O. daily in divided doses.

Adverse reactions

CNS: *drowsiness*, involuntary motor activity. **GI:** *dry mouth*. **Local:** marked discomfort at site of I.M. injection.

Interactions

Alcohol, other CNS depressants: increased CNS depression. Avoid concomitant use.

Nursing diagnoses

- Anxiety related to patient's underlying condition.
- Altered oral mucous membrane related to hydroxyzine-induced dry mouth.
- Knowledge deficit related to hydroxyzine therapy.

Nursing interventions

- *Contraindicated* in patients with hypersensitivity to the drug, in patients in shock or comatose states, and during acute asthmatic attacks.
- *Use cautiously* in patients with angle-closure glaucoma, prostatic hypertrophy, COPD, asthma, hyperthyroidism, or CV disease.
- Dosage should be reduced in elderly or debilitated patients.
- Warn patient to avoid hazardous activities that require alertness and good psychomotor coordination until CNS effects of the drug are known.
- Warn patient not to combine drug with alcohol or other depressants.
- Observe for excessive sedation due to potentiation with other CNS drugs.
- Used perioperatively as an antiemetic and anxiolytic. Its sedative and antihistamine properties make it especially useful to treat pruritus that prevents sleep.
- Used in psychogenically induced allergic conditions, such as chronic urticaria and pruritus.
- Parenteral form (hydroxyzine hydrochloride) for I.M. use only. Never administer I.V. (Z-track injection is preferred.)
- Aspirate injection carefully to prevent inadvertent intravascular injection. Inject deep into a large muscle.
- Suggest sugarless hard candy or gum to relieve dry mouth.
- Hydroxyzine may cause false elevations of urine 17-hydroxycorticosteroids, depending on test method used.

General
Classification: antineoplastic (progestin). **Pregnancy risk category:** X.

Mechanism of action
Changes the tumor's hormonal environment and alters the neoplastic process.

Indications and dosage
- Breast cancer. **Women:** 40 mg P.O. q.i.d.
- Endometrial cancer. **Women:** 40 to 320 mg P.O. daily in divided doses.

Adverse reactions
GU: dysfunctional uterine bleeding when drug is discontinued. **Other:** weight gain, increased appetite, carpal tunnel syndrome, thrombophlebitis, alopecia, hirsutism, breast tenderness.

Interactions
None significant.

Nursing diagnoses
- Impaired physical mobility related to drug-induced adverse reaction.
- Body image disturbance related to drug-induced masculinizing adverse effects.
- Knowledge deficit related to megestrol therapy.

Nursing interventions
- *Contraindicated* in patients with hypersensitivity to the drug, to progestins, with history of thromboembolic disorder, severe hepatic disease, undiagnosed abnormal vaginal bleeding, and in pregnant or breast-feeding women.
- *Use cautiously* in patients with history of thrombophlebitis, cardiac or renal disease, seizure disorder, or migraine. Also, use caution in administering to diabetic patients because decreased glucose tolerance may occur, or to patients with a history of mental depression.
- Megestrol is a relatively nontoxic drug with a low incidence of adverse effects.
- Adequate trial is 2 months. Reassure patient that therapeutic response isn't immediate.
- Monitor effectiveness by evaluating prothrombin and bleeding times and by noting the results of follow-up diagnostic tests and overall physical status.
- Monitor for signs of thrombophlebitis.
- Monitor patient's menstrual cycle; drug may cause dysfunctional uterine bleeding when drug is discontinued.
- Teach patient signs and symptoms of thrombophlebitis, and to report any to the doctor immediately.

General

Classification: antimuscarinic, GI antispasmodic (anticholinergic). **Pregnancy risk category:** C.

Mechanism of action

Competitively blocks acetylcholine, which decreases GI motility and inhibits gastric acid secretion.

Indications and dosage

• GI tract disorders caused by spasm; adjunctive therapy for peptic ulcers. **Adults:** 0.125 to 0.25 mg P.O. or S.L. t.i.d. or q.i.d. before meals and h.s.; 0.375 mg P.O. sustained-release form q 8 hours; or 0.25 to 0.5 mg (1 or 2 ml) I.M., I.V., or S.C. b.i.d. to q.i.d. (Substitute oral medication when symptoms are controlled.) **Children 2 to 10 years:** half of adult dose P.O., not to exceed 1.5 mg daily.

Adverse reactions

CNS: headache, insomnia, drowsiness, dizziness, *confusion or excitement in elderly patients,* nervousness, weakness. **CV:** *palpitations,* tachycardia. **EENT:** *blurred vision,* mydriasis, increased ocular tension, cycloplegia, photophobia. **GI:** *dry mouth,* dysphagia, *constipation,* heartburn, loss of taste, nausea, vomiting, *paralytic ileus.* **GU:** *urinary hesitancy, urine retention,* impotence. **Skin:** urticaria, decreased sweating or possible anhidrosis, other dermal manifestations. **Other:** fever, allergic reactions. **Overdose:** headache, drowsiness, visual disturbances; possible curare-like symptoms.

Interactions

Amantadine, antihistamines, antiparkinsonian agents, disopyramide, glutethimide, meperidine, phenothiazines, procainamide, quinidine: additive adverse effects. Avoid concomitant use. **Ketoconazole:** anticholinergics may interfere with ketoconazole absorption. Avoid concomitant use. **Methotrimeprazine:** anticholinergics may enhance risk of extrapyramidal reactions. Avoid concomitant use.

Nursing diagnoses

• Pain related to patient's underlying condition.
• Urinary retention related to adverse drug reaction.
• Knowledge deficit related to hyoscyamine therapy.

Nursing interventions

• *Contraindicated* in narrow-angle glaucoma, obstructive uropathy, obstructive disease of GI tract, severe ulcerative colitis, myasthenia gravis, hypersensitivity to anticholinergics, paralytic ileus, intestinal atony, unstable CV status in acute hemorrhage, or toxic megacolon.
• *Use cautiously* in autonomic neuropathy, hyperthyroidism, coronary artery disease, cardiac arrhythmias, CHF, hypertension, hiatal hernia associated with reflux esophagitis, hepatic or renal disease, and ulcerative colitis or in patients over 40 years because of the increased incidence of glaucoma. Also use cautiously in hot or humid environments. Drug-induced heatstroke can develop.
• Injection contains sodium metabisulfite, which may cause allergic reaction in some patients.
• Give 30 minutes to 1 hour before meals and at bedtime.
• Monitor patient's vital signs and urine output.
• Instruct patient to avoid driving and other hazardous activities if he is drowsy or dizzy or has blurred vision; to drink plenty of fluids to help prevent constipation; and to report any rash or skin eruption.
• Gum or sugarless hard candy may relieve dry mouth.

General

Classification: antimalarial (quinine derivative).
Pregnancy risk category: C.

Mechanism of action

Exact mechanism unknown. Mefloquine is a structural analog of quinine. Antimalarial activity may be related to its ability to form complexes with hemin.

Indications and dosage

- Treatment of acute malaria infections caused by mefloquine-sensitive strains of *Plasmodium falciparum* or *P. vivax*. **Adults:** 1,250 mg P.O. as a single dose. Patients with *P. vivax* infections should receive subsequent therapy with primaquine or other 8-aminoquinolines to avoid relapse after treatment of the initial infection.
- Malaria prophylaxis. **Adults:** 250 mg P.O. once weekly. Initiate prophylaxis 1 week before entering endemic area, and continue prophylaxis for 4 weeks after return from such areas. When returning to an area without malaria after a prolonged stay in an endemic area, prophylaxis ends after three doses.

Adverse reactions

CNS: dizziness, syncope, headache, transient emotional disturbances (rare). **CV:** extrasystoles. **EENT:** tinnitus. **GI:** loss of appetite, vomiting, *nausea,* loose stools, diarrhea, GI discomfort. **Skin:** rash. **Other:** fatigue, fever, chills.

M

Interactions

Quinine, chloroquine: increased risk of seizures. **Quinine, quinidine, beta-adrenergic blocking agents:** ECG abnormalities and cardiac arrest may occur. **Valproic acid:** decreased valproic acid blood levels and loss of seizure control at start of mefloquine therapy. Monitor anticonvulsant blood levels.

Nursing diagnoses

- High risk for injury related to ineffective dosage regimen.
- High risk for fluid volume deficit related to mefloquine-induced adverse GI reactions.
- Knowledge deficit related to mefloquine therapy.

Nursing interventions

- *Contraindicated* in patients with hypersensitivity to mefloquine or related compounds.
- *Use cautiously* in patients with cardiac disease.
- Advise the patient to take the drug on the same day of the week when using it for prophylaxis.
- Tell the patient not to take the drug on an empty stomach and always to take it with a full glass (at least 8 oz [240 ml]) of water.
- Because the health risks from concomitant administration of quinine and mefloquine are great, mefloquine therapy should not begin sooner than 12 hours after the last dose of quinine or quinidine.
- Advise patients to use caution when performing hazardous activities that require alertness and good coordination because there have been reports of dizziness, a disturbed sense of balance, and neuropsychiatric reactions.
- In cases of suspected overdose, induce vomiting and seek medical advice immediately because there is potential for cardiotoxicity. Animal studies reveal that mefloquine has cardiac actions similar to quinidine and quinine.
- Patients taking mefloquine prophylaxis should discontinue the drug if they notice signs or symptoms of unexplained anxiety, depression, confusion, or restlessness. These symptoms may indicate impending toxicity.
- Periodic ophthalmic examinations are recommended in patients undergoing long-term therapy because ocular lesions have been noted in laboratory animals.
- Periodic liver function tests are recommended.
- Patients with infections caused by *P. vivax* are at high risk for relapse because the drug does not eliminate the hepatic phase (exoerythrocytic parasites). Follow-up therapy is advisable.

General

Classification: nonnarcotic analgesic, antipyretic (NSAID). **Pregnancy risk category:** B (D in 3rd trimester).

Mechanism of action

Produces anti-inflammatory, analgesic, and antipyretic effects, possibly through inhibition of prostaglandin synthesis.

Indications and dosage

- Mild to moderate pain, arthritis, primary dysmenorrhea, gout, postextraction dental pain. **Adults:** 200 to 800 mg P.O. t.i.d. or q.i.d., not to exceed 3.2 g/day.
- Juvenile arthritis. **Children:** 20 to 40 mg/kg P.O. daily in three or four divided doses.
- Fever. **Adults:** 200 to 400 mg P.O. q 4 to 6 hours. Do not exceed 1.2 g daily or take longer than 3 days. **Children 1 to 12 years:** if fever is below 102.5° F (39.2° C), the recommended dose is 5 mg/kg P.O. q 6 to 8 hours. Treat higher fevers with 10 mg/kg q 6 to 8 hours. Do not exceed 40 mg/kg daily.

Adverse reactions

Blood: prolonged bleeding time. **CNS:** *headache, drowsiness, dizziness,* aseptic meningitis. **CV:** *peripheral edema.* **EENT:** visual disturbances, *tinnitus.* **GI:** *epigastric distress, nausea, occult blood loss, peptic ulceration.* **GU:** reversible renal failure. **Hepatic:** elevated enzymes. **Skin:** pruritus, rash, urticaria. **Other:** ***bronchospasm,*** edema.

Interactions

Aspirin: may decrease serum levels of ibuprofen. Avoid concomitant use. **Furosemide, thiazide diuretics:** ibuprofen may decrease the effectiveness of diuretics. **Oral anticoagulants, lithium:** ibuprofen may increase plasma levels or pharmacologic effects of these agents. Monitor for toxicity.

Nursing diagnoses

- Pain related to the patient's underlying condition.
- High risk for trauma related to possible drowsiness or dizziness from adverse CNS reaction to ibuprofen.
- Knowledge deficit related to ibuprofen therapy.

Nursing interventions

- *Contraindicated* in patients with hypersensitivity to the drug, other NSAIDs, or aspirin.
- *Use cautiously* in GI disorders, history of peptic ulcer disease, angioedema, asthma with nasal polyps, hepatic or renal disease, cardiac decompensation, or known intrinsic coagulation defects.
- Tell patient that full therapeutic effect for arthritis may be delayed for 2 to 4 weeks. Analgesic effect occurs at low dosage levels. However, anti-inflammatory effect does not occur at dosages below 400 mg q.i.d.
- Check renal and hepatic function periodically in long-term therapy. Stop drug if abnormalities occur.
- Serious GI toxicity can occur at any time in patients on long-term NSAID therapy. Teach patient signs and symptoms of GI bleeding, and tell patient to report these to the doctor immediately.
- Give with meals or milk to reduce adverse GI reactions.
- Concomitant use with aspirin, alcohol, or steroids may increase the risk of adverse GI reactions.
- Drug is available OTC in several brands (200-mg strength). Instruct patient not to exceed 1.2 g daily, or self-medicate for extended periods without consulting doctor.
- Ibuprofen should not be given to children under age 12 without a doctor's prescription.
- Because of their antipyretic and anti-inflammatory actions, NSAIDs may mask the signs and symptoms of infection.

General

Classification: nonnarcotic analgesic, antipyretic, anti-inflammatory (NSAID). **Pregnancy risk category:** C.

Mechanism of action

Produces anti-inflammatory, analgesic, and antipyretic effects, possibly through inhibition of prostaglandin synthesis.

Indications and dosage

- Mild to moderate pain, dysmenorrhea. **Adults and children over 14 years:** initially, 500 mg P.O., then 250 mg q 6 hours, p.r.n. Maximum therapy 1 week.

Adverse reactions

Blood: leukopenia, thrombocytopenia, *agranulocytosis, aplastic anemia.* **CNS:** *drowsiness, dizziness,* nervousness, headache. **CV:** edema. **EENT:** blurred vision, eye irritation. **GI:** nausea, vomiting, *diarrhea,* ***peptic ulceration,*** hemorrhage. **GU:** dysuria, hematuria, ***nephrotoxicity.*** **Hepatic:** ***hepatotoxicity.*** **Skin:** rash, urticaria.

Interactions

Oral anticoagulants, sulfonylureas, and other drugs that are highly protein-bound: increased risk of toxicity.

M

Nursing diagnoses

- Pain related to patient's underlying condition.
- High risk for trauma related to drowsiness or dizziness caused by CNS reactions to mefenamic acid.
- Knowledge deficit related to mefenamic acid therapy.

Nursing interventions

- *Contraindicated* in GI ulceration or inflammation.
- *Use cautiously* in hepatic or renal disease, CV disease, blood dyscrasias, diabetes mellitus, and a history of peptic ulcer disease and in asthmatics with nasal polyps.
- Serious GI toxicity can occur at any time in patients taking chronic NSAID therapy. Teach patient signs and symptoms of GI bleeding, and tell patient to report these to the doctor immediately.
- Concomitant use with aspirin, alcohol, or steroids may increase the risk of adverse GI reactions.
- Warn patient against hazardous activities that require alertness until CNS effects of the drug are known.
- Severe hemolytic anemia may occur with prolonged use. Monitor CBC every 4 to 6 months or as indicated.
- Stop drug if rash, visual disturbances, or diarrhea develops.
- Should not be administered for more than 1 week at a time because risk of toxicity increases.
- Administer with food to minimize adverse GI reactions.
- Because of their anti-inflammatory and antipyretic actions, NSAIDs may mask the signs and symptoms of infection.
- False-positive reactions for urine bilirubin using the diazo tablet test have been reported.

General

Classification: Antineoplastic antibiotic (anthracycline). **Pregnancy risk category:** D.

Mechanism of action

Inhibits nucleic acid synthesis by intercalation and interacts with the enzyme topoisomerase II. Highly lipophilic, resulting in increased rate of cellular uptake.

Indications and dosage

Dosage and indications may vary. Check current literature for recommended protocol.

• Acute myeloid leukemia, including FAB (French-American-British) classifications M1 through M7, in combination with other approved antileukemic agents. **Adults:** 12 mg/m² daily for 3 days by slow I.V. injection (over 10 to 15 minutes) in combination with 100 mg/m² of cytarabine daily for 7 days by continuous I.V. infusion or as a 25 mg/m² bolus followed by 200 mg/m² daily for 5 days by continuous infusion.

A second course may be administered if needed. If patient experiences severe mucositis, delay administration until recovery is complete and reduce dose by 25%. Dosage should also be reduced in patients with hepatic or renal impairment. Idarubicin should not be given if bilirubin level is above 5 mg/dl.

Adverse reactions

Blood: *myelosuppression.* **CNS:** headache, changed mental status, ***seizures.*** **CV:** ***CHF,*** atrial fibrillation, chest pain, ***MI,*** asymptomatic decline in left ventricular ejection fraction, ***myocardial insufficiency, arrhythmias,*** *hemorrhage,* myocardial toxicity. **GI:** *nausea, vomiting,* cramps, diarrhea, *mucositis,* ***severe enterocolitis with perforation*** (rare). **GU:** decreased renal function, hyperuricemia. **Skin:** alopecia, rash, urticaria, bullous erythrodermatous rash on palms and soles, hives at injection site. **Other:** *infection,* fever, changes in hepatic function, local tissue necrosis (if extravasation occurs), allergic reactions.

Interactions

Heparin, alkaline solutions: incompatible. Idarubicin should not be mixed with other drugs unless specific compatibility data is available.

Nursing diagnoses

• High risk for infection secondary to immunosuppressant effect of idarubicin.

• Altered nutrition: Less than body requirements, related to idarubicin-induced nausea, vomiting, and mucositis.

• Knowledge deficit related to idarubicin therapy.

Nursing interventions

• *Contraindicated* in patients with severe myelosuppression, preexisting cardiac disease, severe hemorrhagic conditions, or overwhelming infection.

• *Use with extreme caution* in hepatic or renal impairment; dosage reduction is necessary.

• Monitor hepatic and renal function frequently. Frequent CBCs are also recommended.

• Hyperuricemia may result from rapid lysis of leukemic cells; take appropriate preventive measures (including adequate hydration) before starting treatment. Allopurinol may be ordered.

• Control systemic infections before therapy.

• Antiemetics may be used to prevent or treat nausea and vomiting.

• **I.V. use:** Reconstitute to a final concentration of 1 mg/ml using 0.9% sodium chloride solution without preservatives. Add 5 ml to the 5-mg vial or 10 ml to the 10-ml vial. *Do not use bacteriostatic saline solution.* Vial is under negative pressure.

• Administer over 10 to 15 minutes into a free-flowing I.V. infusion of 0.9% sodium chloride solution or D_5W that is running into a large vein.

• If signs of extravasation occur, discontinue infusion immediately and notify doctor. Treat with intermittent ice packs—½ hour immediately, then ½ hour four times daily for 4 days.

• Instruct patient to recognize signs and symptoms of extravasation and to call doctor or nurse if these occur.

General

Classification: progestin, antineoplastic (progestin). **Pregnancy risk category:** X.

Mechanism of action

Suppresses ovulation, possibly by inhibiting pituitary gonadotropin secretion. Also forms a thick cervical mucus.

Indications and dosage

- Abnormal uterine bleeding due to hormonal imbalance. **Women:** 5 to 10 mg P.O. daily for 5 to 10 days beginning on the 16th day of menstrual cycle. If patient has received estrogen, give 10 mg P.O. daily for 10 days beginning on 16th day of cycle.
- Secondary amenorrhea. **Women:** 5 to 10 mg P.O. daily for 5 to 10 days.
- Endometrial or renal carcinoma. **Adults:** 400 to 1,000 mg/week I.M.
- Contraception. **Women:** 150 mg I.M. once q 3 months.

Adverse reactions

CNS: dizziness, migraine headache, lethargy, depression. **CV:** hypertension, thrombophlebitis, ***pulmonary embolism,*** edema. **GI:** nausea, vomiting, abdominal cramps. **GU:** breakthrough bleeding, dysmenorrhea, amenorrhea, cervical erosion, or abnormal secretions, uterine fibromas, vaginal candidiasis. **Hepatic:** cholestatic jaundice. **Metabolic:** hyperglycemia. **Skin:** melasma, rash. **Local:** pain, induration, sterile abscesses. **Other:** breast tenderness, enlargement, or secretion; decreased libido.

Interactions

Aminoglutethimide, rifampin: decreased progestin effects. Monitor for diminished therapeutic response. If medroxyprogesterone is used as a contraceptive, patient should use a nonhormonal contraceptive during therapy with these drugs. **Bromocriptine:** may cause amenorrhea, interfering with the effects of bromocriptine. Avoid concomitant use.

Nursing diagnoses

- Sexual dysfunction related to the patient's underlying condition.
- Fluid volume excess related to medroxyprogesterone-induced edema.
- Knowledge deficit related to medroxyprogesterone therapy.

Nursing interventions

- *Contraindicated* in thromboembolic disorders, breast cancer, undiagnosed abnormal vaginal bleeding, missed abortion, and hepatic dysfunction or in pregnant women.
- *Use cautiously* in diabetes mellitus, seizure disorder, migraine, cardiac or renal disease, asthma, and mental illness.
- I.M. injection may be painful. Monitor sites for evidence of sterile abscess. Rotate injection sites to prevent muscle atrophy.
- FDA regulations require that, before receiving first dose, patients read package insert explaining possible progestin adverse reactions. Provide verbal explanation also. Patient should report any unusual symptoms immediately and should stop drug and call doctor if visual disturbances or migraine headache occurs.
- Don't use as test for pregnancy; drug may cause birth defects and masculinization of female fetus.
- Teach patient how to perform a monthly breast self-examination.
- Drug has a prolonged but reversible contraceptive effect. Studies have shown that the median time to conception after discontinuation of drug is 10 months (range 4 to 31 months) in 93% of women; median time to conception is not related to duration of use of drug.
- Has been used effectively to treat obstructive sleep apnea.

General

Classification: antiviral agent (halogenated pyrimidine). **Pregnancy risk category:** C.

Mechanism of action

Interferes with DNA synthesis.

Indications and dosage

• Herpes simplex keratitis. **Adults and children:** instill 1 drop of solution into conjunctival sac q 1 hour during day and q 2 hours at night, or apply ointment to conjunctival sac q 4 hours or 5 times daily, with last dose at bedtime. A response should be seen in 7 days; if not, discontinue and begin alternate therapy. Therapy should not be continued longer than 21 days.

Adverse reactions

Eye: temporary visual haze; blurred vision (with ointment); irritation, pain, burning, or inflammation of eye; mild edema of eyelid or cornea; photophobia; small punctate defects in corneal epithelium; corneal ulceration; slowed corneal wound healing (with ointment). **Other:** hypersensitivity.

Interactions

Boric acid: precipitate formation; increased risk of ocular toxicity.

Nursing diagnoses

• Altered protection related to ocular infection.
• Sensory/perceptual alterations (visual) related to idoxuridine-induced visual blurring.
• Knowledge deficit related to idoxuridine therapy.

Nursing interventions

• *Contraindicated* in deep ulceration.
• Not for long-term use.
• Idoxuridine should not be mixed with other topical eye medications.
• Don't use old solution; causes ocular burning and has no antiviral activity.
• Warn patient to avoid sharing washcloths and towels with family members during infection.
• Tell patient to watch for signs of sensitivity, such as itching lids, swelling, or constant burning. Patient who develops such signs should stop drug and notify doctor immediately.
• Teach patient how to instill drug. Advise him to wash hands before and after administering, and warn him not to touch dropper or tip to eye or surrounding tissue. Tell him to apply light finger pressure on lacrimal sac for 1 minute after drops are instilled.
• Remove excessive exudate from eye area before application. Stress importance of compliance with recommended therapy.
• Refrigerate idoxuridine 0.1% solution. Store in tightly closed, light-resistant container.
• Tell patient not to share eye medications with family members. If a family member develops the same symptoms, instruct him to contact the doctor.
• If photophobia develops, patient should wear sunglasses and avoid prolonged exposure to sunlight.
• Also known as IDU.

General

Classification: nonnarcotic analgesic, antipyretic, anti-inflammatory (NSAID). **Pregnancy risk category:** B (D in 3rd trimester).

Mechanism of action

Produces anti-inflammatory, analgesic, and antipyretic effects, possibly through inhibition of prostaglandin synthesis.

Indications and dosage

- Rheumatoid arthritis and osteoarthritis. **Adults:** 200 to 400 mg/day P.O. in three or four equally divided doses.
- Mild to moderate pain. **Adults:** 50 to 100 mg P.O. q 4 to 6 hours. Maximum dose is 400 mg/day.

Adverse reactions

Blood: leukopenia, thrombocytopenia, ***agranulocytosis, aplastic anemia.*** **CNS:** fatigue, malaise, insomnia, *dizziness*, nervousness, *headache.* **CV:** edema. **EENT:** blurred vision, eye irritation. **GI:** *abdominal pain, flatulence,* ***peptic ulceration,*** nausea, vomiting, *diarrhea,* hemorrhage. **GU:** dysuria, hematuria, nephrotoxicity. **Hepatic:** ***hepatotoxicity.*** **Skin:** rash, urticaria.

Interactions

Alcohol, other NSAIDs, or steroids: increased risk of adverse GI reactions. Monitor patient closely. **Aspirin:** decreased plasma levels of meclofenamate. **Oral anticoagulants:** enhanced anticoagulant effect. Monitor for toxicity.

Nursing diagnoses

- Pain related to patient's underlying condition.
- High risk for trauma related to adverse CNS reactions.
- Knowledge deficit related to meclofenamate therapy.

Nursing interventions

- *Contraindicated* in GI ulceration or inflammation.
- *Use cautiously* in hepatic or renal disease, CV disease, blood dyscrasia, diabetes mellitus, and a history of peptic ulcer disease; in asthmatics with nasal polyps; and in elderly patients, who are more likely to experience adverse reactions.
- Serious GI toxicity can occur at any time in patients taking chronic NSAID therapy. Teach patient signs and symptoms of GI bleeding, and tell patient to report these to the doctor immediately.
- Warn patient against activities that require alertness until CNS effects of drug are known.
- Stop drug if rash, visual disturbances, or diarrhea develops.
- Administer with food to minimize adverse GI reactions.
- False-positive reactions for urine bilirubin using the diazo tablet test have been reported.
- Patients taking drug long-term should test CBC and renal and hepatic function every 6 months or as indicated.
- Because of their anti-inflammatory and antipyretic actions, NSAIDs may mask the signs and symptoms of infection.

General

Classification: antineoplastic (halogenated pyrimidine). **Pregnancy risk category:** D.

Mechanism of action

Cross-links strands of cellular DNA and interferes with RNA transcription, causing an imbalance of growth that leads to cell death. Cell cycle-nonspecific.

Indications and dosage

• Testicular cancer. **Adults:** 1.2 g/m²/day I.V. for 5 consecutive days. Treatment is repeated every 3 weeks or after the patient recovers from hematologic toxicity.

Adverse reactions

Blood: ***leukopenia, thrombocytopenia, myelosuppression.*** **CNS:** *lethargy, somnolence, confusion, depressive psychosis, coma.* **CV:** supraventricular arrhythmias. **GI:** *nausea, vomiting.* **GU:** *hemorrhagic cystitis (dose-limiting adverse reaction occurring in up to 50% of patients), hematuria,* nephrotoxicity. **Hepatic:** elevated liver enzymes. **Other:** *alopecia.*

Interactions

Allopurinol: may produce excessive ifosfamide effect by prolonging half-life. Monitor for enhanced toxicity. **Barbiturates, phenytoin:** induce hepatic enzymes, hastening the formation of toxic metabolites. Ifosfamide toxicity may be increased. **Corticosteroids:** may inhibit hepatic enzymes, reducing ifosfamide's effect. Monitor for enhanced ifosfamide toxicity if concurrent corticosteroid dosage is suddenly reduced or discontinued. **Myelosuppressants:** enhanced hematologic toxicity. Dosage adjustment may be necessary.

Nursing diagnoses

• High risk for infection related to leukopenia and myelosuppression.
• Pain related to drug-induced hemorrhagic cystitis.
• Knowledge deficit related to ifosfamide therapy.

Nursing interventions

• *Contraindicated* in patients with severely depressed bone marrow function.
• *Use cautiously* in renal or hepatic impairment.
• Ifosfamide should be administered with a protecting agent (mesna) to prevent hemorrhagic cystitis. Adequate fluid intake (2 liters/day, either P.O. or I.V.) is essential.
• Obtain a urinalysis before each dose. If microscopic hematuria is present, the patient should be evaluated for hemorrhagic cystitis. Dosage adjustments of mesna may be necessary.
• Bladder irrigation with 0.9% sodium chloride solution may decrease the possibility of cystitis.
• Avoid giving the drug at bedtime because infrequent voiding during the night may increase the possibility of cystitis. Stop the drug if patient develops cystitis.
• Avoid all I.M. injections when platelet count is below 100,000/mm³.
• Use anticoagulants and aspirin products cautiously. Watch closely for signs of bleeding. Instruct patient to avoid OTC products containing aspirin.
• Administering antiemetics before ifosfamide may help decrease nausea.
• Assess patient for changes in mental status and cerebellar dysfunction. Dosage may have to be decreased.
• **I.V. use:** Prepare I.V. solution by reconstituting 1-g vial with 20 ml sterile or bacteriostatic water to yield a solution of 50 mg/ml. This solution may then be further diluted with sterile water, dextrose 2.5% or 5% in water, 0.45% or 0.9% sodium chloride solution, or lactated Ringer's solution. Infusing each dose slowly (over at least 30 minutes) will decrease possibility of cystitis.
• Monitor CBC and renal and liver function tests.
• Monitor patient for CNS changes.
• Parenteral preparation is associated with carcinogenic, mutagenic, and teratogenic risks for personnel. Follow hospital policy to reduce risks.

General

Classification: antiemetic and antivertigo agent (piperazine-derivative antihistamine). **Pregnancy risk category:** B.

Mechanism of action

May affect neural pathways originating in the labyrinth to inhibit nausea and vomiting.

Indications and dosage

- Dizziness. **Adults:** 25 to 100 mg P.O. daily in divided doses. Dosage varies with patient response.
- Motion sickness. **Adults:** 25 to 50 mg P.O. 1 hour before travel, repeated daily for duration of journey.

Adverse reactions

CNS: *drowsiness*, fatigue. **EENT:** blurred vision. **GI:** dry mouth.

Interactions

CNS depressants: increased drowsiness.

Nursing diagnoses

- High risk for fluid volume deficit related to nausea and vomiting induced by motion sickness.
- Altered thought processes related to meclizine-induced drowsiness.
- Knowledge deficit related to meclizine therapy.

Nursing interventions

- *Contraindicated* in patients with hypersensitivity to the drug.
- *Use cautiously* in glaucoma and GU or GI obstruction and in elderly males with possible prostatic hypertrophy.
- Warn patient against driving and other hazardous activities that require alertness until CNS effects of the drug are known.
- This antihistamine has a slower onset and longer duration of action than other antihistamine antiemetics.
- Know that meclizine may mask symptoms of ototoxicity, brain tumor, or intestinal obstruction.

General

Classification: antibiotic (carbapenem, beta-lactant). **Pregnancy risk category:** C.

Mechanism of action

Imipenem is bactericidal and inhibits bacterial cell wall synthesis. Cilastatin inhibits the enzymatic breakdown of imipenem in the kidneys, making it effective in the urinary tract.

Indications and dosage

• Serious infections of the lower respiratory and urinary tracts, intra-abdominal and gynecologic infections, bacterial septicemia, bone and joint infections, skin and soft-tissue infections, and endocarditis. Most known microorganisms are susceptible: *Staphylococcus, Streptococcus, Escherichia coli, Klebsiella, Proteus, Enterobacter, Pseudomonas aeruginosa,* and *Bacteroides,* including *B. fragilis.* **Adults:** 250 mg to 1 g by I.V. infusion q 6 to 8 hours. Maximum daily dosage is 4 g/day.

Adverse reactions

CNS: *seizures,* dizziness. **CV:** hypotension. **GI:** nausea, vomiting, diarrhea, *pseudomembranous colitis.* **Skin:** rash, urticaria, pruritus. **Local:** *thrombophlebitis, pain at injection site.* **Other:** ***hypersensitivity.***

Interactions

Ganciclovir: risk of seizures. Avoid concomitant use.

Nursing diagnoses

• High risk for injury related to ineffectiveness of imipenem/cilastatin in eradicating the infection.
• High risk for fluid volume deficit related to adverse GI reactions caused by imipenem/cilastatin.
• Knowledge deficit related to imipenem/cilastatin.

Nursing interventions

• *Use cautiously* in patients allergic to penicillins or cephalosporins because this drug is chemically similar. Ask patient if he's had a hypersensitivity reaction to either of these drugs before administering first dose of imipenem/cilastatin.
• *Also use cautiously* in patients who have a history of seizure disorders, especially if they also have compromised renal function. If patient develops seizures that persist despite anticonvulsant therapy, notify doctor. The drug should then be discontinued.
• **I.V. use:** Don't administer by direct I.V. bolus injection. Each 250- or 500-mg dose should be given by I.V. infusion over 20 to 30 minutes. Each 1-g dose should be infused over 40 to 60 minutes. If nausea occurs, the infusion may be slowed.
• When reconstituting powder, shake until the solution is clear. Solutions may range from colorless to yellow; variations of color within this range don't affect the drug's potency. After reconstitution, solution is stable for 10 hours at room temperature and for 48 hours when refrigerated.
• Imipenem/cilastatin has the broadest antibacterial spectrum of any available antibiotic. The drug is most valuable for empiric treatment of infections and for mixed infections that would otherwise require a combination of antibiotics, often including an aminoglycoside.
• Patients with impaired renal function may need lower dosage or longer intervals between doses.
• Obtain specimen for culture and sensitivity tests before first dose. Therapy may begin pending test results.
• Monitor patient for bacterial or fungal superinfections and resistant infections during and after therapy.

General
Classification: anthelmintic (benzimidazole).
Pregnancy risk category: C.

Mechanism of action
Selectively and irreversibly inhibits uptake of glucose and other nutrients in susceptible helminths.

Indications and dosage
- Pinworm. **Adults and children over 2 years:** 100 mg P.O. as a single dose. If infection persists 3 weeks later, repeat treatment.
- Roundworm, whipworm, hookworm. **Adults and children over 2 years:** 100 mg P.O. b.i.d. for 3 days. If infection persists 3 weeks later, repeat treatment.

Adverse reactions
GI: occasional, transient abdominal pain and diarrhea in massive infection and expulsion of worms.

Interactions
None significant.

Nursing diagnoses
- Altered health maintenance related to ineffectiveness of mebendazole.
- Diarrhea related to an adverse GI reaction to mebendazole therapy.
- Knowledge deficit related to mebendazole therapy.

Nursing interventions
- *Contraindicated* in patients with hypersensitivity to the drug.
- Tablets may be chewed, swallowed whole, or crushed and mixed with food.
- No dietary restrictions, laxatives, or enemas are necessary.
- Treat all family members.
- Teach patient about the need for good personal hygiene, especially good handwashing technique. To avoid reinfection, teach him to wash perianal area daily. Change undergarments and bedclothes daily. Wash hands and clean fingernails before meals and after bowel movements. Advise patient to refrain from preparing food during infestation.

General

Classification: TCA (dibenzazepine). **Pregnancy risk category:** D.

Mechanism of action

Increases the amount of norepinephrine or serotonin, or both, in the CNS by blocking their reuptake by the presynaptic neurons. This action allows these neurotransmitters to accumulate.

Indications and dosage

• Depression. **Adults:** 75 to 100 mg P.O. or I.M. daily in divided doses, with 25- to 50-mg increments up to 200 mg. (I.M. route rarely used). Maximum dosage is 300 mg daily. Alternatively, entire dosage may be given h.s. (using pamoate).
• Childhood enuresis. **Children 6 years and over:** 25 mg P.O. 1 hour before bedtime. If no response within 1 week, increase to 50 mg if the child is under 12 years; increase to 75 mg for children 12 years and over. In either case, do not exceed 2.5 mg/kg/day.

Adverse reactions

CNS: *drowsiness, dizziness,* excitation, tremor, weakness, confusion, headache, nervousness, EEG changes, ***seizures,*** extrapyramidal reactions. **CV:** *orthostatic hypotension, tachycardia, ECG changes,* hypertension. **EENT:** *blurred vision,* tinnitus, mydriasis. **GI:** *dry mouth, constipation,* nausea, vomiting, anorexia, paralytic ileus. **GU:** *urine retention.* **Skin:** rash, urticaria, photosensitivity. **Other:** *sweating,* allergy. **After abrupt withdrawal of long-term therapy:** nausea, headache, malaise (does not indicate addiction).

Interactions

Barbiturates: decrease TCA blood levels. Monitor for decreased antidepressant effect. **Cimetidine:** may increase imipramine serum levels. Monitor for increased adverse reactions. **Epinephrine, norepinephrine:** increase hypertensive effect. Use with caution. **MAO inhibitors:** may cause severe excitation, hyperpyrexia, or seizures, usually with high dose. Use together cautiously. **Methylphenidate:** increases TCA blood levels. Monitor for enhanced antidepressant effect.

Nursing diagnoses

• Ineffective individual coping related to the patient's underlying condition.
• High risk for injury related to imipramine-induced adverse CNS and cardiovascular reactions.
• Knowledge deficit related to imipramine therapy.

Nursing interventions

• *Contraindicated* during acute recovery phase of MI, in prostatic hypertrophy, and in patients with history of seizure disorders.
• *Use with extreme caution* in cardiovascular disease, urine retention, narrow-angle glaucoma or increased intraocular pressure, thyroid disease, blood dyscrasias, or impaired hepatic function; in patients who are at risk for suicide; and in those receiving electroconvulsive therapy, thyroid medication, or elective surgery. Injectable form contains sulfites, which may precipitate allergic reactions in certain individuals with hypersensitivity.
• Do not withdraw drug abruptly.
• Reduce dosage in elderly or debilitated persons, adolescents, and patients with aggravated psychotic symptoms.
• If psychotic signs increase, dosage should be reduced. Record mood changes. Watch for suicidal tendencies. To lessen suicide risk, provide only minimum supply of tablets.
• Check for urine retention and constipation. Increase fluids to lessen constipation. Suggest stool softener, if needed.
• Warn patient to avoid hazardous activities that require alertness and good psychomotor coordination until CNS effects of drug are known. Drowsiness and dizziness usually subside after a few weeks.
• Expect delay of 2 weeks or more before noticeable effect; 4 weeks or more before full effect.
• Dry mouth may be relieved with sugarless hard candy or gum. Saliva substitutes may be necessary.

General

Classification: viral vaccine (live, attenuated). **Pregnancy risk category:** X.

Mechanism of action

Promotes immunity to measles virus by inducing production of antibodies.

Indications and dosage

- Immunization. **Adults and children 15 months or over:** 0.5 ml (1,000 units) S.C. A two-dose schedule is recommended, with the first dose given at 15 months (12 months in high-risk areas) and the second dose given at the entry of school (kindergarten or first grade).
- Measles outbreak control. **Children:** if cases are occurring in children under 1 year, vaccinate children as young as 6 months. All students and their siblings should be revaccinated if they are without documentation of measles immunity. **Adults:** school personnel born in or after 1957 should be revaccinated if they are without proof of measles immunity. If the outbreak is in a medical facility, all workers born in or after 1957 should be revaccinated if they are without proof of immunity. Revaccination should be considered for persons born before 1957 as well.

Adverse reactions

Local: erythema, swelling, tenderness. **Skin:** rash. **Systemic:** fever, lymphadenopathy, ***anaphylaxis,*** febrile seizures in susceptible children, anorexia, leukopenia.

Interactions

Immune serum globulin, whole blood, plasma: antibodies in serum may interfere with immune response. Don't use vaccine within 3 months of transfusion. **Tuberculin skin test:** may temporarily decrease response to test. Defer skin testing.

Nursing diagnoses

- Altered protection related to lack of immunity to measles virus.
- Decreased cardiac output related to vaccine-induced anaphylactic shock.
- Knowledge deficit related to vaccine therapy.

Nursing interventions

- *Contraindicated* in immunosuppression, cancer, blood dyscrasias, corticosteroid or radiation therapy, gamma globulin disorders, or active, untreated tuberculosis; and in fever.
- *Use cautiously* in patients with hypersensitivity to neomycin, chickens, eggs, or feathers. Defer in acute illness or after administration of blood or plasma.
- Warn patient to avoid pregnancy for 3 months after vaccination.
- Do not give I.V.
- Obtain history of allergies, especially to eggs, and reaction to immunization.
- Keep epinephrine 1:1,000 available.
- Store in refrigerator and protect from light. Solution may be used if red, pink, or yellow, but must be clear (with no precipitation).
- Use only diluent supplied. Discard 8 hours after reconstituting.
- May be given with oral poliovirus vaccine.
- Because of a recent rise in the incidence of measles, the Immunization Practices Advisory Committee recommends that colleges and other post-high school educational institutions, as well as medical institutions employing health care providers, obtain documentation of the receipt of two doses of vaccine after age 1 (or other proof of immunity, such as infection, documented by a doctor). Combined measles, mumps, and rubella (MMR) vaccine is preferred.
- The CDC recommends that, during a measles outbreak in a health care facility, susceptible personnel exposed to the measles virus (whether or not they received measles vaccine or immunoglobulin) avoid patient contact for days 5 through 21 after such exposure. If they become ill, they should avoid patient contact for at least 7 days after developing rash.

General

Classification: immune serum. **Pregnancy risk category:** C.

Mechanism of action

Provides passive immunity by increasing antibody titer. The primary component is IgG.

Indications and dosage

- Agammaglobulinemia or hypogammaglobulinemia. **Adults:** 30 to 50 ml I.M. (Gamastan, Gammar) monthly. Alternatively, administer 100 mg/kg I.V. (Gamimune N) monthly. Infuse at 0.01 to 0.02 ml/kg/minute for 30 minutes. For Sandoglobulin, administer 200 mg/kg I.V. monthly. Infuse at 0.5 to 1 ml/minute. After 15 to 30 minutes, increase infusion rate to 1.5 to 2.5 ml/minute. **Children:** 20 to 40 ml I.M. monthly.
- Hepatitis A exposure. **Adults and children:** 0.02 to 0.04 ml/kg I.M. as soon as possible after exposure. Up to 0.1 ml/kg may be given after prolonged or intense exposure.
- Posttransfusion hepatitis B. **Adults and children:** 10 ml I.M. within 1 week after transfusion and 10 ml I.M. 1 month later.
- Measles exposure. **Adults and children:** 0.02 ml/kg I.M. within 6 days after exposure.
- Modification of measles. **Adults and children:** 0.04 ml/kg I.M. within 6 days after exposure.
- Measles vaccine complications. **Adults and children:** 0.02 to 0.04 ml/kg I.M.
- Poliomyelitis exposure. **Adults and children:** 0.3 to 0.4 ml/kg I.M. within 7 days after exposure.
- Chicken pox exposure. **Adults and children:** 0.2 to 1.3 ml/kg I.M. as soon as exposed.
- Rubella exposure in first trimester of pregnancy. **Women:** 0.2 to 0.4 ml/kg I.M. as soon as exposed.
- Prophylaxis in primary immunodeficiencies. **Adults and children:** 100 mg/kg by I.V. infusion monthly (Gamimune N only). Infusion rate is 0.01 to 0.02 ml/kg/minute for 30 minutes. Rate can then be increased to 0.04 ml/minute for remainder of infusion.
- Idiopathic thrombocytopenic purpura. **Adults:** 0.4 g/kg Gamimune N or Sandoglobulin I.V. for 5 consecutive days; or 1,000 mg/kg Gammagard. Additional doses may be given based on response. Give up to three doses (every other day) if necessary. Or give 500 mg/kg Venoglobulin-I daily for 2 to 7 days.

Adverse reactions

Skin: urticaria. **Systemic:** angioedema, headache, malaise, fever, nephrotic syndrome, ***anaphylaxis.*** **Local:** pain, erythema, muscle stiffness.

Interactions

Live virus vaccines: don't administer within 3 months after administration of immune globulin.

Nursing diagnoses

- Altered protection related to lack of or decreased immunity.
- Ineffective breathing pattern related to immunization-induced anaphylaxis.
- Knowledge deficit related to immune globulin immunization.

Nursing interventions

- *Contraindicated* in patients with hypersensitivity to the drug.
- Most adverse effects are related to a rapid rate of infusion.
- Obtain history of allergies and reactions to immunizations.
- Have drugs available for anaphylactic reaction.
- When giving I.M., inject into different sites, preferably anterolateral aspect of thigh or deltoid muscle for adults and anterolateral aspect of thigh for neonates and children under 3 years. Do not inject more than 3 ml per injection site.
- Do not give for hepatitis A exposure if 6 weeks or more have elapsed since exposure or after onset of clinical illness.
- **I.V. use:** Know that I.V. products are not interchangeable. Gamimune-N, Gammar-IV, Sandoglobulin, and Venoglubulin-I do not require an in-line filter. Gammagard and Iveegam require filters, which are supplied by the manufacturer.

General

Classification: viral vaccine (live, attenuated). **Pregnancy risk category:** X.

Mechanism of action

Promotes immunity to measles and rubella virus by inducing production of antibodies.

Indications and dosage

• Immunization. **Children 15 months to puberty:** 1 vial (1,000 units) S.C.

Adverse reactions

Skin: rash. **Systemic:** fever, lymphadenopathy, ***anaphylaxis.***

Interactions

Immune serum globulin, whole blood, plasma: antibodies in serum may interfere with immune response. Don't use vaccine within 3 months of transfusion. **Tuberculin skin test:** may temporarily decrease response to test. Defer skin testing.

Nursing diagnoses

• Altered protection related to lack of immunity to measles (rubeola) and rubella virus.
• Decreased cardiac output related to vaccine-induced anaphylactic shock.
• Knowledge deficit related to live, attenuated measles and rubella virus vaccine therapy.

Nursing interventions

• *Contraindicated* in immunosuppression, cancer, blood dyscrasias, corticosteroid or radiation therapy, gamma globulin disorders, fever, or active, untreated tuberculosis.
• *Use cautiously* in patients with hypersensitivity to neomycin, chickens, ducks, eggs, or feathers; when there is a history of febrile seizures; or in cerebral injury. Defer immunization in acute illness.
• Do not give within 1 month of other live virus vaccines, except oral poliovirus vaccine.
• Allow an interval of at least 3 weeks between bacillus Calmette-Guérin and rubella vaccines.
• Store in refrigerator and protect from light. Solution may be used if red, pink, or yellow, but must be clear (with no precipitation).
• Use only diluent supplied. Discard 8 hours after reconstituting.
• Inject in outer aspect of upper arm. Don't inject I.V.
• Keep epinephrine 1:1,000 available.

General
Classification: antihypertensive, diuretic (thiazide). **Pregnancy risk category:** B.

Mechanism of action
Inhibits sodium reabsorption in the cortical diluting site of the nephron. Also has a direct vasodilating effect that may be a result of calcium channel-blocking action.

Indications and dosage
• Edema, hypertension. **Adults:** 2.5 mg P.O. daily as a single dose taken in the morning. Dosage may be increased to 5 mg daily.

Adverse reactions
CNS: headache, irritability, nervousness. **CV:** volume depletion and dehydration, orthostatic hypotension. **GI:** anorexia, nausea, pancreatitis. **Metabolic:** hypokalemia; asymptomatic hyperuricemia; fluid and electrolyte imbalances, including dilutional hyponatremia and hypochloremia; metabolic alkalosis; gout. **Skin:** dermatitis, photosensitivity, rash. **Other:** muscle cramps and spasms.

Interactions
Diazoxide: increased antihypertensive, hyperglycemic, and hyperuricemic effects. Use together cautiously. **NSAIDs:** decreased diuretic effectiveness. Avoid concomitant use.

Nursing diagnoses
• Fluid volume excess related to the patient's underlying condition as evidenced by edema.
• Altered urinary elimination related to indapamide therapy.
• Knowledge deficit related to indapamide therapy.

Nursing interventions
• *Contraindicated* in anuria or hypersensitivity to other sulfonamide-derived drugs.
• *Use cautiously* in severe renal disease, impaired hepatic function, and progressive hepatic disease.
• Monitor intake and output, weight, blood pressure, and serum electrolytes.
• Consult with doctor and dietitian to provide high-potassium diet. Foods rich in potassium include citrus fruits, tomatoes, bananas, dates, and apricots. Watch for symptoms of hypokalemia (such as muscle weakness and cramps). Indapamide may be used with a potassium-sparing diuretic to prevent potassium loss. Patients also receiving a digitalis glycoside have an increased risk of digitalis toxicity from the potassium-depleting effects of this diuretic.
• Monitor serum creatinine and BUN regularly. Drug is not as effective if these levels are more than twice normal.
• Monitor blood uric acid level, especially in patients with a history of gout.
• Check insulin requirements in patients with diabetes. May treat severe hyperglycemia with oral antidiabetic agents.
• Give in the morning to prevent nocturia.
• In hypertension, therapeutic response may be delayed several days.
• Elderly patients are especially susceptible to excessive diuresis.
• Thiazides and thiazide-like diuretics should be stopped before tests for parathyroid function are performed.
• Advise patient to avoid sudden postural changes and to rise slowly to avoid orthostatic hypotension.
• Advise patient to use a sunscreen.

General

Classification: viral vaccine. **Pregnancy risk category:** X.

Mechanism of action

Promotes immunity to measles, mumps, and rubella virus by inducing production of antibodies.

Indications and dosage

• Routine vaccination. **Children:** administer 1 vial S.C. A two-dose schedule is recommended, with the first dose given at 15 months (12 months in high-risk areas) and the second dose given at the entry of school (kindergarten or first grade).
• Measles outbreak control. **Children:** if occurring in children under 1 year, vaccinate as young as 6 months. All students and their siblings should be revaccinated if they lack documentation of measles immunity. **Adults:** school personnel born in or after 1957 should be revaccinated if they lack proof of measles immunity. If the outbreak is in a medical facility, all workers born in or after 1957 should be revaccinated if they lack proof of immunity. Revaccination should be considered for persons born before 1957 as well.

Adverse reactions

Skin: rash, urticaria. **Systemic:** fever, regional lymphadenopathy, ***anaphylaxis.*** **Local:** erythema.

Interactions

Immune serum globulin, whole blood, plasma: antibodies in serum may interfere with immune response. Don't use vaccine within 3 months of transfusion.

Nursing diagnoses

• Altered protection related to lack of immunity to measles, mumps, and rubella virus.
• Hyperthermia related to vaccine-induced fever.
• Knowledge deficit related to live measles, mumps, and rubella virus vaccine therapy.

Nursing interventions

• *Contraindicated* in immunosuppression, cancer, blood dyscrasias, corticosteroid or radiation therapy, gamma globulin disorders, fever, or active, untreated tuberculosis.
• *Use cautiously* in patients with hypersensitivity to neomycin, chickens, ducks, eggs, or feathers. Defer immunization in acute illness.
• Incidence of adverse effects is low (0.5 to 4%).
• Presence of maternal antibodies may prevent response in children under 12 months.
• Treat fever with antipyretics, such as acetaminophen.
• Store in refrigerator; protect from light. Solution may be used if red, pink, or yellow, but must not be cloudy.
• Use only diluent supplied. Discard 8 hours after reconstituting.
• Obtain history of allergies, especially to ducks, rabbits, antibiotics, and reaction to immunization.
• Inject in outer aspect of upper arm. Don't give I.V.
• Keep epinephrine 1:1,000 available.
• Because of a recent rise in the incidence of measles, the Immunization Practices Advisory Committee recommends that colleges and other post-high school educational institutions, as well as medical institutions employing health care providers, obtain documentation of the receipt of two doses of vaccine after age 1 (or other proof of immunity, such as infection, documented by a doctor). Combined measles, mumps, and rubella (MMR) vaccine is preferred.
• The CDC recommends that, during a measles outbreak in a health care facility, susceptible personnel exposed to the measles virus (whether or not they received measles vaccine or immunoglobulin) avoid patient contact for days 5 through 21 after such exposure. If they become ill, they should avoid patient contact for at least 7 days after developing rash.
• In clinical trials, vitamin A supplementation (100,000 to 400,000 IU daily) was shown to reduce morbidity and mortality in children with measles.

General

Classification: nonnarcotic analgesic, antipyretic (NSAID). **Pregnancy risk category:** B (D in 3rd trimester).

Mechanism of action

Produces anti-inflammatory, analgesic, and antipyretic effects, possibly through inhibition of prostaglandin synthesis.

Indications and dosage

- Moderate to severe arthritis, ankylosing spondylitis. **Adults:** 25 mg P.O. or P.R. b.i.d. or t.i.d.; may increase dosage by 25 mg daily q 7 days up to 200 mg daily. Alternatively, 75 mg sustained-release capsules P.O. in the morning or h.s., followed, if necessary, by 75 mg b.i.d.
- Acute gouty arthritis. **Adults:** 50 mg P.O. t.i.d. Reduce dose as soon as possible, then discontinue. Don't use sustained-release capsules.
- Closing a hemodynamically significant patent ductus arteriosus in premature infants. **Neonates under 48 hours:** 0.2 mg/kg I.V. (sodium trihydrate) followed by two doses of 0.1 mg/kg at 12- to 24-hour intervals. **Neonates 2 to 7 days:** 0.2 mg/kg I.V. followed by two doses of 0.2 mg/kg at 12- to 24-hour intervals. **Neonates over 7 days:** 0.2 mg/kg I.V. followed by two doses of 0.25 mg/kg at 12- to 24-hour intervals.

Adverse reactions

Blood: ***hemolytic anemia, aplastic anemia, agranulocytosis,*** leukopenia, thrombocytopenic purpura, iron deficiency anemia; decreased platelet aggregation (*I.V. form only*). **CNS:** *headache, dizziness,* depression, drowsiness, confusion, peripheral neuropathy, seizures, psychic disturbances, syncope, *vertigo.* **CV:** hypertension, *edema.* **EENT:** *blurred vision, corneal and retinal damage,* hearing loss, tinnitus. **GI:** *nausea, vomiting,* anorexia, *diarrhea, peptic ulceration,* ***GI bleeding.*** **GU:** hematuria, ***acute renal failure; renal dysfunction*** *(I.V. only).* **Hepatic:** elevated enzymes. **Metabolic:** ***hyponatremia, hyperkalemia, hypoglycemia*** *(all I.V. only).* **Skin:** pruritus, urticaria, ***Stevens-Johnson syndrome.*** **Other:** hyperkalemia, hypersensitivity (shocklike symptoms, rash, respiratory distress, ***angioedema).***

Interactions

Alcohol, corticosteroids: increased risk of GI toxicity. **Aminoglycosides, cyclosporine, methotrexate:** indomethacin may enhance the toxicity of these agents. **Antihypertensive agents:** reduced antihypertensive effect. Monitor closely. **Aspirin:** decreased blood levels of indomethacin. **Diflunisal, probenecid:** decrease indomethacin excretion; watch for increased incidence of adverse reactions. **Digoxin:** indomethacin may prolong half-life of digoxin. **Lithium:** increased plasma lithium levels. Monitor for toxicity. **Thiazide diuretics, furosemide:** impaired response to both drugs. **Triamterene:** possible nephrotoxicity.

Nursing diagnoses

- Pain related to the patient's underlying condition.
- High risk for trauma related to possible adverse CNS reactions.
- Knowledge deficit related to indomethacin therapy.

Nursing interventions

- *Contraindicated* in patients with hypersensitivity to the drug, other NSAIDs, and in active peptic ulcer disease; in infants with untreated infection, active bleeding, coagulation defects or thrombocytopenia, necrotizing enterocolitis, or impaired renal function *(I.V. form only).*
- *Use cautiously* in seizure disorders, coagulation disorders, parkinsonism, hepatic or renal disease, cardiovascular disease, infection, and history of mental illness and in elderly patients.
- Monitor for bleeding in patients receiving anticoagulants, patients with coagulation defects, and neonates and for reduced urine output (*I.V. only*).
- Don't administer second or third scheduled dose if anuria or marked oliguria is evident (*I.V. only*).
- Used as prophylaxis for gout when colchicine is not well tolerated.

General

Classification: antidepressant (tricyclic antidepressant). **Pregnancy risk category:** B.

Mechanism of action

Increases the amount of norepinephrine or serotonin, or both, in the CNS by blocking their reuptake by presynaptic neurons.

Indications and dosage

• Depression. **Adults:** initially, 75 mg P.O. daily for patients with mild to moderate depression, then increased as required to 150 mg daily. Maximum dosage is 225 mg in patients who are not hospitalized. Severely depressed, hospitalized patients may receive up to 300 mg daily.

Adverse reactions

CNS: *drowsiness, dizziness,* excitation, ***seizures,*** tremor, weakness, confusion, headache, nervousness, extrapyramidal reactions. **CV:** *orthostatic hypotension, tachycardia, ECG changes.* **EENT:** blurred vision, tinnitus, mydriasis. **GI:** *dry mouth, constipation,* nausea, vomiting, anorexia, paralytic ileus. **GU:** *urine retention.* **Skin:** rash, urticaria, photosensitivity. **Other:** *sweating,* allergy. **After abrupt withdrawal of long-term therapy:** nausea, headache, malaise (does not indicate addiction).

Interactions

Barbiturates: decrease maprotiline blood levels. Monitor for decreased antidepressant effect. **Cimetidine:** may increase maprotiline serum levels. Monitor for increased adverse reactions. **Epinephrine, norepinephrine:** increase hypertensive effect. Use with caution. **MAO inhibitors:** may cause severe excitation, hyperpyrexia, or seizures, usually with high dose. Use together cautiously. **Methylphenidate:** increases maprotiline blood levels. Monitor for enhanced antidepressant effect.

Nursing diagnoses

• Altered individual coping related to the patient's underlying condition.
• Constipation related to maprotiline-induced adverse GI reactions.
• Knowledge deficit related to maprotiline therapy.

Nursing interventions

• *Contraindicated* during acute recovery phase of MI and in prostatic hypertrophy.
• *Use cautiously* in CV disease, urine retention, narrow-angle glaucoma, thyroid disease or medication, blood dyscrasias, and impaired hepatic function; in patients with a history of seizures; in patients who are at risk for suicide; and in those receiving electroshock therapy or elective surgery.
• Expect delay of 2 weeks or more before noticeable effect; 4 weeks or more before full effect.
• Do not withdraw drug abruptly.
• If psychotic signs increase, reduce dosage. Record mood changes. Monitor closely for suicidal tendencies. To lessen suicide risk, allow minimum supply of tablets. Reduce dosage in elderly or debilitated patients and adolescents.
• Check for urine retention and constipation. Increase fluids to lessen constipation. Suggest stool softener, if needed.
• Warn patient to avoid hazardous activities that require alertness and good psychomotor coordination until CNS effects of the drug are known. Drowsiness and dizziness usually subside after a few weeks.
• Dry mouth may be relieved with sugarless hard candy or gum, but maprotiline usually has a low potential for inducing anticholinergic effects.
• Whenever possible, patient should take full dose at bedtime.
• Advise patient not to take any other medication (prescription or OTC) without first checking with the doctor.
• Discontinue TCAs several days before surgery to prevent hypertensive episodes from occurring during surgery.
• Advise patient to use a sunscreen, wear protective clothing, and avoid prolonged exposure to sunlight to prevent photosensitivity reactions.

General

Classification: viral vaccine (vaccine). **Pregnancy risk category:** C.

Mechanism of action

Promotes immunity to influenza by inducing production of antibodies.

Indications and dosage

• Influenza prophylaxis. **Adults and children over 12 years:** 0.5 ml whole or split virus I.M. (one dose). **Children 9 to 12 years:** 0.5 ml split virus I.M. (one dose). **Children 3 to 8 years:** 0.5 ml split virus I.M. Repeat dose in 4 weeks unless child has been vaccinated previously. **Children 6 to 35 months:** 0.25 ml split virus I.M. Repeat dose in 4 weeks unless child has been previously vaccinated.

Adverse reactions

Local: erythema, induration, soreness at injection site. Fever and malaise reactions occur most often in children and others not exposed to influenza viruses. Severe reactions and paralysis associated with Guillain-Barré syndrome are rare; paralysis has only been associated with 1976 vaccine. **Systemic:** fever, malaise, myalgia, ***anaphylaxis.***

Interactions

Theophylline, warfarin: impaired clearance.

Nursing diagnoses

• Altered protection related to lack of immunity to influenza virus.
• Hyperthermia related to vaccine-induced fever.
• Knowledge deficit related to vaccine.

Nursing interventions

• *Contraindicated* in patients allergic to eggs. Defer in acute respiratory or other active infection.
• *Use cautiously* in patients with a history of sulfite allergy. Also obtain immunization history.
• Pregnancy isn't a contraindication for influenza vaccination according to the CDC. Vaccination shouldn't be postponed, regardless of the stage of pregnancy, in women who have high-risk conditions and who will be in the first trimester of pregnancy when the flu season begins.
• Patients with immunodeficiency may receive two doses 1 month apart; however, there is little evidence to suggest that booster doses improve the immunogenic response to the vaccine. Chemoprophylaxis with amantadine may be helpful.
• Vaccinations should be given in November because outbreaks of influenza generally don't occur until December. Try not to give the vaccine too early because antibody titers may begin to decline before flu season. Vaccines can be given to children and adults throughout the flu season, even as late as April; children age 12 and under should receive second dose in December, if possible.
• Leftover supplies of 1992-1993 vaccine must not be used to immunize patients for the 1993-1994 flu season, even though the 1993-1994 antigen is the same. Vaccination using the current vaccine is necessary because immunity to influenza decreases in the year after an injection.
• Thoroughly agitate vial just before administration to restore suspension.
• Give injections for adults and older children in deltoid muscle; for infants and children under 3 years, in anterolateral aspect of thigh.
• Keep epinephrine 1:1,000 available.
• Influenza vaccine is available as whole virus, split virus, and purified surface antigen preparations. Split virus and purified surface antigen vaccines cause somewhat fewer adverse reactions than whole virus in children.
• Children should not be given pertussis vaccine within 3 days of influenza virus vaccine. However, they may receive Haemophilus b conjugate vaccine, oral polio vaccine, measles-mumps-rubella vaccine, or pneumococcal vaccine at the same time. Injections should be made at different sites.
• Despite little information regarding influenza in HIV-infected patients, these patients should receive the vaccine. Persons with advanced disease may exhibit a low response; there is no evidence that a booster dose will improve the immune response.

General

Classification: diuretic (osmotic). **Pregnancy risk category:** C.

Mechanism of action

Increases the osmotic pressure of glomerular filtrate, inhibiting tubular reabsorption of water and electrolytes. Also elevates blood plasma osmolality, resulting in enhanced flow of water into extracellular fluid.

Indications and dosage

- Test dose for marked oliguria or suspected inadequate renal function. **Adults and children over 12 years:** 200 mg/kg or 12.5 g as a 15% or 20% solution I.V. over 3 to 5 minutes. Response adequate if 30 to 50 ml urine/hour is excreted over 2 to 3 hours.
- Treatment of oliguria. **Adults and children over 12 years:** 50 to 100 g I.V. as a 15% to 20% solution over 90 minutes to several hours.
- Prevention of oliguria or acute renal failure. **Adults and children over 12 years:** 50 to 100 g I.V. of a concentrated (5% to 25%) solution. Exact concentration is determined by fluid requirements.
- Edema. **Adults and children over 12 years:** 100 g I.V. as a 10% to 20% solution over 2 to 6 hours.
- Reduction of intraocular or intracranial pressure. **Adults and children over 12 years:** 1.5 to 2 g/kg as a 15% to 25% solution I.V. over 30 to 60 minutes.
- To promote diuresis in drug intoxication. **Adults and children over 12 years:** up to 200 g of 5% to 10% solution by continuous I.V. infusion, while maintaining 100 to 500 ml urine output/hour and a positive fluid balance.
- Irrigating solution during transurethral resection of prostate. **Men:** 2.5% to 5% solution p.r.n.

Adverse reactions

CNS: rebound increase in intracranial pressure 8 to 12 hours after diuresis, headache, confusion. **CV:** transient expansion of plasma volume during infusion causing circulatory overload and ***pulmonary edema***, tachycardia, chest pain. **EENT:** blurred vision, rhinitis. **GI:** thirst, nausea, vomiting. **GU:** urine retention. **Metabolic:** fluid and electrolyte imbalance, water intoxication, cellular dehydration.

Interactions

None significant.

Nursing diagnoses

- Fluid volume excess related to the patient's underlying condition as evidenced by edema.
- Altered urinary elimination related to diuretic therapy.
- Knowledge deficit related to mannitol therapy.

Nursing interventions

- *Contraindicated* in anuria, severe pulmonary congestion, frank pulmonary edema, severe CHF, severe dehydration, metabolic edema, progressive renal disease or dysfunction, progressive heart failure during administration, or active intracranial bleeding except during craniotomy.
- Monitor vital signs and intake and output hourly. Monitor weight, renal function, fluid balance, and serum and urine sodium and potassium levels daily.
- Solution often crystallizes. To redissolve, warm bottle in hot water bath; shake vigorously; then cool to body temperature. Concentrations above 15% have greater tendency to crystallize. Do not use solution with undissolved crystals.
- **I.V. use:** Always use an in-line filter and an infusion pump. Direct injection is not recommended. Administer as intermittent or continuous infusion at prescribed rate. Check I.V. line patency at infusion site before and during administration.
- Avoid infiltration; if it occurs, observe for inflammation, edema, and necrosis.
- For maximum intraocular pressure reduction before surgery, give 1 to 1½ hours preoperatively.
- Urethral catheter is inserted in comatose or incontinent patients; use an hourly urometer collection bag to facilitate accurate evaluation.
- When used as an irrigating solution, use concentrations of at least 3.5% to avoid hemolysis.

General

Classification: antidiabetic agent (pancreatic hormone). **Pregnancy risk category:** B.

Mechanism of action

Increases glucose transport across muscle and fat cell membranes to reduce blood glucose level. Promotes conversion of glucose to its storage form, glycogen.

Indications and dosage

• Diabetic ketoacidosis (use regular insulin only). **Adults:** 25 to 150 units I.V. immediately; additional doses may be given q 1 hour based on blood glucose level. **Children:** 0.1 unit/kg by I.V. bolus, then 0.1 unit/kg hourly by continuous I.V. infusion; additional dosage based on blood glucose level.

• Type I (insulin-dependent) diabetes mellitus, ketosis-prone diabetics, diabetes mellitus inadequately controlled by diet and oral antidiabetics. **Adults and children:** therapeutic regimen prescribed by doctor and adjusted according to patient's blood and urine glucose concentrations.

Adverse reactions

Metabolic: ***hypoglycemia,*** hyperglycemia. **Skin:** urticaria. **Local:** *lipoatrophy, lipohypertrophy,* itching, swelling, redness, stinging, warmth at site of injection. **Other:** ***anaphylaxis.***

Interactions

Alcohol, beta blockers, clofibrate, fenfluramine, guanethidine, MAO inhibitors, salicylates, tetracycline: prolonged antidiabetic effect. Monitor blood glucose level. **Corticosteroids, epinephrine, dextrothyroxine, thiazide diuretics:** diminished insulin response. Monitor for hyperglycemia.

Nursing diagnoses

• Altered nutrition: More than body requirements, related to inability to produce insulin to maintain blood glucose at normal levels.

• High risk for injury related to insulin-induced hypoglycemia.

• Knowledge deficit related to insulin therapy.

Nursing interventions

• Use only regular insulin in patients with circulatory collapse, diabetic ketoacidosis, or hyperkalemia. Do not use regular insulin concentrated (500 units/ml) I.V. Do not use intermediate or long-acting insulins for coma or other emergency requiring rapid drug action.

• *Use cautiously* in surgery and in patients with high fever, thyroid disease, severe infections, trauma, impaired hepatic or renal function, eating disorders, nausea, vomiting, or diarrhea.

• Accuracy of measurement is very important.

• Lente, semilente, and ultralente insulins may be mixed in any proportion. Regular insulin may be mixed with NPH or lente insulins in any proportion.

• Advise patient not to alter order of mixing insulins or change model or brand of syringe or needle.

• Note that switching from separate injections to a prepared mixture may alter patient's response. Whenever NPH or lente is mixed with regular insulin in the same syringe, be sure to administer immediately to avoid binding.

• Instruct patients on proper use of equipment for performing self-monitoring of blood glucose.

• Press but do not rub site after injection. Rotate injection sites and document them to avoid overuse of one area. However, unstable diabetics may achieve better control if injection site is rotated within same anatomic region.

• To mix insulin suspension, swirl vial gently or rotate between palms or between palm and thigh. Don't shake vigorously: This causes bubbling and air in syringe.

General

Classification: anticonvulsant (mineral/electrolyte). **Pregnancy risk category:** B.

Mechanism of action

May decrease acetylcholine released by nerve impulses; its anticonvulsant mechanism is unknown.

Indications and dosage

- Hypomagnesemic seizures. **Adults:** 1 to 2 g (as 10% solution) I.V. over 15 minutes, then 1 g I.M. q 4 to 6 hours, based on patient response and blood magnesium levels.
- Seizures secondary to hypomagnesemia in acute nephritis. **Children:** 0.2 ml/kg of 50% solution I.M. q 4 to 6 hours, p.r.n. or 100 mg/kg of 10% solution I.V. very slowly. Titrate dosage according to blood magnesium levels and seizure response.
- Prevention or control of seizures in preeclampsia or eclampsia. **Women:** initially, two doses of 4 g I.V. in 250 ml D_5W or 4 g deep I.M. in each buttock; then 4 g deep I.M., alternating buttocks q 4 hours, p.r.n. Alternatively, 4 g I.V. loading dose followed by 1 to 4 g hourly as an I.V. infusion.
- Management of paroxysmal atrial tachycardia. **Adults:** 3 to 4 g I.V. given over 30 seconds.
- Management of life-threatening ventricular arrhythmias, such as sustained ventricular tachycardia or torsades de pointes. **Adults:** 2 to 6 g I.V. given over several minutes, followed by a continuous infusion of 3 to 20 mg/minute for 5 to 48 hours. Dosage and duration of therapy depend on patient response and serum magnesium levels.

Adverse reactions

CNS: *sweating,* drowsiness, *depressed reflexes,* flaccid paralysis, hypothermia. **CV:** *hypotension, flushing,* ***circulatory collapse,*** depressed cardiac function, ***heart block.*** **Other:** ***respiratory paralysis,*** hypocalcemia.

Interactions

Anesthetics, CNS depressants: may cause additive CNS depression. Use cautiously. **Neuromuscular blockers:** may cause increased neuromuscular blockade. Use cautiously.

Nursing diagnoses

- High risk for injury related to the underlying seizure disorder or seizure possibility.
- Ineffective breathing pattern related to magnesium sulfate-induced respiratory depression.
- Knowledge deficit related to magnesium sulfate therapy.

Nursing interventions

- *Use cautiously* in patients with arrhythmias, impaired renal function, myocardial damage, and heart block and in women in labor.
- Drug can decrease the frequency and force of uterine contractions. Has been used as a tocolytic agent (suppresses uterine contractions) to inhibit premature labor.
- If used to treat seizures, institute appropriate seizure precautions.
- Keep I.V. calcium gluconate available to reverse magnesium intoxication; however, use cautiously in patients undergoing digitalization because of danger of arrhythmias.
- **I.V. use:** Monitor vital signs every 15 minutes when giving drug I.V.
- Watch for respiratory depression and signs of heart block. Respirations should be approximately 16 breaths/minute before each dose given.
- Monitor intake and output. Urine output should be 100 ml or more in 4-hour period before each dose.
- Check blood magnesium levels after repeated doses. Disappearance of knee-jerk and patellar reflexes is a sign of pending magnesium toxicity.
- Maximum infusion rate is 150 mg/minute.
- Observe neonates for signs of magnesium toxicity (including neuromuscular or respiratory depression), especially when given I.V. to toxemic mothers within 24 hours before delivery.
- Signs of hypermagnesemia begin to appear at blood levels of 4 mEq/liter.

General

Classification: antineoplastic (biological response modifier). **Pregnancy risk category:** C.

Mechanism of action

May have direct antiproliferative action against tumor cells or viral cells. Also may modulate host immune response.

Indications and dosage

• Hairy-cell leukemia. **Adults:** for induction, give 3 million units S.C. or I.M. daily for 16 to 24 weeks. For maintenance, 3 million units S.C. or I.M. three times a week.
• AIDS-related Kaposi's sarcoma. **Adults:** for induction, give 36 million units S.C. or I.M. daily for 10 to 12 weeks. For maintenance, 36 million units S.C. or I.M. three times a week.

Adverse reactions

Blood: ***leukopenia,*** *mild thrombocytopenia.* **CNS:** *dizziness,* confusion, paresthesia, numbness, lethargy, depression, nervousness, difficulty thinking or concentrating, insomnia, sedation, apathy, anxiety, irritability, fatigue, vertigo, gait disturbances, poor coordination. **CV:** hypotension, chest pain, arrhythmias, palpitations, syncope, ***CHF,*** hypertension, edema. **EENT:** visual disturbances, dryness or inflammation of the oropharynx, rhinorrhea, sinusitis, conjunctivitis, earache, eye irritation, rhinitis. **GI:** *anorexia, nausea, diarrhea,* vomiting, abdominal fullness or pain, constipation, hypermotility, gastric distress, dysgeusia. **GU:** transient impotence. **Hepatic:** ***hepatitis.*** **Respiratory:** ***bronchospasm,*** coughing, dyspnea, tachypnea. **Skin:** *rash,* dryness, *pruritus,* partial alopecia, urticaria, flushing. **Other:** *flulike syndrome,* diaphoresis, hot flashes, excessive salivation, cyanosis.

Interactions

Aminophylline: may reduce the clearance of aminophylline. **CNS depressants:** enhanced CNS depression.

Nursing diagnoses

• Altered protection related to proliferation of tumor or viral cells.
• Altered cardiopulmonary tissue perfusion related to interferon-induced CHF.
• Knowledge deficit related to interferon therapy.

Nursing interventions

• *Use cautiously* in severe hepatic or renal function impairment, seizure disorders, compromised CNS function, cardiac disease, or myelosuppression.
• Neurotoxicity and cardiotoxicity are more common in elderly patients.
• Use with blood dyscrasia-causing medications, bone marrow suppressant therapy, or radiation therapy may increase bone marrow suppressant effects. Dosage reduction may be required.
• Obtain allergy history. Drug contains phenol as a preservative and serum albumin as a stabilizer.
• Administer S.C. in patients whose platelet count is below 50,000/mm^3.
• Flulike symptoms at start of therapy tend to diminish with continued therapy.
• Patients should be well hydrated, especially during initial stages of treatment.
• Severe adverse reactions may require reduction of dosage by 50% or discontinuation of therapy until reactions subside.
• Advise patient that laboratory tests will be performed before and periodically during therapy.
• Instruct patient in proper oral hygiene during treatment.
• Warn patient not to have any immunization without doctor's approval and to avoid contact with persons who have taken oral polio vaccine.

General
Classification: antacid, saline laxative (magnesium salt). **Pregnancy risk category:** B.

Mechanism of action
Neutralizes and buffers stomach acid and produces an osmotic effect in the small intestine by drawing water into the intestinal lumen.

Indications and dosage
• Constipation, to evacuate bowel before surgery. **Adults and children over 6 years:** 15 to 60 ml milk of magnesia P.O. or 10 to 20 ml concentrated milk of magnesia P.O. **Children 2 to 6 years:** 5 to 15 ml milk of magnesia P.O.
• Antacid. **Adults:** 5 to 15 ml milk of magnesia P.O. t.i.d. or q.i.d. or 1 to 2 tablets chewed before swallowing q.i.d., usually after meals and h.s.
• Laxative. **Adults:** 30 to 60 ml milk of magnesia P.O., usually h.s.

Adverse reactions
GI: *abdominal cramping, nausea, diarrhea.* **Metabolic:** fluid and electrolyte disturbances if used daily. **Other:** laxative dependence in long-term or excessive use.

Interactions
None significant.

Nursing diagnoses
• Constipation related to interruption of normal pattern of elimination characterized by infrequent or absent stools.
• Pain related to drug-induced abdominal cramping.
• Knowledge deficit related to magnesium hydroxide therapy.

Nursing interventions
• *Contraindicated* in abdominal pain, nausea, vomiting, or other symptoms of appendicitis or acute surgical abdomen and in myocardial damage, heart block, imminent delivery, fecal impaction, rectal fissures, intestinal obstruction or perforation, or renal disease.
• *Use cautiously* in rectal bleeding.
• Shake suspension well; give with large amount of water when used as laxative. When administering through nasogastric tube, make sure tube is placed properly and is patent. After instilling, flush tube with water to ensure passage to stomach and maintain tube patency.
• For short-term therapy; don't use longer than 1 week.
• When used as laxative, don't give oral drugs 1 to 2 hours before or after administration.
• As a saline laxative, drug produces watery stool in 3 to 6 hours. Time drug administration so that it doesn't interfere with scheduled activities or sleep.
• Before giving for constipation, determine if patient has adequate fluid intake, exercise, and diet. Tell him that dietary sources of bulk include bran and other cereals, fresh fruit, and vegetables.
• Magnesium may accumulate in renal insufficiency.
• Monitor serum electrolytes during prolonged use.
• Frequent or prolonged use as a laxative may cause dependence.

General

Classification: antineoplastic (biological response modifier). **Pregnancy risk category:** C.

Mechanism of action

May exert direct antiproliferative action against tumor cells or viral cells and may modulate host immune response.

Indications and dosage

- Hairy-cell leukemia. **Adults:** 2 million units/m^2 I.M. or S.C. three times a week.
- Condylomata acuminata (genital or veneral warts). **Adults:** 1 million units/lesion intralesionally three times a week for 3 weeks.
- AIDS-related Kaposi's sarcoma. **Adults:** 30 million units/m^2 S.C. or I.M. three times a week.
- Chronic hepatitis B. **Adults:** 5 million units S.C. daily for up to 4 months.

Adverse reactions

Blood: ***leukopenia,*** mild thrombocytopenia. **CNS:** migraine, dizziness, confusion, paresthesia, lethargy, depression, difficulty in thinking or concentrating, insomnia, sedation, anxiety, *fatigue,* hypoesthesia, amnesia, agitation, weakness. **CV:** hypotension, chest pain. **EENT:** visual disturbances, hearing disorders, sty, pharyngitis, nasal congestion, sinusitis, rhinitis. **GI:** *anorexia, nausea,* diarrhea, vomiting, abdominal pain, dyspepsia, constipation, loose stools, eructation, dry mouth, dysgeusia. **GU:** transient impotence, gynecomastia, stomatitis, gingivitis. **Respiratory:** dyspnea, coughing. **Skin:** rash, dryness, pruritus, partial alopecia, urticaria, moniliasis, flushing, dermatitis. **Other:** *flulike symptoms, arthralgia,* asthenia, rigors, leg cramps, arthrosis, bone disorders, back pain, increased sweating, decreased libido, hypertonia, thirst.

Interactions

CNS depressants: enhanced CNS depression.

Nursing diagnoses

- Altered protection related to proliferation of tumor or viral cells.
- Altered nutrition: Less than body requirements, related to interferon-induced anorexia and nausea.
- Knowledge deficit related to interferon therapy.

Nursing interventions

- *Use cautiously* in patients with history of cardiovascular disease, pulmonary disease, diabetes mellitus, coagulation disorders, or severe myelosuppression.
- Neurotoxicity and cardiotoxicity are more common in elderly patients.
- Administer S.C. in patients whose platelet count is below 50,000/mm^3.
- Flulike symptoms at start of therapy tend to diminish with continued therapy. Premedicate with acetaminophen to minimize flulike symptoms.
- Patients should be well hydrated, especially during initial stages of treatment.
- Advise patient that laboratory tests will be performed before and periodically during therapy.
- Teach patient to practice meticulous oral hygiene during treatment.
- When administering interferon for condylomata acuminata, use only 10-million-IU vial since dilution of other strengths required for intralesional use results in a hypertonic solution. Do not reconstitute 10-million-IU vial with more than 1 ml of diluent.
- Monitor for adverse CNS reactions.
- Warn patient not to have any immunization without doctor's approval and to avoid contact with persons who have taken oral polio vaccine.

General

Classification: antiulcer agent, antacid (magnesium/aluminum salt). **Pregnancy risk category:** C.

Mechanism of action

Reduces total acid load in the GI tract and elevates gastric pH to reduce pepsin activity. Also strengthens the gastric mucosal barrier and increases esophageal sphincter tone.

Indications and dosage

- Antacid. **Adults:** 540 to 1,080 mg (5 to 10 ml) suspension P.O. between meals and h.s. with water; or 480 to 960 mg (1 to 2 tablets) P.O. with water between meals and h.s.; 480 to 960 mg (1 to 2 tablets) P.O. chewed before swallowing, between meals and h.s.

Adverse reactions

GI: mild constipation or diarrhea.

Interactions

Allopurinol, antibiotics (including quinolones and tetracyclines), diflunisal, digoxin, iron, isoniazid, penicillamine, phenothiazines, quinidine: decreased pharmacologic effect because absorption may be impaired. Separate administration times.

Nursing diagnoses

- Pain related to gastric hyperacidity.
- Constipation related to adverse reactions to magaldrate.
- Knowledge deficit related to magaldrate therapy.

Nursing interventions

- *Contraindicated* in severe renal disease.
- *Use cautiously* in elderly patients, especially those with decreased GI motility (those receiving antidiarrheals, antispasmodics, or anticholinergics), dehydration, fluid restriction, and mild renal impairment.
- Record amount and consistency of stools.
- Shake suspension well; give with a little water to ensure passage to stomach. When giving through nasogastric tube, be sure tube is placed properly and is patent. After instilling, flush tube with water to ensure passage to stomach and maintain tube patency.
- Monitor serum magnesium in patients with mild renal impairment. Symptomatic hypermagnesemia usually occurs only in severe renal failure.
- Not usually used in renal failure (although it contains aluminum) to help control hypophosphatemia because it contains magnesium, which may accumulate in renal failure.
- Good for patient on restricted sodium intake; very low sodium content.
- Warn patient not to take magaldrate indiscriminately and not to switch antacids without doctor's advice.
- May cause enteric-coated drugs to be released prematurely in stomach. Separate doses by 1 hour.

General
Classification: antiviral (biological response modifier). **Pregnancy risk category:** C.

Mechanism of action
A naturally occurring antiviral agent derived from human leukocytes, interferon alfa-n3 attaches to membrane receptors and causes cellular changes, including increased protein synthesis.

Indications and dosage
- Condylomata acuminata (genital or venereal warts). **Adults:** 0.05 ml per wart by intralesional injection. Treatment usually continues twice weekly for 8 weeks. Dosage should not exceed 0.5 ml (2.5 million units) per session.

Adverse reactions
CNS: dizziness, light-headedness. **GI:** dyspepsia, heartburn, vomiting, nausea. **Other:** *acute hypersensitivity reaction with mild to moderate flulike syndrome (myalgia, fever, headache), arthralgia, back pain, malaise.*

Interactions
None reported.

Nursing diagnoses
- Impaired skin integrity related to lesions induced by condylomata acuminata.
- Pain related to interferon-induced headache, backache, and arthralgia.
- Knowledge deficit related to interferon alfa-n3 therapy.

Nursing interventions
- *Contraindicated* in patients hypersensitive to interferon alfa and in patients with a history of anaphylactic reactions to murine immunoglobulin, egg protein, or neomycin.
- *Use cautiously* in patients with debilitating illnesses (uncontrolled CHF, unstable angina, severe pulmonary disease, coagulation disorders, seizure disorders, severe myelosuppression, or diabetes mellitus with ketoacidosis) because of the association of interferon with a flulike syndrome.
- Although anaphylaxis hasn't been reported, be prepared to treat acute hypersensitivity reactions. Teach patients how to recognize symptoms of hypersensitivity (hives, tightness of the chest, wheezing, shortness of breath). Tell patients to report such symptoms immediately.
- Flulike symptoms may be relieved with acetaminophen.
- Explain to the patient that the warts will continue to disappear after the 8 weeks of therapy are complete and the drug has been discontinued.
- The drug should be injected into each lesion at the base of the wart using a 30G needle.

General

Classification: antidiuretic hormone (posterior pituitary hormone). **Pregnancy risk category:** B.

Mechanism of action

Increases the permeability of the renal tubular epithelium to adenosine monophosphate and water; the epithelium promotes reabsorption of water and produces a concentrated urine (antidiuretic hormone effect).

Indications and dosage

• Nonnephrogenic diabetes insipidus. **Adults and children:** 1 or 2 sprays (approximately 2 USP posterior pituitary pressor units/spray) in either or both nostrils q.i.d. and an additional dose h.s., if needed, to prevent nocturia. If usual dosage is inadequate, increase frequency rather than number of sprays.

Adverse reactions

CNS: headache, dizziness. **EENT:** nasal congestion or ulceration, irritation, pruritus of nasal passages, rhinorrhea, conjunctivitis. **GI:** heartburn due to drip of excess spray into pharynx, abdominal cramps, frequent bowel movements. **GU:** possible transient fluid retention from overdose. **Other:** hypersensitivity reaction.

L

Interactions

None significant.

Nursing diagnoses

• Fluid volume deficit related to increased urine output.
• Impaired tissue integrity related to drug-induced nasal congestion or ulceration.
• Knowledge deficit related to lypressin therapy.

Nursing interventions

• *Contraindicated* in patients with hypersensitivity to the drug.
• *Use cautiously* in patients with coronary artery disease, hypertension, allergic rhinitis, or upper airway infection.
• Patients should understand that the drug is for topical application to the nasal mucosa. It should not be inhaled.
• Instruct patient to clear nasal passage before administering drug.
• Inadvertent inhalation of spray may cause tightness in chest, coughing, and transient dyspnea.
• To administer a uniform, well-diffused spray, hold bottle upright with patient in vertical position holding head upright.
• Particularly useful if diabetes insipidus is unresponsive to other therapy or if antidiuretic hormones of animal origin cause adverse effects.
• Nasal congestion, allergic rhinitis, or upper respiratory infections may diminish drug absorption and require larger dose or adjunctive therapy.
• Test patients sensitive to antidiuretic hormone for sensitivity to lypressin.
• Instruct the patient to carry the medication with him at all times because of its fairly short duration.
• Instruct patient to wear medical alert identification.

General

Classification: antineoplastic (biological response modifier). **Pregnancy risk category:** C.

Mechanism of action

Acts as an interleukin-type lymphokine. It has potent phagocyte-activating properties and enhances the oxidative metabolism of tissue macrophages.

Indications and dosage

• Chronic granulomatous disease. **Adults with a body surface area greater than 0.5 m²:** 50 mcg/m² (1.5 million units/m²) I.M. three times weekly, preferably h.s. The preferred injection site is the deltoid muscle or anterior thigh. **Adults with a body surface area less than 0.5 m²:** 1.5 mcg/kg/dose three times weekly.

Adverse reactions

Blood: ***myelosuppression*** (at high doses). **CNS:** *headache,* fatigue, decreased mental status, gait disturbance. **GI:** nausea, vomiting, diarrhea. **Metabolic:** *elevated hepatic enzymes (at high doses).* **Skin:** rash. **Local:** erythema or tenderness at the injection site. **Other:** fever, myalgia, arthralgia, *chills (flulike syndrome).*

Interactions

Myelosuppressive agents: possible increased myelosuppression. Use together with caution. **Zidovudine:** increased plasma levels of zidovudine. Dosage adjustments are necessary.

Nursing diagnoses

• Hyperthermia associated with interferon gamma-1b-induced fever.
• Pain associated with interferon gamma-1b-induced flulike symptoms.
• Knowledge deficit related to interferon gamma-1b therapy.

Nursing interventions

• *Contraindicated* in patients hypersensitive to the drug or to genetically engineered products derived from *Escherichia coli.*
• *Use cautiously* in patients with cardiac disease, including arrhythmias, ischemia, or CHF. The flulike syndrome commonly seen at high doses of the drug can exacerbate these conditions. Also use cautiously in patients with compromised CNS function or seizure disorders. CNS adverse reactions that may occur at high doses of the drug can exacerbate these conditions.
• Ensure that patient who will self-administer the drug has a copy of the patient information leaflet, which will aid the safe and effective use of the medication. Be sure patient understands the correct methods of drug administration and of disposal of medical waste.
• Note that discomfort from the flulike syndrome commonly associated with this drug may be minimized by taking the drug at bedtime. Acetaminophen may be useful in treating these symptoms.
• Refrigerate drug immediately. Vials must be stored in a refrigerator (36° to 46° F [2° to 8° C]); do not freeze. Do not shake the vial; avoid excessive agitation. Discard vials that have been left at room temperature for a total period of more than 12 hours.
• Each vial is for single dose only. Because the drug does not contain a preservative, discard the unused contents.

General

Classification: antipsychotic (dibenzoxazepine).
Pregnancy risk category: C.

Mechanism of action

Blocks postsynaptic dopamine receptors in the brain.

Indications and dosage

• Psychotic disorders. **Adults:** 10 mg P.O. or I.M. (hydrochloride) b.i.d. to q.i.d., rapidly increasing to 60 to 100 mg P.O. daily for most patients; dosage varies from patient to patient.

Adverse reactions

Blood: transient leukopenia. **CNS:** *extrapyramidal reactions (moderate incidence), sedation (moderate incidence), tardive dyskinesia,* pseudoparkinsonism, EEG changes, dizziness. **CV:** *orthostatic hypotension,* tachycardia, ECG changes. **EENT:** *blurred vision.* **GI:** *dry mouth, constipation.* **GU:** *urine retention,* dark urine, menstrual irregularities, gynecomastia. **Skin:** *mild photosensitivity,* dermal allergic reactions. **Other:** weight gain; increased appetite; rarely, ***neuroleptic malignant syndrome*** (fever, tachycardia, tachypnea, profuse diaphoresis).

Interactions

Alcohol, other CNS depressants: increased CNS depression. Avoid concomitant use.

Nursing diagnoses

• Impaired thought processes related to the patient's underlying condition.
• Urinary retention related to adverse reactions.
• Knowledge deficit related to loxapine therapy.

Nursing interventions

• *Contraindicated* in coma, severe CNS depression, or drug-induced depressed states.
• *Use cautiously* in seizure disorder, CV disorders, glaucoma, urine retention, suspected intestinal obstruction or brain tumor, and renal damage.
• Tardive dyskinesia may occur after prolonged use. It may not appear until months or years later and may disappear spontaneously or persist for life despite discontinuation of drug.
• Neuroleptic malignant syndrome is rare, but frequently fatal. It is not necessarily related to length of drug use or type of neuroleptic, but over 60% of affected patients are men. Watch for symptoms.
• Acute dystonic reactions may be treated with I.V. diphenhydramine.
• Warn against activities that require alertness and good psychomotor coordination until CNS effects of the drug are known. Drowsiness and dizziness usually subside after first few weeks.
• Obtain baseline measures of blood pressure before starting therapy and monitor regularly. Advise patient to get up slowly to avoid orthostatic hypotension.
• Dilute liquid concentrate with orange or grapefruit juice just before giving.
• Dry mouth may be relieved by sugarless gum, sour hard candy, or rinsing with mouthwash.
• Periodic eye examinations are recommended.
• Tricyclic dibenzoxazepine; the only dibenzoxazepine derivative.
• Dose of 10 mg is therapeutic equivalent of 100 mg chlorpromazine.

General
Classification: amebicide (iodine derivative).
Pregnancy risk category: C.

Mechanism of action
Precise mechanism of action is unknown.

Indications and dosage
• Intestinal amebiasis. **Adults:** 630 to 650 mg P.O. t.i.d. after meals for 20 days. Total daily dosage should not exceed 2 g. **Children:** usual dosage 30 to 40 mg/kg of body weight daily in two to three divided doses for 20 days.

Additional courses of iodoquinol therapy should not be repeated before a resting interval of 2 to 3 weeks.

Adverse reactions
Blood: ***agranulocytosis.*** **CNS:** neurotoxicity (dose-related), dysesthesia, weakness, vertigo, malaise, headache, agitation, retrograde amnesia, ataxia, *peripheral neuropathy.* **EENT:** *optic neuritis,* optic atrophy, loss of vision. **GI:** anorexia, nausea, vomiting, abdominal cramps, diarrhea, increased motility, constipation, epigastric burning and pain, gastritis, anal irritation and itching. **Skin:** pruritus, papular and pustular eruptions, urticaria, discoloration of hair and nails. **Other:** thyroid enlargement, fever, chills, generalized furunculosis, alopecia.

Interactions
None significant.

Nursing diagnoses
• High risk for injury related to ineffectiveness of iodoquinol to alleviate infection.
• Altered nutrition: Less than body requirements, related to anorexia, nausea, and vomiting.
• Knowledge deficit related to iodoquinol therapy.

Nursing interventions
• *Contraindicated* in patients with hypersensitivity to 8-hydroxyquinoline derivatives or iodine-containing preparations. Iodoquinol causes hepatic damage in such patients. Also contraindicated in hepatic or renal disease or preexisting optic neuropathy.
• Patient should have periodic ophthalmologic examinations during treatment.
• Give after meals. Crush tablets and mix with applesauce or chocolate syrup.
• Record intake and output and color and amount of stools. Send warm specimens to laboratory for analysis.
• Watch for diarrhea during the first 2 or 3 days of treatment. Notify doctor if it continues past 3 days.
• Advise patient not to discontinue the medication prematurely. Tell him to notify doctor if rash occurs.
• May interfere with thyroid function tests for up to 6 months after discontinuation of drug.
• To help prevent reinfestation, teach patient about the need for good personal hygiene, especially hand-washing technique. Patient should refrain from preparing food until stools are negative.

General

Classification: cholesterol-lowering agent (lactone). **Pregnancy risk category:** X.

Mechanism of action

Lovastatin inhibits 3-hydroxy-3-methylglutaryl-coenzyme A (HMG-CoA) reductase. This enzyme is an early (and rate-limiting) step in the synthetic pathway of cholesterol.

Indications and dosage

• Reduction of low-density lipoprotein (LDL) and total cholesterol levels in patients with primary hypercholesterolemia (types IIa and IIb). **Adults:** initially, 20 mg P.O. once daily with the evening meal. For patients with severely elevated cholesterol levels (for example, over 300 mg/dl), the initial dose should be 40 mg. The recommended range is 20 to 80 mg in single or divided doses.

Adverse reactions

CNS: headache, dizziness. **EENT:** blurred vision, dysgeusia. **GI:** constipation, diarrhea, dyspepsia, flatus, abdominal pain or cramps, heartburn, nausea. **Metabolic:** elevated serum transaminase levels, abnormal liver test results. **Skin:** rash, pruritus. **Other:** peripheral neuropathy, muscle cramps, myalgia, myositis, ***rhabdomyolysis***.

Interactions

Cholestyramine, clofibrate: enhanced lipid-reducing effects. **Immunosuppressive agents, gemfibrozil:** possible increased risk of polymyositis and rhabdomyolysis. Maximum recommended lovastatin dosage is 20 mg daily; monitor patient closely.

Nursing diagnoses

• High risk for injury related to ineffectiveness of lovastatin to lower LDL and total cholesterol levels.
• Sensory/perceptual alterations (visual) related to adverse drug reaction.
• Knowledge deficit related to lovastatin therapy.

Nursing interventions

• *Contraindicated* in patients with hypersensitivity to the drug, active liver disease, or conditions associated with unexplained persistent elevations of serum transaminase; in pregnant and breast-feeding women; and in women of childbearing age unless there is no risk of pregnancy.
• Initiate lovastatin only after diet and other nonpharmacologic therapies have proven ineffective. Patient should be on a standard low-cholesterol diet during therapy.
• Give lovastatin with the evening meal; absorption is enhanced and cholesterol biosynthesis is greater in the evening.
• Therapeutic response occurs in about 2 weeks, with maximum effects in 4 to 6 weeks. Effects of long-term use are unknown.
• Watch for signs of myositis.
• Liver function tests should be performed frequently at start of therapy and periodically thereafter.
• Store tablets at room temperature in a light-resistant container.
• Tell patient to restrict alcohol intake.
• Tell patient to advise doctor of any adverse reactions, particularly muscle aches and pains.
• Advise patient to have periodic eye examinations.
• Teach patient about proper dietary management, weight control, and exercise. Explain their importance in controlling elevated serum lipids.

General
Classification: emetic (alkaloid). **Pregnancy risk category:** C.

Mechanism of action
Induces vomiting by acting locally on the gastric mucosa and centrally on the chemoreceptor trigger zone.

Indications and dosage
- To induce vomiting in poisoning. **Adults and children over 12 years:** 30 ml P.O., followed by 200 to 300 ml of water. **Children 1 year or older:** 15 ml P.O., followed by about 200 ml of water or milk. **Children under 1 year:** 5 to 10 ml P.O., followed by 100 to 200 ml of water or milk. May repeat dose once after 20 minutes, if necessary.

Adverse reactions
CNS: depression. **CV:** ***arrhythmias, bradycardia, hypotension, atrial fibrillation, or fatal myocarditis after ingestion of excessive dose.*** **GI:** diarrhea.

Interactions
Activated charcoal: neutralized emetic effect. Don't give together but may give activated charcoal after vomiting has occurred.

Nursing diagnoses
- High risk for injury related to ingestion of poisonous substance.
- Decreased cardiac output related to ipecac syrup-induced cardiac arrhythmias.
- Knowledge deficit related to the use of ipecac syrup.

Nursing interventions
- *Contraindicated* in semicomatose or unconscious patients, or those with severe inebriation, seizures, shock, or loss of gag reflex. Don't give after ingestion of petroleum distillates (for example, kerosene or gasoline) or volatile oils; retching and vomiting may cause aspiration and lead to bronchospasm, pulmonary edema, or aspiration pneumonitis. Vegetable oil will delay absorption of these substances. Don't give after ingestion of caustic substances such as lye; additional injury to the esophagus and mediastinum can occur.
- Clearly indicate "ipecac syrup," not single word "ipecac," to avoid confusion with fluidextract. Fluidextract is 14 times more concentrated and, if inadvertently used instead of syrup, may cause death. This is unlikely in the United States because fluidextract is no longer commercially available.
- Induces vomiting within 30 minutes in more than 90% of patients; average time usually less than 20 minutes.
- Stomach is usually emptied completely; vomitus may contain some intestinal material as well.
- In antiemetic toxicity, ipecac syrup is usually effective if less than 1 hour has passed since ingestion of antiemetic.
- Recommend that 1 oz (30 ml) of syrup be readily available in the home when child becomes 1 year old for immediate use in case of emergency.
- No systemic toxicity with doses of 30 ml or less.
- If two doses do not induce vomiting, gastric lavage is necessary.
- Be aware that ipecac syrup is commonly abused by bulimics who practice binging and purging.

General
Classification: anxiolytic (benzodiazepine). **Pregnancy risk category:** D. **Controlled substance schedule:** IV.

Mechanism of action
Depresses the CNS at the limbic and subcortical levels of the brain.

Indications and dosage
- Anxiety, tension, agitation, irritability, especially in anxiety neuroses or organic (especially GI or CV) disorders. **Adults:** 2 to 6 mg P.O. daily in divided doses. Maximum dosage is 10 mg daily.
- Insomnia. **Adults:** 2 to 4 mg P.O. h.s.
- Premedication before operative procedure. **Adults:** 0.05 mg/kg I.M. or slow I.V. injection (< 2 mg/minute). Total dose should not exceed 4 mg.

Adverse reactions
CNS: *drowsiness, lethargy, hangover,* fainting. **CV:** transient hypotension. **GI:** dry mouth, abdominal discomfort.

Interactions
Alcohol, other CNS depressants: increased CNS depression. Avoid comcomitant use. **Cigarette smoking:** increased clearance of benzodiazepines. Monitor for lack of effect. **Digoxin:** benzodiazepines may increase serum levels of digoxin, increasing risk of toxicity. Monitor closely.

Nursing diagnoses
- Anxiety related to the patient's underlying condition.
- High risk for injury related to drug-induced CNS reactions.
- Knowledge deficit related to lorazepam therapy.

Nursing interventions
- *Contraindicated* in acute narrow-angle glaucoma, psychoses, or mental depression.
- *Use cautiously* in organic brain syndrome, myasthenia gravis, and pulmonary, renal, or hepatic impairment.
- Dosage should be reduced in elderly or debilitated patients. Preoperative I.V. dose should not exceed 2 mg in patients over 50.
- Possibility of abuse and addiction exists. Do not withdraw drug abruptly after long-term use; withdrawal symptoms may occur.
- When administering I.M., inject deep into muscle mass. Don't dilute.
- **I.V. use:** Give I.V. slowly, at rate not exceeding 2 mg/minute. Dilute with an equal volume of sterile water for injection, 0.9% sodium chloride injection, or dextrose 5% injection.
- Monitor respirations every 5 to 15 minutes and before each repeated I.V. dose. Have emergency resuscitation equipment and oxygen at bedside.
- If lorazepam overdose occurs, flumazenil (a specific benzodiazepine antagonist) may be useful. Know that the duration of action of lorazepam is longer than that of flumazenil, and resedation is possible.
- Store parenteral form in refrigerator to prolong shelf-life.
- Used as a premedication before surgery, lorazepam provides substantial preoperative amnesia. Therefore, patient teaching requires extra care to ensure adequate recall. Provide written materials or inform a family member if possible.
- Warn patient to avoid hazardous activities that require alertness or good psychomotor coordination until CNS effects of the drug are known.
- Warn patient not to combine drug with alcohol or other depressants.
- Caution patient against giving medication to others.
- Drug should not be prescribed regularly for everyday stress.
- Fewer cumulative effects than other benzodiazepines because of short half-life.
- Periodic hepatic, renal, and hematopoietic function studies should be performed in patients receiving repeated or prolonged therapy.

ipratropium bromide

Atrovent

General

Classification: bronchodilator (anticholinergic).
Pregnancy risk category: B.

Mechanism of action

Inhibits vagally mediated reflexes by antagonizing acetylcholine.

Indications and dosage

- Maintenance treatment of bronchospasm associated with chronic obstructive pulmonary disease. **Adults:** 2 inhalations (26 mcg) q.i.d. Additional inhalations may be needed, but total inhalations should not exceed 12 in 24 hours.

Adverse reactions

CNS: nervousness, dizziness, headache. **CV:** palpitations. **EENT:** cough, blurred vision. **GI:** nausea, GI distress, dry mouth. **Skin:** rash.

Interactions

Anticholinergics: increased anticholinergic effects. Avoid concomitant use. **Cromolyn sodium:** will form a precipitate if mixed in the same nebulizer. Don't use together.

Nursing diagnoses

- Ineffective airway clearance related to patient's underlying condition.
- Sensory/perceptual alterations (visual) related to adverse reactions to ipratropium.
- Knowledge deficit related to ipratropium therapy.

Nursing interventions

- *Contraindicated* in patients with hypersensitivity to the drug.
- *Use cautiously* in patients with narrow-angle glaucoma, prostatic hypertrophy, and bladder-neck obstruction.
- Warn patient that this drug is not effective in the treatment of acute episodes of bronchospasm where rapid response is required.
- Teach patient to perform oral inhalation correctly. Give the following instructions for using a metered-dose inhaler:
  - Clear nasal passages and throat.
  - Breathe out, expelling as much air from lungs as possible.
  - Place mouthpiece well into mouth as dose from inhaler is released, and inhale deeply.
  - Hold breath for several seconds, remove mouthpiece, and exhale slowly.
- If more than one inhalation is ordered, the patient should wait at least 2 minutes before repeating the procedure for a second dose.
- Tell patient who is also using a steroid inhaler to use ipratropium first, then wait about 5 minutes before using the steroid. This allows the bronchodilator to open air passages for maximum effectiveness.
- Tell patient to avoid accidentally spraying into eyes. Temporary blurring of vision may result.
- Ipratropium is the first anticholinergic bronchodilator available as an aerosol. Works by a different mechanism from either the adrenergics or theophylline compounds.
- Patient may experience a dry mouth or throat. Suggest using sugarless hard candy or gum, or use a saliva substitute.
- Tell patient to take a missed dose as soon as possible. If it's almost time for the next dose, he should skip the missed dose. Tell him not to double-dose.

General

Classification: antiallergy agent (antihistamine).
Pregnancy risk category: B.

Mechanism of action

Blocks the effects of histamine at H_1 receptors. Loratadine is a nonsedating antihistamine; its chemical structure prevents entry into the CNS.

Indications and dosage

- Symptomatic treatment of seasonal allergic rhinitis. **Adults and children 12 years and over:** 10 mg P.O. daily. Patients with hepatic failure should start therapy with 10 mg every other day.

Adverse reactions

CNS: headache, somnolence, fatigue. **GI:** dry mouth.

Interactions

None reported.

Nursing diagnoses

- Ineffective airway clearance related to the patient's underlying condition.
- Knowledge deficit related to loratadine therapy.

Nursing interventions

- *Contraindicated* in patients with hypersensitivity to the drug.
- *Use cautiously* and in lower dosages in patients with liver failure to prevent accumulation of drug and its active metabolites. Also use cautiously with drugs that are known to impair hepatic drug metabolism. Studies to rule out drug interactions have not been performed.
- Because trace amounts of drug are found in human breast milk, use cautiously in breast-feeding women.
- Although administration with food has been observed to cause only small changes in drug absorption, the manufacturer recommends that loratadine be taken on an empty stomach. Instruct patient to take drug at least 2 hours after a meal and to avoid eating for at least 1 hour after dosing.
- Be sure patient understands that drug should be taken only once daily. If symptoms persist or worsen, he should contact the doctor.
- Warn patient to stop taking drug 4 days before allergy skin tests to preserve accuracy of tests.

General

Classification: hematinic (parenteral iron supplement). **Pregnancy risk category:** C.

Mechanism of action

Provides elemental iron, an essential component in the formation of hemoglobin; 1 ml iron dextran provides 50 mg elemental iron.

Indications and dosage

• Iron deficiency anemia. **Adults:** I.M. or I.V. injections of iron are advisable only for patients for whom oral administration is impossible or ineffective. Test dose (0.5 ml) required before administration.

–I.M. (by Z-track): inject 0.5 ml test dose. If no reaction, next daily dose should ordinarily not exceed 0.5 ml (25 mg) for infants under 5 kg; 1 ml (50 mg) for children under 9 kg; 2 ml (100 mg) for patients under 50 kg; or 5 ml (250 mg) for patients over 50 kg.

–I.V. push: inject 0.5 ml test dose. If no reaction, within 2 to 3 days the dosage may be raised to 2 ml daily I.V., 1 ml/minute undiluted and infused slowly until total dose is achieved. No single dose should exceed 100 mg.

–I.V. infusion: dosages are expressed in terms of elemental iron. Dilute in 250 to 1,000 ml of 0.9% sodium chloride solution; dextrose increases local vein irritation. Infuse test dose of 25 mg slowly over 5 minutes. If no reaction occurs in 5 minutes, infusion may be started. Infuse total dose slowly over approximately 6 to 12 hours.

Adverse reactions

CNS: headache, transitory paresthesia, arthralgia, myalgia, dizziness, malaise, syncope. **CV:** *hypotensive reaction, peripheral vascular flushing with overly rapid I.V. administration, tachycardia.* **GI:** nausea, vomiting, metallic taste, transient loss of taste perception. **Skin:** rash, urticaria. **Local:** *soreness and inflammation at injection site (I.M.), brown skin discoloration at injection site (I.M.), local phlebitis at injection site (I.V.),* sterile abscess, necrosis, atrophy, fibrosis. **Other:** ***anaphylaxis, bronchospasm,*** delayed sensitivity reactions.

Interactions

None significant.

Nursing diagnoses

• Activity intolerance related to iron deficency.
• Altered tissue perfusion (renal, cerebral, cardiopulmonary, GI, peripheral) related to iron dextran therapy.
• Knowledge deficit related to iron dextran therapy.

Nursing interventions

• *Contraindicated* in all anemias except iron deficiency anemia.
• *Use with extreme caution* in patients with impaired hepatic function or rheumatoid arthritis and in infants.
• Monitor vital signs for drug reaction.
• Inject deeply into upper outer quadrant of buttock – never into arm or other exposed area – with a 2″ to 3″, 19G or 20G needle. Use Z-track technique to avoid leakage into subcutaneous tissue and staining of skin.
• Skin staining may be minimized by using a separate needle to withdraw the drug from its container.
• Monitor hemoglobin concentration, hematocrit, and reticulocyte count.
• **I.V. use:** Check hospital policy before administering I.V. Some hospitals do not permit infusion method because its safety is controversial.
• After I.V. iron dextran infusion, flush vein with 10 ml of 0.9% sodium chloride solution.
• Drug not removed by hemodialysis.

General

Classification: antibiotic (synthetic beta-lactam antibiotic of the carbacephem class). **Pregnancy risk category:** B.

Mechanism of action

Inhibits cell wall synthesis, promoting osmotic instability. Similar to second-generation cephalosporins. Usually bactericidal.

Indications and dosage

- Secondary bacterial infections of acute bronchitis. **Adults:** 200 to 400 mg P.O. q 12 hours for 7 days.
- Acute bacterial exacerbations of chronic bronchitis. **Adults:** 400 mg P.O. q 12 hours for 7 days.
- Pneumonia. **Adults:** 400 mg P.O. q 12 hours for 14 days.
- Pharyngitis, tonsillitis, sinusitis. **Adults:** 200 to 400 mg P.O. q 12 hours for 10 days. **Children:** 15 mg/kg P.O. daily in divided doses q 12 hours for 10 days.
- Acute otitis media. **Children:** 30 mg/kg (oral suspension) P.O. daily in divided doses q 12 hours for 10 days.
- Uncomplicated skin and skin structure infections. **Adults:** 200 mg P.O. q 12 hours for 7 days.
- Impetigo. **Children:** 15 mg/kg P.O. daily in divided doses q 12 hours for 7 days.
- Uncomplicated cystitis. **Adults:** 200 mg P.O. daily for 7 days.
- Uncomplicated pyelonephritis. **Adults:** 400 mg P.O. q 12 hours for 7 days.

Adverse reactions

Blood: transient thrombocytopenia, leukopenia, eosinophilia. **CNS:** headache, somnolence, nervousness, insomnia, dizziness. **CV:** vasodilation. **GI:** diarrhea, nausea, vomiting, abdominal pain, anorexia, pseudomembranous colitis. **GU:** vaginal candidiasis or moniliasis, transient increases in BUN and creatinine levels. **Hepatic:** transient elevations in AST, ALT, and alkaline phosphatase levels. **Skin:** rash, urticaria, pruritus, ***erythema multiforme.*** **Other:** hypersensitivity reactions, including ***anaphylaxis.***

Interactions

Probenecid: decreases excretion of loracarbef, causing increased plasma levels. Monitor for toxicity.

Nursing diagnoses

- High risk for injury related to ineffectiveness of loracarbef to eradicate the infection.
- High risk for fluid volume deficit related to adverse GI reactions to loracarbef.
- Knowledge deficit related to loracarbef therapy.

Nursing interventions

- *Contraindicated* in patients with hypersensitivity to cephalosporins and in patients with diarrhea caused by pseudomembranous colitis.
- *Use cautiously* in pregnant or breast-feeding women. Also use cautiously and with dosage adjustments in patients with renal failure. Safety and efficacy not established in infants under 6 months.
- Tell patient to take drug on an empty stomach, at least 1 hour before or 2 hours after eating.
- Beta-lactam antibiotics may trigger seizures in susceptible patients, especially when given without dosage modification to those with renal impairment. If seizures occur, discontinue drug and notify doctor. Administer anticonvulsants as ordered.
- For otitis media, the more rapidly absorbed oral suspension produces higher peak plasma levels than the capsules.
- Oral suspension is stable for 14 days at room temperature (59° to 86° F [15° to 30° C]). Tell patient to discard unused portion after 14 days.

General

Classification: antidepressant (MAO inhibitor).
Pregnancy risk category: C.

Mechanism of action

Promotes accumulation of neurotransmitters by inhibiting MAO.

Indications and dosage

- Depression. **Adults:** 30 mg P.O. daily in divided doses. Reduce to 10 to 20 mg daily when condition improves. Not recommended for children under 16 years.

Adverse reactions

CNS: *dizziness,* vertigo, weakness, headache, overactivity, hyperreflexia, tremors, muscle twitching, mania, *insomnia,* confusion, memory impairment, fatigue. **CV:** *orthostatic hypotension,* ***arrhythmias,*** paradoxical hypertension. **EENT:** blurred vision. **GI:** dry mouth, *anorexia,* nausea, diarrhea, constipation. **Skin:** rash. **Other:** peripheral edema, sweating, weight changes, altered libido.

Interactions

Alcohol, barbiturates, and other sedatives; narcotics; dextromethorphan; TCAs: unpredictable interaction. Use with caution and in reduced dosage. **Amphetamines, antihistamines, ephedrine, levodopa, meperidine, metaraminol, methotrimeprazine, methylphenidate, phenylephrine, phenylpropanolamine, sympathomimetics:** pressor effects of these drugs are enhanced by isocarboxazid. Avoid concomitant use. **Insulin, oral antidiabetic agents:** isocarboxazid may alter requirements for antidiabetic medications.

Nursing diagnoses

- Ineffective individual coping related to the patient's underlying condition.
- High risk for injury related to isocarboxazid-induced adverse reactions.
- Knowledge deficit related to isocarboxazid therapy.

Nursing interventions

- *Contraindicated* in elderly or debilitated patients; severe hepatic or renal impairment; CHF; pheochromocytoma; hypertensive, cardiovascular, or cerebrovascular disease; severe or frequent headaches; with foods containing tryptophan or tyramine; during therapy with other MAO inhibitors or within 10 days of such therapy; and within 10 days of elective eye surgery requiring general anesthetic, cocaine, or local anesthetic containing sympathomimetic vasoconstrictors.
- *Use cautiously* with other psychotropic drugs or with spinal anesthetic; in hyperactive, agitated, or schizophrenic patients; in patients at risk for suicide; and in patients with Parkinson's disease, diabetes, or seizure disorders.
- Avoid combining with alcohol or other depressants.
- Because MAO inhibitors may alleviate chest pain in patients with angina, warn such patients to moderate activities and avoid overexertion.
- If patient develops symptoms of overdosage, hold dose and notify doctor.
- Monitor closely for suicidal tendencies.
- Do not withdraw drug abruptly.
- Weigh patient biweekly. Teach patient how to check for edema and urine retention.
- Warn patient to avoid foods high in tyramine or tryptophan and large amounts of caffeine.
- Warn patient not to take any other medications without first checking with the doctor.
- Have phentolamine (Regitine) available to counteract severe hypertension.
- Continue precautions for 10 days after discontinuation of the drug.
- Obtain baseline blood pressure readings, heart rate, CBC, and liver function tests before therapy, and continue to monitor during treatment.

loperamide hydrochloride

Imodium, Imodium A-D ◊

General

Classification: antidiarrheal (piperidine derivative). **Pregnancy risk category:** B.

Mechanism of action

Inhibits peristaltic activity, prolonging transit of intestinal contents.

Indications and dosage

- Acute, nonspecific diarrhea. **Adults:** initially, 4 mg P.O., then 2 mg after each unformed stool. Maximum 16 mg daily. **Children 8 to 12 years:** 10 ml t.i.d. P.O. on first day. (Subsequent doses of 5 ml/10 kg of body weight may be administered after each unformed stool.) **Children 5 to 8 years:** 10 ml P.O. b.i.d. on first day. **Children 2 to 5 years:** 5 ml P.O. t.i.d. on first day.
- Chronic diarrhea. **Adults:** initially, 4 mg P.O., then 2 mg after each unformed stool until diarrhea subsides. Adjust dosage to individual response.

Adverse reactions

CNS: drowsiness, fatigue, dizziness. **GI:** dry mouth; abdominal pain, distention, or discomfort; *constipation;* nausea; vomiting. **Skin:** rash.

Interactions

None significant.

Nursing diagnoses

- Diarrhea related to interruption of normal pattern of elimination characterized by frequent loose stools.
- Colonic constipation related to excessive use of loperamide.
- Knowledge deficit related to loperamide therapy.

Nursing interventions

- *Contraindicated* in acute diarrhea resulting from poison until toxic material is removed from GI tract, in acute diarrhea caused by organisms that penetrate intestinal mucosa, and when constipation must be avoided.
- *Use cautiously* in severe prostatic hypertrophy, hepatic disease, and history of narcotic dependence.
- Stop drug immediately if abdominal distention or other symptoms develop in acute colitis.
- In acute diarrhea, discontinue drug and seek medical attention if no improvement occurs within 48 hours; in chronic diarrhea, discontinue drug if no improvement occurs after giving 16 mg daily for at least 10 days.
- Warn patient not to exceed recommended dosage.
- Produces antidiarrheal action similar to diphenoxylate hydrochloride but without as many adverse CNS effects.

General

Classification: bronchodilator (adrenergic). **Pregnancy risk category:** C.

Mechanism of action

Relaxes bronchial smooth muscle by acting on beta$_2$-adrenergic receptors.

Indications and dosage

• Bronchial asthma and reversible bronchospasm that may occur with bronchitis and emphysema. **Adults:** 3 to 7 undiluted inhalations by hand nebulizer; or 0.5 ml diluted 1:3 with 0.9% sodium chloride solution by oxygen aerosolization; or 0.5 ml diluted 1:3 with 0.9% sodium chloride solution by IPPB (hydrochloride). Or 1 to 2 inhalations (mesylate). Occasionally, more may be required.

Adverse reactions

CNS: *tremor, headache,* dizziness, excitement. **CV:** *palpitations,* increased heart rate. **GI:** nausea, vomiting.

Interactions

Propranolol and other beta blockers: blocked bronchodilating effect of isoetharine. Monitor patient carefully if used together. **Digitalis glycosides, levodopa, halogenated inhalational anesthetics, cyclopropane:** increased risk of cardiac arrhythmias. Monitor closely.

Nursing diagnoses

• Ineffective airway clearance related to patient's underlying respiratory condition.
• Pain related to isoetharine-induced headache.
• Knowledge deficit related to isoetharine therapy.

Nursing interventions

• *Contraindicated* in patients with tachyarrhythmias, tachycardia caused by digitalis toxicity, narrow-angle glaucoma, or shock; and in those receiving general anesthesia with cyclopropane or halogenated inhalational anesthetics.
• *Use cautiously* in hyperthyroidism, hypertension, or coronary disease and in patients with sensitivity to sympathomimetics.
• Also use cautiously in patients receiving general anesthetics that sensitize the myocardium to sympathomimetic drugs.
• Excessive use can lead to decreased effectiveness.
• Monitor for severe paradoxical bronchoconstriction after excessive use. Discontinue immediately if bronchoconstriction occurs.
• Teach patient to perform oral inhalation correctly. Give the following instructions for using a metered-dose inhaler:
 – Clear nasal passages and throat.
 – Breathe out, expelling as much air as possible.
 – Place mouthpiece well into mouth as dose from inhaler is released, and inhale deeply.
 – Hold breath for several seconds, remove mouthpiece, and exhale slowly.
• If more than one inhalation is ordered, the patient should wait at least 2 minutes before repeating the procedure for a second dose.
• Tell patient who is also using a steroid inhaler to use isoetharine first, then wait about 5 minutes before using the steroid. This allows the bronchodilator to open air passages for maximum effectiveness.
• Because drug oxidizes when diluted with water, pink sputum mimicking hemoptysis may occur after inhaling isoetharine solution. Tell patient not to be concerned.

General

Classification: antineoplastic (alkylating agent, nitrosourea). **Pregnancy risk category:** D.

Mechanism of action

Cross-links strands of cellular DNA and interferes with RNA transcription, causing an imbalance of growth that leads to cell death. Cell cycle-non-specific.

Indications and dosage

• Brain tumors, Hodgkin's disease. **Adults and children:** 130 mg/m^2 P.O. as single dose q 6 weeks. Reduce dosage according to degree of bone marrow suppression. Repeat doses should not be given until WBC count above 4,000/mm^3 and platelet count is above 100,000/mm^3.

Adverse reactions

Blood: ***anemia, leukopenia,*** *delayed up to 6 weeks, lasting 1 to 2 weeks;* ***thrombocytopenia,*** *delayed up to 4 weeks, lasting 1 to 2 weeks.* **GI:** *nausea and vomiting beginning within 4 to 5 hours, lasting 24 hours;* stomatitis. **GU:** nephrotoxicity, progressive azotemia.

Interactions

None significant.

Nursing diagnoses

• High risk for infection related to adverse reactions to lomustine.
• Altered nutrition: Less than body requirements, related to prolonged episodes of nausea and vomiting.
• Knowledge deficit related to lomustine therapy.

Nursing interventions

• *Contraindicated* in patients with hypersensitivity to the drug.
• *Use cautiously.* Dosage modification may be required in patients with decreased platelets, leukocytes, or erythrocytes and in patients receiving other myelosuppressive drugs.
• Give 2 to 4 hours after meals. Lomustine will be more completely absorbed if taken when the stomach is empty. To avoid nausea, give antiemetic before administering.
• May be useful in cancer involving CNS, since CSF level equals 30% to 50% of plasma level 1 hour after administration.
• Monitor CBC weekly. Usually not administered more often than every 6 weeks; bone marrow toxicity is cumulative and delayed.
• Warn patient to watch for signs of infection (fever, sore throat, fatigue) and bleeding (easy bruising, nosebleeds, bleeding gums, melena). Take temperature daily.
• Periodically monitor liver function.
• Avoid all I.M. injections when platelets are below 100,000/mm^3.
• Anticoagulants and aspirin products should be used cautiously. Watch closely for signs of bleeding. Instruct patient to avoid OTC products containing aspirin.
• Therapeutic effects are often accompanied by toxicity.

isoniazid (INH)

DOW-Isoniazid, Isotamine†, Laniazid-C.T., Nydrazid**, PMS-Isoniazid†

General

Classification: antitubercular (isonicotinic acid hydrazine). **Pregnancy risk category:** C.

Mechanism of action

Inhibits cell wall biosynthesis by interfering with lipid and DNA synthesis (bactericidal).

Indications and dosage

• Primary treatment against actively growing tubercle bacilli. **Adults:** 5 mg/kg P.O. or I.M. daily in single dose, up to 300 mg/day, continued for 6 months to 2 years. **Infants and children:** 10 to 20 mg/kg P.O. or I.M. daily in single dose, up to 300 to 500 mg/day, continued for 18 months to 2 years. Concomitant administration of at least one other effective antitubercular drug is recommended.

• Preventive therapy against tubercle bacilli in those closely exposed or those with positive skin test whose chest X-rays and bacteriologic studies are consistent with nonprogressive tuberculous disease. **Adults:** 300 mg P.O. daily in single dose, continued for 1 year. **Infants and children:** 10 mg/kg P.O. daily in single dose, up to 300 mg/day, continued for 1 year.

Adverse reactions

Blood: ***agranulocytosis, hemolytic anemia, aplastic anemia,*** eosinophilia, leukopenia, neutropenia, thrombocytopenia, methemoglobinemia, pyridoxine-responsive hypochromic anemia. **CNS:** *peripheral neuropathy,* usually preceded by paresthesia of hands and feet; psychosis. **GI:** nausea, vomiting, epigastric distress, constipation, dry mouth. **Hepatic:** ***hepatitis (may be severe or fatal).*** **Metabolic:** hyperglycemia, metabolic acidosis. **Local:** irritation at I.M. injection site. **Other:** rheumatic syndrome and lupus-like syndrome; hypersensitivity.

Interactions

Aluminum-containing antacids and laxatives: may decrease the rate and amount of isoniazid absorbed. Give isoniazid at least 1 hour before antacid or laxative. **Carbamazepine:** increased risk of isoniazid hepatotoxicity. Use together very cautiously. **Corticosteroids:** may decrease therapeutic effectiveness. Monitor need for larger isoniazid dose. **Disulfiram:** neurologic symptoms may develop; avoid concomitant use.

Nursing diagnoses

• High risk for injury related to ineffectiveness of isoniazid in eradicating the infection.

• Sensory/perceptual alterations (tactile) related to isoniazid-induced peripheral neuropathy.

• Knowledge deficit related to isoniazid therapy.

Nursing interventions

• *Contraindicated* in acute hepatic disease or isoniazid-associated hepatic damage.

• *Use cautiously* in chronic non-isoniazid-associated hepatic disease, seizure disorders, severe renal impairment, chronic alcoholism, and in elderly patients.

• Monitor hepatic function. Tell patient to notify doctor immediately if symptoms of hepatic impairment occur.

• Advise against alcohol use, which may increase risk of isoniazid-related hepatitis.

• Isoniazid pharmacokinetics may vary among patients because metabolism occurs in the liver by genetically controlled acetylation.

• Pyridoxine should be given to prevent peripheral neuropathy, especially in malnourished patients.

• Warn patient against discontinuing drug without doctor's consent. Encourage patient to fully comply with treatment.

• Advise patient to take with food if GI irritation occurs.

General

Classification: antimanic (alkali metal). **Pregnancy risk category:** D.

Mechanism of action

Alters chemical transmitters in the CNS by interfering with ionic pump mechanisms.

Indications and dosage

- Prevention or control of mania. **Adults:** 300 to 600 mg P.O. up to q.i.d., increasing on the basis of blood levels to achieve optimal dosage. Recommended therapeutic lithium blood levels: 1 to 1.5 mEq/liter (acute mania); 0.6 to 1.2 mEq/liter (maintenance); and 2 mEq/liter (maximum).

Adverse reactions

Blood: *leukocytosis of 14,000 to 18,000/mm*^{3} (reversible). **CNS:** tremor, drowsiness, headache, confusion, restlessness, dizziness, psychomotor retardation, stupor, lethargy, ***coma,*** blackouts, epileptiform seizures, EEG changes, worsened organic brain syndrome, impaired speech, ataxia, muscle weakness, incoordination, hyperexcitability. **CV:** *reversible ECG changes,* ***arrhythmias,*** hypotension, peripheral circulatory collapse, allergic vasculitis, ankle and wrist edema. **EENT:** tinnitus, impaired vision. **GI:** nausea, vomiting, anorexia, diarrhea, dry mouth, *thirst,* metallic taste. **GU:** *polyuria,* glycosuria, incontinence, renal toxicity with long-term use. **Metabolic:** transient hyperglycemia, goiter, hypothyroidism (lowered T_3, T_4, and protein-bound iodine, but elevated ^{131}I uptake), hyponatremia. **Skin:** pruritus, rash, diminished or lost sensation, drying and thinning of hair.

Interactions

Aminophylline, sodium bicarbonate, sodium chloride: these salts increase lithium excretion. Avoid salt loads and monitor lithium levels. **Carbamazepine, probenecid, indomethacin, methyldopa, piroxicam:** increased lithium effect. Monitor for lithium toxicity. **Diuretics:** increased reabsorption of lithium by kidneys (possible toxicity) Use with extreme caution, and monitor lithium and electrolyte levels **Haloperidol, thioridazine:** encephalopathic syndrome. Watch for syndrome and stop drug if it occurs. **Neuromuscular blockers:** lithium may cause prolonged paralysis or weakness. Monitor patient closely. **Thyroid hormones:** lithium may induce hypothyroidism.

Nursing diagnoses

- Altered thought processes related to patient's underlying psychiatric disorder.
- High risk for trauma related to adverse CNS reactions to lithium therapy.
- Knowledge deficit related to lithium therapy.

Nursing interventions

- *Contraindicated* if therapy cannot be closely monitored.
- *Use cautiously* in elderly or debilitated patients and in thyroid disease, seizure disorder, renal or CV disease, brain damage, severe debilitation or dehydration, and sodium depletion.
- Monitor baseline ECG, thyroid, and renal studies, and electrolyte levels. Monitor lithium blood levels 8 to 12 hours after first dose, two or three times weekly first month, then weekly to monthly on maintenance.
- Beneficial effects aren't seen for 1 to 3 weeks.
- Warn patient and family to watch for signs of toxicity and to expect transient nausea, polyuria, thirst, and discomfort during first few days. If toxic symptoms appear, he should withhold one dose and call doctor, but not stop drug abruptly.
- Weigh patient daily; check for edema and weight gain. Check fluid intake and output. Adjust fluid and salt ingestion if excessive fluid loss occurs.
- Perform thyroid and renal function tests biannually. Palpate thyroid to check for enlargement.
- Warn patient to avoid activities requiring alertness until CNS effects of the drug are known.
- Give after meals with plenty of water.
- Tell patient not to switch brands of lithium or to take other drugs without doctor's guidance.

General

Classification: antimuscarinic, GI antispasmodic (anticholinergic). **Pregnancy risk category:** C.

Mechanism of action

Competitively blocks acetylcholine, reducing GI motility and gastric acid secretion.

Indications and dosage

• Adjunctive therapy for peptic ulcer and irritable bowel syndrome. **Adults and children over 12 years:** 5 mg P.O. q 12 hours. Some patients may require 10 mg or more b.i.d. Individualize dosage according to patient's need.

Adverse reactions

CNS: headache, insomnia, drowsiness, dizziness, *confusion or excitement in elderly patients,* nervousness, weakness. **CV:** *palpitations,* tachycardia. **EENT:** *blurred vision,* mydriasis, increased ocular tension, cycloplegia, photophobia. **GI:** *dry mouth,* dysphagia, heartburn, loss of taste, nausea, vomiting, *constipation, paralytic ileus.* **GU:** *urinary hesitancy, urine retention,* impotence. **Skin:** urticaria, decreased sweating or anhidrosis, iodine-induced rash, other dermal manifestations. **Other:** fever, allergic reactions. **Overdose:** possible curare-like symptoms.

Interactions

Amantadine, antihistamines, antiparkinsonian agents, disopyramide, glutethimide, meperidine, phenothiazines, procainamide, quinidine: additive adverse effects. Avoid concomitant use. **Ketoconazole:** anticholinergics may interfere with ketoconazole absorption. Avoid concomitant use. **Methotrimeprazine:** anticholinergics may enhance risk of extrapyramidal reactions. Avoid concomitant use.

Nursing diagnoses

• Pain related to the patient's underlying condition.
• Urinary retention related to isopropamide-induced adverse GU reactions.
• Knowledge deficit related to isopropamide therapy.

Nursing interventions

• *Contraindicated* in hypersensitivity to iodine or anticholinergics, narrow-angle glaucoma, obstructive uropathy, obstructive disease of GI tract, severe ulcerative colitis, myasthenia gravis, paralytic ileus, intestinal atony, unstable cardiovascular status in acute hemorrhage, or toxic megacolon.
• *Use cautiously* in autonomic neuropathy, hyperthyroidism, coronary artery disease, cardiac arrhythmias, CHF, hypertension, hiatal hernia associated with reflux esophagitis, hepatic or renal disease, and ulcerative colitis, or in patients over age 40 because of increased incidence of glaucoma. Use cautiously in hot or humid environments.
• Give 30 minutes to 1 hour before meals and at bedtime. Bedtime dose can be larger; give at least 2 hours after the last meal of the day.
• Monitor patient's vital signs and urine output.
• Instruct patient to avoid hazardous activities if he is drowsy or dizzy or has blurred vision, to drink extra fluids to prevent constipation, and to report any rash or skin eruption.
• Tell patient that gum or sugarless hard candy may relieve dry mouth.
• Single dose produces 10- to 12-hour antisecretory effect and GI antispasmodic effect.
• Because isopropamide interferes with the 24-hour ^{131}I uptake test and may interfere with determinations of protein-bound iodine, discontinue it 1 week before thyroid function tests.

lisinopril
Prinivil, Zestril

General
Classification: antihypertensive (ACE inhibitor). **Pregnancy risk category:** C (D in 2nd and 3rd trimesters).

Mechanism of action
Inhibits angiotensin-converting enzyme (ACE), preventing conversion of angiotensin I to angiotensin II, a potent vasoconstrictor. This decreases peripheral arterial resistance and aldosterone secretion, thereby reducing sodium and water retention and blood pressure.

Indications and dosage
- Mild to severe hypertension. **Adults:** initially, 10 mg P.O. daily. Most patients are well controlled on 20 to 40 mg daily as a single dose.

Adverse reactions
Blood: neutropenia. **CNS:** *dizziness, headache, fatigue,* depression, somnolence, paresthesia. **CV:** hypotension, *orthostatic hypotension,* chest pain. **EENT:** *nasal congestion.* **GI:** *diarrhea,* nausea, dyspepsia, dysgeusia. **GU:** impotence. **Metabolic:** hyperkalemia. **Skin:** rash. **Other:** *upper respiratory symptoms, cough, muscle cramps,* ***angioedema,*** decreased libido.

Interactions
Diuretics: excessive hypotension. **Indomethacin:** attenuated hypotensive effect. **Insulin, oral antidiabetic agents:** risk of hypoglycemia, especially at initiation of lisinopril therapy. Monitor closely. **Potassium-sparing diuretics, potassium supplements, potassium-containing sodium substitutes:** possible hyperkalemia.

Nursing diagnoses
- Altered tissue perfusion (renal, cerebral, cardiopulmonary, and peripheral) related to the patient's underlying condition.
- High risk for injury related to lisinopril-induced adverse reactions.
- Knowledge deficit related to lisinopril therapy.

Nursing interventions
- *Contraindicated* during pregnancy because ACE inhibitors can cause fetal and neonatal injury or death. These problems have not been detected when fetal exposure has been limited to the first trimester. When pregnancy is detected, ACE inhibitors should be discontinued as soon as possible.
- Lower dosage is necessary in patients with impaired renal function.
- Lisinopril absorption is unaffected by food.
- Lisinopril attenuates potassium loss of thiazide diuretics. If patient is taking a diuretic, the diuretic should be discontinued 2 to 3 days before lisinopril therapy, or lisinopril dosage should be reduced to 5 mg once daily.
- If drug does not adequately control blood pressure, diuretics may be added.
- Teach patient about his disease and therapy. Explain the importance of taking this drug as prescribed, even when he's feeling well. Tell outpatient not to discontinue drug suddenly, but to call the doctor if unpleasant adverse reactions occur.
- Instruct patient to check with doctor or pharmacist before taking OTC medications.
- Review WBC and differential counts before treatment every 2 weeks for 3 months, and periodically thereafter.
- Beneficial effects of lisinopril may require several weeks of therapy.
- Tell patient to report light-headedness, especially in first few days of treatment, so dose can be adjusted; signs of infection such as sore throat or fever because drugs may decrease WBC count; facial swelling or difficulty breathing because drug may cause angioedema; and loss of taste, which may necessitate discontinuation of drug.
- Advise patient to avoid sudden postural changes to minimize orthostatic hypotension.
- Has been used investigationally in the treatment of CHF.

General

Classification: bronchodilator, cardiac stimulant (adrenergic). **Pregnancy risk category:** C.

Mechanism of action

Relaxes bronchial smooth muscle by acting on beta$_2$-adrenergic receptors. As a cardiac stimulant, acts on beta$_1$-adrenergic receptors in the heart.

Indications and dosage

• Bronchial asthma and reversible bronchospasm. **Adults:** (hydrochloride) 10 to 20 mg S.L. q 6 to 8 hours. **Children over 6 years:** (hydrochloride) 5 to 10 mg S.L. q 6 to 8 hours.
• Bronchospasm. **Adults and children:** (sulfate) for acute dyspneic episodes, 1 inhalation initially; may repeat if needed after 2 to 5 minutes. Maintenance dosage is 1 to 2 inhalations q.i.d. up to 6 times daily. May repeat once more 10 minutes after second dose, but don't give more than three doses for each attack.
• Heart block and ventricular arrhythmias. **Adults:** (hydrochloride) initially, 0.02 to 0.06 mg I.V., then 0.01 to 0.2 mg I.V. or 5 mcg/minute I.V. Or 0.2 mg I.M. initially, then 0.02 to 1 mg, p.r.n. **Children:** (hydrochloride) may give half of initial adult dose.
• Shock. **Adults and children:** (hydrochloride) 0.5 to 5 mcg/minute by continuous I.V. infusion. Usual concentration is 1 mg (5 ml) in 500 ml dextrose 5% in water. Adjust rate according to heart rate, central venous pressure, blood pressure, and urine flow.

Adverse reactions

CNS: *headache,* mild tremor, weakness, dizziness, nervousness, insomnia. **CV:** *palpitations, tachycardia, anginal pain, blood pressure changes.* **GI:** nausea, vomiting. **Metabolic:** hyperglycemia. **Other:** sweating, flushing of face, ***bronchial edema and inflammation.***

Interactions

Epinephrine: increased risk of arrhythmias. **Propranolol and other beta blockers:** blocked bronchodilating effect of isoproterenol. Monitor patient carefully if used together.

Nursing diagnoses

• Ineffective airway clearance related to patient's underlying respiratory condition.
• Pain related to isoproterenol-induced adverse CV reactions.
• Knowledge deficit related to isoproterenol therapy.

Nursing interventions

• *Contraindicated* in tachycardia caused by digitalis toxicity, in preexisting arrhythmias, and in recent MI.
• *Use cautiously* in coronary insufficiency, diabetes, or hyperthyroidism.
• Doses sufficient to increase the heart rate to more than 130 beats/minute may induce ventricular arrhythmias.
• If precordial distress or anginal pain occurs, stop drug immediately.
• **I.V. use:** When administering isoproterenol I.V. for shock, closely monitor blood pressure, central venous pressure, ECG, arterial blood gas measurements, and urine output.
• Teach patient how to take sublingual tablet properly. Instruct patient to rinse mouth with water between doses.
• If possible, don't give at bedtime because drug interrupts sleep patterns.
• Observe patient closely for adverse reactions.
• Tell patient to discontinue the drug if it causes an increase in chest tightness or dyspnea.
• Warn against overuse to avoid drug tolerance.

General

Classification: thyroid hormone replacement agent (thyroid hormone). **Pregnancy risk category:** A.

Mechanism of action

Stimulates the metabolism of all body tissues by accelerating the rate of cellular oxidation.

Indications and dosage

Dosages are expressed in thyroid equivalents and must be individualized to approximate the deficit in the patient's thyroid secretion.

• Hypothyroidism. **Adults and children:** initially, 15 to 30 mg P.O. daily, increasing by 15 to 30 mg q 1 to 2 weeks to desired response; increments in children's dosage q 2 weeks. **Adults over 65 years:** initially, 15 to 30 mg P.O. Usual adult dosage doubled q 6 to 8 weeks to desired response.

Adverse reactions

Adverse reactions of thyroid hormones are extensions of their pharmacologic properties and reflect patient sensitivity to them.

CNS: hyperirritability, *nervousness, insomnia,* twitching, *tremor.* **CV:** *tachycardia,* **arrhythmias,** angina pectoris, increased blood pressure, ***cardiac decompensation and collapse.*** **GI:** diarrhea, abdominal cramps, vomiting. **Other:** weight loss, menstrual irregularities, heat intolerance, hyperhidrosis; infants and children—accelerated rate of bone maturation.

Interactions

Cholestyramine and colestipol: liotrix absorption impaired. Separate doses by 4 to 5 hours. **I.V. phenytoin:** free thyroid released. Monitor for tachycardia. **Oral anticoagulants:** change in PT. Monitor PT; dosage adjustments may be necessary. **Oral antidiabetic agents:** change in serum glucose levels. Monitor blood glucose levels. **Sympathomimetics such as epinephrine:** increased risk of coronary insufficiency. Monitor closely.

Nursing diagnoses

• Decreased cardiac output related to liotrix-induced adverse CV reactions.
• High risk for activity intolerance related to ineffective dosage of liotrix.
• Knowledge deficit related to liotrix therapy.

Nursing interventions

• *Contraindicated* in MI, thyrotoxicosis (except with antithyroid drugs), or uncorrected adrenal insufficiency (thyroid hormones may cause acute adrenal crisis).
• *Use with extreme caution* in angina pectoris, hypertension, or other CV disorders; renal insufficiency; and ischemic states.
• Rapid replacement in arteriosclerosis may precipitate angina, coronary occlusion, or stroke. *Use cautiously* in these patients. Also use cautiously in myxedema.
• In patients with coronary artery disease, observe carefully for possible coronary insufficiency. Also observe during surgery; drug may precipitate cardiac arrhythmias.
• Potentially dangerous; not indicated to relieve vague symptoms, such as sluggishness, irritability, depression, and ill-defined pains; to treat obesity in euthyroid persons; to treat metabolic insufficiency not associated with thyroid insufficiency; or to treat menstrual disorders or male infertility, unless associated with hypothyroidism.
• Tell patient to take thyroid hormones at the same time each day, preferably before breakfast, to maintain constant hormone levels.
• Warn patient to tell doctor at once if chest pain, palpitations, sweating, nervousness, or other signs of overdosage occur; if any signs of aggravated CV disease develop (chest pain, dyspnea, and tachycardia); or if unusual bleeding and bruising occur.
• Monitor pulse rate and blood pressure.
• Thyroid hormones alter thyroid function test results.

General

Classification: antianginal (nitrate). **Pregnancy risk category:** C.

Mechanism of action

Reduces cardiac oxygen demand by decreasing left ventricular end-diastolic pressure and, to a lesser extent, systemic vascular resistance. Also increases blood flow through the collateral coronary vessels.

Indications and dosage

• Acute anginal attacks (sublingual and chewable tablets); prophylaxis in situations likely to cause anginal attacks; treatment of chronic ischemic heart disease (by preload reduction). **Adults:**
– Sublingual form: 2.5 to 10 mg for prompt relief of anginal pain, repeated q 5 to 10 minutes (maximum of three doses per 30-minute period). For prophylaxis, 2.5 to 10 mg q 2 to 3 hours.
– Chewable form: 5 to 10 mg p.r.n. for acute attack or q 2 to 3 hours for prophylaxis, but only after initial test dose of 5 mg to determine risk of severe hypotension.
– Oral form: 5 to 30 mg P.O. q.i.d. for prophylaxis only (use smallest effective dose); 40 mg P.O. (sustained-release form) q 6 to 12 hours.

Adverse reactions

CNS: *headache, sometimes with throbbing; dizziness;* weakness. **CV:** *orthostatic hypotension, tachycardia, palpitations, ankle edema, syncope.* **GI:** nausea, vomiting. **Skin:** cutaneous vasodilation, *flushing.* **Local:** sublingual burning. **Other:** hypersensitivity reactions.

Interactions

Antihypertensives: possibly increased antihypertensive effects. Monitor closely.

Nursing diagnoses

• Pain related to patient's underlying condition.
• High risk for injury related to isosorbide dinitrate-induced dizziness or orthostatic hypotension.
• Knowledge deficit related to isosorbide dinitrate therapy.

Nursing interventions

• *Contraindicated* in head trauma, cerebral hemorrhage, severe anemia, or hypersensitivity to nitrates.
• *Use cautiously* in hypotension.
• Monitor blood pressure and intensity and duration of response to drug.
• May cause headaches, especially at first. Treat headache with aspirin or acetaminophen. Dosage may need to be reduced temporarily, but tolerance usually develops.
• Tell patient to take medication regularly, even long-term if ordered, and to keep it easily accessible at all times.
• Tell patient taking isosorbide dinitrate to take additional dose before anticipated stress or at bedtime if angina is nocturnal.
• Advise patient to avoid alcoholic beverages.
• To minimize orthostatic hypotension, patient should change to upright position slowly. He should go up and down stairs carefully, and lie down at the first sign of dizziness.
• Teach patient to take sublingual tablet at first sign of attack. Dose may be repeated every 10 to 15 minutes for a maximum of three doses. If no relief, patient should call doctor or go to hospital emergency room.
• Warn patient not to confuse sublingual with oral form.
• Warn patient not to discontinue drug abruptly.
• Store in cool place away from light.
• Don't confuse isosorbide dinitrate with isosorbide mononitrate (another antianginal agent) or isosorbide (an antiglaucoma agent and osmotic diuretic).

General

Classification: thyroid hormone replacement agent. **Pregnancy risk category:** A.

Mechanism of action

Stimulates the metabolism of all body tissues by accelerating the rate of cellular oxidation.

Indications and dosage

- Cretinism. **Children 3 years and older:** 50 to 100 mcg P.O. daily. **Children under 3 years:** 5 mcg P.O. daily, increased by 5 mcg q 3 to 4 days until desired response occurs.
- Myxedema. **Adults:** initially, 5 mcg P.O. daily, increased by 5 to 10 mcg q 1 or 2 weeks. Maintenance dosage is 50 to 100 mcg daily.
- Nontoxic goiter. **Adults:** initially, 5 mcg P.O. daily; may be increased by 12.5 to 25 mcg daily q 1 to 2 weeks. Usual maintenance dosage is 75 mcg daily. **Adults over 65 years and children:** initially, 5 mcg P.O. daily, increased by 5-mcg increments at weekly intervals until desired response.
- Thyroid hormone replacement. **Adults:** initially, 25 mcg P.O. daily, increased by 12.5 to 25 mcg q 1 to 2 weeks until satisfactory response. Usual maintenance dosage is 25 to 75 mcg daily.
- T_3 suppression test to differentiate hyperthyroidism from euthyroidism. **Adults:** 75 to 100 mcg P.O. daily for 7 days.

Adverse reactions

Adverse reactions to thyroid hormones are extensions of their pharmacologic properties and reflect patient sensitivity to them.

CNS: hyperirritability, *nervousness, insomnia,* twitching, *tremor,* headache. **CV:** increased cardiac output, *tachycardia,* ***arrhythmias,*** angina pectoris, increased blood pressure, ***cardiac decompensation and collapse.*** **GI:** diarrhea, abdominal cramps, vomiting. **Other:** weight loss, heat intolerance, hyperhidrosis, menstrual irregularities; in infants and children—accelerated rate of bone maturation.

Interactions

Cholestyramine and colestipol: liothyronine absorption impaired. Separate doses by 4 to 5 hours. **I.V. phenytoin:** free thyroid released. Monitor for tachycardia. **Oral anticoagulants:** change in PT. Monitor PT, and adjust dosage as necessary. **Oral antidiabetic agents:** change in serum glucose levels. Monitor blood glucose levels. Adjust dosage as necessary. **Sympathomimetics such as epinephrine:** increased risk of coronary insufficiency. Monitor closely.

Nursing diagnoses

- High risk for activity intolerance related to ineffective dosage of liothyronine.
- Altered cardiopulmonary tissue perfusion related to liothyronine-induced angina pectoris.
- Knowledge deficit related to liothyronine therapy.

Nursing interventions

- *Contraindicated* in MI, thyrotoxicosis (except with antithyroid drugs), or uncorrected adrenal insufficiency.
- *Use with extreme caution* in angina pectoris, hypertension, or other CV disorders; renal insufficiency; and ischemic states.
- *Use cautiously* in arteriosclerosis; rapid replacement may precipitate angina, coronary occlusion, or stroke. Observe for coronary insufficiency in those with coronary artery disease. Also use cautiously in myxedema; these patients are unusually sensitive to thyroid hormone.
- Tell patient not to change product brands.
- Warn patient (especially elderly patients) to tell doctor at once if chest pain, palpitations, sweating, nervousness, or other signs of overdosage occur; if signs of aggravated CV disease develop; or if unusual bleeding or bruising occurs.
- Tell patient to take thyroid hormones at the same time each day, preferably before breakfast.
- Monitor pulse rate, blood pressure, and PT.
- Stop drug 7 to 10 days before radioactive iodine uptake studies.

General

Classification: antiacne agent, keratinization stabilizer (retinoic acid derivative). **Pregnancy risk category:** X.

Mechanism of action

Normalizes keratinization, decreases the size of sebaceous glands, and alters the composition of sebum to a less viscous form that's less likely to cause follicular plugging.

Indications and dosage

- Severe cystic acne unresponsive to conventional therapy. **Adults and adolescents:** 0.5 to 2 mg/kg P.O. daily given in two divided doses and continued for 15 to 20 weeks.

Adverse reactions

Blood: anemia, elevated platelet count. **CNS:** headache, fatigue, *pseudotumor cerebri.* **EENT:** *conjunctivitis,* corneal deposits, dry eyes. **Endocrine:** hyperglycemia. **GI:** nonspecific GI symptoms, gum bleeding and inflammation. **Hepatic:** elevated AST, ALT, and alkaline phosphatase. **Skin:** *cheilosis, rash, dry skin,* peeling of palms and toes, skin infection, photosensitivity. **Other:** *hypertriglyceridemia, musculoskeletal pain,* thinning of hair.

Interactions

Abrasives, acne preparations containing peeling agents, medicated soaps and cleansers, topical alcohol preparations: cumulative irritation of skin or excessive drying of skin. Use together cautiously. **Alcohol:** increased risk of hypertriglyceridemia. **Tetracyclines:** increased risk of pseudotumor cerebri. **Vitamin A and vitamin supplements containing vitamin A:** increase in isotretinoin's toxic effects. Don't use together without doctor's permission.

Nursing diagnoses

- Impaired skin integrity related to underlying condition.
- Impaired tissue integrity related to adverse effects of the drug.
- Knowledge deficit related to isotretinoin therapy.

Nursing interventions

- *Contraindicated* in women of childbearing age unless the patient has had a negative serum pregnancy test within 2 weeks before beginning therapy; will begin drug therapy on the 2nd or 3rd day of the next menstrual period; and will comply with stringent contraceptive measures for 1 month before therapy, during therapy, and for at least 1 month after therapy. Severe fetal abnormalities may occur if used during pregnancy.
- *Also contraindicated* in patients hypersensitive to parabens, which are used as preservatives.
- If used with other photosensitivity-inducing agents, may have additive effect. Tell patient to avoid prolonged exposure to the sun and to use sunscreen.
- Tell patient to immediately report any visual disturbances and bone or skeletal pain.
- Patients who experience headache, nausea and vomiting, or visual disturbances should be screened for papilledema. If signs and symptoms of pseudotumor cerebri occur, stop drug at once and provide prompt neurologic intervention.
- Perform serum lipid studies and liver function tests before therapy begins and then at regular intervals until response to drug is established.
- Monitor blood glucose regularly.
- Monitor creatine phosphokinase levels in patients who undergo vigorous physical activity.
- Warn patient that contact lenses may feel uncomfortable during isotretinoin therapy.
- If a second course of therapy is needed, don't start it until at least 8 weeks after completion of the first course because improvement may continue after withdrawal of the drug.
- Most adverse reactions are reversible when therapy is discontinued or dosage is reduced.
- Advise patient to take drug with or shortly after meals to ensure adequate absorption.

General

Classification: Class Ib ventricular antiarrhythmic (amide derivative). **Pregnancy risk category:** B.

Mechanism of action

Depresses phase 0 and shortens the action potential. All class I drugs have membrane stabilizing effects.

Indications and dosage

- Ventricular arrhythmias from MI, cardiac manipulation, or digitalis glycosides; ventricular tachycardia. **Adults:** 50 to 100 mg (1 to 1.5 mg/kg) I.V. bolus at 25 to 50 mg/minute. Give half this amount to elderly patients or patients under 50 kg and to those with CHF or hepatic disease. Repeat bolus q 3 to 5 minutes until arrhythmias subside or adverse reactions develop. Don't exceed 300-mg total bolus during a 1-hour period. Simultaneously, begin constant infusion of 20 to 50 mg/kg/minute (1 to 4 mg/minute). If single bolus has been given, repeat smaller bolus 15 to 20 minutes after start of infusion to maintain therapeutic serum level. After 24 hours of continuous infusion, decrease rate by half. *I.M. administration*—200 to 300 mg in deltoid muscle only. **Children:** 1 mg/kg by I.V. bolus, followed by infusion of 30 mcg/kg/minute.

Adverse reactions

CNS: *confusion, tremor,* lethargy, somnolence, *stupor, restlessness,* slurred speech, euphoria, depression, *light-headedness,* paresthesia, muscle twitching, ***seizures.*** **CV:** *hypotension,* bradycardia, ***new or worsened arrhythmias.*** **EENT:** *tinnitus, blurred or double vision.* **Other:** ***anaphylaxis,*** soreness at injection site, sensations of cold, diaphoresis.

Interactions

Cimetidine, beta blockers: decreased metabolism of lidocaine. Monitor for toxicity. **Phenytoin, procainamide, propranolol or quinidine:** additive cardiac depressant effects. Monitor carefully.

Nursing diagnoses

- Decreased cardiac output related to ineffectiveness of lidocaine therapy.
- Altered thought processes related to lidocaine-induced confusion.
- Knowledge deficit related to lidocaine therapy.

Nursing interventions

- *Contraindicated* in patients allergic to related local anesthetics of the amide type, such as Nupercaine, and with epinephrine (for local anesthesia) to treat arrhythmias. Don't use for ventricular escape beats; use atropine instead.
- *Use cautiously* and with reduced dosage in complete or second-degree heart block or sinus bradycardia and in elderly patients; in those with CHF, or renal or hepatic disease; or in those who weigh less than 50 kg.
- If toxic signs (such as dizziness) occur, stop drug at once and notify doctor. Continued infusion could lead to seizures and coma. Give oxygen via nasal cannula, if not contraindicated. Keep oxygen and CPR equipment readily available.
- **I.V. use:** Patients receiving infusions must be attended *at all times* and be on a cardiac monitor. Use an infusion pump for administering infusion precisely. Do not exceed an infusion rate of 4 mg/minute (greatly increases risk of toxicity).
- Monitor patient's response, especially blood pressure and serum electrolyte, BUN, and creatinine levels. Notify doctor promptly if abnormalities develop.
- Discontinue infusion and notify doctor if arrhythmias worsen or ECG changes are evident.
- A bolus dose not followed by infusion will have a short-lived effect.
- A patient who has received lidocaine I.M. will show a sevenfold increase in serum CK level. Such CK originates in the skeletal muscle, not the heart. Test isoenzymes if using I.M. route.

General
Classification: peripheral vasodilator (beta-adrenergic agonist). **Pregnancy risk category:** C.

Mechanism of action
Stimulates beta receptors and may be a direct-acting peripheral vasodilator.

Indications and dosage
• Adjunct for relief of symptoms associated with cerebrovascular insufficiency, peripheral vascular diseases (such as arteriosclerosis obliterans, thromboangiitis obliterans, and Raynaud's disease). **Adults:** 10 to 20 mg P.O. t.i.d. or q.i.d.

Adverse reactions
CV: tachycardia, orthostatic hypotension. **GI:** vomiting, abdominal distress, abdominal hypotension. **Skin:** severe rash.

Interactions
None significant.

Nursing diagnoses
• Altered cerebral and peripheral tissue perfusion related to the patient's underlying condition.
• Impaired skin integrity related to adverse reactions.
• Knowledge deficit related to isoxsuprine therapy.

Nursing interventions
• *Contraindicated* in immediate postpartum period and in patients with arterial bleeding.
• *Use with caution* in CV or cerebrovascular disease.
• Safe use in pregnancy and lactation not established, although drug has been used to inhibit contractions in premature labor.
• Isoxsuprine has also been used to minimize cramping in patients with severe primary dysmenorrhea.
• Discontinue if rash develops.
• Instruct patient to avoid sudden position changes to minimize the risk of orthostatic hypotension.

General

Classification: thyroid hormone replacement agent. **Pregnancy risk category:** A.

Mechanism of action

Stimulates the metabolism of all body tissues by accelerating the rate of cellular oxidation.

Indications and dosage

• Cretinism. **Children under 1 year:** initially, 0.025 to 0.05 mg P.O. daily, increased by 0.05 mg q 2 to 3 weeks to total daily dosage of 0.1 to 0.4 mg.

• Myxedema coma. **Adults:** 0.4 mg I.V., then 0.1 to 0.3 mg I.V. daily. After condition is stabilized, gradually decrease dosage to 0.05 to 0.1 mg daily. Switch to oral maintenance as soon as possible.

• Thyroid hormone replacement. **Adults:** initially, 0.025 to 0.1 mg P.O. daily, increased by 0.05 to 0.1 mg q 1 to 4 weeks until desired response. Maintenance dosage is 0.1 to 0.4 mg daily. May be given I.V. or I.M. when P.O. ingestion is precluded for long periods. **Adults over 65 years:** 0.025 mg P.O. daily, increased by 0.025 mg q 3 to 4 weeks, depending on response. **Children:** initially, maximum 0.05 mg P.O. daily, increased by 0.025 to 0.05 mg q 1 to 4 weeks until desired response is achieved.

Adverse reactions

Adverse reactions of thyroid hormones are extensions of their pharmacologic properties and reflect patient sensitivity to them.

CNS: nervousness, insomnia, tremor. **CV:** *tachycardia, palpitations, **arrhythmias**, angina pectoris,* hypertension. **GI:** appetite change, nausea, diarrhea. **Other:** headache, leg cramps, weight loss, sweating, heat intolerance, fever, menstrual irregularities.

Interactions

Cholestyramine, colestipol: levothyroxine absorption impaired. Separate doses by 4 to 5 hours. **Oral antidiabetic agents:** change in serum glucose levels. Monitor blood glucose levels. Adjust dosage as necessary. **I.V. phenytoin:** free thyroid released. Monitor for tachycardia. **Oral anticoagulants:** change in PT. Monitor PT, and adjust dosage as necessary. **Sympathomimetics such as epinephrine:** increased risk of coronary insufficiency. Monitor closely.

Nursing diagnoses

• High risk for activity intolerance related to the patient's underlying condition.

• Decreased cardiac output related to high risk for adverse CV reactions.

• Knowledge deficit related to levothyroxine therapy.

Nursing interventions

• *Contraindicated* in MI, thyrotoxicosis (except with antithyroid drugs), or uncorrected adrenal insufficiency.

• *Use with extreme caution* in angina pectoris, hypertension, or other CV disorders; renal insufficiency; and ischemic states.

• *Use cautiously* in arteriosclerosis; rapid replacement may precipitate angina, coronary occlusion, or stroke. Also use cautiously in myxedema; patients are unusually sensitive to thyroid hormone.

• Prepare I.V. dosage just before injection. Don't mix with other solutions. Inject into vein over 1 to 2 minutes.

• Observe for coronary insufficieny in patients with coronary artery disease.

• Tell patient not to change product brands.

• Warn patient to tell doctor at once if chest pain, palpitations, sweating, nervousness, shortness of breath, or other signs of overdosage or aggravated CV disease or unusual bleeding or bruising occur.

• Tell patient to take thyroid hormones at the same time each day, preferably before breakfast.

• Monitor pulse rate, blood pressure, and PT.

• Stop drug 4 weeks before radioactive iodine uptake studies.

General

Classification: antihypertensive (calcium channel blocker). **Pregnancy risk category:** C.

Mechanism of action

Inhibits calcium ion influx across cardiac and smooth muscle cells, thus decreasing arteriolar resistance and reducing blood pressure.

Indications and dosage

- Essential hypertension. **Adults:** initially, 2.5 mg P.O. b.i.d given alone or with a thiazide diuretic. Adjust dosage based on tolerance and response to a maximum of 20 mg daily.

Adverse reactions

CNS: dizziness. **CV:** edema, flushing, palpitations, tachycardia. **GI:** nausea, diarrhea. **GU:** frequent urination. **Skin:** rash. **Other:** dyspnea.

Interactions

Fentanyl anesthesia: severe hypotension has been reported with concomitant use of a beta blocker and a calcium channel blocker. Be sure to inform anesthesiologist that the patient is taking a calcium channel blocker.

Nursing diagnoses

- Altered tissue perfusion (renal, cerebral, cardiopulmonary, and peripheral) related to the patient's underlying condition.
- High risk for injury related to isradipine-induced hypotension and adverse CNS reactions.
- Knowledge deficit related to isradipine therapy.

Nursing interventions

- *Contraindicated* in patients with hypersensitivity to the drug.
- *Use cautiously* in patients with CHF, especially if combined with a beta blocker.
- Isradipine has diuretic activity; the mechanism is not fully understood. Patients may note an increased need to void.
- Like other calcium channel blockers, isradipine is known to cause symptomatic hypotension; however, syncope and severe dizziness have not been reported. Most adverse reactions are mild and transient and related to vasodilation (dizziness, edema, flushing, palpitations, and tachycardia).
- Initial therapy produces antihypertensive effect in 2 to 3 hours; however, maximal response usually develops after 2 to 4 weeks of continuous therapy.
- Increase dosage by gradual titration. If response is inadequate after first 2 to 4 weeks, increase dosage to 5 mg b.i.d. Continue increasing at 5-mg/day intervals every 2 to 4 weeks to a maximum of 10 mg b.i.d. Most patients show no additional response at dosages over 10 mg daily (5 mg b.i.d.).
- The bioavailability of isradipine is increased in elderly patients and those with impaired hepatic function. However, the starting dosage should still be 2.5 mg b.i.d.
- Teach patient to take his blood pressure.

General

Classification: analgesic, adjunct to anesthesia (opioid). **Pregnancy risk category:** B (D for prolonged use or high doses at term). **Controlled substance schedule:** II.

Mechanism of action

Binds with opiate receptors at many sites in the CNS (brain, brain stem, and spinal cord), altering both perception of and emotional response to pain through an unknown mechanism.

Indications and dosage

- Moderate to severe pain. **Adults:** 2 to 3 mg P.O. or S.C. q 6 to 8 hours, p.r.n. or around the clock.

Adverse reactions

CNS: *sedation, somnolence, clouded sensorium,* dizziness, *euphoria,* seizures with large doses. **CV:** *hypotension,* bradycardia. **GI:** *nausea, vomiting, constipation,* ileus. **GU:** urine retention. **Other:** ***respiratory depression,*** physical dependence.

Interactions

Alcohol, CNS depressants: additive effects. Use together cautiously.

Nursing diagnoses

- Pain related to patient's underlying condition.
- Ineffective breathing pattern related to levorphanol-induced respiratory depression.
- Knowledge deficit related to levorphanol therapy.

Nursing interventions

- *Contraindicated* in patients with hypersensitivity to the drug or other opiate analgesics, acute alcoholism, bronchial asthma, increased intracranial pressure, respiratory depression, and anoxia.
- *Use with extreme caution* in hepatic or renal disease, hypothyroidism, Addison's disease, seizures, head injury, severe CNS depression, brain tumor, COPD, and shock and in elderly or debilitated patients.
- Warn ambulatory patient to avoid hazardous activities that require mental alertness and physical coordination.
- Monitor circulatory and respiratory status and bowel function.
- Protect from light.
- Keep narcotic antagonist (naloxone) available.
- Use with general anesthetics, other narcotic analgesics, tranquilizers, sedatives, hypnotics, alcohol, tricyclic antidepressants, or MAO inhibitors increases CNS depression. Reduce levorphanol dose. Use together with extreme caution. Monitor patient response.
- For better analgesic effect, give before patient has intense pain.
- When used postoperatively, encourage turning, coughing, and deep breathing to prevent atelectasis.
- Warn patient that drug has bitter taste.

General

Classification: antibiotic (aminoglycoside). **Pregnancy risk category:** D.

Mechanism of action

Inhibits protein synthesis by binding directly to the 30S ribosomal subunit. Generally bactericidal.

Indications and dosage

- Serious infections caused by sensitive *Escherichia coli, Proteus, Enterobacter aerogenes, Klebsiella pneumoniae, Serratia marcescens, or Acinetobacter.* **Adults and children with normal renal function:** 15 mg/kg daily divided q 8 to 12 hours deep I.M. into upper outer quadrant of buttocks or I.V. infusion (diluted 500 mg/200 ml of 0.9% sodium chloride solution or D_5W infused at 60 to 80 drops/minute). Maximum daily dosage is 1.5 g. **Neonates:** 15 mg/kg daily I.M. or I.V. divided q 12 hours.
- Adjunctive treatment in hepatic coma. **Adults:** 8 to 12 g daily P.O. in divided doses.
- Preoperative bowel sterilization. **Adults:** 1 g P.O. q 1 hour for four doses, then q 4 hours for four doses; or 1 g P.O. q 1 hour for four doses, then q 6 hours for 36 to 72 hours.
- Intraperitoneal irrigation. 500 mg in 20 ml sterile distilled water instilled via catheter into wound after patient is fully recovered from anesthesia and neuromuscular blocker effects.
- Wound irrigation. Up to 2.5 mg/ml in 0.9% sodium chloride solution irrigant.

Adverse reactions

CNS: headache, lethargy, ***neuromuscular blockade.*** **EENT:** *ototoxicity (tinnitus, vertigo, hearing loss).* **GU:** *nephrotoxicity (cells or casts in the urine, oliguria, proteinuria, decreased creatinine clearance, increased BUN and serum creatinine levels).* **Other:** ***hypersensitivity reactions.***

Interactions

Cephalothin: increases nephrotoxicity. Use together cautiously. **Dimenhydrinate:** may mask symptoms of ototoxicity. Use with caution. **General anesthetics, neuromuscular blocking agents:** may potentiate neuromuscular blockade. **I.V. loop diuretics (such as furosemide):** increase ototoxicity. Use cautiously. **Other aminoglycosides, amphotericin B, cisplatin, methoxyflurane:** increase nephrotoxicity. Don't use together. **Parenteral penicillins (such as carbenicillin and ticarcillin):** kanamycin inactivation in vitro. Don't combine in I.V. line.

Nursing diagnoses

- High risk for injury related to ineffectiveness of kanamycin to eradicate the infection.
- Altered urinary elimination related to kanamycin-induced nephrotoxicity.
- Knowledge deficit related to kanamycin therapy.

Nursing interventions

- *Contraindicated* for oral use in intestinal obstruction and treatment of systemic infection.
- *Use cautiously* in patients with impaired renal function and in elderly patients.
- Obtain specimen for culture and sensitivity tests before first dose, but begin therapy pending results.
- Weigh patient and obtain baseline renal function studies before therapy.
- **I.V. use:** Dilute 500 mg of the drug per 200 ml of 0.9% sodium solution or D_5W, and infuse at 60 to 80 drops/minute.
- Monitor renal function carefully, and notify doctor of signs of decreasing renal function.
- Keep patient well hydrated while taking drug to minimize irritation of the renal tubules.
- Evaluate patient's hearing before and during therapy. Notify doctor if patient complains of tinnitus, vertigo, or hearing loss.
- Watch for superinfection (continued fever and other signs of new infection, especially of upper respiratory tract).
- If no response in 3 to 5 days, stop therapy and obtain specimens for culture and sensitivity tests.
- Peak blood levels over 30 mcg/ml and trough levels over 10 mcg/ml may be associated with increased incidence of toxicity.

General

Classification: contraceptive (progestin). **Pregnancy risk category:** X.

Mechanism of action

Slowly releases the synthetic progestin levonorgestrel into the bloodstream. How progestins provide contraception is not fully understood, but they alter the mucus covering the cervix, prevent implantation of the egg, and in some patients prevent ovulation.

Indications and dosage

• Prevention of pregnancy. **Women:** six capsules implanted subdermally in the midportion of the upper arm during the first 7 days of the onset of menses. Contraceptive efficacy lasts for 5 years.

Adverse reactions

CNS: headache, nervousness, dizziness, change of appetite. **GI:** nausea, *abdominal discomfort.* **GU:** *amenorrhea, many bleeding days or prolonged bleeding, spotting, irregular onset of bleeding, frequent onset of bleeding, scanty bleeding, cervicitis, vaginitis, leukorrhea.* **Skin:** dermatitis, acne, hirsutism, hypertrichosis, scalp hair loss. **Local:** infection at implant site, transient pain or itching at implant site. **Other:** adnexal enlargement, mastalgia, weight gain, *musculoskeletal pain, removal difficulty, breast discharge.*

Interactions

Carbamazepine, phenytoin, rifampin: may reduce efficacy of levonorgestrel implants.

Nursing diagnoses

• Pain related to levonorgestrel-induced abdominal and musculoskeletal discomfort.
• Impaired tissue integrity related to high risk for levonorgestrel-induced cervicitis and vaginitis.
• Knowledge deficit related to levonorgestrel therapy.

Nursing interventions

• *Contraindicated* in patients with thrombophlebitis or thromboembolic disorders, undiagnosed abnormal genital bleeding, acute liver disease, malignant or benign liver tumors, breast carcinoma, and known or suspected pregnancy.
• *Use cautiously* in patients with a history of depression (drug can worsen depression); in diabetic and prediabetic patients (drug may alter carbohydrate metabolism); and in patients with hyperlipidemias (drug may alter lipid metabolism).
• Most patients develop variations in menstrual bleeding patterns, including irregular bleeding, prolonged bleeding, spotting, and amenorrhea. These irregularities usually diminish over time.
• Irregular bleeding may mask symptoms of cervical or endometrial cancer.
• Warn patients that missed menstrual periods are not an accurate indicator of early pregnancy because the drug may induce amenorrhea. Advise patients that 6 weeks or more of amenorrhea (after a pattern of regular menstrual periods) could indicate pregnancy. If pregnancy is confirmed, the implants must be removed.
• The implants should be removed if the patient develops active thrombophlebitis or thromboembolic disease or will be immobilized for a significant length, such as from illness.
• Closely monitor patients with conditions that may be aggravated by fluid retention because steroid hormones may cause fluid retention.
• Encourage annual physical examinations.
• Tell patient to report to the doctor immediately if any implant capsules fall out (before the skin heals). Contraceptive efficacy may be impaired.
• Patients with sudden unexplained vision problems, including users of contact lenses who develop vision changes or changes in lens tolerance, should be immediately evaluated by an ophthalmologist.
• Laboratory tests for sex hormone-binding globulin and thyroxine concentrations may show decreased values; for triiodothyronine uptake, increased values.

kaolin and pectin mixtures

Donnagel-MB*†, Kao-Con†, Kaopectate◇, Kaopectate Concentrate◇, Kao-tin◇, Kapectolin◇

General

Classification: antidiarrheal (absorbent). **Pregnancy risk category:** C.

Mechanism of action

Decrease the stools' fluid content, although *total* water loss seems to remain the same.

Indications and dosage

- Mild, nonspecific diarrhea. **Adults:** 60 to 120 ml P.O. after each bowel movement. **Children over 12 years:** 60 ml P.O. after each bowel movement. **Children 6 to 12 years:** 30 to 60 ml P.O. after each bowel movement. **Children 3 to 6 years:** 15 to 30 ml P.O. after each bowel movement.

Adverse reactions

GI: drug absorption of nutrients, drugs, and enzymes; fecal impaction or ulceration in infants and elderly or debilitated patients after chronic use; constipation.

Interactions

Orally administered drugs: adsorption may occur. Separate administration times of other orally administered drugs.

Nursing diagnoses

- Diarrhea related to interruption in normal pattern of elimination characterized by frequent loose stools.
- Colonic constipation related to chronic use of kaolin and pectin mixtures.
- Knowledge deficit related to therapy with kaolin and pectin mixtures.

Nursing interventions

- *Contraindicated* in suspected obstructive bowel lesions.
- Don't use for more than 2 days.
- Don't use in place of specific therapy for underlying cause.
- Be aware that drug is a GI absorbent and may reduce absorption of other orally administered drugs, requiring dosage adjustments.

General

Classification: antiparkinsonian agent (precursor of dopamine). **Pregnancy risk category:** C.

Mechanism of action

Levodopa is decarboxylated to dopamine, countering the depletion of striatal dopamine in extrapyramidal centers, which is thought to produce parkinsonism.

Indications and dosage

• Idiopathic parkinsonism, postencephalitic parkinsonism, and symptomatic parkinsonism after carbon monoxide or manganese intoxication; or in association with cerebral arteriosclerosis. **Adults and children over 12 years:** initially, 0.5 to 1 g P.O. daily, given b.i.d., t.i.d., or q.i.d. with food; increase by no more than 0.75 g daily q 3 to 7 days, until usual maximum of 8 g is reached. Carefully adjust dosage to individual requirements, tolerance, and response. Higher dosage requires close supervision.

Adverse reactions

Blood: ***hemolytic anemia,*** leukopenia. **CNS:** *choreiform, dystonic, and dyskinetic movements, involuntary grimacing, head movements, myoclonic body jerks, ataxia, tremors, muscle twitching, bradykinetic episode, psychiatric disturbances, aggressive behavior, memory loss, mood changes, nervousness, anxiety, disturbing dreams, euphoria, malaise, fatigue, severe depression, suicidal tendencies, dementia, delirium, hallucinations (may necessitate reduction or withdrawal of drug).* **CV:** *orthostatic hypotension,* cardiac irregularities, flushing, hypertension, phlebitis. **EENT:** blepharospasm, blurred vision, diplopia, mydriasis or miosis, widening of palpebral fissures, activation of latent Horner's syndrome, oculogyric crises, nasal discharge. **GI:** *nausea, vomiting, anorexia,* weight loss, constipation, flatulence, diarrhea, epigastric pain, hiccups, sialorrhea, dry mouth, bitter taste. **GU:** urinary frequency, retention, incontinence; darkened urine; excessive and inappropriate sexual behavior; priapism. **Hepatic:** hepatotoxicity. **Other:** dark perspiration, hyperventilation.

Interactions

Antacids: increased absorption of levodopa. **Antihypertensives:** additive hypertensive effect. **High-protein foods:** decreased absorption of levodopa. **Metoclopramide:** accelerated gastric emptying of levodopa. **Papaverine, phenothiazines and other antipsychotics, phenytoin:** watch for decreased levodopa effect. **Pyridoxine (vitamin B_6):** reduced efficacy of levodopa. Examine vitamin preparations and nutritional supplements for content of pyridoxine. **Sympathomimetics:** increased risk of cardiac arrhythmias.

Nursing diagnoses

• Impaired physical mobility related to underlying parkinsonian syndrome.
• Altered thought processes related to adverse CNS reactions to levodopa.
• Fluid volume deficit related to high risk of adverse GI reactions.
• Knowledge deficit related to levodopa therapy.

Nursing interventions

• *Contraindicated* in narrow-angle glaucoma, melanoma, or undiagnosed skin lesions.
• *Use cautiously* in cardiovascular, renal, hepatic, and pulmonary disorders; peptic ulcer; psychiatric illness; MI with residual arrhythmias; bronchial asthma; emphysema; or endocrine disease.
• Muscle twitching and blepharospasm may be early signs of drug overdose; report immediately.
• Patients receiving long-term treatment should be tested regularly for diabetes and acromegaly and should have periodic tests of renal, hepatic, and hematopoietic function.
• Patient who must undergo surgery should continue levodopa as long as oral intake is permitted, generally until 6 to 24 hours before surgery. Drug should be resumed as soon as patient is able to take oral medication.

General

Classification: antifungal (imidazole derivative).
Pregnancy risk category: C.

Mechanism of action

Inhibits purine transport and DNA, RNA, and protein synthesis; increases cell wall permeability, making the fungus more susceptible to osmotic pressure.

Indications and dosage

- Systemic candidiasis, chronic mucocandidiasis, oral thrush, candiduria, coccidioidomycosis, histoplasmosis, chromomycosis, and paracoccidioidomycosis; severe cutaneous dermatophyte infections resistant to therapy with topical or oral griseofulvin. **Adults and children over 40 kg:** initially, 200 mg P.O. daily as single dose. Dosage may be increased to 400 mg once daily in patients who don't respond to lower dosage. **Children 2 years and over:** 3.3 to 6.6 mg/kg P.O. daily.

Adverse reactions

CNS: headache, nervousness, dizziness. **GI:** *nausea, vomiting,* abdominal pain, diarrhea, constipation. **Hepatic:** elevated liver enzymes, ***fatal hepatotoxicity.*** **Skin:** itching. **Other:** gynecomastia with breast tenderness in males.

Interactions

Antacids, anticholinergics, H_2 blockers: decreased absorption of ketoconazole. Wait at least 2 hours after ketoconazole dose before administering these drugs. **Isoniazid, rifampin:** increase ketoconazole metabolism. Monitor for decreased antifungal effect.

Nursing diagnoses

- High risk for injury related to ineffectiveness of ketoconazole in eradicating the fungal infection.
- High risk for fluid volume deficit related to ketoconazole-induced adverse GI reactions.
- Knowledge deficit related to ketoconazole therapy.

Nursing interventions

- *Contraindicated* in patients with hypersensitivity to the drug.
- *Use cautiously* in patients with hepatic disease and in those who are taking other hepatotoxic drugs.
- Because of the risk of serious hepatotoxicity, ketoconazole should not be used for less serious conditions, such as fungal infections of the skin or nails.
- Ketoconazole is not effective in patients with achlorhydria because drug requires acidity for dissolution and absorption. Instruct such patients to dissolve each tablet in 4 ml aqueous solution of 0.2 N hydrochloric acid and, to avoid contact with teeth, to sip the mixture through a straw (glass or plastic). Tell patient to follow with a glass of water.
- Make sure patient understands that treatment should be continued until all clinical and laboratory tests indicate that active fungal infection has subsided. If drug is discontinued too soon, infection will recur. Minimum treatment period for candidiasis is 7 to 14 days. Minimum treatment period for other systemic fungal infections is 6 months. Minimum treatment period for resistant dermatophyte infections is 4 weeks.
- Reassure patient that, although nausea is common early in therapy, it will subside. To minimize nausea, you may (with doctor's permission) divide the daily dosage into two doses. Taking drug with meals also helps to decrease nausea.
- Monitor for elevated liver enzymes, nausea that does not subside, unusual fatigue, jaundice, dark urine, or pale stools. These may be signs of hepatotoxicity.
- Much larger doses (up to 800 mg/day) can be used to effectively treat fungal meningitis and intracerebral fungal lesions.

levamisole hydrochloride

Ergamisol

General

Classification: antineoplastic (immunomodulator). **Pregnancy risk category:** C.

Mechanism of action

Unknown. Drug's effects on immune system are complex. It appears to restore depressed immune function and may potentiate actions of monocytes and macrophages and enhance T-cell responses.

Indications and dosage

- Adjuvant treatment of Dukes' stage C colon cancer (with fluorouracil) after surgical resection. **Adults:** 50 mg P.O. q 8 hours for 3 days. Therapy should begin no sooner than 7 days and no later than 30 days after surgery, if patient is out of the hospital, ambulating, and maintaining normal oral nutrition; has well-healed wounds; and has recovered from any postoperative complications. Fluorouracil (450 mg/m²/day I.V.) is given daily for 5 days, starting 21 to 34 days after surgery. Maintenance dosage 50 mg P.O. q 8 hours for 3 days, q 2 weeks for 1 year. Given with fluorouracil maintenance therapy (450 mg/m²/day by rapid I.V. push, once a week beginning 28 days after the initial 5-day course) for 1 year.

Adverse reactions

Blood: ***agranulocytosis, leukopenia, thrombocytopenia, granulocytopenia.*** **CNS:** *dizziness, headache, paresthesia, somnolence, depression, nervousness, insomnia, anxiety, fatigue, fever.* **CV:** chest pain, edema. **EENT:** blurred vision, conjunctivitis. **GI:** *nausea, diarrhea, stomatitis, vomiting, anorexia, abdominal pain, constipation, flatulence, dyspepsia.* **Metabolic:** hyperbilirubinemia. **Skin:** *dermatitis, alopecia,* ***exfoliative dermatitis,*** *pruritus, urticaria.* **Other:** rigors, *infection, dysgeusia, altered sense of smell, arthralgia, myalgia.*

Interactions

Alcohol: may precipitate a disulfiram-like (Antabuse) reaction. Avoid concomitant use. **Phenytoin:** plasma levels may be elevated when administered with levamisole and fluorouracil.

Nursing diagnoses

- Altered protection related to the patient's underlying condition.
- High risk for injury related to hematologic effects of levamisole.
- Knowledge deficit related to levamisole therapy.

Nursing interventions

- Monitor hematologic status closely because drug is associated with agranulocytosis, especially at higher doses, which may be fatal. Neutropenia is usually reversible when therapy is discontinued.
- If levamisole therapy begins 7 to 20 days after surgery, fluorouracil should be started with the second course of therapy, beginning no sooner than 21 days and no later than 35 days after surgery. If levamisole is deferred until 21 to 30 days after surgery, fluorouracil therapy should begin with the first course of levamisole.
- If stomatitis or diarrhea develops during initial course of fluorouracil therapy, discontinue drug, then begin weekly fluorouracil therapy 28 days after start of initial course. If stomatitis or diarrhea develops during weekly doses of fluorouracil, defer fluorouracil therapy until these symptoms subside. Then restart fluorouracil therapy, reducing dosage by 20%.
- Dosage modifications are based on hematologic parameters. If WBC count is 2,500/mm³ to 3,500/mm³, don't administer fluorouracil until WBC count is above 3,500/mm³. When fluorouracil is restarted, reduce dosage by 20%. If WBC count stays below 2,500/mm³ for over 10 days after fluorouracil is withdrawn, discontinue levamisole.
- If platelet count is below 100,000/mm³, discontinue both fluorouracil and levamisole therapy.
- Baseline CBC with differential and platelets and electrolyte and liver function studies are necessary immediately before starting therapy. Then, a CBC with differential and platelets should be performed at weekly intervals before treatment with fluorouracil. Electrolyte and liver function studies should be repeated every 3 months for 1 year.

General

Classification: nonnarcotic analgesic, antipyretic (NSAID). **Pregnancy risk category:** B (D in 3rd trimester).

Mechanism of action

Produces anti-inflammatory, analgesic, and antipyretic effects, possibly through inhibition of prostaglandin synthesis.

Indications and dosage

- Rheumatoid arthritis and osteoarthritis. **Adults:** 150 to 300 mg P.O. in three or four divided doses. Usual dosage is 75 mg t.i.d. Maximum dosage is 300 mg/day. Or, 100 mg P.R. b.i.d. or 1 suppository h.s. (in conjunction with oral ketoprofen during the day).
- Mild to moderate pain; dysmenorrhea. **Adults:** 25 to 50 mg P.O. q 6 to 8 hours p.r.n.

Adverse reactions

Blood: prolonged bleeding time. **CNS:** *headache,* dizziness, *CNS inhibition or excitation.* **EENT:** tinnitus, visual disturbances. **GI:** *nausea, abdominal pain, diarrhea, constipation, flatulence,* ***peptic ulceration,*** anorexia, vomiting, stomatitis. **GU:** ***nephrotoxicity,*** *elevated BUN.* **Hepatic:** elevated enzymes. **Skin:** rash.

Interactions

Hydrochlorothiazide, other diuretics: decreased diuretic effectiveness. Monitor for lack of effect. **Lithium, methotrexate:** increased levels of these drugs, leading to toxicity. Monitor closely. **Oral anticoagulants:** increased risk of bleeding. Monitor closely. **Aspirin, probenecid:** decreased plasma levels of ketoprofen. Avoid concomitant use.

Nursing diagnoses

- Pain related to patient's underlying condition.
- High risk for trauma related to possible adverse CNS reactions.
- Knowledge deficit related to ketoprofen therapy.

Nursing interventions

- *Contraindicated* in patients with hypersensitivity to ketoprofen, aspirin, or other NSAIDs.
- *Use cautiously* in patients with history of peptic ulcer disease or renal dysfunction.
- Serious GI toxicity can occur at any time in patients on long-term NSAID therapy. Teach such patients signs and symptoms of GI bleeding, and tell them to report these to the doctor immediately.
- Tell patient to report visual or auditory adverse reactions immediately.
- Concomitant use with aspirin, alcohol, or steroids may increase the risk of adverse GI reactions.
- Tell patient that full therapeutic effect may be delayed for 2 to 4 weeks.
- Check renal and hepatic function every 6 months or as indicated during long-term therapy.
- Give dose 30 minutes before or 2 hours after meals. If adverse GI reactions occur, give with milk or meals.
- Ketoprofen may interfere with some laboratory determinations of blood glucose and serum iron levels, depending on the testing method used.
- Because of their antipyretic and anti-inflammatory actions, NSAIDs may mask the signs and symptoms of infection.

General

Classification: antineoplastic (gonadotropic hormone). **Pregnancy risk category:** X.

Mechanism of action

Initially stimulates but then inhibits the release of follicle-stimulating hormone and luteinizing hormone. This results in testosterone suppression.

Indications and dosage

- Management of advanced prostate cancer. **Men:** 1 mg S.C. daily. Alternatively, give 7.5 mg I.M. (depot injection) monthly.
- Endometriosis. **Women:** 3.75 mg I.M (depot injection only) as a single injection once a month for up to 6 months.

Adverse reactions

CNS: dizziness, depression, headache. **CV:** arrhythmias, angina, MI. **Endocrine:** *hot flashes.* **GI:** nausea, vomiting. **Local:** skin reactions at injection site. **Other:** pulmonary embolus, peripheral edema, decreased libido, elevated liver enzymes, transient bone pain during first week of treatment.

Interactions

None significant.

Nursing diagnoses

- High risk for impaired skin integrity related to drug-induced skin reactions.
- Sexual dysfunction related to drug-induced decreased libido.
- Knowledge deficit related to leuprolide therapy.

Nursing interventions

- *Contraindicated* in patients with hypersensitivity to the drug or to other gonadotropin-releasing hormone analogues, during pregnancy, and in women with undiagnosed vaginal bleeding.
- *Use cautiously* in patients hypersensitive to benzyl alcohol.
- Never administer by I.V. injection.
- Leuprolide is a nonsurgical alternative to orchiectomy for prostate cancer.
- Studies show that leuprolide is therapeutically equivalent to diethylstilbestrol in "medical castration" palliative treatment but has significantly milder and fewer adverse effects.
- Reassure patient who has had undesirable effects from other endocrine therapies that leuprolide is much easier to tolerate.
- When treating prostate cancer, symptoms (bone pain, difficulty urinating, neurologic symptoms) may worsen when therapy is initiated. Reassure patient that these effects are transient and will disappear after about 1 week.
- If patient is going to self-administer S.C. injection, teach him proper administration techniques and advise him to use only the syringes provided by the manufacturer. If another syringe must be substituted, a low-dose insulin syringe (U-100, 0.5 ml) may be an appropriate choice.
- Advise patient to store the drug at room temperature, protected from light and sources of heat.
- Once-monthly depot injections should be administered under medical supervision. Use supplied diluent to reconstitute drug. Draw 1 ml into a syringe with a 22G needle (extra diluent is provided and should be discarded). Inject into vial, then shake well. Suspension will appear milky. Although the suspension is stable for 24 hours after reconstitution, it contains no bacteriostat. Use immediately.

General
Classification: analgesic (NSAID). **Pregnancy risk category:** B.

Mechanism of action
Acts by inhibiting the synthesis of prostaglandins.

Indications and dosage
• Short-term management of pain. **Adults:** initially, give 30 or 60 mg I.M as a loading dose, followed by half of the loading dose (15 or 30 mg) I.M. q 6 hours on a regular schedule or p.r.n. Subsequent dosage should be based on patient response. If pain returns before 6 hours, dosage may be increased by as much as 50% (up to 60 mg); if pain relief continues for 8 to 12 hours, increase interval between doses to q 8 to 12 hours, or reduce dose. The recommended maximum dosage is 150 mg I.M. on the first day and 120 mg daily thereafter.

Alternatively, the drug may be given orally on a short-term basis. Give 10 mg P.O. q 4 to 6 hours p.r.n. Do not give more than 40 mg daily, and use the drug *only* for a short time.

Adverse reactions
CNS: *drowsiness,* dizziness, headache, sweating. **CV:** edema. **GI:** *nausea, dyspepsia, GI pain,* diarrhea. **Local:** pain at the injection site.

Interactions
Lithium: NSAIDs increase lithium levels. Monitor closely. **Methotrexate:** NSAIDs decrease methotrexate clearance and increase its toxicity. Don't use together. **Salicylates, warfarin:** ketorolac may increase the levels of free (unbound) salicylates or warfarin in the blood. Clinical significance is unknown.

Nursing diagnoses
• Pain related to the patient's underlying condition.
• High risk for trauma related to possible adverse CNS reactions to ketorolac.
• Knowledge deficit related to ketorolac therapy.

Nursing interventions
• *Contraindicated* in patients with hypersensitivity to the drug and in patients with the complete or partial triad syndrome: nasal polyps, angioedema, and bronchospasm after use of other NSAIDs or aspirin.
• *Use cautiously* in patients with hepatic or renal impairment. Also use cautiously in patients with cardiac disease or hypertension because NSAIDs can cause fluid retention and edema.
• This drug is intended solely for short-term management of pain. The rate and severity of adverse reactions should be less than that observed in patients taking NSAIDs on a long-term basis.
• When switching patients from injectable to oral ketorolac, do not exceed a total dose of 120 mg of drug on the day of transition, including the maximum of 40 mg P.O.
• Carefully observe patients with coagulopathies and those who are taking anticoagulants. Ketorolac inhibits platelet aggregation and can prolong bleeding time. This effect will disappear within 48 hours of discontinuing the drug. It will not alter platelet count, partial thromboplastin time, or PT.
• I.M. administration may cause pain at the injection site. Holding pressure over the site for 15 to 30 seconds after the injection may minimize local effects.
• GI ulceration, bleeding, and perforation can occur at any time, with or without warning, in any patient taking NSAIDs on a long-term basis. Teach patients the signs and symptoms of GI bleeding.
• Use lower initial doses in patients who are over age 65 or who weigh less than 110 lb (50 kg).
• Because of their antipyretic and anti-inflammatory actions, NSAIDs may mask the signs and symptoms of infection.
• Trace amounts of the drug have been detected in breast milk. Use with caution in breast-feeding women.

General

Classification: vitamin, antidote (folic acid derivative). **Pregnancy risk category:** C.

Mechanism of action

A reduced form of folic acid that is readily converted to other folic acid derivatives.

Indications and dosage

- Overdose of folic acid antagonist. **Adults and children:** P.O., I.M., or I.V. dose equivalent to the weight of the antagonist given.
- Leucovorin rescue after high methotrexate dose in treatment of cancer. **Adults and children:** dose given at doctor's discretion within 6 to 36 hours of last dose of methotrexate.
- Toxic effects of methotrexate used to treat severe psoriasis. **Adults and children:** 4 to 8 mg I.M. 2 hours after methotrexate dose.
- Hematologic toxicity caused by pyrimethamine therapy. **Adults and children:** 5 mg P.O. or I.M. daily.
- Hematologic toxicity caused by trimethoprim therapy. **Adults and children:** 400 mcg to 5 mg P.O. or I.M. daily.
- Megaloblastic anemia caused by congenital enzyme deficiency. **Adults and children:** 3 to 6 mg I.M. daily, then 1 mg P.O. daily for life.
- Folate-deficient megaloblastic anemia. **Adults and children:** up to 1 mg I.M daily. Duration of treatment depends on hematologic response.

Adverse reactions

Skin: allergic reactions (rash, pruritus, erythema). **Other:** ***allergic bronchospasms.***

Interactions

None significant.

Nursing diagnoses

- Altered protection related to the patient's underlying condition.
- Ineffective breathing pattern related to adverse respiratory reactions.
- Knowledge deficit related to leucovorin therapy.

Nursing interventions

- *Contraindicated* in treating undiagnosed anemia since it may mask pernicious anemia.
- *Use cautiously* in pernicious anemia; a hemolytic remission may occur while neurologic manifestations remain progressive.
- Also known as citrovorum factor and folinic acid; do not confuse folinic acid with folic acid.
- Follow leucovorin rescue schedule and protocol closely to maximize therapeutic response. Generally, leucovorin should not be administered simultaneously with systemic methotrexate.
- When treating overdose of folic acid antagonists, administer leucovorin within 1 hour if possible; drug is usually ineffective after 4-hour delay.
- Protect from light and heat, especially reconstituted parenteral preparations.
- Allergic reactions have been reported with folic acid. Consider the possibility of allergic reactions to leucovorin.

General

Classification: antihypertensive (alpha- and beta-adrenergic blocking agent). **Pregnancy risk category:** C.

Mechanism of action

Blocks response to alpha and beta stimulation and depresses renin secretion.

Indications and dosage

- Hypertension. **Adults:** 100 mg P.O. b.i.d. with or without a diuretic. Dosage may be increased to 200 mg b.i.d. after 2 days. Further dosage increases may be made q 1 to 3 days until optimum response is reached. Usual maintenance dosage is 200 to 400 mg b.i.d.
- Severe hypertension and hypertensive emergencies. **Adults:** dilute 200 mg to 200 ml with D_5W. Infuse at 2 mg/minute until satisfactory response is obtained. Then stop the infusion. May repeat q 6 to 8 hours.

Alternatively, administer by repeated I.V. injection: Initially, give 20 mg I.V. slowly over 2 minutes. May repeat injections of 40 to 80 mg q 10 minutes until maximum dose of 300 mg is reached.

Adverse reactions

CNS: vivid dreams, fatigue, headache. **CV:** *orthostatic hypotension and dizziness*, peripheral vascular disease, bradycardia. **EENT:** nasal stuffiness. **Endocrine:** hypoglycemia without tachycardia. **GI:** nausea, vomiting, diarrhea. **GU:** sexual dysfunction, urine retention. **Skin:** rash. **Other:** increased airway resistance, transient scalp tingling.

Interactions

Cimetidine: may enhance labetalol's effect. Give together cautiously. **Halothane:** additive hypotensive effect. **Insulin, oral antidiabetic drugs:** can alter dosage requirements in previously stabilized diabetics. Observe patient carefully.

Nursing diagnoses

- Altered tissue perfusion (renal, cerebral, cardiopulmonary, and peripheral) related to the patient's underlying condition.
- High risk for injury related to labetalol-induced adverse reactions.
- Knowledge deficit related to labetalol therapy.

Nursing interventions

- *Contraindicated* in bronchial asthma.
- *Use cautiously* in CHF, hepatic failure, chronic bronchitis, emphysema, preexisting peripheral vascular disease, and pheochromocytoma.
- Monitor blood pressure frequently.
- Teach patient about his disease and therapy. Explain the importance of taking this drug as prescribed, even when he's feeling well. Tell outpatient not to discontinue this drug suddenly; abrupt discontinuation can exacerbate angina and MI. Tell patient to call doctor if unpleasant adverse reactions occur.
- Instruct patient to check with doctor or pharmacist before taking OTC medications.
- This drug may mask common signs of shock and hypoglycemia.
- Unlike other beta blockers, labetalol does not decrease heart rate or cardiac output.
- Dizziness is the most troublesome adverse reaction and tends to occur in early stages of treatment, in patients also receiving diuretics, and in patients receiving higher dosages. Inform patient that dizziness can be minimized by rising slowly and avoiding sudden position changes. Taking a dose at bedtime or taking smaller doses t.i.d. will also help minimize this reaction. Discuss changes in medication schedule with doctor.
- **I.V. use:** Labetalol injection should be administered with a controlled infusion pump. Monitor blood pressure closely: q 5 minutes for 30 minutes, then q 30 minutes for 2 hours, then hourly for 6 hours. Patient should remain supine for 3 hours after infusion.
- When administered I.V. for hypertensive emergencies, labetalol produces a rapid, predictable fall in blood pressure within 5 to 10 minutes.

General

Classification: laxative (disaccharide). **Pregnancy risk category:** B.

Mechanism of action

Produces an osmotic effect in the colon. Resultant distention promotes peristalsis. Also decreases blood ammonia, probably as a result of bacterial degradation, which decreases the pH of colon contents.

Indications and dosage

• Constipation. **Adults:** 15 to 30 ml P.O. daily.
• Prevention and treatment of hepatic encephalopathy, including hepatic precoma and coma in patients with severe hepatic disease. **Adults:** initially, 20 to 30 g P.O. (30 to 45 ml) t.i.d. or q.i.d., until two or three soft stools are produced daily. Usual dosage is 60 to 100 g daily in divided doses. Can also be given by retention enema in at least 100 ml of fluid.

Adverse reactions

GI: abdominal cramps, belching, diarrhea, gaseous distention, flatulence. **Metabolic:** hypernatremia.

Interactions

Antacids, antibotics, orally administered neomycin: decreased effectiveness of lactulose. Avoid concomitant use.

Nursing diagnoses

• Constipation related to interruption of normal pattern of elimination.
• Pain related to abdominal cramping.
• Knowledge deficit related to lactulose therapy.

Nursing interventions

• *Contraindicated* in low-galactose diet.
• *Use cautiously* in diabetes mellitus.
• Reduce dosage if diarrhea occurs. Replace fluid loss.
• Monitor serum sodium for possible hypernatremia, especially when giving higher doses to treat hepatic encephalopathy.
• Minimize drug's sweet taste by diluting with water or fruit juice or giving with food.
• Store at room temperature, preferably below 86° F (30° C). Don't freeze.